MATERNAL AND CHILD HEALTH

Programs, Problems, and Policy in Public Health

Third Edition

Edited by
Jonathan B. Kotch, MD, MPH, FAAP
The University of North Carolina at Chapel Hill
Chapel Hill, North Carolina

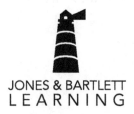

JONES & BARTLETT
LEARNING

World Headquarters
Jones & Bartlett Learning
5 Wall Street
Burlington, MA 01803
978-443-5000
info@jblearning.com
www.jblearning.com

Jones & Bartlett Learning books and products are available through most bookstores and online booksellers. To contact Jones & Bartlett Learning directly, call 800-832-0034, fax 978-443-8000, or visit our website, www.jblearning.com.

Production Credits
Publisher: Michael Brown
Editorial Assistant: Kayla Dos Santos
Editorial Assistant: Chloe Falivene
Production Manager: Tracey McCrea
Senior Marketing Manager: Sophie Fleck Teague
Manufacturing and Inventory Control Supervisor: Amy Bacus
Composition: Cenveo Publisher Services
Cover Design: Scott Moden
Cover Image: Baby: © Hunta/ShutterStock, Inc.; Kids playing ball: © stefanolunardi/ShutterStock, Inc.;
Boy reading with mother: © Jenkedco/ShutterStock, Inc.; Girl with mother: © Studio 1One/ ShutterStock, Inc.
Printing and Binding: Edwards Brothers Malloy
Cover Printing: Edwards Brothers Malloy

Library of Congress Cataloging-in-Publication Data
Maternal and child health : programs, problems, and policy in public health / edited by Jonathan B. Kotch. — 3rd ed.
   p. ; cm.
 Includes bibliographical references and index.
 ISBN 978-1-4496-1159-0 (pbk.)
 I. Kotch, Jonathan.
 [DNLM: 1. Child Health Services—United States. 2. Maternal Health Services—United States. 3. Child Welfare—United States. 4. Maternal Welfare—United States. WA 310 AA1]

 362.198'92000973—dc23
                          2011039513

6048

Printed in the United States of America
16   10 9 8 7 6 5 4 3

Dedicated in honor of Dr. C. Arden Miller, Chair, Dean, Vice Chancellor, whose exemplary vision, enduring leadership, and unwavering advocacy has improved the health and welfare of generations of families, parents, women, children, and communities in the United States through sound policies and programs.

CONTENTS

Foreword

Herbert Peterson, MD, FACOG

With the 100th anniversary of the Children's Bureau in 2012 and the approaching target date of 2015 for achieving the Millennium Development Goals (MDG), we celebrate the achievements in global Maternal and Child Health (MCH) to date and renew our commitments to the challenges ahead. While the approximately 30% decrease in maternal mortality since 1990 is greatly encouraging, the associated annual rate of decline of 2.3% is less than half of that needed to achieve MDG 5, and approximately 1000 women still die each day from complications of pregnancy and childbirth—with 99% of these deaths in developing countries (WHO, 2010). Likewise, we've seen a one-third decrease in under-5 child mortality since 1990 with about half of deaths in 2009 occurring in only five countries (You, et al., 2010), yet 63% of these child deaths are preventable (Jones, et al., 2003). The proportion of child deaths that are in the neonatal period has increased to 41%, and a 2011 report on trends in neonatal mortality highlights the challenges remaining in the United States, which now ranks behind 40 countries including Cuba, Malaysia, and Poland (Oestergaard, et al., 2011).

Since the second edition of this book was published, there have been remarkable and encouraging new forces and dynamics around family planning. Globally, the Reproductive Health Supplies Coalition launched a campaign in 2010 to reduce unmet need for family planning in support of the United Nations Secretary-General's Global Strategy for Women's and Children's Health. The Campaign's goal is to have 100 million new users of modern contraception by 2015 and, thereby, meet the needs of 80% of women in low-middle income countries. Domestically, there is a reason to hope for greater availability and access to contraceptives as well through the Department of Health and Human Services' decision in 2011 to make contraceptives available as a preventive health service at no additional cost through the Affordable Care Act.

This third edition thus comes at an important time for both global and domestic MCH as the MCH leaders of tomorrow are trained. The success of the first two editions of this text contributed to this effort and the third will surely follow. It reflects the way MCH is taught at UNC-Chapel Hill and brings together the stages of the cycle of MCH, including reproductive health, maternal and infant health, child and adolescent health, and women's health, through a state, national, and global lens. This edition includes updates and enhancements to chapters from the second edition and have highlighted the life course perspective on MCH. This new edition will be helpful as we move forward together in preparing to seize the opportunities and address the challenges ahead.

References

Jones, G., Steketee, S. W., Black, R. E., Zulfiqar, Z. A., Morris, S. S., et al. (2003). How many child deaths can we prevent this year? *Lancet, 362,* 65–71.

Oestergaard, M. Z., Inoue, M., Yoshida, S., Mahanani, W. R., Gore, F. M., Cousens, S., et al. (2011). Neonatal mortality levels for 193 countries in 2009 with trends since 1990: A systematic analysis of progress, projections, and priorities. *PLOS Medicine, 8*(8), e1001080. doi:10.1371/journal.pmed.1001080.

World Health Organization. Trends in maternal mortality: 1990 to 2008. Estimates developed by WHO, UNICEF, UNFPA and the World Bank. 2010. Available at: http://whqlibdoc.who.int/publications/2010/9789241500265_eng.pdf. Retrieved September 1, 2011.

You, D., Jones, G., Hill, K., Wardlaw, T., Chopra, M. (2010). Levels and trends in child mortality, 1990-2009. *Lancet, 376,* 931–933.

INTRODUCTION[i]

Women, children, and families have had their ups and downs in the six years since the second edition of this textbook was published. Infant mortality and low birthweight have improved slightly, whereas racial and ethnic disparities have not.[1] Teen pregnancy went down, but so did children's participation in physical education classes.[2] Although children in poverty has increased, health insurance coverage among children has not decreased, thanks to public health insurance programs such as Medicaid and the Child Health Insurance Program.[3] Internationally, although under-five deaths continue to decline, that decline is slowest in the countries with the highest child mortality rates.[4] In the developed world, the biggest child health problem is obesity.

During the course of writing and editing the second edition, I had the pleasure of discussing and corresponding with the late Dr. Greg Alexander, Chair of the Department of Maternal and Child Health of the School of Public Health, University of Alabama at Birmingham at the time. We had each discovered on our own that there was no definition of MCH in the first edition of *Maternal and Child Health: Programs, Problems, and Policies in Public Health.* Greg was gracious enough to share his definition:

> *MCH is the professional and academic field that focuses on the determinants, mechanisms and systems that promote and maintain the health, safety, well-being and appropriate development of children and their families in communities and societies, in order to enhance the future health and welfare of society and subsequent generations.*[5]

The above definition I would characterize as linear, that is, it starts with "determinants, mechanisms and systems", and ends with the "future health and welfare of society", a goal no one can argue with. I prefer a more circular approach, captured in Figure I.1, a contribution of the late Earl Siegel and affectionately known to his students as "Siegel's Circles." One can hop on board this life cycle-go-round at any point, and find common ground with colleagues in women's health, perinatal health, reproductive health, and children's health. The means to achieving optimal health and well-being for all children and women of reproductive age are just as important as the ends.

---

[i]The author would like to thank Dr. Helen M. Wallace for her review of this Introduction.

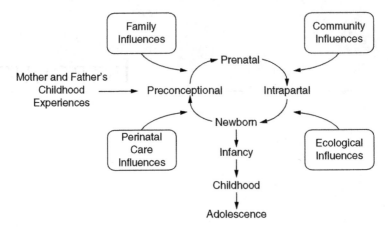

Figure I.1 A Longitudinal/Life Cycle Perspective of Child Health and Development

Maternal and Child Health (MCH) is a profession rather than a discipline. It is a big tent, characterized by a multidisciplinary cast of characters who share a commitment to a vulnerable population. While a source of strength, the focus on a specific population rather than a theory or methodology can be a weakness in an academic setting, placing MCH training programs on the defensive. Are MCH programs training public health practitioners or future faculty and MCH researchers?

The answer, of course, is that we need to train all of the above, academics, researchers, and MCH practitioners, in order to improve the health status of women, children, and families. In doing so, MCH borrows from many health and social science disciplines, but increasingly MCH is developing a set of knowledge and skills of its own, including life course theory as a unifying paradigm. (See Chapter 4.) It was as recently as 1993, for example, that the Association of Schools of Public Health (ASPH) and the Association of Teachers of Maternal and Child Health (ATMCH) (1993) first developed the competencies that MCH training programs across the country are striving to implement.[6] These have been revised in February, 2001.[7]

This book is an attempt to present, in a consolidated form, the way one such MCH training program, the Department of Maternal and Child Health of the UNC Gillings School of Global Public Health, approaches the task of educating Master's students in the core material necessary for entering the field of MCH. With a few important exceptions, all of the contributors to this edited volume are faculty (current or former), students, or alumni of The University of North Carolina at Chapel Hill (UNC-CH). The chapters by and large correspond with courses that students at UNC-CH must take to satisfy the requirements of the Master of Public Health degree or the Master of Science in Public Health degree in MCH. As such, the scope of this book is not intended to be comprehensive, nor is any individual topic pursued in depth. Rather, this book is an introduction to MCH for students, hopefully with some prior health training or experience, approaching formal training in MCH for the first time.

The structure of the book is straightforward. The first two chapters, which cover children's rights and MCH history, provide the ethical and philosophical underpinnings without which MCH would be a mechanical exercise at best. The chapter on families provides background to the changing social context affecting the health and development of all children. The fourth chapter on the life course perspective is a new look at how life course theory informs the study and the practice of MCH. The next five chapters follow the developmental cycle, beginning with family planning and proceeding through maternal and infant health, preschool, school-age and adolescent health. In these chapters, to the extent possible, the authors have followed a similar, but not identical, outline, from demography to history to epidemiology, to programs, policy, and current or future issues.

The next seven chapters deal with issues which cross-cut the developmental stages of the previous five chapters and are more idiosyncratic in structure as befits the various topics – health disparities, women's health, children with special needs, children's environmental health (new), nutrition, oral health (new), and global MCH. Finally, the last four chapters present public health skills no MCH professional should leave home without, namely, MCH research, planning, monitoring and evaluation (new, with a global focus), and MCH advocacy. While necessarily succinct, these chapters should inspire readers to seek hands-on experience to complement the didactic presentations herein.

As with any edited text, there are bound to be a variety of styles, but the faculty of the UNC-CH Department of MCH and the other contributors have provided material of uniformly high quality, making my job as editor that much easier. It is a credit to the Department, both to those currently in residence and to those who have since moved on, that such a book can be produced almost entirely from within.

Because the focus of the book is on how MCH is taught at UNC-CH (with additional contributions from colleagues at other institutions), there are many important areas which, in another format, would deserve chapters, indeed whole books, of their own. Injuries, HIV/AIDS, immunizations, mental health, and other key public health issues overlap with core MCH areas and are discussed, to a greater or lesser extent, within one or more chapters. Yet none of these topics is unique to MCH. To do them justice, one would have to call upon the skills of disciplines such as health behavior, epidemiology, health policy and management, to name a few. In fact, this is exactly how courses in these areas are offered at UNC, sometimes with, and sometimes without, MCH faculty participation. There are only so many of us to go around.

At the end of the day, we hope we have produced a readable introduction to MCH problems, programs and policies for the beginning graduate student. If some of our readers go on to careers which promote and protect the health of women and children, then this effort will have been a success.

Jonathan B. Kotch

References

1. Forum on Child and Family Statistics. (2011). America's Children. Key National Indicators of Well-being, 2011. Accessed Oct. 18, 2011, from http://www.childstats.gov/index.asp.
2. US Department of Health and Human Services/Health Resources and Services Administration/Maternal and Child Health Bureau. (2010). Child Health USA 2010. Rockville, MD:Author
3. Forum, op. cit.
4. UNICEF. The State of the World's Children, 2008. Executive Summary. Accessed Oct. 18, 2011, from http://www.unicef.org/publications/files/SOWC_2008_Exec_Summary_EN_042908.pdf.
5. Alexander GR. (2002). Maternal and Child Health (MCH). In, Encyclopedia of Health Care Management. M.J. Stahl (Ed.). Thousand Oaks, CA: Sage Publications, Inc.
6. Association of Teachers of Maternal and Child Health/Association of Schools of Public Health-MCH Council (1993). *Competencies for Education in Maternal and Child Health*. Arlington, VA: National Center for Education in Maternal and Child Health, November.
7. Association of Teachers of Maternal and Child Health. February, 2001. *Maternal and Child Health Competencies*. [available] http://www.atmch.org/mchcomps.PDF [cited] October 18, 2011.

CONTRIBUTORS

Sara E. Benjamin Neelon, PhD, MPH, RD
Assistant Professor
Department of Community and
Family Medicine
Duke University Medical Center and
Duke Global Health Institute
Duke University
Durham, North Carolina

Shelah S. Bloom, MA, SM, ScD
Research Assistant Professor
Department of Maternal and Child Health
Gillings School of Global Public Health
The University of North Carolina at Chapel Hill
Chapel Hill, North Carolina

Dorothy C. Browne, DrPH, MSW, MPH
Dean and Professor
The Ethelyn R. Strong School of Social Work
Norfolk State University
Norfolk, Virginia

Sara Buckelew, MD, MPH
Assistant Clinical Professor of Pediatrics
Department of Pediatrics
University of California, San Francisco
San Francisco, California

Diane Calleson, PhD
Clinical Associate Professor
Public Health Leadership Program
Gillings School of Global Public Health
The University of North Carolina at Chapel Hill
Chapel Hill, North Carolina

Theresa D. Chapple-McGruder, MPH, PhD
Director
Office of Maternal and Child Health
Epidemiology
Georgia Department of Public Health
Atlanta, Georgia

Sheryl L. Coley, MPH
Doctoral Candidate
Department of Public Health Education
Center for Social, Community and Health
Research and Evaluation
The University of North Carolina at Greensboro
Greensboro, North Carolina

Paula Hudson Collins, MHDL, RHEd
Chief Health and Community Relations Officer
North Carolina Department of Public Instruction
Raleigh, North Carolina

Sian Curtis, MSc, PhD
Research Associate Professor
Department of Maternal and Child Health
Gillings School of Global Public Health
The University of North Carolina at Chapel Hill
Chapel Hill, North Carolina

Pamela A. Dickens, MPH
Women's Health Coordinator
FPG Child Development Institute
The University of North Carolina at Chapel Hill
Chapel Hill, North Carolina

Anita M. Farel, MSW, DrPH
Clinical Professor
Associate Chair for Graduate Studies
Department of Maternal and Child Health
Gillings School of Global Public Health
The University of North Carolina at Chapel Hill
Chapel Hill, North Carolina

Siobán D. Harlow, PhD
Professor
Department of Epidemiology
School of Public Health
University of Michigan
Ann Arbor, Michigan

Bethany Hendrickson, MPH
Study Coordinator
The Center for Health and Community
The Center for Obesity Assessment, Study
    and Treatment (COAST)
University of California, San Francisco
San Francisco, California

Catherine A. Hess, MSW
Managing Director
National Academy for State Health Policy
Washington, DC

Margaret Hicken, PhD, MPH
Robert Wood Johnson Foundation Health &
    Society Scholar
Department of Epidemiology
School of Public Health
University of Michigan
Ann Arbor, Michigan

Jon M. Hussey, PhD, MPH
Research Assistant Professor
Department of Maternal and Child Health
Gillings School of Global Public Health
The University of North Carolina at Chapel Hill
Chapel Hill, North Carolina

Laili Irani, MD, MPH
Doctoral Candidate
Department of Maternal and Child Health
Gillings School of Global Public Health
The University of North Carolina at Chapel Hill
Chapel Hill, North Carolina

David Janicke, PhD
Associate Professor
Department of Clinical and Health Psychology
College of Public Health and Health Professions
University of Florida
Gainesville, Florida

Jill Kerr, DNP, MPH, NCSN
Instructor
Associate Degree Nursing
College of the Albemarle
Elizabeth City, North Carolina

Russell S. Kirby, PhD, MS, FACE
Professor and Marrell Endowed Chair
Department of Community and Family Health
College of Public Health
University of South Florida
Tampa, Florida

David Knopf, LCSW, MPH
Assistant Clinical Professor of Pediatrics
Research and Policy Center on Middle
    Childhood and Adolescence
Department of Pediatrics
University of California, San Francisco
San Francisco, California

Jonathan B. Kotch, MD, MPH, FAAP
Carol Remmer Angle Distinguished Professor
    of Children's Environmental Health
Department of Maternal and Child Health
Gillings School of Global Public Health
The University of North Carolina at Chapel Hill
Chapel Hill, North Carolina

Milton Kotelchuck, PhD, MPH
Senior Scientist in Maternal and Child Health
MGH Center for Child and Adolescent
    Health Policy
MassGeneral Hospital for Children, and
Visiting Professor of Pediatrics
Harvard Medical School
Boston, Massachusetts

Barbara A. Laraia, PhD, MPH, RD
Associate Professor
Department of Medicine, and Co-Director,
The Center for Obesity Assessment, Study
    and Treatment (COAST)
University of California, San Francisco
San Francisco, California

Jessica Y. Lee, DDS, MPH, PhD
Associate Professor
Department of Pediatric Dentistry
School of Dentistry
The University of North Carolina at Chapel Hill
Chapel Hill, North Carolina

Jack K. Leiss, PhD
Adjunct Associate Professor
Department of Maternal and Child Health
Gillings School of Global Public Health
The University of North Carolina at Chapel Hill
Chapel Hill, North Carolina, and
Director, Epidemiology Research Program
Cedar Grove Institute for Sustainable
    Communities
Mebane, North Carolina

Lewis Margolis, MD, MPH
Associate Professor
Department of Maternal and Child Health
Gillings School of Global Public Health
The University of North Carolina at Chapel Hill
Chapel Hill, North Carolina

Dara D. Mendez, PhD, MPH
Postdoctoral Scholar
Departments of Psychiatry and Epidemiology
School of Medicine and Graduate School of
    Public Health
University of Pittsburgh
Pittsburgh, Pennsylvania

C. Arden Miller, MD
Professor Emeritus and Chair Emeritus
Department of Maternal and Child Health
Gillings School of Global Public Health
The University of North Carolina at Chapel Hill
Chapel Hill, North Carolina

Mary D. Peoples-Sheps, MS, DrPH
Associate Professor
Senior Associate Dean for Public Health
College of Public Health and Health
    Professions
University of Florida
Gainesville, Florida

Donna J. Petersen, MHS, ScD
Professor and Dean
College of Public Health
University of South Florida
Tampa, Florida

Herbert B Peterson, MD, FACOG
Kenan Distinguished Professor and Chair,
Department of Maternal and Child Health,
Gillings School of Global Public Health, and
Professor, Department of Obstetrics and
    Gynecology,
School of Medicine
The University of North Carolina at Chapel Hill
Chapel Hill, North Carolina

Linda Piccinino, MPS (ID)
Senior Researcher
Public Health Research
Social & Scientific Systems, Inc.
Silver Spring, Maryland

Liana Janine Richardson, PhD, MPH
Postdoctoral Scholar
Department of Sociology and Carolina
    Population Center
The University of North Carolina at Chapel Hill
Chapel Hill, North Carolina

Diane L. Rowley, MD, MPH
Professor of the Practice
Department of Maternal and Child Health
Gillings School of Global Public Health
The University of North Carolina at Chapel Hill
Chapel Hill, North Carolina

Ghazaleh Samandari, PhD
Adjunct Assistant Professor
Public Health Leadership Program
Gillings School of Global Public Health
The University of North Carolina at Chapel Hill
Chapel Hill, North Carolina

Renee Schwalberg, MPH
Co-Director, Center for Women, Children,
    and Adolescents
Altarum Institute
Portland, ME

Kavita Singh, PhD, MPH
Research Assistant Professor
Department of Maternal and Child Health
Gillings School of Global Public Health
The University of North Carolina at Chapel Hill
Chapel Hill, North Carolina

Ilene S. Speizer, PhD
Research Associate Professor
Department of Maternal and Child Health
Gillings School of Global Public Health
The University of North Carolina at Chapel Hill
Chapel Hill, North Carolina

David Steffen, DrPH, MSN
Clinical Assistant Professor, and
Director, Leadership Concentration
Public Health Leadership Program
Gillings School of Global Public Health
The University of North Carolina at Chapel Hill
Chapel Hill, North Carolina

Kelly L. Strutz, MPH
Doctoral Candidate
Department of Maternal and Child Health
Gillings School of Global Public Health
The University of North Carolina at
    Chapel Hill
Chapel Hill, North Carolina

Joseph Telfair, DrPH, MSW, MPH
Professor
Public Health Research and Practice, and
Director, Center for Social, Community and
    Health Research and Evaluation
The University of North Carolina at
    Greensboro
Greensboro, North Carolina

Amy O. Tsui, PhD
Professor
Department of Population, Family and
    Reproductive Health, and
Director, Bill and Melinda Gates Institute for
    Population and Reproductive Health
Bloomberg School of Public Health
The Johns Hopkins University
Baltimore, Maryland

Anjel Vahratian, PhD, MPH
Chief, Data Analysis and Quality
    Assurance Branch
Division of Health Interview Statistics
National Center for Health Statistics
Hyattsville, Maryland

William F. Vann, Jr., DMD, PhD
Research Professor
Department of Pediatric Dentistry
School of Dentistry
The University of North Carolina at Chapel Hill
Chapel Hill, North Carolina

Karen Williams, BA
MPH Candidate
Department of Health Care Organization
    and Policy
Maternal and Child Health Concentration
School of Public Health
The University of Alabama at Birmingham
Birmingham, Alabama

Martha S. Wingate, MPH, DrPH
Associate Professor
Maternal and Child Health Program Director
Department of Health Care Organization
    and Policy
School of Public Health
The University of Alabama at Birmingham
Birmingham, Alabama

B. Cecilia Zapata, MPH, DrPH
Professor and Director
Office of Equity and Inclusion
State University of New York
SUNY Oneonta
Oneonta, New York

ABOUT THE EDITOR

Jonathan B. Kotch, Carol Remmer Angle Distinguished Professor of Children's Environmental Health in the Department of Maternal and Child Health of the UNC Gillings School of Global Public Health, is a public health pediatrician who is Board Certified in both Pediatrics and Preventive Medicine. He attended Columbia University, Stanford University, the University of North Carolina at Chapel Hill, and King's College. Cambridge. He has been recognized as a national leader in Maternal and Child Health by the American Public Health Association, which awarded him the Martha May Eliot Award in 2008, and by the Association of Maternal and Child Health Programs, which named him its John MacQueen lecturer in 2007. His campus-wide affiliations include the Injury Prevention Research Center and the FPG Child Development Institute. Through these affiliations Dr. Kotch has pursued innovative research projects including a longitudinal study, now in its 21st year, of children at risk of child maltreatment, and studies of health, safety, nutrition, and social and emotional health among children in out of home child care. He has published over 80 scientific articles and edited the first two editions of this textbook.

FOUNDATIONS OF MATERNAL AND CHILD HEALTH

CHILDREN'S RIGHTS AND DISTRIBUTIVE JUSTICE IN MATERNAL AND CHILD HEALTH

Lewis Margolis and Jonathan Kotch

Remember that the human being is the most important of all products to turn out. I am eagerly anxious to do everything I can to wake up our people to the need of protecting the soil, protecting the forests, protecting the water; but first and foremost, protect the people. If you do not have the right kind of citizens in the future, you cannot make any use of the natural resources. Protect the children—protect the boys; still more, protect the girls; because the greatest duty of this generation is to see to it that the next generation is of the proper kind to continue the work of this nation.

(President Theodore Roosevelt, 1911)

INTRODUCTION

In 1988, the Institute of Medicine (IOM) published *The Future of Public Health*, a study and critique of the state of the public health field, accompanied by recommendations to enhance its effectiveness as the nation moves into the 21st century. The authors of the report articulated a definition of public health with three components: the mission, the substance, and the organizational framework. The mission was defined as "the fulfillment of society's interest in assuring the conditions in which people can be healthy" (IOM, 1988, p. 40). The substance was defined as "organized community efforts aimed at the prevention of disease and promotion of health" (IOM, 1988, p. 41). The organizational framework of public health encompasses "both activities undertaken within the formal structure of government and the associated efforts of private and voluntary organizations and individuals" (IOM, 1988, p. 42). Each component of this definition reflects the central

dynamic or tension in the field of public health, that is, balancing the rights of individuals to pursue their private interests with the needs of communities to control the hazards that inevitably arise when groups of people pursue those interests (Beauchamp & Steinbock, 1999; Gostin, 2000; Jennings, Kahn, Mastroianni, & Parker, 2003).

It is only since the evolution of the recognition of children as individuals with interests and rights, potentially separate from those of their parents, that communities and nations have justified and conferred special protections and benefits on children through assorted public health, welfare, and education programs. In the United States, for example, the early-20th-century movement to ban child labor recognized that a child's right to an education was in conflict with the rights of employers to use child labor and the rights of parents to insist that their children go to work, especially if the family needed the income. Today's child advocates continue the tradition that argues that children should never be treated as means to an end. Rather, optimal health, growth, and development in childhood are ends in themselves. This chapter explores ethical principles underlying maternal and child health and relates those principles to advocacy for services on behalf of mothers and children.

RIGHTS

Rights are defined as valid claims (Feinberg, 1978) that imply a reciprocal duty. Such claims must be validated by rules obligating someone to respond. In the case of moral rights, such claims must be validated by moral rules. Similarly, legal rights are validated by legal rules. Although moral rights may make claims on religion and social conscience, only legal rights are enforceable by the legal apparatus of the state.

Rights are classified as positive or negative according to whether reciprocating a claimed right may require the transfer of resources. Therefore, positive rights are also referred to as subsistence rights or welfare rights, requiring some people to give up something of economic value in order to satisfy the legitimate claims of others. Negative rights, on the other hand, are option rights or rights of forbearance. A positive right is a right to something tangible, whereas a negative right is a right to be left alone.

Philosophers have argued about which came first, positive or negative rights. Historically, negative rights appeared in the U.S. Constitution and the French Declaration of the Rights of Man before positive rights were codified in the United Nations' charter and the constitution of the Soviet Union, but Bandman (1977) claimed that logically some assurance of human subsistence must have preceded liberty, citing the biblical tale of the gleaners, who benefited from the harvesters' moral obligation to leave behind some produce in the fields after the harvest.

The distinction between positive and negative rights may not always be clear cut, especially in the case of children. For example, the Bill of Rights of the U.S. Constitution articulates negative rights in that Congress is prohibited from passing laws that restrict freedom of speech, freedom of assembly, and the free exercise of religion. These are rights to be left alone, not rights to economic resources. However, the ability of children to exercise negative rights is, more so than for adults, a direct function of education, housing, nourishment, and health care. Satisfying children's valid claims to these goods and services would involve their recognition by society as positive rights. Positive and negative rights are enumerated in the United Nations Convention on the Rights of the Child (Melton, 1991), ratified by the United Nations in 1989. Examples of positive rights are rights to:

- The highest attainable standard of health and access to medical services,   ·
- Access to information and material from a diversity of sources,
- An adequate standard of living,
- Education, and
- Leisure, play, and participation in cultural and artistic activities.

Examples of negative rights are rights to:

- Respect for parents or guardians to provide direction to the child in the exercise of his or her rights,
- Legal protection against arbitrary or unlawful interference with privacy, family, home, or correspondence or attacks on honor and reputation,
- Freedom of association,
- Express an opinion in matters affecting the child and to have that opinion heard, and
- Practice any belief.

Obligations to satisfy rights may clash with one another. For example, participation in cultural activities may conflict with the right to practice any belief. Respect for parents to provide direction may conflict with access to information.

The issue of children's rights is further complicated by the fact that they cannot make claims on their own behalf. In other words, if children are to have rights at all, someone else must claim those rights for them. In fact, a child's first claims are against its own parents, and the rights of parents in their own child derive from a prior duty to satisfy the legitimate needs of that child (Blackstone, 1968). Unlike the case with adults' rights, which require a reciprocal obligation on the part of another, a parent's right in a child requires an obligation on the part of that same parental rights holder. "Parents' rights" therefore imply "parents' duties." Parents who do not satisfy their child's need for subsistence and, indeed, for love and affection as well, risk losing their rights in that child, as in the case of the state's removal of a neglected child from his or her home.

A parent, however, has not been required to act in the best interests of the child until recent history. Many ancient cultures codified aspects of the parent–child relationship by institutionalizing the absolute authority of the parent. Greek city-states condoned infanticide and even required it in the case of unwanted, illegitimate, and deformed children. In classical Sparta, a defective child could be thrown from a cliff without penalty. In the Roman Empire, a father had absolute legal authority over the life and death of his children (and, for that matter, his wife). In Egypt, the Middle East, China, and the Scandinavian countries, children were routinely sold into slavery or, if without value on the open market, strangled, drowned, "thrown from a high place," or abandoned. European laws supported the right of parents to use lethal force in controlling adolescents, who were sometimes flogged or even executed for disobedience. Unwanted European newborns were discarded without penalty. There are accounts of infants left to die on trash heaps and dung heaps or buried alive in the foundations of bridges and buildings for "good luck" (DeMause, 1974; Leiby, 1976; Williams, 1983).

Children were not even depicted in archival art until after the 11th century. The historian Barbara Tuchman has written that medieval illustrations show people in every contemporary human activity—making love and dying, sleeping and eating, being in bed and in the bath, praying, hunting, dancing, plowing, participating in games and in combat, trading, traveling, reading and writing—yet rarely with children. When children did appear, they were portrayed as miniature adults in adult clothing. The concept of childhood as a developmental continuum simply did not exist, and children were pushed into adulthood as quickly as possible. Tuchman surmises that it just was not worth investing in individuals who were apt to die before they could actively participate in the adult struggle to survive. "Owing to the high infant mortality rate of the times, estimated at one or two in three, the investment of love in a young child may have been so unrewarding that by some ruse of nature . . . it was suppressed. Perhaps also the frequent childbearing put less value on the product. A child was born and died and another took its place" (Tuchman, 1978, p. 50).

Intermittently, children came under official protection. The Code of Hammurabi made it a crime for a mother to murder her newborn, and Tiberius ordered the death penalty for those caught sacrificing children to non-Roman gods. In 13th-century England, sleeping parents smothered so many infants that it was made illegal to "bed with a swaddling child" (Pfohl, 1976; Williams, 1983). Furthermore, by the 16th century, there was a dawning recognition of the unique identity and developmental status of children. Christian reformers such as Martin Luther had for some time advocated for social concern and intervention, and there was a trend among contemporary secular philosophers and commentators to romanticize childhood. However, in the main, children were regarded as innately evil little adults or the playthings of adults. There are accounts from the medical literature of injuries resulting from the popular pastime of "child tossing," and the violent control of children by parents continued largely unabated (DeMause, 1974; Williams, 1983). Since the promulgation of Elizabethan Poor Laws, English tradition has vested ultimate guardianship over those incapable of acting on their own behalf in the sovereign (i.e., the king or queen). In the United States, the states, rather than the federal government, have this power. Hence, the states are ultimately responsible for public education, child welfare, and child protection. The early 20th century saw the passage of a number of child welfare and child labor laws during what has since become known as the Progressive Era in U.S. history. When enacted at the federal level, some of these, such as the National Child Labor Law, ultimately were declared unconstitutional. Although subsequently enacted during the depression of the 1930s, in 1918 the Supreme Court ruled that the federal government had no jurisdiction to intervene in a decision (to make a child go to work instead of school) best left to parents (*Hammer v. Dagenhart,* 1918).

Nevertheless, the children's rights movement continued to gain momentum. The 1930 White House Conference on Children promulgated the Children's Charter, which declared, among other things, that every child should have "health protection from birth through adolescence, including: periodic health examinations and, where needed, care of specialists and hospital treatment; regular dental examinations and care of the teeth; protective and preventive measures among communicable diseases; the insuring of pure food, pure milk, and pure water" (U.S. Department of Health, Education, and Welfare, 1976). Recent Supreme Court decisions established certain constitutional rights of children, such as the right to due process in adult court (*Kent v. US,* 1966) and the same rights as adults in criminal court (*In Re Gault,* 1967), rights that even parents may not overrule (*Planned Parenthood of Central Missouri v. Danforth,* 1976).

Legislation at the federal level has recognized some rights of children. Child abuse and neglect legislation, for example, establishes that children must be protected from abuse and that parents may be prosecuted for failing to provide necessary food, clothing, shelter, education, medical care, and even love and affection, as determined by state governments (Child Abuse Treatment and Prevention Act, 1973). Protection from abuse corresponds with a negative right, whereas protection from neglect corresponds with the child's positive right to subsistence. Other rights established at the federal level include the right to a free, public education for all handicapped children (Education for All Handicapped Children Act, 1975) and the right to a barrier-free environment for children and adolescents with disabilities, as found in the Americans with Disabilities Act (1990).

Satisfying positive rights to, for example, health care or education requires the expenditure of resources. In the face of limited resources, societies need rules for the fair allocation of resources. Such rules are called the principles of distributive justice.

THEORIES OF JUSTICE

From the perspective of social policy, it is necessary to justify taking or redistributing resources legitimately earned by one person in order to purchase health care or any other good for another, or in this case, for the child of another. For the purposes of analyzing and assessing distributive justice for children, it is useful to consider two basic theories of justice (for an excellent discussion of ethical frameworks for professionals, see Applebaum & Lawton, 1990). One theory is based on the principle of utility that Jeremy Benthem and John Stuart Mill developed. This theory assumes that individuals act to maximize their own happiness or utility. A just allocation of resources within a community, therefore, derives from the calculation and balancing of positive and negative utilities for each of the individuals in the group. If the total of the positive utilities or benefits exceeds the total of the negative utilities or costs, then that allocation is deemed to be just or fair. Utilitarian theory is the basis for cost–benefit analysis as a common and powerful tool in policy analysis.

In the United States, the market is the mechanism for maximizing utility. To the extent that it rewards effort, merit, and social contribution, the market is the primary determinant of how healthcare resources are allocated (Arrow, 1963; Epstein, 1997). Economists note, however, that under certain circumstances, markets may not be the most efficient way to distribute resources. For example, markets may result in a distribution of income and other resources that leaves some individuals incapable of meeting their needs (Stiglitz, 2000). Under such circumstances, the distributive principle of need argues that people who are ill or even at risk of becoming ill should have access to more medical care resources (Beauchamp & Childress, 2001; Buchanan, 1984). Public support for health insurance for low-income individuals through the Medicaid program, supplemental security income for people with disabilities, or targeted services for children with special healthcare needs may be considered examples of redistribution of health care according to the principle of need. Another condition that leads to market failure is that of public goods, items for which it does not cost anything for an additional individual to participate in the benefits, and it is impossible to exclude individuals from the benefits. Although children represent the products of private reproductive decisions and parents reap the benefits of children—pleasure, support in old age—to some extent, all members of a community benefit from healthy children. Children grow up to be economically productive, cultivating the resources needed to produce the goods and services that sustain societies in general. Therefore, another justification for redistributing resources to children or to families with children is that as public goods the market may not allocate to them very efficiently.

A second basic theory, articulated by Immanuel Kant, is based on rules or duties. Unlike utilitarian theory that focuses on the consequences of resource allocation, Kant's focus is on fundamental duties. Kant asserted, "Act in such a way that you treat humanity, whether in your own person or in the person of any other, never simply as a means, but always at the same time as an end" (Applebaum & Lawton, 1990, p. 16). Kantian theory would emphasize individual need or perhaps merit as allocation principles.

Building on the work of Kant, Rawls (1969), in *A Theory of Justice*, described a thought experiment to explain one way that fair rules of distributive justice might be derived. In the "original position," rational adults come together behind a "veil of ignorance" for the sole purpose of making the rules that govern the distribution of goods and benefits. In such a position, with the decision makers ignorant of their statuses and roles in society, Rawls posited that all would agree with the following: that basic political liberties would be guaranteed, that desirable statuses and roles would be equally accessible to all, and that unequal distribution of resources would be tolerated to the extent that such inequalities benefit the least well off. One implication of this theory, however, is that it is necessary to take resources from those who are "well off"; that is, the effort of some individuals would be used as a means to make others better off, an apparent contradiction of the Kantian view.

Rawls' formulation provides one test of social policy: Does such policy benefit the least well off? Take the case of infant mortality. For as long as race/ethnicity has been recorded for infant mortality, a marked disparity has existed between white and black rates of infant death. Nevertheless, the rates for both groups have consistently declined, suggesting that the medical, social, and public health resources affecting infant mortality have been distributed in a just manner. On the other hand, one could argue that when disparity increases, that is, infant mortality rates diverge or decline at different rates, then in the interest of justice resources should be distributed differently.

Building on the work of Rawls, Green (1976) argued that society cannot withhold from children their fair share of healthcare resources. Because children are not considered "rational" from a developmental and legal perspective, they cannot participate in the original position. What would then be a child's "fair share"? Certainly a child's fair share of health care can be no less than that necessary for him or her to grow and develop to be able to exercise fully those political liberties and human rights guaranteed to all.

SOCIAL JUSTICE AND SOCIAL POLICY

Richard Titmuss (1975), the architect of the British National Health Service, has described three models of social policy that reflect the spectrum of political views at play in discussions of the well-being of children and families. One, the Residual Welfare Model, postulates that there are two legitimate ways to meet people's needs—through the family and through the free market. When one or the other breaks down, social institutions temporarily provide the necessary resources to individuals. Under this model, "the object of the welfare state is to teach people to do without it," and beneficiaries are expected to accept society's judgment that in some way or ways they have failed. This view prevailed in the passage of welfare reform in 1996. The transformation of welfare in the United States from an entitlement to a more incentive-based system has been associated with a marked decline in the proportion of children in poverty, especially those children at greatest risk of poverty (Blank & Haskins, 2001; Finegold & Wherry, 2004), although the severe recession of 2007–2009 (and high unemployment continuing into 2011) has seen a return of poverty among children to late 1990s levels.

The second model, Industrial Achievement-Performance, exemplified by the former communist societies and currently represented by North Korea and Cuba, garners little political support in the United States. This model offers the social welfare system as an adjunct to the economy. Benefits are putatively distributed on the basis of need, but political decisions end up allocating welfare benefits based on one's status in the government, civil service, or military bureaucracy.

Third, Titmuss describes the Industrial-Redistributive model, which offers universal services outside of the market economy. Resources are distributed according to the principle of equity based on need, that is, disproportionately more social benefits are allocated to the least well off. Under this model, social welfare is not viewed as short-term charity for individuals, but as an instrument of a social policy that provides for the needs of society as a whole. For Titmuss, this orientation is exemplified by the British National Health Service itself, although this respected institution in Great Britain has been the object of continuous political debate, especially as Britain grapples with the same challenges to health care—aging population, increasing use of technology, and medical cost inflation—that are at play in the United States (Klein, 2001).

Generous support for the older population in Europe and the United States is based on the view that the past social contributions of seniors entitle them to current social benefits. The United States and many European countries have increasingly relied on debt to fund these benefits, especially in response to the severe economic decline beginning in 2008. But as David Walker, former comptroller general of the United States and head of the Government Accountability Office has explained, the current strategy of using debt is unsustainable (Walker, 2010). As of the third quarter of 2010, the debt to GDP ratio for the United States was over 90% (Bureau of Economic Analysis, 2010; U.S. Treasury, 2010) and greater than 50% of this debt is now held by foreign lenders. As Walker emphasizes, however, these debt figures do not include the unfunded liabilities stemming from entitlement obligations for Social Security, Medicare, and Medicaid to the future demands of retiring Baby Boomers. By Walker's estimates, as of September 30, 2009, the total obligation of debt plus these unfunded liabilities approximated $63 trillion.

Such staggering fiscal projections pose significant challenges for the field of maternal and child health. Promoting justice for children by securing their rights and distributing resources based on children's needs will be central to assuring the well-being of children and their families. The future of children is dependent on active and vibrant advocacy that articulates the unique value that the children's cause brings to political and economic analysis and policy development.

References

American Academy of Pediatrics. (2009). AAP advocacy guide. Elk Grove Village, IL: Author.

American Academy of Pediatrics, Government Affairs Committee. (1981). *Pediatricians and the legislative process: A potent prescription for children.* Washington, DC: American Academy of Pediatrics, Office of Government Liaison.

Americans with Disabilities Act, US Code Vol. 104, sec. 12101. Pub. L. 101-336 (1990).

Applebaum, D., & Lawton, S. V. (1990). *Ethics and the professions.* Englewood Cliffs, NJ: Prentice Hall.

Arrow, K. (1963). Uncertainty and the welfare economics of medical care. *American Economic Review, 53,* 941–973.

Bandman, B. (1977). Some legal, moral, and intellectual rights of children. *Educational Theory, 17,* 169–178.

Beauchamp, T., & Childress, J. F. (2001). *Principles of biomedical ethics.* New York: Oxford University Press.

Beauchamp, D., & Steinbock, B. (Eds.). (1999). *New ethics for the public's health.* New York: Oxford University Press.

Blackstone, W. (1968). Blackstone on children and the rights and duties of parents. In G. Abbott (Ed.), *The child and the state: Legal status in the family, apprenticeship and child labor* (Vol. 1, pp. 9–13). New York: Greenwood Press.

Blank, R., & Haskins, R. (Eds.). (2001). *The new world of welfare.* Washington, DC: Brookings Institution Press.

Buchanan, A. (1984). The right to a decent minimum of health care. *Philosophy and Public Affairs, 13,* 54–78.

Bureau of Economic Analysis. (2010). Gross domestic product: Third quarter 2010 (second estimate). Corporate profits: Third quarter 2010 (preliminary). Retrieved December 17, 2010 from http://www.bea.gov/newsreleases/national/gdp/2010/pdf/gdp3q10_2nd.pdf.

Child Abuse Treatment and Prevention Act, Pub. L. 93-247 (1973).

Children's Defense Fund. (1991). *An advocate's guide to lobbying and political activity for nonprofits: What you can and can't do.* Washington, DC: Author.

DeMause, L. (1974). The evolution of childhood. In L. deMause (Ed.), *The history of childhood.* New York: Psychohistory Press.

Education for All Handicapped Children Act. Pub. L. 94-142 (1975).

Epstein, R. (1997). *Mortal peril: Our inalienable right to health care?* Reading, MA: Addison Wesley Publishing Company.

Feinberg, J. (1978). Rights. In T. Beauchamp & L. Walters (Eds.), *Contemporary issues in bioethics* (pp. 38–43). Encino, CA: Dickerson Publishing Co.

Finegold, K., & Wherry, L. (2004). *Race, ethnicity, and economic well-being: Snapshots of America's families* (No. 19). Washington, DC: Urban Institute.

Gostin, L. (2000). *Public health law: Power, duty, restraint.* Berkeley, CA: University of California Press.

Green, R. (1976). Health care and justice in contract theory perspective. In R. M. Veatch & R. Branson (Eds.), *Ethics and health policy.* Cambridge, MA: Ballinger.

Hammer v. Dagenhart, 247 US Reports 251, 268 (1918).

Hill, I. T. (1992). The role of Medicaid and other government programs in providing medical care for children and pregnant women. *Future of Children, 2*, 134–153.

In Re Gault, 387 US 1 (1967).

Institute of Medicine. (1988). *The future of public health*. Washington, DC: National Academy Press.

Jennings, B., Kahn, J., Mastroianni, A., & Parker, L. (Eds.). (2003). *Ethics and public health: Model curriculum*. Rockville, MD: Health Services and Resources Administration.

Kent v. US, US 383 541, 16 LE 2d 84, 86 S. Ct. 1045 (1966).

Klein, R. (2001). What's happening to Britain's national health service? *New England Journal of Medicine, 345*, 305–308.

Kopelman, L., & Palumbo, M. (1997). The U.S. health care delivery system: Inefficient and unfair to children. *American Journal of Law and Medicine, 28*, 319–337.

Leiby, J. (1976). History of social welfare. In A. Minahan (Ed.), *Encyclopedia of social work* (18th ed., Vol. 1). Silver Spring, MD: National Association of Social Workers.

Melton, G. B. (1991). Preserving the dignity of children around the world: The UN Convention on the rights of the child. *Child Abuse and Neglect, 15*, 343–350.

Michigan Council for Maternal and Child Health. (n.d.). *From vision to action: A citizens' guidebook to grass roots advocacy*. Lansing, MI: Michigan Council for Maternal and Child Health.

Pfohl, S. J. (1976). The "discovery" of child abuse. *Social Problems, 24*, 310–323.

Planned Parenthood of Central Missouri v. Danforth, 428 US 52, 96 S. Ct. 2831 (1976).

Preston, S. H. (1984). Children and the elderly: Divergent paths for America's dependents. *Demography, 21*, 435–457.

Rawls, J. (1969). *A theory of justice*. Cambridge, MA: Harvard University Press.

Roosevelt, T. (1971). The conservation of childhood. In R. Bremner (Ed.), *Children and youth in America* (Vol. 2, pp. 653–654). Washington, DC: American Public Health Association.

Specter, M. (1998, July 10). Population implosion worries a graying Europe. *New York Times*.

Stiglitz, J. (2000). *Economics of the public sector*. New York: W. W. Norton.

Titmuss, R. (1975). *Social policy: An introduction*. New York: Pantheon Books.

Tuchman, B. W. (1978). *A distant mirror*. New York: Alfred A. Knopf.

U.S. Department of Health, Education, and Welfare, Office of Child Development, Children's Bureau, National Center on Child Abuse and Neglect. (1976). *Child abuse and neglect: The problem and its management. Vol. 1: An overview of the problem*. Washington, DC: Author.

U.S. Treasury. (2010). The debt to the penny and who holds it. Retrieved December 17, 2010 from http://www.treasurydirect.gov/NP/NPGateway.

Walker, D. M. (2010). *Comeback America*. New York: Random House, Inc..

Williams, G. J .R. (1983). Child protection: A journey into history. *Journal of Clinical Child Psychology, 12*, 236–243.

2

Tracing the Historical Foundations of Maternal and Child Health to Contemporary Times

Lewis Margolis and Jonathan B. Kotch

These questions of child health and protection are a complicated problem requiring much learning and action. And we need have great concern over this matter. Let no one believe that these are questions which should not stir a nation; that they are below the dignity of statesman or governments. If we could have but one generation of properly born, trained, educated, and healthy children, a thousand other problems of government would vanish.

(Herbert Hoover, 1931)

INTRODUCTION

Policy development to address the needs of mothers and children has played out in the unique political and social context of the United States. Three attributes in particular have influenced and continue to influence the development of maternal and child health (MCH) policies. One attribute is federalism, that is, the fact that there are two major governmental entities—federal and state—that vie for influence within the structure outlined in the U.S. Constitution. This federal–state relationship is further complicated by the fact that there are thousands of county and city jurisdictions, each of which relates to both the federal government and its own state. The relative influence of these partners has waxed and waned since the onset of local and state government interest in the population of mothers and children at the close of the 19th century.

A second attribute is the independent judiciary that has served as the interpreter and upholder of the basic values infused in the Constitution. Although the interpretation of certain constitutional limits has varied over the years, any given legislative action must pass judicial muster. The third attribute of the U.S. political and social scene is the high value placed on individualism, the free enterprise economic system, and the dominant role of the private sector. Governmental influence in many spheres of life in the United States is generally justified in response to market failures rather than as a fundamental aspect of the social framework (Epstein, 2003; Gostin & Blocke, 2003).

This chapter characterizes three phases in the development of U.S. health policy for mothers and children. First, the chapter reviews the origins of local, state, and federal participation in health care for mothers and children. Next, the discussion focuses on the emergence of the federal government as a major force in public MCH program development, with particular attention to the federal role in addressing equity.

The chapter then concludes with consideration of the current political tensions and efforts to return power and responsibility for MCH policies, once again, to the states. Table 2–1 presents a chronology of the development of selected MCH services in the United States.

ORIGINS OF GOVERNMENTAL PARTICIPATION IN THE CARE OF MOTHERS AND CHILDREN

The three attributes of social policy began to interact in prominent ways with regard to mothers and children after the Civil War.

Table 2–1 Chronology of MCH Services in the United States

1855	Founding of the Children's Hospital of Philadelphia
1869	State board of health established in Massachusetts
1879	Formation of a Section on Diseases of Children of the American Medical Association
1888	The American Pediatric Society founded to promote scientific inquiry into children's diseases
1893	First milk station established in New York City
1904	National Child Labor Committee organized to monitor effects of child labor on health and development
1907	First Bureau of Child Hygiene established in New York City
1909	First White House Conference on Children called by President Theodore Roosevelt
1912	Congress established the Children's Bureau
1921	First Maternity and Infancy Act (Sheppard-Towner)
1930	American Academy of Pediatrics founded
1935	Social Security Act, including grants to states for aid for dependent children and maternal and child welfare (Titles IV and V, respectively), enacted
1943	Emergency Maternity and Infant Care Act
1944	Association of Maternal and Child Health Programs founded as the Association of Directors of State and Territorial Maternal and Child Health and Crippled Children's Services
1951	American College of Obstetricians and Gynecologists founded
1954	Special appropriation to MCH programs for community services for children with mental retardation
1963	Special project grants for Maternity and Infant Care
1965	Title XVIII (Medicare) and Title XIX (Medicaid) added to the Social Security Act; amendments to Title V establish maternity care and children's projects; first Neighborhood Health Center grant awarded
1967	Office of Child Development created as a home for Head Start; functions of the Children's Bureau distributed among four federal agencies
1968	Amendments to Title V and Title XIX authorizing the creation of Early and Periodic Screening, Diagnosis, and Treatment (EPSDT)
1972	Special Supplemental Food Program for Women, Infants, and Children (WIC) established

(continues)

Table 2–1 (Continued)

1974	Child Abuse Prevention and Treatment Act enacted
1981	Maternal and Child Health Services Block Grant amendments to Title V enacted
1984	Beginning of a series of amendments to expand access to Medicaid
1989	Title V amended to increase accountability
1991	Healthy Start funded in 15 communities
1996	The Personal Responsibility and Work Opportunity Reconciliation Act
1997	Title XXI (State Child Health Insurance Program) added to the Social Security Act
2010	Patient Protection and Affordable Care Act (P.L. 111-148) to expand health insurance coverage is signed into law

A series of developments prompted increased attention to the particular needs of children. In the field of medicine, Dr. Abraham Jacobi and others began to articulate that the therapeutic needs of children differed from those of adults. Developments in the field of sanitation provided new understanding of determinants of infant mortality (Meckel, 1990). Fundamental discoveries in bacteriology and the prevention and control of infectious diseases provided a dramatic opportunity to demonstrate the possibilities of preventing infant deaths (Lesser, 1985). Although the discovery of the germ theory of disease gave public health a technological base, it became clear that prevention was not simply a medical research issue. Effective health promotion also demanded social mechanisms, the most important of which was public health education (Tratner, 1974).

In 1874, Henry Bergh, founder of the New York Society for the Prevention of Cruelty to Animals, personally intervened on behalf of a child who had been physically abused, bringing her situation to the attention of local authorities in New York City. Outrage over the absence of laws to protect children from such treatment prompted New York and other cities to enact laws prohibiting child cruelty and giving private agencies police authority to intervene in abusive situations (Williams, 1983). In New York, the new Society for the Prevention of Cruelty to Children assumed this responsibility.

Throughout history, children have been expected to provide menial or hazardous labor for their parents. The intense industrialization of the late 19th century drew many children into factories and mines, raising the concerns of child advocates and social reformers about the effects of working conditions on the health and education of children. Industrialization led to the creation of labor-intensive, low-paid jobs in mills, mines, and factories. Coupled with the high Civil War mortality experienced by working-aged males, especially in the South, this situation resulted in the widespread employment of children in a number of out-of-home occupations (Schmidt & Wallace, 1988). By 1900, one in six 10- to 15-year-olds was employed, 40% in industry, 60% in agriculture, and children as young as 7 years were employed in poor or hazardous work environments (Schmidt & Wallace, 1988).

In 1916 the Keating–Owen Act prohibited interstate commerce of goods produced by children. This legislation was controversial because of the necessity for children from poor families to work, and it was overturned by the Supreme Court in a 1918 case, *Hammer v. Dagenhart*, from textile-producing North Carolina (Berger & Johansson, 1980). It was not until the Depression forced unemployed adults to take jobs previously reserved for children that child labor was permanently constrained (Miller, 1988).

As immigrants poured into cities seeking new opportunities, the unmet health and educational needs of their children, as well as the potential threat to public health through the transmission of infectious diseases, became the subject of concern for reformers and politicians. The institutionalization of vital records keeping provided the first real evidence of the social impact of infant mortality. Infant death records revealed that in the United States in 1900, infant mortality averaged 150 per 1,000 births and was as high as 180/1,000 in some industrial cities. Death claimed as many as 50% of the infants that had been abandoned or orphaned to the foundling hospitals that proliferated as a result of urbanization and immigration (Schmidt & Wallace, 1988). In this context, late 19th- and early 20th-century social workers and public health officials joined forces. As social workers recognized that poverty and social dislocation engendered ill health and that ill health caused poverty by creating economic burdens, they used their particular skills to combat poverty by promoting good health. They mobilized the lay leaders and residents of the community for the control of disease (Tratner, 1974). For example, recognizing the risk to infants of consuming spoiled milk, and the heightened risk for poor infants because of the lack of adequate storage facilities, public health advocates urged municipalities and private individuals to fund milk stations where poor families could collect fresh milk (Grotberg, 1977).

The evolving concept of childhood as a "special" period of growth, socialization, and development provided a rational context for advocacy, whereas child labor, infant mortality, and child maltreatment provided highly visible targets for reform. A coalition of female reformers, the driving force behind the women's suffrage movement, lent energy, motivation, and critical mass to the ranks of settlement house workers, social

workers, and public health nurses engaged in child advocacy. The first Bureau of Child Hygiene was established in 1907 in New York City under the leadership of Dr. S. Josephine Baker. She had entered the New York City Health Department after prejudice against female physicians had limited her ability to advance in academic medicine and private practice (Baker, 1994). One of the main strategies undertaken by Baker was to send public health nurses to visit the tenement homes of newborn babies in order to educate mothers about how to care for their new infants. The bureau became involved in the health care of school children, the supervision of midwives, and the regulation of children's institutions.

The convergence of social, economic, and political forces at the turn of the century resulted in the call for a federal role in promoting, if not ensuring, the well-being of children. In 1909, President Theodore Roosevelt convened the first White House Conference on Children. Emerging from the conference were calls for service programs and financial aid to protect the home environment and recommendations that the federal government take responsibility for gathering information on problems of infant and child health and welfare (Lesser, 1985; Schmidt & Wallace, 1988; Skocpol, 1992; Tratner, 1974). These recommendations gave rise to the Mother's Aid Movement and the American Association for the Study and Prevention of Infant Mortality. The former group drew attention to the benefits of keeping children in the family while pointing out the detrimental effects of dehumanizing institutions. The latter group drew attention to the unacceptably high rate of infant deaths (Lesser, 1985; Schmidt & Wallace, 1988; Tratner, 1974).

With advocacy from education, psychology, medicine, public health, labor, and social work, and over the opposition of groups opposing federal meddling in the private domain of parents, Congress followed another of the conference's recommendations and enacted legislation establishing the Children's Bureau. Legislation for such an agency had been first introduced in 1906, but intense debate centering on the question of whether child welfare was a federal or state responsibility stalled its passage until 1912. Assigned to the Department of Commerce and Labor, reflecting the roots of the bureau in concern over labor conditions for children, the act charged the Children's Bureau to "investigate and report . . . upon all matters pertaining to the welfare of children and child life among all classes of our people, and . . . especially investigate the questions of infant mortality, the birth rate, orphanages, juvenile courts, desertion, dangerous occupations, accidents and diseases of children, employment, and legislation affecting children in the several States and Territories" (U.S. Congress, 1912). The tension between public and private responsibility for children was reflected in the legislation that stated, "No official, or agent, or representative of said bureau shall, over the objection of the head of the family, enter any house used exclusively as a family residence."

Under the leadership of its first chief, Julia Lathrop, the Children's Bureau embarked on an active portfolio of investigations into the conditions of children. For example, the bureau conducted a longitudinal study of the relationship between income and infant mortality (Lathrop, 1919). Other studies addressed child labor, working mothers, children's nutrition, services for crippled children, and juvenile delinquency. In 1915, as the result of bureau studies that concluded that birth registration is "the starting point for the reduction of infant mortality by identifying infants at risk for health problems, or dying," the National Birth Registry was established.

Although the mandate of the bureau was to investigate and report, its leaders began to develop a legislative agenda to address identified problems. In 1918, Representative Jeanette Rankin of Montana introduced legislation to provide federal funds to the states to establish preventive health programs for mothers and infants (Wilson, 1989). This legislation was strongly supported by the suffragettes, but was opposed by the medical community because it would place responsibility for a healthcare program under the "nonmedical" Children's Bureau (Lesser, 1985). In the midst of the debate over the legislation, the Second White House Conference on Children in 1919 issued recommendations for minimum standards of MCH care.

By 1920, sponsorship of the bill was assumed by Senator Morris Sheppard of Texas and Representative Horace Towner of Iowa. Partially in recognition that the United States was not doing particularly well in responding to problems of maternal and infant health, Congress passed the Maternity and Infancy Act (also known as the Sheppard-Towner Act) in November 1921 (Schmidt & Wallace, 1988).

The Sheppard-Towner Act authorized grants paid "to the several States for the purpose of cooperating with them in promotion the welfare and hygiene of maternity and infancy as hereinafter provided" (Bremner, 1970). Under the act, each state that elected to receive these funds was required to establish a child welfare or child hygiene agency, representing the first federal effort to develop an MCH infrastructure within the states. The monies were allocated as a grant in two parts. Under the first part, each state received an equal share of a $480,000 appropriation. Under the second part, totaling $1,000,000, each state received $5,000, plus an amount proportionate to that state's population in the census of 1920. States were required to match the funds provided under the second part of the act. Funds were distributed in response "to detailed plans for carrying out the provisions of this Act within such State." Although the Sheppard-Towner Act did not regulate the content of these plans beyond "promoting the welfare and hygiene of maternity and infancy," the legislation was quite explicit in what states were not permitted to do. Continuing the attention to individual liberty instilled in the Children's Bureau authorization, the act asserted the following:

No official, agent, or representative of the Children's Bureau shall by virtue of this

Act have any right to enter any home over the objection of the owner thereof, or to take charge of any children over the objection of the parents, or either of them, or of the person standing in loco parentis or having custody of such child. Nothing in this Act shall be construed as limiting the power of a parent or guardian or person standing in loco parentis to determine what treatment or correction shall be provided for a child or the agency or agencies to be employed for such purpose. Second, states were not permitted to spend monies on buildings or payment of any maternity or infancy pension, stipend, or gratuity.

The Congressional debate over the Sheppard-Towner Act replicated the heated encounters that occurred over the establishment of the Children's Bureau. On one side were those who argued for a federal role in promoting the welfare of mothers and children. This argument was presented in economic terms, that is, that the federal government plays a role in agricultural and commercial activities in order to promote economic development and that children represent no less valuable a resource. The opposition to Sheppard-Towner was argued on several grounds. Some were opposed to any governmental role, that is, interference, in the relationship between children and their parents. In this view, the family was a private domain, and the responsibility for children resided with their parents or local family members or charities. Another source of opposition was organized medicine through the American Medical Association (AMA). Exploiting the uncertainty and fear stemming from the Communist revolution in Russia in 1917, the AMA decried the law as an "imported socialistic scheme unsuited to our form of government." Furthermore, the AMA sought to protect practitioners from what was perceived as the potential for governmental interference or control over the practice of medicine, despite the fact that Sheppard-Towner support for primary care (as opposed

to preventive care) was expressly forbidden. The bill was also assailed by conservatives as "a move toward eliminating racial discrimination" because it required services to be available to all citizens.

The debate within the AMA over Sheppard-Towner spawned the birth of the American Academy of Pediatrics (Hughes, 1980). During the 1922 meeting of the AMA, the Pediatric Section debated and endorsed Sheppard-Towner, concluding that it was in the best interests of mothers and children. The AMA House of Delegates, however, not only condemned the act, but also repudiated the Pediatric Section for its endorsement without the approval of the governing House. Recognizing that the AMA was not prepared to speak for the welfare of children, pediatricians met over the next 8 years and finally convened the first meeting of the American Academy of Pediatrics in Detroit in 1930, becoming a powerful and consistent supporter of MCH policies and programs (Lesser, 1985; Schmidt & Wallace, 1988).

The Sheppard-Towner Act ended up passing handily in 1921, in part because of uncertainty over how newly enfranchised women would vote, coming as it did shortly after the incorporation the previous year of the 19th amendment, granting women the right to vote (Lemons, 1969). Another factor that facilitated its passage was the effort to assuage organized medicine by emphasizing the preventive nature of this legislation in an attempt to avoid a conflict with the private practice of medicine. Whereas physicians were viewed as the appropriate source of care for sick infants and parturient women, the educational and screening activities envisioned in the bill were presented as complements and enhancements of traditional medical care. Nevertheless, opposition intensified throughout the 1920s. Physicians began to recognize the competitive potential that the provision of preventive services had for the development of their practices. Opposition also grew within the Catholic Church, fearful of a governmental role in the provision of historically church-based charitable services. A third source of protest came from within the Public Health Service, annoyed at the dissemination of health services through this program of the Department of Commerce and Labor. As a result, the act was not renewed after 1929. In succumbing, the Maternity and Infancy Act established the hegemony of both the medical community and the medical model in MCH policy development and established the publicly funded use of private providers as the preferred method of healthcare delivery.

The accomplishments of the Sheppard-Towner Act were reviewed in the Eighteenth Annual Report of the Children's Bureau. Birth registration increased from 30 states, covering 72% of the births in 1922, to 46 states, representing 95% of the population. By 1920, child hygiene bureaus had been established in 28 states, 16 of them in 1919 alone, as a result of Children's Bureau leadership. After the implementation of the act, another 19 states established such bureaus. Hundreds of maternal and/or child health consultation centers were established, often in conjunction with local health agencies. Even after expiration of the appropriation, 19 states continued to fund the efforts implemented under the act.

THE EMERGENCE OF THE FEDERAL GOVERNMENT IN COMMUNITY ASSESSMENT, POLICY DEVELOPMENT, AND ASSURANCE FOR MOTHERS AND CHILDREN

With the descent into the Great Depression in 1929, many states and local communities were confronted by the challenge of rising health needs in the face of catastrophic levels of unemployment and devastated budgets as state and local governments witnessed the decimation of their tax bases. State programs for indigent parents and children existed, but without Maternity and Infancy Act funds, health services for mothers and infants were drastically reduced. By 1934, "23 states appropriated virtually no MCH funds" for such

services (Lesser, 1985, p. 592). The Depression impoverished 40% of the population, including a good number of citizens of good moral credentials. Therefore, the link between indigency and immorality was weakened.

After his election in 1932, President Franklin D. Roosevelt recommended legislation designed to provide temporary assistance to the "deserving" poor and ongoing economic insurance to those who were making it but might need help in the future (Guyer, 1987). He charged the Economic Security Committee to address "security for men, women and children . . . against several of the great disturbing factors of life—especially those which relate to unemployment and old age" (Grotberg, 1977, p. 87). Consultation with Grace Abbott and other representatives of the Children's Bureau resulted in the incorporation of bureau plans into the Social Security Act of 1935. The bureau proposed three major sets of activities: (1) aid to dependent children, (2) welfare services for children needing special care, and (3) MCH services including services for crippled children. These were incorporated into the Social Security Act, enacted on August 14, 1935 (Hutchins, 1994). Title IV provided cash payments to mothers who had lost fathers' support for their children. Responsibility for this title was given to the newly created Social Security Board, rather than the Children's Bureau. Title V consisted of four parts. Part 1, Maternal and Child Health Services, represented an expansion of the programs established under the Sheppard-Towner Act. Part 2, Services for Crippled Children, enabled states to improve services for locating crippled children and "for providing medical, surgical, corrective, and other services and care, and facilities for diagnosis, hospitalization, and aftercare, for children who are crippled or who are suffering from conditions which lead to crippling" (U.S. Congress, 1935, p. 631). Part 3, Child-Welfare Services, enabled states to provide services for "the protection and care of homeless, dependent, and neglected children, and children in danger of becoming delinquent" (U.S. Congress, 1935, p. 633). Part 4, Vocational Rehabilitation, enabled states to strengthen programs of vocational rehabilitation of people with physical disabilities, although the administration of this part was not under the Children's Bureau.

A broad base of public support existed for the child health, welfare, and economic security components of the Social Security Act. Support for Titles IV and V was especially strong, with leading women's organizations of the country present at the Congressional hearings to express their support. Opposition to Titles IV and V, which might have been expected given the history of the Maternity and Infancy Act, did not materialize. The AMA was preoccupied with the broader issue of blocking any possibility of national health insurance (Witte, 1963).

Unlike Title IV, which was an entitlement, funding for Title V was discretionary and had several components. One set of funds sent an equal share to each state. A second set was distributed on the basis of live births and required a dollar for dollar match. A third set of funds was allocated based on financial need and the number of live births, without a required match. Finally, Crippled Children's funds provided an equal share as well as an allotment based on the number of children served, building an incentive to locate and treat children. The Secretary of Labor (as the original home department for the Children's Bureau and Title V) retained up to 15% of the appropriation for training, research, and demonstrations, including Special Projects of Regional and National Significance (SPRANS).

The onset of World War II created a new challenge in addressing the health needs of mothers and children. With the mobilization of millions of soldiers, many military wives who relocated from their homes were in need of maternity care. Although the bureau attempted to provide support for medical care and hospitalization of these women through Title V funds, the amounts were inadequate. In 1943, Congress appropriated additional funds for the Emergency Maternity and Infant Care Program. These funds, allocated from general revenues and distributed through the states with no required match, paid for medical care for the wives of servicemen in the lowest four pay grades. By the time the program was phased out in 1949, it had provided care in 1.5 million maternity cases, approximately one of every seven births in the United States at its peak (Grotberg, 1977).

Federal initiatives after World War II were rather limited. Although Title V secured and encouraged the development of MCH agencies within state health departments, the federal government directed its efforts mainly at the support of research and services for particular diseases. For example, the Crippled Children's Program adopted many conditions beyond the orthopedic problems that were its first targets. Epilepsy, congenital and rheumatic heart disease, hearing impairments, premature newborn care, and other conditions were incorporated into state programs (Lesser, 1985).

After the Second World War, the Children's Bureau began a slow but steady decline from its position of prominence in the national health and welfare arena. At its founding in 1912, the director of the bureau reported directly to the Secretary of Commerce and Labor and then, after the department split in 1913, to the Secretary of Labor. Although arguments were raised about the appropriateness of the bureau within Labor as opposed to the Public Health Service, the early leaders of the bureau maintained its leadership role in a wide range of maternal and child interests. During the 1930s, consideration was given to dividing the health, education, and welfare activities of the bureau among various agencies, but the political pressure both within and outside the federal bureaucracy was not sufficient to effect this change until the late 1940s. The bureau was moved to the newly created Federal Security Administration in 1945. Although it did retain control, temporarily, of the various grant-in-aid programs that it had developed and administered, this move marked the beginning of the decline of the influence of the Children's Bureau.

SOCIAL ACTIVISM, EQUITY, AND THE DEVELOPMENT OF MATERNAL AND CHILD HEALTH POLICY IN THE 1960S

Special Projects under Title V of the Social Security Act

President Kennedy's interest in mental retardation, stirred in part by the efforts of his parents to provide for their mentally retarded daughter, provided the bureau with the opportunity to launch new initiatives. Arguing that mental retardation could be prevented, in part, by adequate prenatal care, the administration developed a program of special grants through Title V. Different from the traditional Bureau focus on preventive services, these maternity and infant care (M & I) projects, authorized by PL 88-156 in 1963, were designed to provide comprehensive medical services including prenatal, intrapartum, and postpartum care and hospitalization. By 1969, 53 projects had served 100,000 impoverished women and their infants nationwide (Lesser, 1985). Not only did the scope of supported activities change with the introduction of these projects, but also the administration of bureau activities changed. Rather than allocating funds through state health agencies, the bureau distributed M & I funds directly to the service agencies. Furthermore, funds for these demonstration projects could be allocated to private, nonprofit institutions. Comparable projects for children and youth (C & Y) were inaugurated in 1965. By 1969, 58 C & Y projects had provided preventive and primary medical care to 335,000 children (Lesser, 1985). Funded as "demonstration" projects, the M & I projects in particular reported notable improvements in infant health (Sokol, Woolf, Rosen, & Weingarden, 1980). Special projects for neonatal intensive care, family planning, and dental care followed. The M & I and C & Y projects expanded in number during the 1960s and early 1970s but were never extended beyond their demonstration status to become the general policy.

Public Health and Child Protection

The period from 1960 to 1974 was much like the earlier era of social reform in its public expression of social malcontent and institutional mistrust. Civil rights advocates established that otherwise disenfranchised adults and children had rights that could be enforced by legal and administrative means. Furthermore, by gaining legal access to bureaucratic decision making, those same advocates challenged the complacency of professionals who purportedly "served" disenfranchised adults and children.

At the same time, medical and public health professionals were challenged to reconsider the relationship of child health and social phenomena. In 1946, John Caffey, a pediatric radiologist, published an article describing traumatic long bone fractures in infants. In 1953, an article by Silverman, also a radiologist, discussed the possibility that such fractures might be induced by "parental carelessness." In 1955, Wooley and Evans concluded that infants suffering from repeated fractures often come from homes with aggressive, immature, or emotionally ill adults. In 1957, Caffey recapitulated his earlier findings, adding a commission to physicians to consider parental abuse when diagnosing injured infants (Pfohl, 1976).

However, it was not until 1962, with the publication of Henry Kempe's article, "The Battered Child Syndrome," that the phenomenon of physically abused children seen in the nation's hospitals caught the attention of child health professionals and the public everywhere. "The Battered Child Syndrome" challenged the belief that parental abuse "was a deplorable fact of antiquity." It also documented the medical community's unwillingness to implicate parents in diagnosing abuse (Pfohl, 1976; Williams, 1983).

The public health community's response to the "discovery" of child abuse was immediate and dramatic, and within a decade, child protection had become a national priority. In 1962, the Children's Bureau prepared and disseminated a model child abuse reporting law, and the Social Security Amendments of 1962 required each state to make child welfare services available to all children, including the abused child. In 1963, 18 bills to protect abused children were introduced in Congress, 11 of which passed, and "throughout the 1960s and into the early 1970s, states developed or expanded their capacities to investigate and treat reports of child abuse." By 1967, all states had child abuse reporting laws (Pfohl, 1976; Williams, 1983).

In 1973, widely publicized hearings were chaired by Senator Walter Mondale (Democrat from Minnesota) on proposed legislation to establish federal leadership in child protection. In 1974, with the support of virtually every children's advocacy group and the AMA, the Child Abuse Prevention and Treatment Act was passed, creating a structure for responding to the problem of child maltreatment much like the original Children's Bureau had been a structure for responding to MCH needs (Williams, 1983).

Title XVIII (Medicare) and Title XIX (Medicaid)

Culminating 3 decades of debate over the nature of the federal role in providing health insurance, Congress enacted Medicare, Title XVIII of the Social Security Act, in 1965. Unique among industrialized nations with national health insurance, the United States limits its coverage to the older population. Medicare provides coverage for short-term hospitalization and medical services. Hospitalization is financed through employment taxes, and physician services are financed jointly through premiums (approximately 25% of the actuarial cost) and general federal revenues (the remaining cost). Unlike Title V, states play no role in the financing, administering, or standard setting for this program.

Because the political struggle over the federal role in health care was waged in the arena of Medicare, the accompanying legislation to establish Medicaid, a program of health insurance assistance for the poor, was shielded from controversy. Enacted as Title XIX of the Social Security Act, the structure of the Medicaid program built on earlier federal support to the states for low-income older persons. Although an entitlement like Medicare, the Medicaid program involves joint federal–state financing and state development of standards within guidelines established by the federal government. A third characteristic of Medicaid (a characteristic that has gradually changed through a series of alterations during the 1980s) was the linkage of eligibility for Medicaid to eligibility for Aid for Families with Dependent Children (AFDC). Consistent with the state–federal partnership, criteria for welfare eligibility are established by the states so that state welfare regulations had a direct effect on eligibility for the federal Medicaid program. The welfare eligibility requirement severely limited eligibility for Medicaid. As Davis and Schoen (1978) noted in *Health and the War on Poverty*, a majority of states limited AFDC to families without a father in the home. The income and assets requirements further limited access to the program. For example, in 1985, the cutoff for eligibility for Medicaid ranged among states from a low of only 16% of the federal poverty income guidelines to 97% (Rosenbaum & Johnson, 1986).

Soon after the implementation of Medicaid, it became apparent that its focus on acute medical care rather than preventive services impeded its effectiveness for children. Social Security amendments submitted by President Lyndon Johnson in 1967 modified Medicaid and the Title V Crippled Children's Programs to include a new benefit, the Early and Periodic Screening, Diagnosis, and Treatment (EPSDT) program. Building on language in the original Crippled Children's legislation of 1935, the EPSDT program has been described as "potentially the most comprehensive child health care program the government had ever undertaken" (Foltz, 1975, p. 35). The program called for specific services such as physical and developmental exams, vision and hearing screening, appropriate laboratory tests, dental referral, immunizations, and payment for other services covered by each state's Medicaid program. Furthermore, the services had to be provided according to a periodicity schedule consistent with reasonable standards of care. Finally, states were expected actively to enroll Medicaid-eligible children into their programs.

Unfortunately, the implementation of EPSDT was slowed by several issues. First, the program was cobbled together through changes in programs (Medicaid and Title V) with different missions and different bureaucracies. In particular, the Medicaid program was anchored in the welfare system with its restrictive eligibility criteria, impairing the ability of this bold screening, referral, and treatment program to reach broad groups of children in need. Second, the costs of such an ambitious screening and treatment program were daunting to the states that were required to pay for these new services under the shared financing structure of Medicaid. As Rosenbaum and Johnson (1986) have emphasized, however, the main obstacle to the successful implementation of EPSDT as a program to address the preventive health needs of poor children was the fact that the proportion of poor children who were Medicaid eligible remained low.

In spite of the limitations of the Medicaid program, it did increase access to medical care for poor children. According to a review conducted by the Office of Technology Assessment (U.S. Congress, 1988) and published in *Healthy Children: Investing in the Future*, children with Medicaid were similar to middle-income insured children with regard to general check-ups and immunizations. Furthermore, Medicaid recipients with health problems were more likely to have seen a physician than were uninsured children. Although use of services increased for Medicaid recipients, the sites of care tended to be public health clinics, emergency rooms, and

hospital outpatient departments rather than private physician offices (Orr & Miller, 1981), resulting in the further evolution of a dual system of health care. Studies of the effectiveness of EPSDT in particular suggest that participation in the program decreased the likelihood of referral for specialized care over time (Irwin & Conroy-Hughes, 1982; Keller, 1983). Other studies confirm that this screening and prevention program has not achieved the goals originally envisioned. For example, a review of California's screening program indicated that 30% of the children under age 1 enrolled in Medicaid reported a preventive service, and only 65% of children aged 1 to 4 years were up to date on their immunizations (Yudkowsky & Fleming, 1990).

Neighborhood/Community Health Centers

Although Medicaid quickly became the financial underpinning of medical services for poor mothers and children, several additional health programs arose out of the political and social activism of the early 1960s. The Economic Opportunity Act of 1964 established the Office of Economic Opportunity (OEO). Recognizing medical care as only one of many determinants of health, the OEO funded a series of Neighborhood Health Centers. Although these centers provided comprehensive medical services, including prevention and treatment of physical and mental conditions, their mission was much broader. The Neighborhood Health Centers provided employment opportunities in their low-income catchment areas and served as the focus for other community and economic development activities. In addition to the broad service mandate, several other characteristics made these centers a unique approach to health services for the poor. For example, independent of state and local governments, the centers were supposed to be governed by boards of community members. Furthermore, services were supposed to be without cost to the users.

A key administrative and political aspect of these centers was that their federal support came directly to the local community organizations that had solicited the funds. Unlike the Title V program and Medicaid that allocated funds to states and required a state match, the establishment of Neighborhood Health Centers enabled federal policy makers to leap over potential state-level bureaucratic impediments to addressing local conditions as well as social and political attitudes and prejudices that had disenfranchised the poor people who needed the services provided by these health centers (Sardell, 1988).

As political support for the War on Poverty declined with the election of Richard Nixon in 1968, the legislative base for Neighborhood Health Centers changed. As Sardell (1988) noted, the centers achieved their own authorization under PL 94-63 and were renamed Community Health Centers. Unfortunately, attempts to rationalize the administration and oversight of the centers through the delineation of two types of financial support for (1) required and (2) supplemental services resulted in disproportionate emphasis on required, traditional medical services in contrast to the supplemental services such as health education, social services, and outreach. The appeal of the infrastructure established by the centers was strong, however, and Congress has occasionally appropriated funds for special infant mortality initiatives by them.

Special Supplemental Food Program for Women, Infants, and Children

Created in 1972, the Special Supplemental Food Program for Women, Infants, and Children (WIC) has become a fundamental component of government support for mothers and children. This discretionary program provides supplemental food, nutrition education, and access to medical care. Under eligibility guidelines established by the federal government and through federally appropriated funds, states distribute food (or coupons for

selected, nutritious foods) to low-income pregnant women, nursing mothers, and infants and children considered at nutritional risk. The key economic risk factor is family income under 185% of the federal poverty level. WIC has been associated with health improvements reflected in decreased rates of low birth weight (Rush et al., 1988) and anemia (Yip, Bintin, Fleshood, & Trowbridge, 1987). From a services perspective, however, there has been difficulty in incorporating WIC into other MCH programs. As indicated later in the discussion of major policy changes in the 1980s, administrative efforts are underway to make the supplemental food program a more cohesive part of services for mothers and children. For example, studies of the linkage of the provision of WIC services with immunization have, not surprisingly, shown marked improvement in immunization rates (Kotch & Whiteman, 1982) and use of dental services (Lee, Rozier, Kotch, Norton, & Vann, 2004).

Head Start

Just as Community Health Centers provided sites around which to organize efforts to address the more far-reaching determinants, the period of early childhood offered a time during which key social and economic influences might be altered to promote the later well-being of children. Project Head Start was launched as a summer program in 1965 to provide an intellectually stimulating and healthful environment for preschool children in centers established for that purpose. Proposed for 100,000 children, the popularity was such that over 560,000 children enrolled during that first summer. In spite of controversy over the intellectual benefits of Head Start, this federal effort has grown steadily since its inception. An often overlooked impact of Head Start has been its effect on health. In a review of Head Start studies, Ron Haskins (1989), then a staff analyst with the Committee on Ways and Means of the House of Representatives, noted that children attending Head Start were "more likely to get medical and dental exams, speech and developmental assessments, nutrition evaluations, and vision and hearing screenings." Furthermore, Head Start programs are well targeted toward poor children and provide many jobs as teachers and staff for low-income community members.

With the implementation of Head Start, the Children's Bureau met its functional, if not legislative, demise. The focus of bureau responsibilities had become increasingly in the area of welfare, even though the actual administration of AFDC fell within the purview of another agency. As reviewed by Steiner (1976), there was reluctance to assign a prominent and potentially substantial initiative such as Head Start to the Children's Bureau. Secretary of Health, Education, and Welfare Robert Finch, lacking strong political support for the Children's Bureau, delegated Head Start to a newly created Office of Child Development, also assigning the Children's Bureau, a shell of its former self, to this newly created office. The Title V Maternal and Child Health and Crippled Children's programs were assigned to the Health Services and Mental Health Administration of the Public Health Service. Child Welfare Services and the Juvenile Delinquency Service were assigned to the Social and Rehabilitation Service (Hutchins, 1994). What remained of the Children's Bureau was left with its responsibilities limited to that of a clearinghouse for agency information about children's health and welfare.

REDEFINING THE ROLES OF STATES

The election of Ronald Reagan as President in 1980 was followed by changes in Title V and Medicaid. As part of the Reagan effort to decrease the size of the federal government, reduce federal spending for social programs, and return power to the states, many categorical grants were combined into a series of block grants. The initial proposal by the president was to create two health block grants, converting 11 health services grants and 15

preventive health programs, respectively. Negotiations with Congress resulted in the consolidation of 21 programs into 4 health block grants: (1) alcohol, drug abuse, and mental health; (2) primary care; (3) preventive health; and (4) MCH.

The Maternal and Child Health Services Block Grant consolidated seven programs: Maternal and Child Health Services and Crippled Children's Services under Title V, Supplemental Security Income Disabled Children's Services, Hemophilia, Sudden Infant Death Syndrome, Prevention of Lead-Based Paint Poisoning, Genetic Disease, and Adolescent Health Services. Federal regulations covering the content of the programs in this block grant were minimal, permitting states to establish their own priorities. Funding for the block grant was reduced from $454.9 million in fiscal year 1981 to $373.7 million in fiscal year 1982, under the rationale that reduced federal regulation would enable states to undertake these activities more efficiently (Peterson, Bovbjerg, Davis, Davis, & Durman, 1986). States were permitted, however, to transfer other block grant funds into the MCH block grant, although transfers of funds from MCH were prohibited. As the decade progressed, Congress increased MCH Block Grant funding to a high of $527 million by 1986 (Guyer, 1987). Political forces in the 104th Congress threatened to cut the 1997 appropriation for Title V by 50%, but MCH advocates succeeded in reducing the proposed reduction to 1%.

The allocation formula for Title V funds with the Maternal and Child Health Services Block Grant as their current incarnation has undergone several revisions. The initial formula described previously here was altered in 1963 when Congress authorized that project grants could be distributed directly to local health agencies and various public and nonprofit organizations, providing the funding base for the M & I Projects and the C & Y Projects mentioned previously. As described by Klerman (1981) in her lucid review of the development of Title V, Congress decided in

1967 to reallocate these special project funds back into the basic formula grant. States were required to have a "Program of Projects" in M & I care, neonatal intensive care, family planning, health of C & Y, and dental health of children, although by no means was the intent or expectation that these were to extend statewide, beyond the "demonstration" mode. Funds were provided to ensure that each state undertook these required programs, but states with large urban populations were at risk of receiving smaller allocations than they had received under the previous scheme. The section 516 allotment was added to ensure that no state received less through the formula grants than it had received through its previous formula and project grants.

With the creation of the Maternal and Child Health Services Block Grant in 1981, the allocation formula was again based on previous allocations under the categorical programs. States were held "harmless" in that they would receive the same proportion of funds as under the prior legislation. As excess funds became available, they were to be distributed on the basis of the low-income population, but as the General Accounting Office (GAO) noted in 1990, 90% of the MCH block grants were allocated on the basis of their previous allocations, rather than adjustments for the low-income population. In a provocative study of allocation, the U.S. GAO (1992) examined what allocations would look like if done on the basis of three simple "at-risk" indicators—proportion of low birthweight children, proportion of children living in poverty, and proportion of the state's population under the age of 21 years (compared with the U.S. population). The GAO determined that 14% of the block grant funds would shift from lower risk to higher risk states, with decreases in 37 states and increases in 14.

The Medicaid program also was the object of major change in 1981. Mothers and children were directly affected by adverse changes in the eligibility requirements for AFDC. Because eligibility for AFDC was the major criterion for participation in Medicaid, a loss of AFDC meant a loss of Medicaid coverage, resulting in a decline in the proportion of poor people covered by Medicaid early in the 1980s.

Changes in Title V and Medicaid during the 1980s reflected the ongoing tension between the White House, controlled by Republicans, and the Congress, controlled by Democrats. The back-to-back economic recessions of 1979 through 1982 were accompanied by deterioration in several fundamental MCH indicators. For example, although the national infant mortality rate continued to decline, several states experienced increases or plateauing rates. The proportion of children covered by health insurance declined. Pressured by governors and advocates for mothers and children, Congress turned to the Medicaid program as the structure on which to address some of the glaring gaps in health services for mothers and children. The budget reconciliation process produced the changes shown in Table 2–2. In 1986, Congress severed the link between AFDC and Medicaid by permitting states to enroll pregnant women in Medicaid whose incomes were up to 100% of the federal poverty level even if their incomes were greater than the state income limit. The 1989 Omnibus Budget Reconciliation Act (OBRA) was noteworthy in that it set a national floor for Medicaid eligibility. By April, 1990, states were required to extend Medicaid coverage to all pregnant women and children up to the age of 6 years with family incomes below 133% of the federal poverty level.

The Medicaid expansions of the 1980s were effective in increasing access to care for poor pregnant women and children. As Cartland, McManus, and Flint (1993) have reported, Medicaid added 5 million recipients, half of whom were children. In 1990, 7% of the children enrolled in Medicaid were recipients as a result of the expansions of the 1980s. The proportion of recipients as a result of AFDC eligibility decreased from

Table 2–2 Changes in Medicaid Eligibility Beginning in the 1980s

1984	Required states to provide Medicaid coverage to single pregnant women, women in two-parent unemployed families, and all children born after September 30, 1983, if their incomes would have made them eligible for AFDC, according to each state's income guidelines.
1985	Required states to provide Medicaid coverage to all remaining pregnant women with family incomes below each state's AFDC eligibility levels and immediate coverage of all children under the age of 5 years with AFDC-level income or below.
1986	Allowed states to cover pregnant women, infants up to 1 year old, and, on an incremental basis, children up to 5 years old living in families with incomes above the state's AFDC income levels, but below 100% of the federal poverty level, effectively severing the link between AFDC eligibility and Medicaid eligibility. Also, permitted states to make pregnant women presumptively eligible for prenatal care after application and permitted states to eliminate the assets tests for poverty-related eligible pregnant women and children, allowing shortened application forms.
1987	Permitted states to increase the upper limit on income for pregnant women and infants up to 1 year old from 100 to 185% of the FPL.
1989	Required states to provide Medicaid coverage to all pregnant women and children up to the age of 6 years with family incomes below 133% of the FPL by April 1990.
1990	Increase eligibility level for pregnant women and infants to 185% of the FPL for children ages 1 to 6 years to 133% of the FPL.
2010	Patient Protection and Affordable Care Act expands eligibility to a national floor of 133% of the FPL.

90% in 1979 to 72% in 1990, although this population accounted for 29.8% of the increased costs in contrast to 26.8% by the expansion children. The remaining increased costs were accounted for by children not receiving cash assistance (19.4%) and medically needy (24.0%).

The OBRA of 1989 also mandated changes in the design and implementation of the Maternal and Child Health Services Block Grant. States were required to allocate 30% of the their funds to children's preventive/primary care services and 30% to children with special healthcare needs.[1] For appropriations greater than $600 million, 12.75% was set aside for four targeted initiatives. One set of initiatives expanded maternal and infant home visiting programs as well as enhanced the abilities of states to provide a range of health and social services using the "one-stop shopping" model. A second set of initiatives was aimed at increasing the participation of obstetricians and pediatricians in Medicaid. Third, monies were directed at the enhancement of rural projects for the care of pregnant women and infants and at the development of MCH centers at nonprofit hospitals. The fourth targeted area was to expand outpatient and community-based services (including child care) for children with special health needs. Furthermore, the act required states to undertake a statewide needs assessment and formulate a plan for the use of Title V funds that was based on

---

[1]During the 1980s, the name of the Crippled Children's Program was changed to Children With Special Health Care Needs to reflect the multifaceted aspects of care for these children.

the identified needs. In addition to these specific MCH mandates to improve access to care, OBRA 1989 directed the Secretary of Health and Human Services to develop a uniform, simple application for use by Medicaid, Maternal and Child Health, WIC, Head Start, Migrant and Community Health Centers, and Health Care Programs for the Homeless. A final initiative to promote accessibility required state Title V agencies to coordinate their activities with Medicaid. For example, state Title V agencies were expected to work with Medicaid agencies to achieve specified enrollment goals for the EPSDT program.

OBRA 1989 mandated changes to hold states and the Maternal and Child Health Bureau more accountable for the Block Grant expenditures. Annual reports were required to address progress toward their state goals, particularly as linked to the goals articulated in Healthy People 2000 (U.S. Department of Health and Human Services, 1991). Required reporting elements included a variety of MCH health status indicators by class of individuals (pregnant women, infants up to 1 year old, children with special healthcare needs, and other children less than 22 years of age), provider information, and the numbers served as well as health insurance status, including enrollment to Medicaid. The secretary is also required to provide the House Energy and Commerce and Senate Finance Committees with detailed summaries of states' annual reports, a compilation of national MCH data by health status indicators (including an assessment of progress toward Healthy People 2000 goals), and detailed results of each Special Projects of Regional and National Significance project.

Concern over infant mortality, particularly the persistence of areas of strikingly high rates, prompted President George H. W. Bush to launch a targeted infant mortality initiative of substantial size. The Healthy Start program, administered by the Maternal and Child Health Bureau, selected 15 communities (13 urban and 2 rural) and provided over $200 million dollars annually to facilitate community-driven approaches to infant mortality reduction. Building on the lessons of Sheppard-Towner and M & I projects, Healthy Start has provided social and educational interventions as well as medical services. Employment of community members as outreach workers reflects economic development as yet another component of this substantial initiative. Beginning in 1998, the initiative was expanded so that by 2002, 96 federally funded Healthy Start projects were addressing infant mortality through perinatal health, border health, interconceptional care, perinatal depression, and family violence services with a budget reduced in scale to approximately $97 million. In 2000, Mathematica Policy Research, Inc., completed its evaluation of the first 15 Healthy Start projects, noting associations with improved adequacy of prenatal care, lower preterm birth rates, decreased low and very low birthweight rates only in selected sites, and infant mortality rates that declined significantly, but of the same magnitude as comparable communities (Devaney, Howell, McCormick, & Moreno, 2000).

Since the inception of Title V in 1935, there have been three major motivations behind federal involvement in health services for children. Arising out of the Great Depression, Title V was the first in a series of federal initiatives that attempted to address disparities in health outcomes and services. With the globalization of the economy in the 1970s and 1980s, the motivation shifted to a recognition that a healthy workforce was needed in order to remain competitive. Although Medicaid expansions certainly addressed inequities, the broadening of eligibility represented a strategy to invest in the health of the potential workforce. As healthcare costs continued to grow at an alarming rate, with Medicaid and Medicare in particular escalating at annual rates of 21% and 10%, respectively, the motivating force behind health care reform became cost control. Bill Clinton's election to the presidency in 1992 was motivated, in part, by a growing concern over access to health care, particularly as escalating costs impeded the abilities of employers to offer health care as a benefit, state governments to finance Medicaid and other state healthcare programs, and individuals to purchase needed care.

Soon after his election, President Clinton proposed the Health Security Act, a sweeping reorganization of the healthcare system. The primary goal was to ensure that every citizen would have access to health insurance. Stemming from the work of Enthoven and Kronick (1989), the proposal promoted the concept of managed competition, with a substantial federal role. Large "accountable health partnerships," consisting of providers of health services (physicians, hospitals, etc.) and managers of payment systems (insurance companies, large health maintenance organizations), would compete with one another to offer packages of services to those who pay for services (employers, governments, and individuals). The "managed" part reflects the imposition of standardized packages of services and in some models the requirement that all populations be served. The "competition" takes place among the partnerships, as they would adjust their prices (and to some degree their packages of services within the established guidelines) in order to attract those who pay for services. As Iglehart (1993, p. 1220) explained, "Managed competition is price competition, but the price it focuses on is the annual premium for comprehensive health care services, not the price for each service." Each partnership was required to provide several "packages" from which consumers might choose on the basis of price. The packages were required to include one choice that was without cost to the consumer, for example, a health maintenance organization (HMO) in which costs could be strictly controlled. Other packages could include the equivalent of fee-for-service options in which consumers could choose among physicians, but they would bear the additional cost through premiums.

The complexity of the Health Security Act and the timing of its consideration leading up to the 1994 midterm Congressional elections resulted in the defeat of this initiative. The 1994 elections were a watershed in national and local politics in that the Republicans gained the majority in the House of Representatives for the first time in 50 years and regained the majority in the Senate, which they had maintained from 1981–1986. No Republican incumbent governors lost reelection bids, and Republicans ended up controlling 31 states. Acting on the belief that the role of the federal government must be reduced and that responsibility for health and welfare should return to states and even local communities, the Republicans proposed an end to the entitlement status for AFDC and Medicaid, creating instead block grants to the states to address these issues as they deemed appropriate.

In August 1996, after 2 years of raucous debate, President Clinton signed into law The Personal Responsibility and Work Opportunity Reconciliation Act of 1996 (PRWORA) (P.L. 104-193). This comprehensive reform made welfare a transition to work, enhanced child support enforcement programs, required unmarried teen mothers to live with parent(s) and remain in school, and limited eligibility for noncitizens (Blank & Haskins, 2001). AFDC, the individual cash entitlement, was repealed and replaced with a block grant, Temporary Assistance to Needy Families (TANF), allowing states the flexibility to convert welfare from a cash assistance program to a jobs program. The block grant also provided an incentive to states to assist individuals in the transition from dependence on a government subsidy to reliance on work, because unlike previous policy efforts to encourage work, work requirements were imposed on the state programs. For example, most participants were limited to 2 consecutive years of assistance and 5 years of lifetime assistance, although 20% of the caseload (e.g., people with disabilities) was exempt from this requirement.

The legislation also incorporated sanctions, particularly financial penalties, for states that failed to meet the work requirements. Although the number of families in receipt of AFDC and then TANF benefits has declined from 4,415,000 at the signing of the law in August 1996, to 2,032,157 in June 2003 (Administration for Children and Families, 2004), the scholarly and policy debates about how to measure the effects of this fundamental change in welfare policy continue (Blank & Haskins, 2001). TANF was reauthorized under the Deficit Reduction Act (DRA) of 2005, and required states to increase the work activities of those receiving TANF funds. Congress failed to reauthorize TANF as scheduled in 2010, extending the program through inclusion in the Claims Resolution Act (P.L. 111-291) to await debate in 2011.

In contrast to the successful effort to convert welfare to a block grant, removing the entitlement to cash welfare, parallel proposals to change the entitlement to Medicaid continue to be debated. Overall, the states are responsible for 43% of Medicaid costs, with state contributions ranging from 50% for the wealthier states to 23% for the poorer states (U.S. GAO, 2003). Annual growth of

total Medicaid spending reached 27.1% in 1990–1992, subsided to a more modest 3.2% rate of growth in 1995–1997, gradually accelerated to 12.8% in 2002 (Smith, Ellis, Gifford, & Ramesh, 2002), declined to 4.9% in 2008 and then doubled to 9.0% in 2009, as Medicaid programs increased their expenditures as safety nets in response to rising eligibility from the recession of 2007–2009. By 2009, Medicaid expenditures totaled $373.9 billion (Centers for Medicare and Medicaid Services, n.d.). As an entitlement, Medicaid requires states to generate the funds to cover eligible individuals, thus potentially impinging on discretionary expenditures in state budgets. From the perspective of mothers and children, however, it is important to examine Medicaid expenditures through the lens of Figure 2–1 and Figure 2–2: children comprise approximately 50% of the population of Medicaid recipients but consume only 18% of the expenditures. Coverage of children and pregnant women accounts for a small component of Medicaid's financial demands on state budgets.

Given the large and growing impact of Medicaid on state budgets, governors and state legislatures vigorously have opposed

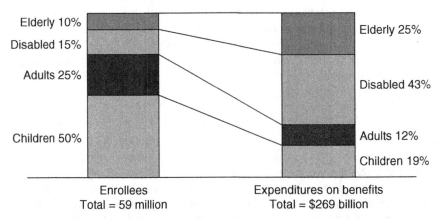

*Expenditure distribution based on CBO data that includes only spending on services and excludes Disproportionate Share Hospitals (DSH), supplemental provider payments, vaccines for children, and administration.

Figure 2–1 *Medicaid Enrollees and Expenditures by Enrollment Group, 2006*
Source: This information was reprinted with permission from the Henry J. Kaiser Family Foundation, a leader in health policy analysis, health journalism and communication, dedicated to filling the need for trusted, independent information on the major health issues facing our nation and its people. The Foundation is a non-profit private operating foundation, based in Menlo Park, California.

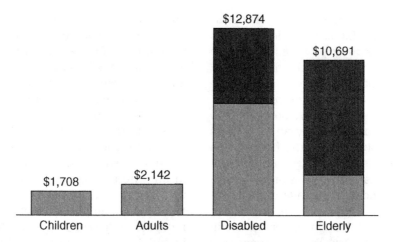

Figure 2–2 Medicaid Expenditures per Enrollee by Acute and Long-Term Care, 2006
Source: This information was reprinted with permission from the Henry J. Kaiser Family Foundation, a leader in health policy analysis, health journalism and communication, dedicated to filling the need for trusted, independent information on the major health issues facing our nation and its people. The Foundation is a non-profit private operating foundation, based in Menlo Park, California.

the reform of Medicaid from an entitlement to a discretionary block grant, with the likely limitation on federal funds inherent in a discretionary grant (Iglehart, 2003). Medicaid has become the infrastructure for many components of the health system—health care for poor, medically needy, and other vulnerable individuals; long-term care for the older population; and maintenance of hospitals and other organizations that serve the population of those eligible for Medicaid—so that even in the face of the fiscal pressures created by the entitlement, states are reluctant to accept the managerial freedom that would be associated with a block grant.

In spite of the ascendancy of the Republicans in the House and the Senate after the 1994 election and their assertion of a political view that would limit the implementation of new major federal expenditures, there was a growing consensus on the appropriateness of providing health insurance to low-income children who were not eligible for Medicaid, even after the expansions that had taken place beginning in the 1980s. As part of the Balanced Budget Act of 1997, Congress created the State Children's Health Insurance Program (SCHIP) to provide $40 billion in additional federal funds over a 10-year period, with a match that is 30% more generous than the Medicaid match. Established as Title XXI of the Social Security Act, SCHIP reflected the prevailing view that responsibility for design and implementation of programs should rest with the states by allowing states to pursue one of three basic options: (1) create a separate child health program, (2) expand Medicaid eligibility, or (3) develop a combination of new insurance and Medicaid expansion. Of the estimated 11 million children without health insurance in 1998, approximately 39.5% were eligible for Medicaid but had not been enrolled; 25.3% had incomes above that required for Medicaid or the new SCHIP insurance, and the remaining 35.2% became the focus of a new health insurance effort. As of July 2002, 16 states had developed separate SCHIP programs, 15 expanded Medicaid, and 19 adopted a combination (Mann, Rowland, & Garfield, 2003). By 2002, the number of uninsured children had declined to approximately 9.2 million (approximately 12% of children under the age of 19 years), with approximately 23.5% covered by Medicaid or SCHIP (Kaiser Commission on Medicaid and the Uninsured,

2003a). For low-income children, however, 25% of children in families with incomes less than 100% of the poverty level and 17% with incomes less than 199% of the poverty level remained without insurance (Kaiser Commission on Medicaid and the Uninsured, 2003b).

The election of George W. Bush in 2000 aligned both the presidency and Congress under the Republicans for the first time in nearly 50 years. Ironically, this alignment resulted in the largest expansion of federal entitlements since the passage of Medicare and Medicaid in 1965, with the creation of the Medicare drug benefit under the Medicare Prescription Drug Improvement and Modernization Act (P.L. 108-173). Originally budgeted at $409.8 billion for the 10-year period from 2004 to 2013, estimates from the Medicare actuaries and the Office of Management and Budget subsequent to the bill's passage and signature in December 2003 were as high as $534 billion (Pear & Andrews, 2004). As an entitlement, the fiscal effects created by the demand for drugs will likely create extraordinary pressure on the entire federal budget in general, especially the discretionary health and social service programs that affect so many families (Iglehart, 2004).

In December 2007, the most severe economic downturn since the Great Depression began, triggered by the bursting of a housing bubble and the collapse of major banks and other financial institutions involved in housing and real estate. Although the National Bureau of Economic Research, using its standard metrics, declared the recession over in June 2009, the unemployment rate of 5% in December 2007 had risen to 9.8% in November of 2010, with a record 30.9% unemployed for 52 weeks or more (U.S. Department of Labor, 2010). According to the Pew Research Center's report *How the Great Recession Has Changed Life in America* (Taylor et al., 2010), in May of 2010, 48% of survey respondents said they were in worse financial shape than before the recession and that household wealth had declined by about

20% from 2007 to 2009. As reported by the U.S. Census Bureau (DeNavas-Walt, Proctor, & Smith, 2010), the official poverty rate in 2009 was 14.3%, up from 13.2% in 2008, and the poverty rate for children under 18 years of age increased from 19.0% in 2008, to 20.7% in 2009.

The election of Barack Obama to the presidency in 2008 was accompanied by the election of substantial Democrat majorities in both houses of Congress. An ambitious political agenda was at first driven by the need for leadership to address the severe recession, reflected in a substantial increase in federal expenditures and authority as a response to the economic crisis. By one estimate, the $787 billion American Recovery and Reinvestment Act of 2009 (ARRA) directed approximately 20% of the total to children's programs (Aber & Chaudry, 2010). According to Aber and Chaudry, ARRA funds supported children through education and early education ($86.3 billion); tax programs ($28.7 billion), including expansion of the Earned Income Tax Credit (EITC); health and nutrition ($4.8 billion) such as Medicaid and Supplemental Nutrition Assistance Program (SNAP) funding; and others totaling $153 billion. To put the magnitude of these expenditures in some perspective, recall that the MCH Services Block Grant in 2010 was $662 million.

The return of Democrat control of the presidency and Congress prompted a renewed effort to establish national health insurance. The first immediate step was to reauthorize the SCHIP (now called CHIP) which had been held up by the Bush administration in a dispute over proper mechanisms to reallocate funds from some states to others when funds were not expended as expected. The Congressional Budget Office (CBO) estimates that the renewed program will cover an additional 6.5 million children in CHIP and Medicaid by 2013. Interestingly, funding is provided by a 62 cent per pack increase in the federal cigarette tax. Thanks to this and other public health insurance programs, insurance coverage for children actually went up from 2007 to 2008, even though the economy was in a serious recession (childstats.gov, 2010).

In March 2010, after 14 months of highly partisan debate and an eventual vote along strict party lines, President Obama signed the Patient Protection and Affordable Care Act (PPACA). As noted by John Iglehart, "On a scale of significant social legislation, the reform bill ranks with Medicare and Medicaid as a fundamental change in federal policy. The Congressional Budget Office has estimated that 95% of legal U.S. residents would have health insurance by 2019, up from 83% today, with about half carrying employer-based coverage and the other half entitled to publicly sponsored insurance through Medicare, Medicaid, the new state-based exchanges, or other government programs. Employer-sponsored insurance would be subject to new federal regulations, such as a ban on denying coverage to workers with a preexisting condition" (Iglehart, 2010, p. e48[3]). Provisions of the PPACA that specifically target mothers and children include home visiting programs, mandatory break time for nursing mothers, expansion of Medicaid, prohibition of preexisting conditions exclusions from health insurance eligibility, elimination of co-pays for prevention and screening services (including immunizations), dependent coverage up to age 26, and grants for school-based health centers, to name a few.

As this textbook goes to press, the implementation of this historic legislation is in active play, because the 2010 midterm elections produced yet another realignment of political power. The Republican Party picked up 63 seats in the House of Representatives for a 242 to 193 majority, added 5 seats in the Senate, reducing the Democrat majority to 51 seats, and added 6 governorships to total 29, results that will slow the momentum toward an increasing federal role in health care. In addition, legal challenges that reflect the attributes described at the beginning of this chapter are proceeding. For example,

while the overall political forces were aligned to enact this particular legislation, it was not politically feasible to pass a single-payer plan or even a tax analogous to the 2.9% payroll tax for Medicare. In order for this private insurance-driven plan to work, it is essential that all eligible participants purchase health insurance, so that the pool of insured is not limited to those in need of health care, but to the entire population as is the case with conventional health insurance. Challenges to the Affordable Care Act's requirement that individuals purchase insurance or face a penalty are working their way through the court system (Hall, 2010).

Readers are encouraged to follow the eventual implementation through very informative websites such as the Kaiser Family Foundation (KFF.org) and the journal *Health Affairs* (healthaffairs.org), and specifically for developments that apply to children and families, the Association of Maternal and Child Health Programs (amchp.org) and the American Academy of Pediatrics (aap.org).

CONCLUSION

Now well into the 21st century, the population of U.S. mothers and children remains at the center of the same debate that raged over the establishment of the Children's Bureau at the beginning of the 20th century. On one side are those that argue that children represent a community resource, a type of public good, the support of which is a responsibility of all citizens. On the other side are those who assert that the care and nurturance of children, although a community resource, are most effectively undertaken by families and their immediate communities. Interestingly, the same debate with regard to the other large dependent population—older persons—seems to have been answered in 1935, again in 1965, and once again in 2003. Namely, it is the federal government, rather than the states, to which we assign responsibility for the older population. Furthermore, benefits for older persons—Social Security

Old Age and Survivors Benefits, Medicare (and the new drug benefit)—are entitlements and are not subject to the same uncertainty of discretionary programs such as Title V, TANF, and CHIP.

With the implementation of TANF as block grants, particularly the elimination of the categorical entitlements to income support for poor, dependent children, states have assumed more responsibility for ensuring minimum health and welfare services for children. Although state and local governments are indeed "closer" to the people whom they serve, it is the federal government through the Congress and the Supreme Court that has traditionally articulated and enforced children's rights to the special services and protections that are the prerequisites of their healthy growth and development. With the devolution of responsibility to the states, it remains to be seen who will ensure, and to what degree, that all children, the most vulnerable and innocent among us, receive the social and health benefits that they need to become productive members of society (Nathan, 1996). Acknowledging and understanding this tension over responsibility for children is especially relevant for the field of maternal and child health as the crisis builds over the ultimate capacity of developed countries to finance the health and welfare benefits that they envision and promise to their citizens, as discussed in the previous chapter on children's rights and distributive justice.

References

Aber, L., & Chaudry A. (2010, January 15). *Low-income children, their families and the Great Recession: What next in policy?* Paper prepared for The Georgetown University and urban Institute Conference on Reducing Poverty and Economic Distress after ARRA.

Administration for Children and Families. (2004). Change in TANF caseloads. Retrieved from http://www.acf.dhhs.gov/news/stats/case-fam.htm.

American Recovery and Reinvestment Act. Pub. L. 111-5 (2009).

Baker, J. P. (1994). Women and the invention of well child care. *Pediatrics, 94,* 527–531.

Berger, L., & Johansson, S. R. (1980). Child health in the workplace: The Supreme Court in Hammer v. Dagenhart (1918). *Journal of Health Politics, Policy and Law, 5,* 81–97.

Blank, R., & Haskins, R. (2001). *The new world of welfare.* Washington, DC: Brookings Institution Press.

Bremner, R. H. (1970). *Children and youth in America.* Cambridge, MA: Harvard University Press.

Cartland, J. D. C., McManus, M. A., & Flint, S. S. (1993). A decade of Medicaid in perspective: What have been the effects on children? *Pediatrics, 91,* 287–295.

Centers for Medicare and Medicaid Services. (n.d.). National health expenditures 2009 highlights. http://www.cms.gov/NationalHealthExpendData/downloads/highlights.pdf.

Childstates.gov. America's children: Key national indicators of well-being, 2011. Retrieved September 24, 2011 from http://www.childstats.gov/americas-children/care.asp.

Davis, K., & Schoen, C. (1978). *Health and the war on poverty.* Washington, DC: Brookings Institution.

DeNavas-Walt, C., Proctor, B. D., & Smith, J. C. (2010). *Income, poverty, and health insurance coverage in the United States: 2009.* Current Population Reports, P60-238. Washington, DC: U.S. Census Bureau.

Devaney, B., Howell, E., McCormick, M., & Moreno, L. (2000). *Reducing infant mortality: Lessons learned from Healthy Start.* Princeton, NJ: Mathematica Policy Research.

Enthoven, A., & Kronick, R. (1989). A consumer-choice health plan for the 1990s. *New England Journal of Medicine, 320,* 29–37.

Epstein, R. (2003). Let the shoemaker stick to his last. *Perspectives in Biology and Medicine, 46,* S138–S159.

Foltz, A. (1975). The development of ambiguous federal policy: Early and Periodic Screening, Diagnosis and Treatment (EPSDT). *Milbank Memorial Fund Quarterly, 53,* 35–64.

Gostin, L. O., & Blocke, M. G. (2003). The politics of public health: A response to Epstein. *Perspectives in Biology and Medicine, 46,* S160–S175.

Grotberg, E. (1977). *200 years of children.* Washington, DC: U.S. Department of Health, Education, and Welfare.

Guyer, B. (1987). [Title V: An overview of its evolution and roles]. Unpublished paper.

Hall, M. A. (2010). Health care reform—what went wrong on the way to the courthouse. *New England Journal of Medicine, 364,* 295–297.

Haskins, R. (1989). Beyond metaphor. *American Psychologist, 44,* 274–282.

Hoover, H. (1931). *White House conference on child health and protection.* New York: Century Company.

Hughes, J. G. (1980). *American Academy of Pediatrics: The first 50 years.* Elk Grove Village, IL: American Academy of Pediatrics.

Hutchins, V. (1994). Maternal and Child Health Bureau: Roots. *Pediatrics, 94,* 695–699.

Iglehart, J. K. (1993). Managed competition. *New England Journal of Medicine, 328,* 1208–1212.

Iglehart, J. K. (2003). The dilemma of Medicaid. *New England Journal of Medicine, 348,* 2140–2148.

Iglehart, J. K. (2004). The new Medicare prescription-drug benefit: A pure power play. *New England Journal of Medicine, 350,* 826–833.

Iglehart, J. K. (2010). Historic passage—reform at last. *New England Journal of Medicine, 362,* e48(1)-(3).

Irwin, P., & Conroy-Hughes, R. (1982). EPSDT impact on health status: Estimates based on secondary analysis of administratively generated data. *Medical Care, 20,* 216–234.

Kaiser Commission on Medicaid and the Uninsured. (2003a). *Coverage in America: 2002 Data update.* Washington, DC: Henry J. Kaiser Foundation.

Kaiser Commission on Medicaid and the Uninsured. (2003b). *Uninsured: A primer.* Washington, DC: Henry J. Kaiser Foundation.

Keller, W. (1983). Study of selected outcomes of the EPSDT program in Michigan. *Public Health Reports, 28,* 110–118.

Klerman, L. (1981). Title V The Maternal and Child Health and Crippled Children's Services Section of the Social Security Act: Problems and opportunities. In Select Panel for the Promotion of Child Health (Ed.), *Better health for our children: A national strategy* (DHHS [PHS] Publication No. 79-55071). Washington, DC: U.S. Department of Health and Human Services.

Kotch, J. B., & Whiteman, D. (1982). Effect of the WIC program on children's clinic activity in a local health department. *Medical Care, 20,* 691–698.

Lathrop, J. (1919). Income and infant mortality. *American Journal of Public Health, 19,* 270–274.

Lee, J. Y., Rozier, R. G., Kotch, J. B., Norton, E. C., & Vann, W. F. Jr. (2004). The effects child WIC participation on use of oral health services. *American Journal of Public Health, 94,* 772–777.

Lesser, A. J. (1985). The origin and development of maternal and child health programs in the United States. *American Journal of Public Health, 75,* 590–598.

Lemons, J. S. (1969). The Sheppard-Towner Act: Progressivism in the 1920s. *Journal of American History, 55,* 776–786.

Mann, C., Rowland, D., & Garfield, R. (2003). Historical overview of children's health care coverage. *Future of Children, 13,* 31–53.

Meckel, R. (1990). *"Saving babies": American public health and the prevention of infant mortality.* Baltimore, MD: The Johns Hopkins University Press.

Miller, C. A. (1988). Development of MCH services and policy in the United States. In: H. M. Wallace, G. M. Ryan, Jr., & A. Oglesby (Eds.), *Maternal and child health practices* (3rd ed.). Oakland, CA: Third Party Publishing Co.

Nathan, R. (1996). *The "devolution revolution."* Rockefeller Institute Bulletin. Albany, NY: The Nelson A. Rockefeller Institute of Government.

Orr, S. T., & Miller, C. A. (1981). Utilization of health services by poor children since advent of Medicaid. *Medical Care, 19,* 583–590.

Pear, R., & Andrews, E. (2004, February 2). White House says Congressional estimate of new Medicare cost was too low. *New York Times.*

Peterson, G. E., Bovbjerg, R. R., Davis, B. A., Davis, W., & Durman, E. (1986). *The Reagan Block Grants: What have we learned?* Washington, DC: Urban Institute Press.

Pfohl, S. J. (1976). The "discovery" of child abuse. *Social Problems, 24,* 310–323.

Rosenbaum, S., & Johnson, K. (1986). Providing health care for low-income children: Reconciling child health goals with child health financing realities. *Milbank Quarterly, 64,* 442–478.

Rush, D., Sloan, N. L., Leighton, J., Alvir, J. M., Horvitz, D. G., Seaver, W. B., Garbowski, G. C., Johnson, S. S., Kulka, R. A., Holt, M., et al. (1988). The national WIC evaluation: Evaluation of the special supplemental food program for women, infants, and children. *American Journal of Clinical Nutrition,* *48,* 389–519.

Sardell, A. (1988). *The U.S. experiment in social medicine.* Pittsburgh, PA: University of Pittsburgh Press.

Schmidt, W. M., & Wallace, H. M. (1988). The development of health services for mothers and children in the U.S. In H. M. Wallace, G. M. Ryan, Jr., & A. Oglesby (Eds.), *Maternal and child health practices* (3rd ed.). Oakland, CA: Third Party Publishing Co.

Skocpol, T. (1992). *Protecting soldiers and mothers: The political origins of social policy in the U.S.* Cambridge, MA: Harvard University Press.

Smith, V., Ellis, E., Gifford, K., & Ramesh, R. (2002). *Medicaid spending growth: Results from a 2002 survey.* Washington, DC: Kaiser Family Foundation.

Sokol, R. J., Woolf, R. B., Rosen, M. G., & Weingarden, K. (1980). Risk, antepartum care, and outcome: impact of a maternity and infant care project. *Obstetrics & Gynecology, 56,* 150–156.

Steiner, G. (1976). *The children's cause.* Washington, DC: Brookings Institution.

Taylor, P., Morin, R., Kochhar, R. et al. (2010). *How the Great Recession has changed life in America.* Washington, DC: Pew Research Center. Retrieved September 24, 2011 from http://pewsocialtrends .org/files/2010/11/759-recession.pdf.

Tratner, W. I. (1974). *The public health movement: from poor laws to welfare state. In: A history of social welfare in America.* New York: The Free Press.

U.S. Congress. (1912). *An act to establish in the Department of Commerce and Labor a bureau to be known as the Children's Bureau.* 37 US Statutes 79.

U.S. Congress. (1935). *Grants to states for maternal and child welfare. Social Security Act.* 49 US Statutes 633, Title V.

U.S. Congress, Office of Technology Assessment. (1988). *Healthy children: Investing in the future* (OTA-H-345). Washington, DC: US Government Printing Office.

U.S. Department of Health and Human Services. (1991). *Healthy people 2000: National health promotion and disease prevention objectives* (DHHS Publication No. [PHS] 91-50212). Washington, DC: Author.

U.S. Department of Labor. (2010, October). *Ranks of those unemployed for a year or more up sharply.* Issues in Labor Statistics. Washington, DC: Author.

U.S. General Accounting Office. (1992, April). *Maternal and child health: Block grant funds should be distributed more equitably* (GAO/HRD-92-5). Washington, DC: Author.

U.S. General Accounting Office. (2003, July). *Medicaid formula: Differences in funding ability among states often are widened* (GAO-03-620). Washington, DC: Author.

Williams, G. J. R. (1983). Child protection: A journey into history. *Journal of Clinical Child Psychology, 12,* 236–243.

Wilson, A. L. (1989). Development of the U.S. federal role in children's health care: A critical appraisal. In L. Kopelman & J. Moskop (Eds.), *Children and health care.* Dordrecht: Kluwer Academic Publishers.

Witte, E. E. (1963). *The development of the Social Security Act.* Madison, WI: University of Wisconsin Press.

Yip, R., Bintin, F., Fleshood, L., & Trowbridge, F. L. (1987). Declining prevalence of anemia among low income children in the U.S. *Journal of the American Medical Association, 258,* 1619–1623.

Yudkowsky, B., & Fleming, G. (1990). Preventive health care for Medicaid children. *Health Care Financing Review,* Suppl, 89–96.

3

FAMILIES AND HEALTH

Joseph Telfair and Sheryl L. Coley

The life of a man is a circle from childhood to childhood, and so it is in everything where power moves. Our tepees were round like the nests of birds, and these were always set in a circle, the nation's hoop, a nest of many nests, where the Great Spirit meant for us to hatch our children.

(Neihardt, 1975)

INTRODUCTION

Historical and ethical concerns with the needs of children are inextricably linked with the family, the social institution most basic to the study and practice of maternal and child health (MCH). A family has been defined as a small, usually kinship-structured group, whose key function is nurturant socialization (Reiss & Lee, 1988). In contrast to the theory that the extended family was the prevalent structure in preindustrial society, in the United States, the predominant family system has always been the nuclear family (i.e., social positions of husband–father, wife–mother, and offspring). Relationships with extended kin had importance, but as mobility of families has increased, accessibility to these relationships has decreased.

The nuclear family, or more appropriately the "nuclear household" (Hareven, 1984), has been the definitive unit of analysis in the social scientific study of kinship relationships of the past several centuries. Much of what we know about the social health and overall well-being of children has come from these household studies, which have portrayed the family as the foundation for understanding human social development in modern U.S. society.

The family is an institution beneficial to both individuals and society; however, it is an institution that is under great stress from the significant changes that have taken place over the last 25 years. The increase in single-parent units, the intensification of economic hardships, the exacerbation of racial disparities, and the rise in rates of divorce and separation are all changes that are shaking the foundation of families as we have come to know them.

With the current political emphasis on "family values" connoting the more idealized "traditional" family unit, it has become necessary for practitioners in the field of MCH to develop an empirical understanding of the reality of the composition of the family in the United States today. It is of value in MCH practice to recognize that, as a system-level foundation for social development, a healthy, nurturing family is essential to a child's as well as a parent's normal physical, emotional, and social development. Consistent, supportive relationships as well as adequate nutrition, safe environments, and healthy lifestyles are as important to the well-being of children and parents as timely access to appropriate medical care (Center for the Future of Children, 1992; Van Dyck & Hogan, 2003).

This chapter describes the characteristics of current American families. As part of these descriptions, there is a discussion of health and health service issues (including emerging trends) as they affect families and whether these services meet their needs. Emerging trends in family services are also examined. For a very thorough review of the topics examined in this chapter, the reader is referred to the edited text by Wallace, Green, and Jaros (2003), *Health and Welfare for Families in the 21st Century* (2nd ed.) and the excellent resource page for the Department of Health and Human Services Administration for Children and Families located at http://www.acf.hhs.gov/acf_policy_planning .html#pubs and the agency's Child Welfare Information Gateway located at http://www .childwelfare.gov/.

FAMILY TRENDS IN THE HISTORICAL CONTEXT

World War I and World War II

Until World War I, the United States was primarily a society of farms and small towns with a few big urban centers. In these early communities, the typical form of household structure was the nuclear family. These were family units consisting of parents and their children, of a childless couple, or of one parent and children. Interestingly, the most important distinguishing feature of the nuclear family was the absence of extended kin. The nuclear *family* should not, however,

be seen as identical to the nuclear *household*, as the latter may have included nonrelatives (Hareven, 1984; Laslett & Wall, 1972).

By the time of the 1920 U.S. Census, the majority of the U.S. population had shifted from rural to urban areas (*World Almanac*, 1990). Before World War II, the nuclear household served the economic purpose of members working together on the farm (in rural areas) or in family businesses or for others (in urban areas). Adult children tended to live near their parents, creating communities with multigenerational kinship ties. There was a continuity of shared values and prescribed family roles. For example, men were seen as the major wage earners, and women remained at home, if possible, with the responsibility of rearing the children. Furthermore, because of the values of close family bonds, mutual support, and the overall well-being of the community, the care of poor children and families was not always seen as a responsibility to be shared by the community and the government. However, the impact of World War II on the economic and social structure of the United States brought significant change to kinship and community relationships on the one hand and government responsibilities on the other.

The continuing urbanization of the United States during and after World War II led to many changes that significantly affected the family unit and its functional roles and responsibilities. The increased mobility of families over the last 3 decades, spurred by the need to seek employment wherever it could be found, led to less spatial and temporal continuity and communal security (McNally, 1980). Furthermore, the lure of opportunity and the need to survive within a rapidly changing society have led to a redefinition of the role of family members and to a new understanding of family structure and family life.

American Family Composition

The makeup of American families has changed significantly since the end of World

War II. There has been an increase in the total number of households from 91.9 million in 1990 to 105 million in 2000 to 113.6 million in 2009 (U.S. Bureau of the Census, 2000, 2010j). The trend over the last 40 years has been a slowed growth rate in the number of family households (households that have at least two members related by birth, marriage, or adoption[1]) per year. Married couples constitute the largest proportion of U.S. households at 55.5 million, followed by the second most common household, people living alone (31 million). Family households increased by 11% from 64.5 million in 1990 to 71.8 million in 2000. However, since 2000 the growth of these households slowed, reaching 75.5 million in 2009, an increase of only 5.1% (Kreider & Elliot, 2009; U.S. Bureau of the Census, 2010j).

The proportion of children living with two biological parents has decreased in each decade since 1960. Whereas 88% of children lived with two biological parents in 1960, 70% of children are currently living with two biological parents as of 2009 (U.S. Bureau of the Census, 2010b). Single-mother families with children under 18 years old increased from approximately 3 million in 1970 to 8.3 million in 2009, whereas the number of single-father families grew from approximately 393,000 to 2.6 million in 2009 (U.S. Bureau of the Census, 2010j). In 1970, 12% of family households with children under 18 years old were headed by single mothers compared with 1% headed by single fathers. In 2009, the proportions of these single-parent households grew to 24% and 7% for mother-headed and father-headed households, respectively (U.S. Bureau of the Census, 2010g & 2010j). This trend illustrates a continual shift in our society from two-parent to one-parent family households, with a larger proportion of births occurring to unmarried women when comparing the 2000s to the 1960s and 1970s. These one-parent households are an outgrowth of several factors, including the delaying or opting out of marriage, which increases the likelihood of nonmarital births. These trends affect a number of programs and policies, which in turn have an overall effect on the well-being of children in single-parent households through changes in work and family life.

Grandparents play a huge role in many children's lives in the United States. Over the past 2 decades, grandparents carried increased responsibility for their grandchildren due to an increase of children living in grandparent households that started in the 1990s. In 2000, the Current Population Survey (CPS) determined that 4 million children (5% of all children) under 18 years old lived with a grandparent. This trend continues as approximately 7 million children (9% of all children) living with at least one grandparent as of 2009, marking an increase of almost 75% in the past decade (U.S. Bureau of the Census, 2010j). Thirty-three percent of children living with a grandparent had both mother and father living with them also. Forty-one percent of children who lived with grandparents lived with a mother and no father, whereas 4% living with grandparents lived also with a father and no mother. The other 22% lived with their grandparents only (U.S. Bureau of the Census, 2010b). Even with one parent present, 12% of children who lived with a single mother and 8% of children living with a single father were living in a household headed by a grandparent. These percentages convey the increasing role that grandparents play in the lives of their adult children. Moreover, 40.3% of the 6.7 million grandparents who live with grandchildren claimed parental responsibility for their grandchildren as of 2009 (U.S. Bureau of the Census, 2010j).

These trends of increased responsibilities of grandparents for their children and grandchildren have significant implications on the

[1]U.S. Bureau of the Census definition, 2010.

children's socioeconomic status. In 2002, children who lived with grandparents without a parent present (30%) were two times as likely to live in a family below the poverty level when compared with children who live with grandparents and a parent (15%) (U.S. Bureau of the Census, 2000). This trend continues as 32% of children who live with grandparents without a parent lived in poverty as of 2008 (Federal Interagency Forum on Child and Family Statistics, 2009). As of 2009, a greater proportion of children living with either single or married grandparents without a parent lived below the poverty level in contrast to children who also live with a single parent (33% vs. 24%) and children who also lived with both parents (9%). The proportion of children who lived with single grandparents without a parent present and who lived below the poverty level was five times higher than children who also lived with both parents (45% vs. 9%) (U.S. Bureau of the Census, 2010b). Overall, approximately 20% of grandparents who raise their grandchildren live in poverty (Children's Defense Fund, 2010). This trend also affects both health insurance coverage and public assistance, with significant differences found when comparing children living with grandparents with and without parents present (Fields, 2003). As of 2009, a greater proportion of uninsured children lived with single or married grandparents without a parent present (22%) in contrast to uninsured children who also live with a single parent (19%) or married parents (12%). This trend particularly affects children who live with single grandmothers. The proportion of uninsured children who lived with single grandmothers without a parent present is significantly greater than the proportion of uninsured children who live with a single parent (25% vs. 15%) and more than three times higher than the proportion of uninsured children who also live with both parents (8%) (U.S. Bureau of the Census, 2010b). These trends illustrate how the pools of resources from parents are a primary source for economic well-being for children because of the likelihood of parents contributing to the household economy and children's health needs when present (Current Population Reports, 2003; Fields, 2003).

Other noteworthy trends in the U.S. family are the growing numbers of extended families and cohabiting parents and the decreasing number of blended families. Blended families are created when remarriages result in stepparents living in the household with their children from previous marriages (in 1996, 17% of all children lived in blended families). However, the percentage of children living with stepparents decreased to 5.7% in 2009 (U.S. Bureau of the Census, 2010b). Extended families are created when a child lives with at least one parent and someone other than his or her own parents or siblings, often an additional relative (in 1996, 14% of all children lived in extended families). As of 2009, this percentage doubled to 28% (U.S. Bureau of the Census, 2010b). Cohabitating parent–child families are defined as when the children's parent is living with at least one nonrelated adult of the opposite sex. This person may or may not be the biological parent of the child; in 1996, 5% of all children were living with one parent and that parent's partner (U.S. Bureau of the Census, 2000). As of 2009, 3% of all children under 18 years old were living with both parents who are not married to each other, and an additional 2.7% of all children were living with a single parent and an unmarried partner (U.S. Bureau of the Census, 2010b).

Family and Household Size

The trend toward smaller families and households began with the end of the postwar baby boom in the mid-1960s, reaching in 1990 a level of 2.63 persons per household, on average, and 3.17 persons per family. This trend continued through 2009 as the average number in a household remains as 2.63 and the average number in a family declined slightly to 3.23 (U.S. Bureau of the

Census, 2010j). The most significant changes in household size occurred in the smallest and largest households. From 1970 to 2007, the smallest (households with one or two persons) increased from 46% to 60% of all households, and largest (households with five or more persons) decreased from 21% to 10% of all households (Kreider & Elliot, 2009). The average sizes of households and families have declined in the last decade because there are fewer children per family, more one-parent families, a growing number of persons living alone, and a growing number of couples choosing to delay having children or not have them at all (U.S. Bureau of the Census, 2000; Ventura, 2003).

During the last 40 years, the overall percentage of families with children less than 18 years old present declined. In 1970, approximately 29 million (56%) of the 51 million families had children less than 18 years old. In 2009, of the 79 million family households, approximately 36 million (45%) had children less than 18 years old, a decrease of 11% (U.S. Bureau of the Census, 2010g). Despite this decrease in the overall percentage of families with children less than 18 years old, the number of one-parent families with children increased significantly. In 1970, there were 3.8 million one-parent family groups, only 13% of the 29 million families with children at that time. By 2009, that proportion had risen to 30%, representing 11 million of the 36 million family households with children under 18[2] (U.S. Bureau of the Census, 2010g). The number of female-headed family households with no husband present but with children rose from 6 million in 1990 to 7.6 million in 2000 to 8.3 million in 2009 (Fields & Casper, 2001; U.S. Bureau of the Census, 2010g). According to 2009 U.S. Census data, 19.4 million children under 18 years old lived with one parent, including 16.9 million children living with a single mother. Out of these children who live with single mothers, the largest

proportion (7.4 million) live with mothers who have never been married (U.S. Bureau of the Census, 2010b).

Several factors have affected the trend in society for the shift from two-parent to one-parent households; one factor is the increased rate of births to unmarried women. Since 1970, this rate grew from 26.4 per 1,000 to 45.2 per 1,000 unmarried women aged 15–44 years in 2000 (Ventura, 2003). By 2007, the birth rate rose significantly to 53 per 1,000. In 2007, unmarried women contributed the highest proportion of all U.S. births ever reported, 40% (Federal Interagency Forum on Child and Family Statistics, 2010). However, the number of births to unmarried women has decreased slightly to 38 per 1,000 unmarried women aged 15–44 years of age as of 2009 (U.S. Bureau of the Census, 2010j).

Family Composition, Race, and Ethnicity

Between 1970 and 2009, the proportion of two-parent family groups has declined for white non-Hispanics, blacks, and persons of Hispanic origin (who may be of any race), whereas father–child and mother–child family groups have increased. In 1970, 90% of white family households had two parents, whereas 64% of black family households had two parents. As of 2008, 71% of all white non-Hispanic children lived with two married parents, in comparison to 36% of black children (U.S. Bureau of the Census, 2010e). The percentage of two-parent households for Hispanic children dropped significantly from 75% in 1980 to 64% of Hispanic children in 2008 (Federal Interagency Forum on Child and Family Statistics, 2009; U.S. Bureau of the Census, 2010h).

The proportion of mother–child family groups has increased most dramatically because of births outside of marriage and the rise in divorce. In 1990, approximately 32% of children who lived with single parents

[2]These data from the U.S. Census include parents who may live with partners unrelated to their children.

were living in homes in which the mother never married. This percentage of children living with never-married single mothers varied by the race of the child, with approximately 53 % of black children, 37 % of Hispanic children (all races), and 22 % of white non-Hispanic children living in family households with never-married mothers between the ages of 14 and 44 years (Lugaila, 1992; U.S. Bureau of the Census, 2000). Possible reasons for the increase for all races during the 1990s have been noted as follows (Donovan, 1995):

1. Increasing sexual activity at earlier ages,
2. Decreasing social stigma associated with out-of-wedlock birth, and
3. The only positive relationships in the woman's life being those with the male partner and the baby.

As of 2009, 44 % of all children living with single mothers had mothers who never married. Within this proportion of children who lived with never-married single mothers, black children still constitute the highest proportion (52 %) in comparison to 26 % of Hispanic children (all races) and 21 % of white non-Hispanic children (U.S. Bureau of the Census, 2010b). In 2009, 31 % of all children in households headed by single mothers lived with mothers who were divorced (U.S. Bureau of the Census, 2010b). More white non-Hispanic children within this population of children lived with single mothers who were divorced (61 %) than black or Hispanic children (19 % and 16 % respectively) (U.S. Bureau of the Census, 2010b).

Current data indicate that racial and ethnic differences also exist regarding children who live without the presence of either parent. As of 2009, more than twice the proportion of black children (8.3 %) lived with neither parent in comparison to white non-Hispanic (3.1 %) and Hispanic (3.9 %) children, and this proportion was more than four times the proportion for Asian children (2 %) (Children's Defense Fund, 2010). More than twice the proportion of black children lives with

their grandparents, other relatives, or nonrelatives than all other racial and ethnic groups (Children's Defense Fund, 2010).

The ethnic composition of American families has been significantly changed by the influx of immigrant families over the past few decades. From 1990 to 2000, the percentage of the foreign-born population increased by 57 % from 19.8 million to 31.1 million (Malone et al., 2003). Since 2000, the Hispanic population has grown to constitute the largest minority group in the United States. The proportion of all American children who are Hispanic has grown from 9 % in 1980 to 22 % in 2008 (Federal Interagency Forum on Child and Family Statistics, 2009). This proportion of children is now higher than the proportion of black non-Hispanic children (15 % in 2008). As of 2008, the majority of family households in the foreign-born population are headed by married couples (55.3 %), and foreign-born households are more likely than native-born households to constitute families of three or more people. Approximately 46.5 % of foreign-born households had three- or four-person families in contrast to 40.3 % of native-born households, and the percentage of foreign-born households that have five or more family members is more than double the percentage for native-born households (Pew Hispanic Center, 2010). In 2009, 22 % of all children under the age of 18 living in the United States had at least one foreign-born parent. This percentage has grown from 15 % in 1994 (Federal Interagency Forum on Child and Family Statistics, 2010).

Marriage, Divorce, and Remarriage

In the decades since World War II, changes in the social and technologic fabric of American society have led to dramatic challenges and changes for families. Opportunities for women to delay (choosing to marry at a later age) or not pursue marriage as the path to having a family have increased dramatically. These opportunities were the result of the changing social perceptions of the role of women. The chance for many more women to pursue higher education and careers rose significantly between 1960 and 1990. Married-couple families dropped from 87% in 1970 to 82% in 1980, 79% in the first quarter of 1990 to 52.8% in 2000 (U.S. Bureau of the Census, 1990, 2000). This decline has continued as the percentage of married-couple families had dropped to 49.1% in 2009, which is less than half of all households in the United States (U.S. Bureau of the Census, 2010j). Between 1970 and 1990, the overall marriage rate has decreased from 76% of all women 15 years of age and older in 1970 to 52.3% of women 15 years of age and older in 1992 (Rawlings, 1993). As of 2009, the percentage of married women 15 years of age and older has dropped to 47.4%, which also accounts for less than half of all women in the United States (U.S. Bureau of the Census, 2010j).

For both men and women, the median ages at first marriage were lowest in the mid-1950s and have been rising since (Lugaila, 1992). In 1970, the median age for marriage for men was 23.2 years and for women was 20.8 years. In 2000, the average age for first marriage increased to 26.8 years for men and 25.1 years for women. This trend continues as the median ages for men and women for first marriage was 28.1 and 25.9 respectively as of 2009 (U.S. Bureau of the Census, 2010i). In 2000, never-married people accounted for 31% of men and 25% of women over 15 years of age. This is an increase since 1970 from 28% and 22%, respectively (Fields & Casper, 2001). The proportions of never-married people continue to grow as 35% of men and 29% of women over 15 years of age have never been married as of 2009 (U.S. Bureau of the Census, 2010j).

Over the past 4 decades, the increasing median age for first marriage and increasing divorce rates (which became level in the 1990s) caused a great demographic shift in the status of marriage in the U.S. population.

Larger numbers of Americans in 2000 were never married or divorced than in 1970, resulting in a decline in the numbers currently married. Just as age at first marriage has been rising, so are the proportions of men and women who have never married. Increases have occurred for each 5-year age group between ages of 20 and 34 years in the proportions who have never married. For women, only 23% had never married in 1960 compared with 63% in 1990. For men, 53% had never married in 1960 compared with 79% in 1990 (Fields & Casper, 2001). However, the proportion of men and women who have never been married has decreased for the 20 to 34 year age groups since 1990. As of 2009, 50% of women between the ages of 20 and 34 years old have never been married, and 62% of men in these age groups have never been married (U.S. Bureau of the Census, 2010b).

Change in social mores and the attenuation of some of the earlier taboos against single parenthood and divorce have allowed both to become more socially acceptable. The discarding of traditional social constraints and the availability of medical methods of contraception led to more acceptance of cohabitation without marriage. In 2009, an estimated 6.7 million couples were reported as cohabiting (Kreider, 2010). Bias decreased against pregnancy out of wedlock, and a trend developed for single mothers to keep their babies rather than placing them for adoption or in long-term child care homes (Schorr & Schorr, 1988). Divorce rates have increased since 1921, with the sharpest increases occurring from the mid-1960s to the late 1970s (Lugaila, 1992; Schorr & Schorr, 1988). The rate of divorce dramatically rose over the last 3 decades from approximately 15% of all marriages in 1960 to a rate of approximately 50% of all marriages in 1990 (i.e., 4.6 of every 10 marriages ends in divorce), and the children of these divorces typically live in one-parent families (Lugaila, 1992). The divorce rate for men over 15 years of age in 1990 was 8.8% and for women 11.7%. As of 2000, approximately 1 in 5 adults (men and women) has ever been divorced. The average duration of marriages that end in divorce was 8 years (Kreider, 2005). An overall increase occurred for divorce in the United States from 1950 to 2000 among persons aged 25 to 34 years from 2% to 6% for men and from 3% to 9% for women. By 2000, the divorce rate for both sexes had risen slightly to 10.1% for men and 12.6% for women. However, as of 2009, the divorce rate had slightly decreased to 8.5% for men and 10.8% for women (U.S. Bureau of the Census, 2010b). According to the most recent marital status report by U.S. Bureau of the Census, the highest rate of divorce is among the age group of 45 to 64 years for both men (14%) and women (17%) as of 2009. The overall divorce rate for women is generally higher because of the trend that ever-divorced men are more likely to be currently married than ever-divorced women (Kreider, 2005). With regards to race and ethnicity, Asians have the lowest divorce rate when compared with whites, African Americans, American Indians and Alaska Natives, Native Hawaiians, or other Pacific Islanders.

Similarly, a high percentage of remarriages fail. In 1991, 37% of remarriages versus 30% of first marriages failed. Studies suggest that children growing up in divorced families and in stepfamilies have greater difficulties in social relationships, achievement, and behavioral adjustment (Hetherington & Jodl, 1994). Researchers caution, however, that the results of these studies have small effect sizes and diversity in outcome. There is considerable variation in the balance of risk and protective factors within family structures, and individual and policy decisions should not be based on these findings alone (Amato, 1994). In 2001, the average duration of second marriages that ended in divorce was 9.2 years for men and 8.1 years for women (Kreider, 2005). According to the 2008 American Community Survey, the highest proportion of men and women who have remarried

were in the 45 to 54 years age group (27.4% of all second marriages) and among white non-Hispanic men and women (77.4%). More women than men have remarried (53.3% vs. 46.7%) (U.S. Bureau of the Census, 2008).

Of children living with two parents in 1996, 88% lived with both biological mother and father, and 9% lived with a stepparent (U.S. Bureau of the Census, 2000). However, these percentages dropped as the number of children who live with only one parent increased. As of 2009, only 62.5% of all children under 18 years old lived with both biological parents, and 5.7% of all children lived with one parent and one stepparent (U.S. Bureau of the Census, 2010b). The vast majority of these stepfamily situations consist of a biological mother and a stepfather combination because children more often remain with their mother after divorce. In the case of unmarried parents, the children also usually remain with the mother. In 1990, the majority of children living with one parent were living with a parent who was divorced or whose spouse was absent (either separated or living elsewhere). The proportion living with a widowed parent declined during the past 40 years from 20% to 3.9%. (U.S. Bureau of the Census, 2010b, 2010e).

Finally, the increased availability of artificial insemination technology and the number of states allowing adoption by same-sex couples provided many single women the chance to have a family without a commitment to marriage. Both of these trends have contributed to the increased proportion of children living with single, never-married mothers from 1970 through 2000. The proportion of children in one-parent families who lived with a never-married mother increased from 7% in 1970 to 32% in 1990 and 43% in 2000 (Fields & Casper, 2001). At the same time, the development of an effective oral contraceptive and the initiation of public policy allowing the use of tax funds to support family planning clinics gave couples the opportunity to avoid pregnancy. The proportion of children in one-parent families who lived with a never-married mother decreased to 38.3% as of 2009 (U.S. Bureau of the Census, 2010e). This decrease may have resulted from the following factors: (1) the decrease of live births to unmarried women, (2) the increase of mothers who have cohabiting partners, and (3) the increase in the proportion of single households headed by men.

Family Income, Wealth, and Employment

The median family income increased by 104% during the 26 years between 1947 and 1973. During this time, the median income of married-couple families increased by 115%. Despite these fluctuations and the increase in wives' labor force participation, by 1990, the median income for all families was only 6% more than in 1973, and the median income for married-couple families was only 11% greater than in 1973. Among families with female householders and no spouse present, the median family income grew by 37% between 1947 and 1973 but increased only by 5% between 1973 and 1990. In 1989, the median family income was $33,585. In 1992, the median family income was $31,553. In 1993, the median family income was $31,241, and in 2000, the median family income was $48,196. This illustrates an increase in median family income of approximately $17,000 over 7 years from 1993 to 2000 (Current Population Survey, 2001). The median family income peaked at $61,355 in 2007 but decreased slightly to $60,088 as of 2009 due to the recession that started in 2007 (U.S. Bureau of the Census, 2010f).

The median family income differs significantly by race. In 1999, the median family income for Asians was reported at $51,908, white non-Hispanics at $45,367, Hispanics at $33,676, and blacks at $29,423 (Welniak & Posey, 2005). By 2009, the median family income reached $74,791 for Asians, $67,341 for white non-Hispanic family households, $39,730 for Hispanics and $38,493 for blacks (U.S. Bureau of the Census, 2010f). The median family income for all racial and ethnic groups declined from 2007 to 2009 with the economic downturn.

As the median income has fluctuated since the early 1980s, the status for families with children has constantly changed. In 2001, more children lived in families with relatively medium incomes (33%) than in other income groups; 22% lived in relatively low-income families, and 29% lived in relatively high-income families (U.S. Bureau of the Census, 2002).[3] However, the percentage of children living in families with relatively medium incomes fell from 41% in 1980 to 33% in 2001, whereas the percentage of children living in families with relatively high incomes rose from 17 to 29% during that same period (Federal Interagency Forum on Child Health and Family Statistics, 2003). These rates had remained relatively the same as more children lived in medium-income families (32%) than in low-income families (21%) or high-income families (30%) as of 2007 (Federal Interagency Forum on Child Health and Family Statistics, 2009).

The rates of low relative income for families with children vary significantly by race. For whites, the proportion of relatively low-income families increased from 13% in 1969 to 15% in 1989. For Hispanics, the increase was from 33% in 1979 to 38% in 1989 (1969 numbers were not available). For blacks, the increase was from 42% in 1974 to 44% in 1989 (1969 numbers were not available) (U.S. Bureau of the Census, 1991b). More recent statistics suggest the same pattern. Subsequently, the low-income rate is much higher for black or Hispanic children than for white, non-Hispanic children.

---

[3]The U.S. Bureau of the Census defines low income as 100–199% of the current poverty level, medium income as 200–399% of the current poverty level, and high income as 400% or above the poverty level.

The 2009 U.S. Census data (2010b) indicate that 31% of Hispanic children and 26% of black children have low-income status in comparison to 17% of white non-Hispanic children.

Women in the Workforce

An increasing number of women have entered the workforce since 1950. The percentage of married mothers with children less than 18 years old in the workforce in 1960 was less than 30%; in 1970 the number was 40%, in 1990 was 59%, and in 2000 was 74%. The percentage of married mothers with children aged 6 to 17 years who were employed rose from less than 30% in 1960 to 49% in 1970 and to 74% in 1990. However, this percentage decreased slightly to 71% in 2000 (U.S. Bureau of the Census, 2000). Among married women with children less than 6 years old, the proportion of those in the labor force doubled from 30% in 1970 to 59% in 1990 (Lugaila, 1992), and a moderate increase occurred through 2000 to 61% (U.S. Bureau of the Census, 2000). These data indicate that labor force participation by married women had increased significantly, especially for those women with children less than 6 years old. According to the 2000 U.S. Census, labor force participation among all women increased between 1990 and 2000 (57 in every 100 to 58 in every 100 women). Yet, women in 2000 were still more likely than men to be outside the workforce (30% women of women compared to 18.1% of men) (Clark & Weismantle, 2003).

The economic downturn that occurred since 2000 had a moderate impact on women in the workforce. Between 2008 and 2009, the number of working women decreased from 74.6 to 73 million, and the number of women working full time within this population decreased from 44.1 to 43.2 million (DeNavas-Walt, Proctor, & Smith, 2010). By 2009, the overall percentage of working married women with children under 18 had slightly decreased to 66%, with the percentage of working mothers with children under

6 decreasing to 58% and the percentage of working mothers with children 6–17 years old decreasing to 68% (U.S. Bureau of the Census, 2010b).

Parents in the Workforce

Among married-couple families with children in 1990, the proportion in which both the husband and wife worked was 70%. A slight decrease occurred between 1990 and 2002, with 68.7% of all children having both parents in the workforce (Fields, 2003). By 2007, 66% of married-couple families with children had both parents in the labor force (Kreider & Elliott, 2009). With regard to single-parent families with children ages 6 to 17 years old, the custodial parent was working in 71% of single-mother families and 85% of single-father families in 2000 (U.S. Department of Education and U.S. Department of Justice, 2000). These trends stayed relatively the same as 81.3% of custodial single parents worked at least in part-time employment as of 2007 (Grall, 2009). However, there were only moderate increases in full-time employment for single parents from 45.6% in 1993 to 53.5% in 2007, and custodial mothers were less likely to have full-time employment than custodial fathers (49.8% vs. 71.7%) (Grall, 2009).

More attention has been given to stay-at-home parents in recent years, particularly mothers who choose to stay at home. In 2002, only 7% of all U.S. households consisted of married couples with children in which only the husband worked. Dual-income families with children made up more than two times as many households. Even families with two incomes and no children outnumbered the traditional family by almost two to one (U.S. Bureau of the Census, 2002). Married couple families with children are more likely to have mothers out of the workforce than fathers (Fields, 2003). By 2009, 5.7 million of 24 million married-couple families with children had a stay-at-home mother, which represents approximately 24% of married-couple families (Kreider &

Elliott, 2010). In contrast, there were only 158,000 stay-at-home dads in 2009 (Bernstein, 2010). Even though white non-Hispanic mothers constitute the majority of the stay-at-home mother population (60.4% of all stay-at-home mothers), stay-at-home mothers are prevalent within Hispanic married-couple households (26.7%) and within foreign-born married-couple households (34%) (Kreider & Elliott, 2009). In addition, stay-at-home mothers were more likely to be younger, as 44% of all stay-at-home mothers are under 35 years old (Kreider & Elliott, 2009).

Means-Tested Cash Assistance

In the year 2002, almost one third of all children lived in families with incomes below $30,000, and 17% were in families below 100% of poverty. Public assistance was received by 5% of children, and 11% received food stamps. In comparison, 49% of all children lived in families with incomes of $50,000 per year or more, and 29% were in families with $75,000 per year.

In the early 1990s, 14% of the population received some form of means-tested cash assistance,[4] with 7.7% of married couple families receiving assistance in comparison to 42.9% of female-headed families with children (Tin, 1996). Sixty-nine percent of poor married couple families had one or more members who worked to earn wages or salaries (Baugher, 1993). Poor, female-headed households with children, on the other hand, were more likely to have received means-tested cash assistance than to have one or more members with income earned through work (67% vs. 49%). Of the total income of poor families, approximately 80% was received from these two sources. The remaining 20% of total income for poor families with children came from other sources, such as Social Security. By the third quarter of 2008, a monthly average of approximately 28.4 million households received at least one type of cash or noncash assistance. This average constitutes about 24% of all U.S. households in contrast to 16% of U.S. households in 1984 (Palumbo, 2010). The most commonly received services were Medicaid, free or reduced-price school meals, and food stamps. A majority of those households that received noncash assistance (54%) participated in two or more programs. About 5.9 million female-headed households with no husband present and children under 18 years old received noncash benefits (Palumbo, 2010). A majority of women who received Temporary Assistance for Needy Families (TANF) in recent years were never married (51%); 28% of TANF-recipient women were widowed, divorced, or separated; and 21% were married (Irving, 2010).

Poverty

Families with children under 18 years of age experienced a decline in poverty from 20.3% in 1959 to 10.8% in 1966. Between 1966 and 1979, the poverty rate remained within 2.5 percentage points of this previous low, varying from 10.8% to 13.3%. Poverty estimates based on the current definition date back to the early 1960s. The poverty rate fell dramatically during the 1960s from 22.2% in 1960 to 12.1% in 1969. From 1970 to 1978, changes in poverty were relatively small, with the poverty rates ranging between 12.6% in 1970 and 11.7% in 1979. The poverty rate in 1983 (15.2%) was the highest since 1965. Although the poverty rate in 1991 (14.2%) was lower than that more recent peak, it remained well above the 1978 level of 11.4%, a recent low point (U.S. Bureau of the Census, 1994). The official poverty rate rose from 11.7% in 2001 to 12.1% in 2002. The number in poverty increased by 1.7 million people to 34.6 million in 2002.

---

[4]Means-tested cash assistance includes public assistance or welfare payments and Supplemental Security Income (SSI).

The official poverty rate for children has fluctuated since the early 1980s. It reached a high of 22% in 1993 but decreased to 16% in 2000 (Federal Interagency Forum on Child Health and Family Statistics, 2003). In contrast, the percentage of children living in families experiencing extreme poverty (families with income below 50% of the poverty threshold)[5] rose from 7% in 1980 to 10% in 1992 and has steadily decreased to 7% in 2001 (U.S. Bureau of the Census, 2002). Overall, child poverty rates have dropped over one quarter within these years, but this decline stopped in 2001.

The U.S. economy has spiraled downward since the recession started in 2007. Subsequently, the U.S. poverty rate grew to 14.3% in 2009, bringing the total number of people living in poverty to 43.6 million (Gould & Shierholz, 2010). This total is the largest since 1959 (DeNavas-Walt, Proctor, & Smith, 2010). The percentage of families in poverty grew to 11.1% in 2009, which represents 8.8 million families. Overall, the poverty rates for all types of families (married couples with and without children, single-parent households) increased during this time (DeNavas-Walt, Proctor, & Smith, 2010). In addition, the child poverty rate grew 2.7%, which represents 2.1 million children (DeNavas-Walt, Proctor, & Smith, 2010). The child poverty rate reached 20.7% in 2009, representing 15.5 million children living at or below the poverty level (Gould & Shierholz, 2010). The 2009 child poverty rate conveys that children comprised more than one third of all persons living in poverty in the United States. Moreover, 1 in 12 children now live in extreme poverty ($11,025 to below $22,050 per year for a family of four) (Children's Defense Fund, 2010).

Downward spirals in the economy often result in policy changes that affect programs for families in low-income levels. As of this writing (2011), the federal poverty level for a family of four is $22,050. The U.S. child poverty rate is higher than those of most other large industrialized nations, frequently two to three times higher.

Poverty and Race

Between 1980 and 1990, the poverty rate for families of all races with children under 18 years of age varied from 14.7% to 17.9%, respectively (Baugher, 1993; Lugaila, 1992). By 2002, 13.9% were below the poverty level among all races (U.S. Bureau of the Census, 2002). During this period, white families consistently had the lowest poverty rates (e.g., 12% in 1990), and black families the highest (e.g., 38% in 1990).[6] Yet, almost half of all families in poverty are white. A little more than one quarter of the families are Hispanic. Slightly less than one quarter are black, and the remainder are Asian or from other groups (Simms, Fortuny, & Henderson, 2009). However, when poverty rates are examined within each racial and ethnic group, whites are less likely than other groups to be poor. In fact, black and Hispanic families are about two to three times more likely to live in poverty than white families (Federal Interagency Forum on Child Health and Family Statistics, 2003; Children's Defense Fund, 2010).

By 2009, 20.1% of all families in the United States with children under 18 years old lived below the poverty line (U.S. Bureau of the Census, 2010c). From 2007 to 2009, the poverty rate for blacks and Hispanics had increased to 25.8% and 25.3% respectively. The rate for white non-Hispanics also increased during this period, but this population still had the lowest poverty rate at 9.4% (DeNavas-Walt, Proctor, & Smith, 2010; Gould & Shierholz, 2010). These trends in poverty rates for families are reflected in the poverty rates for children by race and ethnicity. In 2001, 9% of white, non-Hispanic children

---

[5]U.S. Bureau of the Census definition.
[6]Estimates are for all white and all black families during this time period.

lived in poverty compared with 30% of black children and 27% of Hispanic children (Federal Interagency Forum on Child Health and Family Statistics, 2003). As of 2009, the proportions of black and Hispanic children who live in poverty are still approximately two to three times higher than white non-Hispanic children; 34.7% of black children and 30.6% of Hispanic children are poor in comparison to 15.8% of white non-Hispanic children (Children's Defense Fund, 2010). Moreover, current research conveys that black children are approximately seven times more likely to live persistently in poverty than white non-Hispanic children (Ratcliffe & McKernan, 2010).

Poverty, Race, and Marital Status

Despite a decrease in overall poverty rates since 1966, poverty rates for married-couple families with children for all races have been much lower than corresponding poverty rates for female-headed families with children, from 17% in 1959 to 8% in 1990 for all married-couple families with children versus from 60% in 1959 to 45% in 1990 for female-headed families with children (Lugaila, 1992; U.S. Bureau of the Census, 1990, 1991b). After leveling off in the early 1980s, the proportion of female-householder families among all poor families has grown from 48.1% in 1985 to 54.1% in 1991. In 1991, 40.9% of all poor families were maintained by a married couple, whereas 54% were headed by a female householder, with no spouse present. In contrast, women maintained only 12.7% of nonpoor families. In 2009, families headed by single mothers still constituted the majority of families living in poverty; 3.8 million of the 6.6 million families living in poverty were headed by single mothers (Gould & Shierholz, 2010). Moreover, children in female-headed families are more than four times more likely to be poor than children in married-couple families (Children's Defense Fund, 2010; U.S. Bureau of the Census, 2010b).

Within these two family types, however, the poverty rates for blacks and Hispanics have been substantially higher than for white non-Hispanic families. For example, from 1975 to 1990, the poverty rate for married-couple families has remained stable at 8%, whereas the poverty rate for black married couples has remained stable at 15% (U.S. Bureau of the Census, 1991a).[7] Furthermore, in 1991, female-headed households constituted 78.3% of all poor black families compared with 45.7% of poor Hispanic-origin families and 28.4% of poor white families (Baugher, 1993). The racial and ethnic disparities in poverty rates of these two types of families still remained as of 2009, but the gaps between the rates have decreased. According to U.S. Census data, the poverty rate for poor black married couples has decreased overall between 1990 and 2009 to 11.4%, even though this rate still remains higher than the 8.3% poverty rate for all married-couple families. Also, female-headed households constitute a significantly lower percentage of poor black families (50.3%) than in 1990, whereas this percentage for Hispanic households remained stable at 46% and the percentage for white non-Hispanic households had actually increased to 31.7% (U.S. Bureau of the Census, 2010b).

Poverty, Race, and Educational Attainment

Current Population Survey (CPS) reports track educational level improvement since 1947. The 2000 CPS reported that over four fifths of all adults had completed at least high school. One in four of these adults had attained a bachelor's degree or higher. Eighty-eight percent of white non-Hispanics were high school graduates. Black high

---

[7]The exception in both cases is the increase in the rate of poverty for all families by 5 percentage points from 1975 to 1985.

school graduates increased to 79%, narrowing the difference among high school graduates between whites and blacks. Asian and Pacific Islanders had the greatest proportion of college graduates. When comparing races among individuals 25 years of age and older, Hispanics were the least likely to complete high school or college, although this proportion increased from 51% in 1989 to 57% in 1999. In contrast, 44% of Asian/Pacific Islanders had college degrees or higher compared with 28% of white non-Hispanics, 17% of blacks, and 11% of Hispanics in the 25 years and older age group (U.S. Bureau of the Census, 2000).

Significant improvements in education continued in the past 10 years. By 2009, only 14.7% of people in the United States 25 years of age and older did not have a high school degree or an equivalent, and 27.9% of this population has obtained a bachelor's degree or higher (U.S. Bureau of the Census, 2010j). The educational gaps in high school and college education have decreased with regard to race and ethnicity, particularly for blacks. Approximately 82% of blacks and 60.9% of Hispanics had at least a high school diploma in comparison to 87.5% of white non-Hispanics and 85.8% of Asian/Pacific Islanders as of 2009 (U.S. Bureau of the Census, 2010a). In addition, 23.5% of blacks and 12.6% of Hispanics have at least a bachelor's degree in comparison to 29.3% of white non-Hispanics and 48.8% of Asian/Pacific Islanders (U.S. Bureau of the Census, 2010a).

These trends in educational improvement remain significant because educational attainment influences the wealth status of the American household. White, black, and Hispanic-origin family householders aged 25 years and over with higher educational attainments were each less likely to live in poverty. As of 2009, 24.7% of Americans of all races without a high school diploma live below the poverty level in comparison to 13.8% with only a high school diploma and 4.5% with a college degree (U.S. Bureau of the Census, 2010d). However, the poverty rates for blacks and Hispanics were much greater than for whites within educational levels. For example, the overall poverty rate for white, black, and Hispanics with at least a high school education in 1990 was 9% for high school graduates in 1990. Within this rate, the rate of poverty for Hispanics was 15%, the poverty rate for whites was 7% and for blacks was 26%. As of 2009, the poverty rate for Hispanic high school graduates grew to 19.3% and 10.4% for white non-Hispanics. Black high school graduates still maintained the highest poverty rate of any racial group among high school graduates, but the poverty rate decreased to 24.7% as of 2009 (U.S. Bureau of the Census, 2010d).

Poverty and Work Status

During the era of welfare reform in the late 1990s and early 2000s, the percentage of poor children in working families increased steadily from 32% in 1995 to 43% in 2000 before decreasing to 40% in 2001. This illustrates a reversal of the trend that occurred during a period of recession that resulted in a loss of jobs in the U.S. economy as a whole. Despite this decline, child poverty remained constant at 16% overall. These trends are also evident for children living in single-mother families. Among all children, the percentage of children living in working poor families had stayed constant at 6% to 7% as of 2001. During this year, only one third of poor children had at least one parent in the household employed full time, full year compared with seven of eight nonpoor children. Among poor children, those living with families with two parents were much more likely to have a parent employed full time, full year than children living with only their mother or father (54% compared with 19% and 29%, respectively, in 2001). Among children living in two-parent and father-only families, there is no difference between children less than 6 years old and older children in the percentage who have at least one parent employed full time, full year. For those in single-mother families, however, the difference is substantial, at 38% for those under the age of 6 years versus 53% for those ages 6 to 17 years.

Some of these trends stayed consistent through the late 2000s. However, the percentage of poor children living in families with at least one working householder has increased to 10.8% of all children as of 2009 (U.S. Bureau of the Census, 2010c). The poverty rate among all people in the workforce increased to 6.9%, and this increase was mainly a result of the increase in poverty among workers who worked part time for the full year (DeNavas-Walt, Proctor, & Smith, 2010). In 2007, only 32% of poor children had at least one parent in the household employed full time, full year in comparison to 87% of nonpoor children (Federal Interagency Forum on Child and Family Statistics, 2009). 54% of children who lived in married-couple families and who had at least one parent who worked all year in full-time employment lived below poverty level (Federal Interagency Forum on Child and Family Statistics, 2009). The poverty rate for children who live in female-headed households that have at least one full-time, full-year householder decreased from 19% to 17.6% overall from 2001 to 2009 (U.S. Bureau of the Census, 2010c).

Assistance Programs

Survey results of the Survey of Program Dynamics suggest that levels of participation in Food Stamps (now called the Supplemental Nutrition Assistance Program), housing assistance, energy assistance, and free or reduced-price school lunches declined significantly between 1993 and 1996 for all household types, including married-couple households with children and for other family households with children. Individuals in other family households with children were more likely to participate in these noncash benefit programs than their married-couple counterparts in 1996. Changes in the welfare system were precipitated by the Personal

Responsibility and Work Opportunity Reconciliation Act of 1996, which replaced the Aid for Families of Dependent Children (AFDC) program with TANF (Barr, Lee, & Benjamin, 2003). Although individuals in married-couple households with children were less likely to participate in these programs than those in other family households with children, their relative decline in receipt of Food Stamps and housing assistance between 1993 and 1996 was greater. The two groups experienced similar declines in receipt of energy assistance and free or reduced-price lunches between 1993 and 1996. This has been accelerated with the passage of the welfare law enacted in 1996. That is, the number of individual welfare recipients declined by 56%, and the number of families decreased by 52%, respectively, since 1996 (Parrott, 2002). In 2002, 2.1 million families received cash assistance through TANF (Administration for Children and Families, 2002). In 2002, approximately 5 million individuals and 2 million families received TANF benefits, a decline of 5% and 4%, respectively, from 2001 (U.S. Department of Health and Human Services, 2002). Interestingly, relatives caring for children comprised 9% of the TANF caseload in 2001. Generally, a large proportion of mothers who receive government assistance benefits work at least part time. In 2004, 3.9 million (52%) of the 7.5 million mothers who received any type of government assistance had jobs (Dye, 2008).

The Deficit Reduction Act of 2005 (also known as the TANF Reauthorization) proposed in part to move recipients either out of the TANF program completely or into employment. However, there was no significant change found at the national level in TANF participation nor in the employment status of women who received TANF benefits from 2004 to 2007 (Irving, 2010). The proportion of households that received TANF benefits declined overall to less than 2 million families from 2002 to 2008 (only 1.6% of all U.S. households) (Palumbo, 2010). However, the number of households that received government assistance has increased since the recent economic downturn. More than 40 million people received assistance through the Supplemental Nutrition Assistance Program in April of 2010, with children comprising half of this population (Children's Defense Fund, 2010).

CHILD CARE

Every day, three of five children under school age are in nonparental child care arrangements (Laughlin, 2010). The increased number of parents in the workforce led to schools and other institutions (e.g., organized child care) taking on more of the responsibility for caring for children. The increase in labor force participation among mothers with preschool children was not limited to mothers with older preschoolers. In 1976, the proportion of women with children less than 1 year old who were in the labor force was only 31%. However, the rapid increase in the proportion of women with infants and children under 1 year of age who were in the labor force, jumping to 59% in 1999, has produced a corresponding increase in the demand for child care for children under the age of 1 year. Among the 49 million children living at home with both parents, 29 million had both parents in the workforce. During this time, 14 million children living with single mothers and 2 million with single fathers had their custodial parents in the workforce. Seventeen million children lived with a single mother in the United States, which indicates that more than 75% of these single mothers were working (U.S. Bureau of the Census, 2000).

In 2005, 62.8% of the 20 million children under the age of 5 years were in some form of nonparental care on a regular basis. For the children who were situated in a regular child care arrangement, 41.3% of those under 5 years old were cared for by a relative, and 34.9% were cared for by a nonrelative (Laughlin, 2010); 23.3% of these children were cared for in organized child care facilities (Laughlin, 2010). Families who are in poverty with preschoolers and employed mothers use relative care more often than child care centers. Grandparents and fathers cared for more preschool children during the day than did child care centers in 2005 among families living in poverty with a working mother (Laughlin, 2010). Among preschoolers in general, there is a higher proportion of 3–4 year olds in organized child care facilities (child care, nursery and preschools, and Head Start centers) than 1–2 year olds. This trend may suggest a relationship with age and preparation for school (Laughlin, 2010; Smith, 2002).

School-age children of employed mothers numbered 39.6 million in 2005, and 65% of all children in grade school have employed mothers with whom they are living. Just 6% of these children (5–14 years old) are cared for in organized facilities. The difference between the percentages of organized child care for this age group in comparison to the percentage of children under 5 lies in the percentage of older children enrolled in school (94%). In 2005, 14% percent of the school-aged children took care of themselves outside of school hours without adult supervision, and 14% attended enrichment activities (Laughlin, 2010).

The cost of child care is significant, and the cost has grown significantly over recent years. In 1997, $67 per week was the average payment for child care for 51% of the 12.1 million preschoolers living with mothers (Smith, 2002). By 2005, mothers paid an average of $87 per week for only one child, and mothers with two or more children under age 15 paid an average of $124 per week (Laughlin, 2010). The average cost per week for families paying for child care services under age 15 was $104 according to the last Survey of Income and Program Participation; this cost more than doubled the average weekly cost in 1985 (Laughlin, 2010). School-age children were not as likely to be in paid child care as the under 5s, and the cost of child care per week is also lower for elementary-school children. Mothers with preschool children paid an average of $48 more per week than mothers with school-age children (Laughlin, 2010; Smith, 2002). Overall, the average annual cost of center-based child care for one 4-year-old exceeded the annual in-state tuition of 4-year public colleges and universities in 36 states (Children's Defense Fund, 2010).

As of 2005, there were approximately 32.4 million children less than 15 years old who had regular child care arrangements. Within the past 2 decades, a significant proportion of parents have received assistance with paying for this care. The sources of such assistance are often the government, their parent's employer, the other parent, or another source. In 1997, parents of preschoolers were more likely to receive assistance (7%) when compared with elementary-school-aged children (4%). Although 812,000 children under the age of 15 received assistance from the government in 1997, this proportion is directly related to one's economic level. Nine percent of preschoolers in poverty received this kind of assistance compared with only 5% living just above poverty and only 1% of those preschoolers at 200% of poverty. Fifteen percent of children receiving TANF were also recipients of government assistance for child care. A relationship may exist, with the TANF families having the needed connections to access this kind of assistance for child care (Smith, 2002).

Increased governmental attention had been given in recent years to alleviating some of the burden of child care costs. The federal Child and Dependent Care Tax Credit helped 6.5 million families with child care expenses in 2007. In addition, the Child Care and Development Fund provided assistance to 1.7 million children per month during this year (Children's Defense Fund, 2010).

Even with the availability of child care assistance, disparities continue to exist in the cost of child care by income level and poverty status among children. In 1997, a poor family with a working mother paid an average of $52 per week compared with nonpoor families who paid an average of $77 per week. As a proportion of the family budget, however, poor families spent roughly three times the amount (20%) as did nonpoor families (7%) on child care. As of 2005, poor families paid an average of $94 per week in comparison with nonpoor families that pay an average of $108 per week. Poor families now spend about four times the proportion of their budgets on child care than did nonpoor families (28% vs. 7%) (Laughlin, 2010). These differences in child care costs have persisted in poor and nonpoor families since 1987 (Laughlin, 2010; Smith, 2002).

HEALTH INSURANCE COVERAGE

In contrast to what many believe, access to health care is not primarily a problem of the poor. Historically, a large proportion of uninsured children live in two-parent families in which at least one parent is employed full time and earns an income above the poverty line (Foley, 1991). In previous years, 70% of the uninsured have family incomes above the poverty level (Darman, 1992). As of 2009, 58.5% of uninsured children under 18 live with a full-time, full-year employed family member (Fronstin, 2010). Nevertheless there has been increasing concern that both poor and nonpoor families with children are at risk of having no source of health insurance for their dependents (U.S. Department of Health and Human Services, 2001). The percentage for uninsured individuals under 65 years old had increased to 18.9% in 2009, which is the highest percentage since 1994 (Fronstin, 2010).

Children's health insurance coverage comes from two major sources: private insurance companies and the government. From 1987 through 2007, the proportion of children with some form of health insurance from either source had fluctuated between

85% and 90% (Federal Interagency Forum on Child and Family Statistics, 2009). Due to the expansion of federal and state health insurance, more children obtained coverage under Medicaid. Approximately 7.3 million children enrolled in Medicaid received health insurance coverage under the Children's Health Insurance Program (CHIP) during the 2008 fiscal year, and this number increased to 7.8 million for FY 2009 (Centers for Medicare & Medicaid Services, 2011; Children's Defense Fund, 2010). However, the number of children covered under private insurance programs has decreased through 2009, covering only 60% of all children. This percentage is the lowest percentage on record for private insurance coverage (Child Trends, 2010).

1987–Early 1990s

Between 1987 and 1991, approximately 22.2 million children had no health insurance during some part of each year (Flint, 1992; Short, 1993). Although the number of non-poor children without insurance exceeds that of poor children, in 1990, poor families with children were twice as likely as nonpoor families with children not to be covered by private or public health insurance at any given time during the year (22% vs. 11%) (Lugaila, 1992; Short, 1993; U.S. Bureau of the Census, 1991b). Among nonpoor families with children, those in female-headed household families were about twice as likely as those in married-couple families not to be covered by health insurance at any given time during the year (17% vs. 9%). The reverse held true for poor families with children. It should be noted that some families with children covered by health insurance during 1990 had coverage for only part of the year. Hence, the proportions of families with children not covered at any given time (or at all) during the year are certainly smaller than the proportions that did not have coverage for the full year. In addition, families with children who did not have health insurance coverage may

also differ in the extent to which specific healthcare costs were fully, partially, or not paid by their health insurance (Short, 1993).

At the end of 1990, 87% of Americans were covered at a given point in time by health insurance of all types. Approximately six in eight insured persons were covered by private insurance. Stable full-time employment improved the chances of having continuous coverage (Short, 1993). From mid-1987 to the end of 1990, only 14% of those who worked full time—35 hours or more per week—for 28 months experienced lapses in coverage. In contrast, 43% of those who spent a month or more without a job experienced a lapse in health insurance coverage (Short, 1993). Furthermore, taking into account the changing system of employer-provided dependent coverage, Newson and Harvey (1994; pp. 11–12) point out:

Currently, 60% of all Americans obtain insurance through their own or a family member's employment. This arrangement, however, is seriously threatened. Employers concerned with rising health care costs are either dropping dependent health insurance, reducing the benefit packages, or increasing the employee's share of the premium for dependent coverage. In 1980, 72% of medium-and large-sized firms paid the full cost of health insurance for their workers, and 51% paid the full cost of dependent coverage. By 1991, fully paid individual insurance dropped to 45% of firms, and family coverage to 23%. While employer-provided health insurance is declining, even plans that do cover dependents often fail to meet the health care needs of children, which are not the same as those of adults. Most child health services are provided in an ambulatory setting, and services rendered in such a setting are often not covered by health insurance. Because health insurance plans tend to be designed for adults, children's needs are often addressed inadequately.

Late 1990s – 2002

In the late 1990s, healthcare insurance coverage for children increased somewhat from 85% in 1996 through 1998 to 88% in 2000 and has remained stable through 2002. Medicaid coverage for children increased from 20% in 2000 to 24% in 2002 (Mills & Shailesh, 2003). Government health insurance, which consists primarily of Medicaid but includes several other sources of coverage such as CHIP, covered 27% of all children in 2002 (Holahan, Dubay, & Kenney, 2003). The percentage of children with private insurance decreased from 71% in 2000 to 68% in 2001, remaining at 68% in 2002.

In 2002, 79% of children in single-father families and 86% of children in single-mother families had health insurance coverage compared with 90% of children with married-couple families. The likelihood of being covered by health insurance increases with income. In 2002, 95% of children living in families with incomes of $75,000 or more were covered by health insurance. In contrast, only 81% of children in families with incomes of under $25,000 were covered. U.S. citizens, whether native born or naturalized, are more likely than are noncitizens to have health insurance coverage. The health insurance coverage rates in 2002 for U.S. citizens were 90% for native-born citizens and 81% for naturalized citizens compared with only 59% for noncitizens under the age of 18 years. In general, children belonging to economically advantaged groups are the most likely to have private health insurance, which is largely employment based, whereas children in economically disadvantaged groups are the most likely to have government health insurance, which is most often Medicaid, a needs-tested program.

More attention has been given to racial and ethnic disparities regarding health insurance in the past 2 decades. Private health insurance covered 68% of all children in 2002. However, private health insurance coverage is most common among white non-Hispanic children (79%), children in married-couple families (77%), and children in families with incomes of $75,000 and over (92%). Private health insurance is least common among Hispanic children (43%), black children (50%), children in single-mother families (45%), and noncitizens (37%). Although Medicaid covers only about 24% of the entire population of children, it covers 62% of poor children. Among poor children, Medicaid coverage is highest for black children (70%) and is substantially lower for white non-Hispanics, Hispanics and Asian or Pacific Islanders, with 57%, 61%, and 51%, respectively, receiving coverage (Child Trends, 2003). Hispanic children are much less likely than other children to have any form of health insurance coverage. In 2002, only 77% of Hispanic children had health insurance coverage compared with 88% of Asian children, 86% of black-only children, and 92% of white, non-Hispanic children. A lack of awareness of eligibility, language barriers, enrollment problems, and fear of repercussions for using publicly funded insurance may partially explain why more Hispanic children are uninsured (Holahan, Dubay, & Kenney, 2003).

2003 to present

Due to the economic downturn in 2007, the number of Americans without health insurance has significantly increased. The number of Americans with some form of health insurance decreased by 1.5 million people from 2008 to 2009, which is the first time since 1987 that a decrease occurred (DeNavas-Walt, Proctor, & Smith, 2010). As of 2009, 50.7 million Americans were uninsured, which means that one out of six Americans did not have health insurance (Center on Budget and Policy Priorities, 2010). While the percentage of people who received Medicaid grew from 14.1% to 15.7% from 2008 to 2009, the percentage of people with private healthcare coverage dropped from 66.7% to 63.9% during this time (Center on

Budget and Policy Priorities, 2010; DeNavas-Walt, Proctor, & Smith, 2010). By 2009, the proportion of people covered by private employment-based insurance had dropped to 55.8%, which is the lowest percentage since 1987 (DeNavas-Walt, Proctor, & Smith, 2010).

In 2007, 8.1 million children were uninsured, which constituted approximately 11% of all children during that year (Federal Interagency Forum on Child and Family Statistics, 2009). The ethnic disparities in health insurance coverage persist, as fewer Hispanic children had health insurance than white non-Hispanic or black children. In 2007, 80% of Hispanic children had some form of insurance throughout the year in comparison to 93% of white non-Hispanic and 88% of black children (Federal Interagency Forum on Child and Family Statistics, 2009). These racial and ethnic gaps for uninsured children continued to persist through 2009, but there were slight increases in health insurance coverage for black and Hispanic children (83% Hispanic, 89% black) (Child Trends, 2010). In 2009, foreign-born children who are not naturalized citizens are less likely to have health insurance than children who are native-born or naturalized citizens (68% in comparison to 91% and 89%, respectively) (Child Trends, 2010).

Recent government intervention includes the execution of the Children's Health Insurance Program Reauthorization Act of 2009 (CHIPRA), which purposes to finance the program through fiscal year 2013 and to expand state health insurance coverage for approximately 5 million additional uninsured children. The reauthorization also seeks to increase access for uninsured children in higher incomes and uninsured pregnant women of low-income status (Centers for Medicare and Medicaid Services, 2011). However, this program does not cover children and families of state employees, even though these employees collectively constitute a large proportion of the workforce.

COMMUNITY SERVICES

Historical Background

The most basic social agency available in almost every U.S. community today is the tax-supported public welfare agency. However, voluntary nonprofit agencies have played an important role in the history and current provision of social services in the United States. Because of the greater need, they have flourished mainly in urban areas. Nonetheless, the public welfare agency remains the one resource available nationwide.

The public welfare system of the United States is based on the English poor laws of the 17th century, which placed the responsibility for care of the needy on the local community and stated that the income of persons receiving assistance should not be greater than the lowest income of a self-sufficient person (Reisch, 1995). In the United States, public welfare was administered entirely by local and state agencies until the Social Security Act was passed in 1935. The reason for this change was that there was great inequity in criteria for eligibility and benefits across states. Nevertheless, the belief that the state or local community is better situated to assess the need using a means test and determine the benefits for dependent persons forms the basis for much of current welfare reform policies. Thus, the United States' welfare system is founded on the Residual Welfare Model, and there is still adherence to some of these principles, whereas England and other western European countries have adopted the principles of the Industrial Redistributive Model of social welfare (Kahn, 1973).

In the 18th and early 19th century, the American welfare system also used institutional care for the older population, chronically ill persons, and dependent children, for example, almshouses and orphanages. With the industrial revolution and the wave of immigration, private agencies were developed to help people in their own homes. The Community Organization Societies, which developed into today's Family Service Agencies, and Children's Aid Societies (antecedents of United Way) were major resources offering financial assistance as well as other services in kind. With the onset of the Great Depression in 1929, private organizations found that they were unable to meet the financial needs of the masses of unemployed persons. After the passage of the Social Security Act, private agencies made the policy decision not to provide income maintenance but to provide only counseling and supplementary services. In turn, the original Social Security Act provided only financial assistance, not services (Meyer, 1995).

The Social Security Act established the responsibility of the federal government to provide funds to all states for the support of certain groups and the policy of entitlement, that is, that all persons who met eligibility criteria were entitled to benefits (Reisch, 1995). Originally, the Social Security Act provided funds for three groups in the population: elderly persons (Old Age Assistance), blind individuals (Aid to the Blind), and dependent children (Aid to Dependent Children [ADC]). In 1950, a third group, persons with disabilities (Aid to the Permanently and Totally Disabled), was added. These programs were administered by the states. That is, under general federal guidelines, states established eligibility criteria and benefits. In answer to complaints about the wide variation in benefits according to the economic status of a state, Old Age Assistance, Aid to the Blind, and Aid to the Permanently and Totally Disabled were "federalized" in 1974 under a program named Supplemental Security Income (SSI) (Meyer, 1995). It is administered directly by the Social Security Administration whose primary responsibilities are to (1) set eligibility criteria, (2) establish a basic measure of income maintenance, and (3) mail checks directly to recipients. States can supplement the amount of SSI benefit. States that gave higher benefits before 1974 were required to supplement

the new federal level in order to remain at that level (Meyer, 1995).

The ADC program originally provided benefits only for the children; however, in 1950, funds for the caretaker in the family were added, and the name was changed to AFDC. It was never "federalized" as were the other programs because of the moral and political feelings expressed by communities toward the population group served by this program. "To qualify for assistance, a child in a single parent household must be deprived of support because the parent is deceased, continually absent from the home, or suffering a mental or physical incapacity that is expected to last more than 30 days. Under limited conditions, a two-parent family can receive aid if principal wage earner is unemployed" even with support from other service programs (Abramovitz, 1995, p. 184). In 1935, one of the goals of the Social Security Act was to remove from the labor pool economically dependent persons, thus freeing employment opportunities for the able bodied. In the beginning, mothers of dependent children continued to work because they were not included as recipients of the ADC benefits. They were included in 1950 because of the culture of that era. That is, it was believed to be better for the development of children if the mother remained at home to care for them. Also, the role of women as homemakers was encouraged as a means of removing women from the labor pool after World War II in order to increase opportunities for returning servicemen.

The demographics of AFDC also changed between 1935 and 1990. The AFDC program subsumed the population previously served by Mothers Pensions programs, which states had initiated as a result of the 1909 White House Conference on Children. These programs were focused primarily on widows who otherwise would have had to place their children in orphanages. The proportion of widows with children was high under the original ADC program but diminished as this group became eligible for survivors' benefits under the Social Security insurance program. Currently, the children in the AFDC caseload are primarily those of divorced, separated, or never-married women. The average monthly AFDC family caseload for calendar year 1992 was 4,829,000, up 8.1% from the preceding year (U.S. Department of Health and Human Services, Social Security Administration, 1994). The AFDC recipient count averaged 13,773,000 in 1992. In 1992 payments to AFDC recipients totaled $21.66 billion, an increase of $725.3 million or 3.5% above 1991 (U.S. Department of Health and Human Services, Social Security Administration, 1994). However, the average monthly payment per family was down $16.73 (−4.3%) to $373.71 for 1992 from the 1991 level of $390.44 (Abramovitz, 1995; U.S. Department of Health and Human Services, Social Security Administration, 1994).

The role of public welfare agencies in providing social services not only to its own beneficiaries but also to the general population has varied in recent years. Beginning in 1956, the federal government offered to match a certain percentage of state funds spent on counseling, rehabilitation, and other direct services to persons receiving public welfare benefits. These services were always perceived as services to individual cases for purposes of rehabilitation and oversight of recipients. In the 1960s, in the era of the War on Poverty and the Great Society, there was more of an interest among academicians and policy makers in dealing with the problem of social dependency on a systems basis (Reisch, 1995). A leader in the systems approach was Dr. Alfred J. Kahn, Professor at the Columbia University School of Social Work, who was influenced by the work of Titmuss. He believed that a function of public welfare was the socialization and development of society, regardless of the economic status of individuals. His ultimate goal was the Industrial Redistributive Model, but as an intermediate phase, he recommended that governmental units be responsible for providing "social utilities," that is, services that are needed to meet emerging needs and are generally accepted as representing social infrastructure (Kahn, 1973). Public social utilities may be divided into those available at user options (e.g., museums, community centers) and others by user status (child care, centers for the aged). Kahn stresses that the user is a citizen, not a client or patient (Kahn, 1973).

This concept of public welfare offering services to all citizens was incorporated into Title XX of the Social Security Act passed in 1975. The services of information and referral, family planning, and protective services for children and elderly persons were provided to all families regardless of income. Other developmental services were available to people with incomes up to 115% of a state's median income; persons with 80% to 115% of the state's median income paid a sliding fee for services. Title XX legislation led to many innovative programs with a preventive approach. However, it was an open-ended appropriation. In the 1980s, it was placed in a block grant with all other provisions for social services under the Social Security Act, and a cap was placed on appropriations (Reisch, 1995). Current programs are more limited.

The history of child welfare services for the protection and enhancement of the lives of children has a history similar to income maintenance. Services, such as they were, were provided by the local judicial and welfare system with the use of institutional care. Private nonprofit, including religious, agencies developed protective and custodial care. Until the 1930s, these varied according to the state and locality. The child welfare provisions under Title V of the Social Security Act required each state to have a statewide agency that is responsible for public child welfare services. Originally administered by the Children's Bureau, this program offered mainly guidance and staff training in foster care, adoption, maternity homes, child care centers, and homemaker services. Its relatively small budget was used to try to upgrade the quality of staffs of public child welfare agencies, providing funds for the employment of social workers with master's degrees. It did not provide funds for the payment of foster care or to assist adoptive parents. Studies in the 1970s, which tracked children through their experiences in foster care, documented the inadequacy of foster homes, the agencies' tendencies to "lose children" and not to provide continuous service to the child. It also found that, if children were not returned to their parents within their first 2 years in foster care, they were likely never to be returned.

These findings resulted in the Child Welfare and Adoption Assistance Act in the 1980s. Federal funds were appropriated for payment of foster care. Agencies were required to establish registers and tracking systems. Plans had to be made to review cases by the time the child was in foster care for 18 months to see whether there was potential for the child to be returned to his or her parents or plans made for placement in an adoptive home. Funds were provided to assist adoptive parents with the cost of care of children with special needs.

The original placement of Child Welfare Services and MCH services in the Children's Bureau was a felicitous one in that the two programs had so many areas of mutual concern, such as services to unwed mothers, standards for foster homes, adoption, child care centers, and homemaker services. During the 1960s, they both received funds to expand services for mentally retarded children. The Social Work Section of MCHB was able to work closely with the social workers in the Child Welfare Division on these issues (Kadushin, 1980). Since 1973, when Child Welfare Services was transferred to the Administration for Children and Families and MCH was transferred to the Public Health Service, these two programs have had to collaborate through interagency committees.

When initiated in 1935 the Social Work Section of the Children's Bureau was concerned mainly with the program for Children with Special Health Care Needs (then called the Crippled Children's Program) because many of the states had incorporated social work positions into their clinical services. The impetus for the development of social work positions in state MCH agencies came with the initiation of the Program of Projects in the 1960s. Because of the nature of the programs, the federal administrators of MCH services always insisted on the multidisciplinary approach. Social work positions were created in state health departments to give guidance and supervision to the social workers employed in the special projects. After the end of the Program of Projects with the initiation of block grants to the states in the 1980s, state-level positions for public health social workers remained important in assessing the impact of health and social policy on the health status and social needs of low-income families. For example, data gathered by public health social workers in the southeastern states regarding rates of premature birth and infant death occurring to women not eligible for Medicaid were used in the development of legislation for the expansion of Medicaid to include married women and women with incomes up to 185% of poverty. The provision of payment for case-management services to Medicaid patients led to an increase in the number of social work positions in local public health departments providing MCH services (Schmidt & Wallace, 1994; Watkins, 1993). These public health social workers provide information about and referral to other community resources as well as counseling and follow-up. They work closely with other community agencies in developing new resources for families as well as working to changing policies that may serve as barriers. The trend for states to assign the Medicaid population to managed-care programs has led to a reduction of the availability of public health social work and other "wrap-around" services, which facilitate the accessibility and effectiveness of medical care for low-income populations.

Current Issues

Decreasing support for public social welfare services threatens the health and social resources available to young low-income families. Politicians expressing the need to "reform the welfare system" echo the negative atmosphere that surrounded the AFDC program. After that more socially acceptable group of women, that is, widows, came under the auspices of Survivors Insurance, the politically less socially acceptable group of divorced, separated, and unmarried women emerged as the primary recipients of AFDC. This group of women continues to be targeted for "reform" despite the fact that their numbers reflect a social phenomenon that is occurring in all economic groups. As well, AFDC recipients were perceived negatively because of their high rate of unemployment. Today, greater numbers of women work outside the home, and thus, TANF recipients are today seen as not meeting society's expectations, even though the early intention of supporting the caregivers of dependent children was explicitly to enable mothers to stay home and raise their children. Since the passage of Family Support legislation in 1988, recipients whose children are over 3 years of age have been required to participate in the Job Opportunity and Basic Skills program. However, these efforts did not lead to any greater numbers obtaining employment. Current proposals enshrined in TANF have a more punitive approach, that is, cutting off benefits if the woman does not return to work within a certain time limit (e.g., 2 years) or if she has additional children while receiving benefits.

In 1996 the Personal Responsibility and Work Opportunity Reconciliation Act (U.S. Congress, 1996) replaced AFDC with TANF and gave administration of TANF to the states with minimal federal guidelines, reduced funds, employment requirements, and time limits on assistance, ending entitlements for those most in need. The 2005 Deficit Reduction Act placed further responsibility on the states to increase the number of TANF recipients moving into the labor force; however, the results have varied from state to state (Irving, 2010). Now there is the question whether state legislatures will be willing to raise taxes to replace lost federal revenue in order to meet the new demands of the law (training, employment, child care, etc.). The resources of private organizations are inadequate and too unevenly distributed to meet nationwide needs. Efforts to help recipients enter employment or return to school require training programs and provision of child care services that are not guaranteed by the new legislation.

The proposal to fund Medicaid through block grants to the states would have led to similar problems of inequity in criteria for eligibility and benefits. Mothers and children excluded from TANF assistance may find they are also excluded from a state's Medicaid program. Although converting Medicaid to a block grant was originally considered as part of welfare reform legislation of 1996, it was omitted from the final version of PL 104-193. The 2005 Deficit Reduction Act aimed to reduce $4.8 billion from Medicaid spending by increasing cost sharing and premiums for beneficiaries (Kaiser Family Foundation, 2006). Despite the changes in legislation, the vast majority of TANF recipient women continued to receive Medicaid in recent years, even though a decrease occurred from 98.5% in 2005 to 93.1% in 2007 (Irving, 2010).

The increase in acquired immunodeficiency syndrome, drug abuse, and family violence has placed a great strain on child welfare agencies (Reiss & Lee, 1988). Children in these families often have to be removed from these threatening environments temporarily or permanently. There are insufficient qualified foster homes to meet this demand. A high proportion of caseworkers in child welfare agencies has not had formal social work training and is given responsibility for solving problems in family relationships far beyond their abilities. Turnover in staff is frequent, and children in care often become lost in the system. Also, the policy that a decision must be made either to return the child to his or her biological parents or place him or her in a permanent adoptive home after 18 months in foster care often leads to the child's being returned to the original hazardous environment. Current approaches to remedying this situation include closer case management and monitoring, crisis and long-term family counseling, parental life-skill training, and permanency planning that involves the family's biological and "other kinship/support network."

The Earned Income Tax Credit and Child Tax Credit benefited working families with incomes below $50,000 and helped keep children out of poverty. Working families and individuals received over $48 billion dollars from the EITC and $31 billion in child tax credits in 2007. These programs helped over 25 million families and individuals (Children's Defense Fund, 2010).

The American Recovery and Reinvestment Act was passed in February 2009 to grant income supports in unemployment insurance, nutritional assistance, and tax cuts (Gould & Shierholz, 2010). This act resulted in positive effects in employment. The Congressional Budget Office reported that between 1.3 and 2.7 million jobs (full-time equivalent) were either created or saved as of the end of 2009 (Gould & Shierholz, 2010). According to recent estimates, $28 billion was spent for unemployment insurance benefits, and these benefits provided by the act kept 900,000 Americans out of poverty in 2008 and 3.3 million Americans out of poverty in 2009 (Center on Budget and Policy Priorities, 2010; Gould & Shierholz, 2010).

CONCLUSION

American family life has changed dramatically during the past 3 decades. Age at first marriage for women has increased, as has age at first pregnancy for married women. Since 1970, small families with one or two children increased sharply as a proportion of all families with children. In contrast, there are high rates of divorce and births to unmarried mothers, which are largely responsible for the growing proportion of families headed by single, mostly female, parents. These families are a heterogeneous group in terms of income, education, employment, and race. However, black and Hispanic-origin families are disproportionately represented (Cunningham & Hahn, 1994). Thus, given the continuing high levels of divorce and premarital childbearing, the proportion of children living with a lone parent doubled between 1970 and 1990, reaching approximately 25% (Lugaila, 1992).

There was an increase in the proportion of women in general, particularly mothers, participating in the labor force since 1970. This increase in mothers in the labor force corresponded with the increased need for child care, especially for children under 5 years old. Furthermore, in 1990, nearly 30% of married-couple families had both spouses working year round. Also, the number of parents with at least some college education increased during the 1970s and 1980s. Despite the increases in mothers and married couples in the labor force and higher educational attainment of parents, the overall median family income was only 6% above what it was in 1970. This increase was so small predominantly because of the rise in single-parent households.

The disparity in poverty rates between married and unmarried has increased, with unmarried women being far more likely to have incomes below the poverty level or to be receiving public assistance than married women. Similarly, the disparity in poverty rates between employed and unemployed women with children has also increased. As with many other demographic trends over the last 30 years, blacks and Hispanic-origin women and children were disproportionately represented among the ranks of the poor. The latter is particularly poignant as blacks have much lower median family incomes and higher rates of poverty than whites with similar educational attainment and patterns of work (Lugaila, 1992). The lack of health insurance coverage is often noted as a problem for poor children living in mother-only families, but even among children living in married-couple families, the proportion not covered by health insurance any time during 1990 was 9% for the nonpoor and 3% for the poor.

Stable family relationships and adequate financial support are essential for the healthy development of children. In the United States, changes in family structure and in the economic system are weakening supports for families. Current social systems, such as public assistance, tax-supported medical care, and child welfare services, are being questioned and restructured, possibly placing some families at risk. Public health professionals in the field of MCH are challenged with the tasks of assessing the impact of these proposed changes on the health status of families with children and initiating policies and programs that will promote and protect their well-being.

References

Abramovitz, M. (1995). Aid to families with dependent children. In R. L. Edwards (Ed.-in-Chief), *Encyclopedia of social work* (Vol. 1, 19th ed., pp. 183–194). Washington, DC: National Association of Social Workers.

Administration for Children and Families. (2002). *Temporary assistance for needy families: Total number of families and recipients April–June 2002.* Washington, DC: U.S. Department of Health and Human Services.

Amato, P. R. (1994). The implications of research findings on children in stepfamilies. In A. Booth & J. Dunn (Eds.), *Stepfamilies: Who benefits? Who does not?* (pp. 81–88). Hillsdale, NJ: Lawrence Erlbaum Associates.

Barr, D. A., Lee, P. R., & Benjamin, A. E. (2003). Health care and health care policy in changing world. In H. M. Wallace, G. Green, & K. J. Jaros (Eds.), *Health and welfare for families in the 21st century* (2nd ed., pp. 26–42). Sudbury, MA: Jones and Bartlett Publishers.

Baugher, E. (1993). *Population profile of the U.S. 1993: Poverty.* Current population reports: Population characteristics (Special Studies Series P-23, No. 185). Washington, DC: U.S. Department of Commerce, Economics and Statistics Administration, Bureau of the Census.

Bernstein, R. (2010). "Census Bureau reports families with children increasingly face unemployment." Retrieved May 10, 2011 from http://www.census.gov/newsroom/releases/archives/families_households/cb10-08.html.

Center on Budget and Policy Priorities. (2010). *Statement by Robert Greenstein, Executive Director, on Census 2009 poverty and health insurance data.* Retrieved September 29, 2011 from http://www.cbpp.org/cms/index.cfm?fa=view&id=3292.

Center for the Future of Children. (1992, Winter). *U.S. health care for children* (Vol. 2, No. 2). Los Altos, CA: The David and Lucille Packard Foundation.

Centers for Medicare and Medicaid Services. (2011). Children's Health Insurance Program Reauthorization Act of 2009. Retrieved March 27, 2011 from http://www.cms.gov/CHIPRA/.

Child Trends. (2003). *Health care coverage.* Retrieved from: www.childtrendsdatabank.org/indicators/26healthcarecoverage.cfm.

Child Trends. (2010). *Health care coverage.* Retrieved May 10, 2011 from http://www.childtrendsdatabank.org/?q=node/297.

Children's Defense Fund. (2004). *The state of America's children 2004.* Washington, DC: Children's Defense Fund.

Children's Defense Fund. (2010). *The state of America's children 2010.* Washington, DC: Children's Defense Fund.

Clark, S. L., & Weismantle, M. (2003, August). *Employment status 2000, Census 2000 brief.* Washington, DC: U.S. Department of Commerce, Economics and Statistical Administration, Bureau of the Census.

Cunningham, P. J., & Hahn, B. A. (1994). The changing American family: Implication for children's health insurance coverage and the use of ambulatory care services. *The Future of Children, 4,* 24–42.

Current Population Survey. Annual demographic survey. (2001, March Suppl.). Retrieved May 10, 2011 from http://www.bls.census.gov/cps/ads/sdata.htm.

Darman, R. (1992, January 17). *Comprehensive health reform: Observations about the problem and alternative approaches to solution* (p. 6). Testimony before the U.S. House of Representatives, Committee on Ways and Means, Washington, DC.

DeNavas-Walt, C., Proctor, B. D., & Mills, R. J. (2004). *Income, poverty, and health insurance coverage in the United States: 2003.* Current Population Reports, P60-226. Washington, DC: U.S. Department of Commerce, Economics and Statistical Administration, Bureau of the Census. Retrieved September 29, 2011 from http://www.census.gov/prod/2004pubs/p60-226.pdf.

DeNavas-Walt, C., Proctor, B. D., & Smith, J. C. (2010). *Income, poverty, and health insurance coverage in the United States: 2009.* Current Population Reports, P60-238. Washington, DC: U.S. Department of Commerce, Economics and Statistical Administration, Bureau of the Census.

Donovan, P. (1995). *The politics of blame: Family planning, abortion, and the poor.* New York: Alan Guttmacher Institute.

Dye, J. L. (2008). *Participation of mothers in government assistance programs: 2004.* Current Population Reports, P70-116. Washington, DC: U.S. Department of Commerce, Economics and Statistical Administration, Census Bureau.

Federal Interagency Forum on Child Health and Family Statistics. (2003). *America's children: Key national indicators of well-being, 2003.* Washington, DC: U.S. Government Printing Office.

Federal Interagency Forum on Child and Family Statistics. (2009). *America's Children: Key national indicators of well-being, 2009.* Washington, DC: U.S. Government Printing Office.

Federal Interagency Forum on Child and Family Statistics. (2010). *America's Children in Brief: Key national indicators of well-being, 2010.* Washington, DC: U.S. Government Printing Office.

Fields, J. (2003, June). *Children's living arrangements and characteristics: March 2002, population characteristics.* Washington, DC: U.S. Department of Commerce, Economics and Statistics Administration, Bureau of the Census, Demographic Programs.

Fields, J., & Casper, L. M. (2001, June). *America's families and living arrangements: 2000, Current Population Reports.* Washington, DC: U.S. Department of Commerce, Economics and Statistics Administration, Bureau of the Census, Demographic Programs.

Flint, S. (1992). *Decline in uninsured children registered in 1990: Child health financing report* (Vol. IX, No. 1, p. 5). Elk Grove Village, IL: American Academy of Pediatrics.

Foley, J. D. (1991). *Uninsured in the United States: The nonelderly population without health insurance: Analysis of the March 1990 Current Population Survey* (EBRI Special Report SR-10). Washington, DC: Employee Benefit Research Institute.

Fronstin, P. (2010). *Sources of health insurance and characteristics of the uninsured: Analysis of the March 2010 Current Population Survey.* (EBRI Issue Brief, 347). Washington, DC: Employer Benefit Research Institute. Retrieved March 27, 2011 from http://www.ebri.org/publications/ib/index.cfm?fa=ibDisp&content_id=4643.

Gould, E., & Shierholz, H. (2010). "A lost decade: Poverty and income trends paint a bleak picture for working class families." Washington, DC: Economic Policy Institute. Retrieved May 10, 2011 from http://www.epi.org/publications/entry/a_lost_decade_poverty_and_income_trends/.

Grall, T. S. (2009). *Custodial mothers and fathers and their child support: 2007.* Current Population Reports, P60-237. Washington, DC: U.S. Department of Commerce, Economics and Statistics Administration, Bureau of the Census.

Hareven, T. K. (1984). Themes in the historical development of the family. In R. D. Parke (Ed.), *The review of child development* (Vol. 7, pp. 137–178). Chicago, IL: The University of Chicago Press.

Hetherington, E. M., & Jodl, K. M. (1994). Stepfamilies as settings for child development. In A. Booth & J. Dunn (Eds.), *Stepfamilies: Who benefits? Who does not?* (pp. 55–80). Hillsdale, NJ: Lawrence Erlbaum Associates.

Holahan J., Dubay L., & Kenney G. (2003). Which children are still uninsured and why. *The Future of Children, 13,* 68–70.

Irving, S. (2010). *TANF participation and employment in SIPP (2004–2007).* Washington, DC: U.S. Bureau of the Census.

Kadushin, A. (1980). *Child welfare services* (3rd ed.). New York: Macmillan Publishing.

Kahn, A. J. (1973). *Social policy and social services.* New York: Random House.

Kaiser Family Foundation. (2006). *Deficit Reduction Act of 2005: Implications for Medicaid.* Retrieved September 29, 2011 from http://www.kff.org/medicaid/7465.cfm.

Kreider, R. M. (2005). *Number, timing, and duration of marriages and divorces: 2001*. Current Population Reports, P70-97. Washington, DC: U.S. Department of Commerce, Economics and Statistics Administration, Bureau of the Census.

Kreider, R. M. (2010). *Increase in opposite-sex cohabiting couples from 2009 to 2010 in the Annual Social and Economic Supplement (ASEC) to the Current Population Survey (CPS)*. Working Paper. Washington, DC: U.S. Bureau of the Census, Housing and Household Economic Statistics Division. Retrieved May 10, 2011 from http://www.census.gov/population/www/socdemo/Inc-Opp-sex-2009-to-2010.pdf.

Kreider, R. M. & Elliott, D. B. (2009). *America's families and living arrangements: 2007*. Current Population Reports, P20-561. Washington, DC: U.S. Department of Commerce, Economics and Statistics Administration, Bureau of the Census.

Kreider, R. M. & Elliott, D. B. (2010). *Historical changes in stay-at-home mothers: 1969 to 2009*. Working Paper. Washington, DC: U.S. Bureau of the Census, Housing and Household Economic Statistics Division. Retrieved May 10, 2011 from http://www.census.gov/population/www/socdemo/ASA2010_Kreider_Elliott.pdf.

Laslett, P., & Wall, R. (1972). *Households and families in past times*. Cambridge, UK: Cambridge University Press.

Laughlin, L. (2010). *Who's minding the kids? Child care arrangements: Spring 2005/Summer 2006*. Current Population Reports, Household Economic Studies (Series P70-121). Washington, DC: U.S. Department of Commerce, Economics and Statistics Administration, Bureau of the Census.

Lugaila, T. (1992). Households, families, and children: A 30-year perspective. *Current population reports: Population characteristics* (Special Studies Series P-23, No. 181). Washington, DC: U.S. Department of Commerce, Economics and Statistics Administration, Bureau of the Census.

McNally, S. J. (1980). Historical perspectives on the family. In J. R. Miller & E. H. Janosik (Eds.), *Family focused care* (pp. 16–30). New York: McGraw-Hill.

Meyer, D. (1995). Supplemental Security Income. In R. L. Edwards (Editor-in-Chief), *Encyclopedia of social work* (Vol. 3, 19th ed.). Washington, DC: National Association of Social Workers.

Mills, R. J., & Bhandari, S. (2003). *Health insurance coverage in the United States: 2002. Current Population Reports*, P60-223. Washington, DC: U.S.

Department of Commerce, Economics and Statistics Administration, Bureau of the Census.

Morello, C. (2010). "About 44 million in U.S. lived below poverty line in 2009, census data show." *The Washington Post*. Retrieved September 29, 2010 from http://www.washingtonpost.com/wp-dyn/content/article/2010/09/16/AR2010091602698.html.

Neihardt J. (1975). *Black Elk speaks* (p. 165). New York: Pocket Books.

Newson, G., & Harvey, B. (1994). Assuring access to health care. In H. M. Wallace, R. P. Nelson, & P. J. Sweeney (Eds.), *Maternal and child health practices* (4th ed., pp. 11–17). Oakland, CA: Third Party Publishers.

Palumbo, T. (2010). Economic characteristics of households in the United States: Third quarter 2008. *Current Population Reports* (Household Economic Series, P-70, No. 119). Washington, DC: U.S. Department of Commerce, Economics and Statistics Administration, Bureau of the Census.

Parrott, S. (2002). *The TANF-related provisions in the president's budget*. Washington, DC: Center on Budget and Policy Priorities.

Pew Hispanic Center. (2010). *Statistical portrait of the foreign-born population in the United States, 2008*. (Tables 18 & 19). Retrieved October 13, 2010 from http://pewhispanic.org/factsheets/factsheet.php?FactsheetID=59.

Ratcliffe, C., & McKernan, S. (2010, June). *Childhood poverty persistence: Facts and consequences*. Brief 14. Washington, DC: The Urban Institute. Retrieved May 10, 2011 from http://www.urban.org/uploadedpdf/412126-child-poverty-persistence.pdf.

Rawlings, S. (1993). *Population profile of the U.S. 1993: Households and families*. Current population reports: Population characteristics (Special Studies Series P-23, No. 185). Washington, DC: U.S. Department of Commerce, Economics and Statistics Administration, Bureau of the Census.

Reisch, M. (1995). Public social services. In R. L. Edwards (Ed.-in-Chief), *Encyclopedia of social work* (Vol. 3, 19th ed., pp. 1982–1991). Washington, DC: National Association of Social Workers.

Reiss, I., & Lee, G. (1988). *Family systems in America*. New York: Holt, Rinehart and Winston.

Schmidt, W. M., & Wallace, H. M. (1994). The development of health services for mothers and children in the U.S. In H. M. Wallace, R. P. Nelson, & P. J. Sweeney (Eds.), *Maternal and child health practices*

(4th ed., pp. 103–119). Oakland, CA: Third Party Publishers.

Schorr, L., & Schorr, D. (1988). *Within our reach: Breaking the cycle of disadvantage.* New York: Anchor Doubleday.

Short, E. (1993). *Population profile of the U.S. 1993: Health insurance.* Current population reports: Population characteristics (Special Studies Series P23, No. 185). Washington, DC: U.S. Department of Commerce, Economics and Statistics Administration, Bureau of the Census.

Smith, K. (2002, July). *Who's minding the kids? Child care arrangements: Spring 1997.* Current Population Reports, Household Economic Studies (Series P-70-86). Washington, DC: U.S. Department of Commerce, Economics and Statistics Administration, Bureau of the Census.

Simms, M. C., Fortuny, K., & Henderson, E. (2009). *Racial and ethnic disparities among low-income families.* Washington, DC: Urban Institute. Retrieved May 10, 2011 from http://www.urban.org/uploadedpdf/411936_racialandethnic.pdf.

Tin, J. (1996). *Dynamics of economic well-being: Program participation, 1992–1993: Who gets assistance? Current Population Reports, Household Economic Studies* (Series P70-78). Washington, DC: U.S. Department of Commerce, Economics and Statistics Administration, Bureau of the Census.

U.S. Bureau of the Census. (1990). *How we are changing: Demographic state of the nation: 1990.* Current Population Reports (Special Studies Series P-23, No. 170). Washington, DC: U.S. Department of Commerce.

U.S. Bureau of the Census. (1991a). *Poverty in the U.S.: 1990.* Current Population Reports (Consumer Income Series P-60, No. 175). Washington, DC: U.S. Department of Commerce.

U.S. Bureau of the Census. (1991b). *Trends in relative income: 1964–1989.* Current population reports (Consumer Income Series P-60, No. 177). Washington, DC: U.S. Government Printing Office.

U.S. Bureau of the Census. (1994). *Demographic state of the nation: 1995.* Current Population Reports (Special Studies Series P-23, No. 188). Washington, DC: U.S. Department of Commerce, Bureau of the Census.

U.S. Bureau of the Census. (2000). *Population profile of the United States: 2000, from birth to seventeen: The living arrangements of children, 2000.* Washington, DC: U.S. Department of Commerce, Bureau of the Census. Retrieved September 29, 2011 from http://www.census.gov/population/pop-profile/2000/chap06.pdf.

U.S. Bureau of the Census. (2002). *Age, sex, household relationship, race and Hispanic origin: Poverty status of people by selected characteristics in 2001* (Table 1). Washington, DC: U.S. Department of Commerce.

U.S. Bureau of the Census. (2004). *America's Families and Living Arrangements: 2003. Table MS-2: Estimated Median Age at First Marriage, by Sex: 1890 to Present.* Annual Social and Economic Supplement: 2003 Current Population Survey, Current Population Reports, Series P20-553. Washington, DC: U.S. Department of Commerce, Bureau of the Census. Retrieved September 29, 2011 from http://www.census.gov/population/socdemo/hh-fam/tabMS-2.pdf.

U.S. Bureau of the Census. (2008). 2008 American Community Survey 1-year estimates. Retrieved May 10, 2011 from http://factfinder.census.gov/servlet/DatasetMainPageServlet?_program = ACS&_submenuId = &_lang = en&_ds_name = ACS_2008_3YR_G00_&ts = .

U.S. Bureau of the Census. (2010a). *Current Population Survey, 2009 annual social and economic supplement.* Table 1: Educational attainment of the population 18 years & over by age, sex, race, & Hispanic origin. Retrieved September 29, 2011 from http://www.census.gov/hhes/socdemo/education/data/cps/2009/tables.html.

U.S. Bureau of the Census. (2010b). *Current Population Survey, 2009 Annual Social and Economic Supplement.* Tables A1, C3, C4, C8, C9, FG1, & FG10. Washington, DC: U.S. Bureau of the Census.

U.S. Bureau of the Census. (2010c). *POV21: Related children under 18 by householder's work experience and family structure: 2009.* Retrieved September 29, 2011 from http://www.census.gov/hhes/www/cpstables/032010/pov/new21_000.htm.

U.S. Bureau of the Census. (2010d). POV29: Years of school completed by poverty status, sex, age, nativity and citizenship. Retrieved September 29, 2011 from http://www.census.gov/hhes/www/cpstables/032010/pov/new29_100.htm.

U.S. Bureau of the Census. (2010e). *Table CH-5: Children under 18 years living with mother only, by marital status of mother: 1960 to present.* Retrieved September 29, 2011 from http://www.census.gov/population/www/socdemo/hh-fam.html.

U.S. Bureau of the Census. (2010f). *Table F-5. Race and Hispanic origin of householder—families by median and mean income: 1947 to 2009*. Retrieved September 29, 2011 from http://www.census.gov/hhes/www/income/data/historical/families/index.html.

U.S. Bureau of the Census. (2010g). *Table FM-1. Families, by presence of own children under 18: 1950 to present.* Retrieved September 29, 2011 from http://www.census.gov/population/www/socdemo/hh-fam.html#history.

U.S. Bureau of the Census. (2010h). *Table FM-2. All parent-child situations, by type, race, and Hispanic origin of householder or reference person: 1970 to present.* Retrieved September 29, 2011 from http://www.census.gov/population/www/socdemo/hh-fam.html#history.

U.S. Bureau of the Census. (2010i). *Table MS-2. Estimated median age at first marriage, by sex: 1890 to the present.* Retrieved September 29, 2011 from http://www.census.gov/population/www/socdemo/hh-fam.html#history.

U.S. Bureau of the Census. (2010j). *United States–Selected social characteristics in the United States: 2009.* Washington, DC: U.S. Department of Commerce.

U.S. Congress. (1996). *Personal Responsibility and Work Opportunity Reconciliation Act,* Public Law 104-193.

U.S. Department of Education and U.S. Department of Justice. *(2000). Working for children and families: Safe and smart after-school programs.* Retrieved September 29, 2011 from http://www2.ed.gov/offices/OESE/archives/pubs/parents/SafeSmart/index.html.

U.S. Department of Health and Human Services. (2001). *Trends in the well-being of America's children and youth 2001.* Washington, DC: Office of the Assistant Secretary for Planning and Evaluation. Retrieved September 29, 2011 from http://aspe.hhs.gov/hsp/01trends/contents.htm#HC. (see Tables HC 1.1.A and HC 1.1.C).

U.S. Department of Health and Human Services. (2002, November 1). *Welfare caseloads continue downward trends* (press release). Washington, DC: Author.

U.S. Department of Health and Human Services, Social Security Administration. (1994, August). Annual statistical supplement. *Social Security Bulletin,* SSA Pub. No. 13-71700.

Van Dyck, P., & Hogan, M. D. (2003). Health and social care of women, children, youth and families. In H. M. Wallace, G. Green, & K. J. Jaros (Eds.), *Health and welfare for families in the 21st century* (pp. 5–25). Boston, MA: Jones and Bartlett Publishers.

Ventura, S. J. (2003). Demographic factors affecting fertility patterns in the United States. In H. M. Wallace, G. Green, & K. J. Jaros (Eds.), *Health and welfare for families in the 21st century* (pp. 52–70). Boston, MA: Jones and Bartlett Publishers.

Wallace, H. M., Green, G., & Jaros, K. J. (Eds.). (2003). *Health and welfare for families in the 21st century* (pp. 5–25). Boston, MA: Jones and Bartlett Publishers.

Watkins, E. (1993). The history of maternal and child health: The role of public health social workers. In J. J. Fickling (Ed.), *Social problems with health consequences: Program design, implementation, and evaluation.* Proceedings of the 1990 Bi-Regional Conference for Public Health Social Workers in Regions IV and VI. Columbia, SC: College of Social Work, University of South Carolina.

Welniak, E., & Posey, K. (2005). *Household income: 1999.* Washington, DC: U.S. Bureau of the Census. Retrieved May 10, 2011 from http://www.census.gov/prod/2005pubs/c2kbr-36.pdf.

World Almanac and Book of Facts 1990. (1990). (p. 551). New York: Pharos Books.

4

A LIFE COURSE PERSPECTIVE ON MATERNAL AND CHILD HEALTH

Liana J. Richardson, Jon M. Hussey, and Kelly L. Strutz

It seems likely and biologically plausible that healthy children become healthy adults with reduced risk for a variety of health problems, including reproductive problems. The evidence for this simple principle has been accumulating over the last five decades and, I believe, has been largely ignored in the search for other causal factors that presumably are more amenable to immediate intervention. It does not seem likely that immediate interventions will solve the problems of interest. On the other hand, it appears that the roots of these problems to some extent are laid down in childhood.

(Emanuel, 1986, p. 35)

Historically, the prevailing approach to maternal and child health (MCH) research, policy, and practice has been dominated by a focus on temporally proximate or contemporaneous risk factors. For example, efforts to understand and address perinatal health problems have focused on prenatal exposures, childhood health problems on childhood exposures, and adult health problems on adult exposures. During the past 2 decades, however, several factors—most notably the intractability of key MCH problems in the U.S. and beyond—have contributed to the questioning of this approach and the search for new ways to address these problems.

In the United States, the discrepancy between expenditures and global rankings on key MCH indicators, as well as the persistence and growth of racial/ethnic and socioeconomic disparities in some of the indicators, are chief among the problems for which new answers are needed. Rates of low birth weight, preterm birth, and infant mortality in this country remain considerably

higher than the Healthy People 2010 goals (Hamilton, Martin, & Ventura, 2010; U.S. Department of Health and Human Services, 2000), and nearly double the rates observed in other developed countries (Langhoff-Roos, Kesmodel, Jacobsson, Rasmussen, & Vogel, 2006; Morken et al., 2008). In 2007, the low birth weight rate in the United States ranked 27th worst among the 30 wealthy, industrialized countries of the Organisation for Co-operative Development (OECD, 2009)—a ranking that lies in stark contrast to the fact that the United States is the second wealthiest nation in per capita gross domestic product and spends the most on health care (OECD, 2009; Raphael, 2007). Within-country disparities in infant health are also a prominent feature of the troubling U.S. population health profile. Historically, African Americans have experienced roughly twofold higher rates of adverse birth outcomes than whites (Martin, Osterman, & Sutton, 2010)—a difference that known risk factors, including behavioral, biomedical, and socioeconomic factors, do not fully explain (Gennaro, 2005; Goldenberg, Culhane, Iams, & Romero, 2008; Shiono, Rauh, Park, Lederman, & Zuskar, 1997).

Seemingly intractable problems in global MCH also lead us to reconsider prevailing approaches to understanding and addressing them (World Health Organization [WHO], 2009). Approximately 7.7 million children under 5 years of age, almost half of whom were neonates, died in 2010 (Rajaratnam et al., 2010). In addition, almost 350,000 women succumbed to pregnancy-related deaths in 2008 (Hogan et al., 2010). Although many countries are on target to meet the Millennium Development Goal of reducing under-5 mortality by two thirds from the year 2000 baseline, advancement toward achieving the maternal and neonatal mortality reduction goals has been limited (Bhutta et al., 2010). In addition to high mortality, endemic problems such as undernutrition, gender-based socioeconomic inequalities, and short intervals between births due to unmet need for contraception lead to high prevalence of morbidity in women and children in many countries (WHO, 2009).

If the answers to these problems cannot be found fully in temporally proximate risk factors, where can we find them? By focusing our attention instead on the potential long-term health impact of experiences, exposures, and behaviors over individuals' *entire* life spans, a life course perspective on MCH provides one clear alternative. Among the questions that this perspective prompts us to answer are: To what degree is our health impacted by our life history, our mother's and father's life histories, and the histories of our ancestors? Are exposures that we experienced *in utero* linked to our risk of developing hypertension or diabetes as an adult? Do childhood adversities influence adult health and well-being? How might childhood and adolescent experiences impact our reproductive health during our 20s, 30s, and 40s?

Current attention to these questions and excitement about the life course perspective within the MCH policy, practice, and scientific communities are unprecedented, although the suggestion that early life exposures may have important consequences for future health and well-being, including future reproductive health and pregnancy outcomes, dates back at least 150 years (Meckel, 1990). Recent events contributing to the revival of interest in applying a life course perspective to MCH include: the emergence of life course epidemiology in 1997; the 2003 publication of Michael Lu's and Neil Halfon's seminal conceptual paper, "Racial and Ethnic Disparities in Birth Outcomes: A Life-Course Perspective"; and the growing availability of longitudinal data suitable for evaluating life course hypotheses. The (U.S.) Maternal and Child Health Bureau's use of the life course perspective as a foundation for its next 5-year strategic plan (Van Dyck, 2010) is yet another example of the growing influence of this model on MCH policy and practice (see Figure 4–1).

The growth of interest in life course approaches is also evident in patterns of publication. The number of research articles in which the terms "life course," "lifecourse," or "life-course" appear in the title or abstract has steadily grown since the early 1990s, with even more rapid growth in the past 5 years (see Figure 4–2).

Given this widespread adoption of the life course perspective, it is now imperative for MCH scholars and practitioners to be familiar with it. The goal of this chapter, therefore, is to provide an introductory overview of the perspective and its applications to some of the most active areas of investigation in the MCH field. We begin by tracing the life course perspective to its roots in the social and behavioral sciences and reviewing eight fundamental principles and concepts in life course theory. Second, we discuss the manner in which some of these principles and concepts have been translated into what has been dubbed "life course epidemiology." Third, we trace the emergence of life course scholarship within the MCH field and review three key areas of its contemporary scholarship that are consistent with a life course perspective. We explicate the links between these areas and life course principles and concepts,

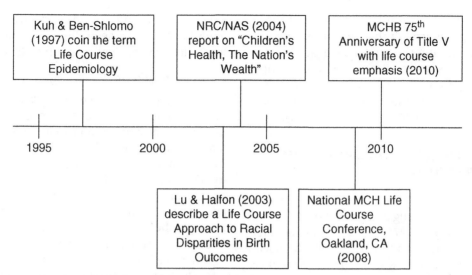

Figure 4–1 Key Events in Life Course MCH since 1995

(*Abbreviations: MCHB, Maternal and Child Health Bureau; NAS, National Academy of Sciences; NRC, National Research Council) Source*: Adapted from Kuh, D., & Ben-Schlomo, Y. (2004). Preface. In D. Kuh, & Y. Ben-Schlomo (Eds.), A life course approach to chronic disease epidemiology (pp. ix–x). Oxford: Oxford University Press, and National Research Council and Institute of Medicine. (2004). Children's Health, the Nation's Wealth: Assessing and Improving Child Health. Committee on Evaluation of Children's Health. Board on Children, Youth, and Families, Division of Behavioral and Social Sciences and Education. Washington, DC: The National Academies Press, and Van Dyck, P. C. Moving from theory to practice: Life course, social determinants and health equity framework in maternal and child health. http://webcast.hrsa.gov/conferences/mchb/TitleV75/rams_transcripts/TheoryToPractice.pdf. Accessed April 4, 2011, and Lu, M. C., & Halfon, N. (2003). Racial and ethnic disparities in birth outcomes: A life-course perspective. Maternal and Child Health Journal, 7(1), 13–30, and Pies, C., Parthasarathy, P., Kotelchuck, M., & Lu, M. (2009). Making a paradigm shift in maternal and child health: A report on the national MCH life course meeting. http://www.citymatch.org/lifecoursetoolbox/documents/NationalMCH-LCMeeting/Meeting%20Report%20Final%2020100709.pdf. Accessed September 20, 2011.

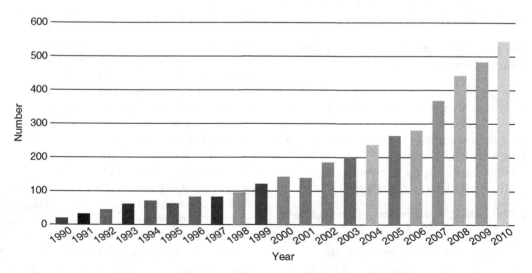

Figure 4–2 Annual Number of Research Articles on Life Course Topics, 1990–2010

Source: Data from ISI Web of Knowledge.

and draw from the latter to identify new research questions that hold the potential for expanding the evidence base. Finally, we address the implications of a life course approach for MCH policy and practice, but conclude with a general discussion about what else is needed to advance this agenda.

FUNDAMENTAL CONCEPTS IN LIFE COURSE THEORY

Sociologist Glen Elder, Jr. has played a leading role in the founding and growth of life course studies (Elder, 1975, 1979). In his seminal work on the changing historical and social contexts of lives and their consequences for human development and aging, the "life course" is both a concept and a theoretical orientation. As a concept, it refers to the sequence of events and roles—age graded, socially defined, and nested within historical time and place—that form our individual biographies (Elder & Shanahan, 2006). At the same time, the life course is a theoretical orientation that can be used to identify questions suitable for scientific inquiry, justify the selection of research variables, and guide the choice of study design and data analysis methods (Elder, Johnson, & Crosnoe, 2004). In the paragraphs that follow, we focus on life course *theory* and describe its components.

The Five Defining Principles of Life Course Theory

Elder (2006) identifies five defining principles and three temporal concepts of life course theory. We describe them here and briefly mention relevant MCH examples. We present a more detailed discussion of three key MCH areas of investigation and their links to life course theory later in the chapter.

1. The Principle of Life Span Development

The *principle of life span development* suggests that health and well-being are lifelong processes. Thus, they can be fully understood only within the context of experiences across one's entire life span. For example,

studies that attempt to link birth weight to adult health outcomes reflect this principle (e.g., Richardson, Hussey, & Strutz, 2011).

2. The Principle of Human Agency

The *principle of human agency* calls attention to the impact of individuals' decisions and actions on their health and well-being. Given that these decisions and actions are influenced by motivations, goals, values, and personality, this principle highlights the central roles of personal control and behavior in health and illness. Another critical assumption of this principle, however, is that human agency is *embedded in social context*. Elder (2006) asserts that, although individuals select themselves into situations and social roles, decisions and actions are made "within the opportunities and constraints of history and circumstance" (p. 2635). Studies that acknowledge the mediating role of behavioral and psychosocial factors between neighborhood socioeconomic conditions and birth outcomes (e.g., Richardson, 2009; Schempf, Strobino, & O'Campo, 2009) are examples of this principle.

3. The Principle of Timing

The *principle of timing* suggests that our health and well-being are shaped not only by *what* happens to us (i.e., the causes and consequences) but also by *when* in the life course (and in history, see Principle #5) it happens, how long it lasts (*duration*), and in what order it occurs relative to other roles and events (*sequencing*; Elder, 1994, 2006). For example, the impact of childbearing on female educational attainment greatly depends on the mother's age at the time of the birth (e.g., teens vs. 30s; Hofferth, Reid, & Mott, 2001). Similarly, the consequences of family instability for a child may depend on his/her age at the onset of such instability (Cavanagh & Huston, 2008). Timing, or more specifically *social* timing, also applies to the goodness of fit between an individual's multiple life course trajectories. Among women, for example, asynchrony between work and fertility trajectories may increase the likelihood of experiencing fertility problems if it causes them to delay childbearing.

With regard to *duration*, life course scholars also invoke the concept of cumulative advantage/disadvantage (hereafter referred to as *cumulative dis/advantage*), particularly to explain inequality. Cumulative dis/advantage, which is traceable to Merton's (1968, 1988) work on the "Matthew effect," refers to the systematic tendency for inequality to widen over time (i.e., with increasing age) due to the social structuring of—and ongoing differences in—risks, resources, opportunities, and returns to resources (Dannefer, 1987; DiPrete & Eirich, 2006; O'Rand, 1996). This tendency may, therefore, explain diverging life and health trajectories (Willson, Shuey, & Elder, 2007). For example, it has been suggested that racial disparities in adverse birth outcomes and their widening with increasing age may be a result of cumulative dis/advantage (Geronimus, 1992).

4. The Principle of Linked Lives

The *principle of linked lives* suggests that our health and well-being are shaped by the social networks to which we belong and, particularly, our relationships with significant others (Elder, 2006). As Elder (1994) notes, "No principle of life course study is more central than the notion of interdependent lives ... The misfortune and the opportunity of adult children, as well as their personal problems, become intergenerational" (p. 6). Within the domain of MCH, an obvious example of this principle is the linkage between maternal and infant health. However, the range of relationships that matter to MCH scholars and practitioners extends well beyond this direct biological connection. The associations between caregiver characteristics and child maltreatment risk (Hussey, Chang, & Kotch, 2006), peer relationships and adolescent risk behaviors (Kreager, 2007), and sexual network characteristics and sexually transmitted infection (STI) risk (Morris, Kurth, Hamilton, Moody, & Wakefield, 2009) are just a few other MCH examples that are consistent with this principle.

5. The Principle of Historical Time and Place

The *principle of historical time and place* highlights the ways in which period, cohort, and contextual factors influence the life course. Historical events, like the Great Depression in the past century or the Great Recession in the current one, may impact the life course in a variety of ways, with both immediate and long-term consequences for health and well-being. For example, economic stress within the household may have an immediate impact on parenting behaviors (Gershoff, Aber, Raver, & Lennon, 2007), which in turn has longer-term implications for a child's health and development (Repetti, Taylor, & Seeman, 2002). It is also important to appreciate that the impact of historical events may vary by place or location (Elder, 2006). The current economic crisis, for instance, may differentially impact women and children by region, state, city, or even neighborhood of residence, and in ways that differ from those created by previous economic recessions.

The link between place (or context) and other principles of the life course also is clear. For example, understanding the impact of place on health and well-being requires that we consider the features of one's current context, as well as the characteristics of the places to which they have been exposed over their entire life course—i.e., the *principle of life span development*. Furthermore, the *principle of timing* suggests that the impact of contextual factors on child and adult outcomes may vary according to the timing, sequencing, and duration of exposure. Context also figures prominently in the *principle of human agency* as a key factor that constrains individual choices and behaviors. Finally, several health-relevant characteristics illustrative of the *principle of linked lives*, such as social networking opportunities (Swaroop & Morenoff, 2006) and exposure to infectious disease (Feldacker, Emch, & Ennett, 2010), vary by context.

Three Key Concepts in Life Course Theory: Trajectories, Transitions, and Turning Points

Elder (2006) also describes three temporal concepts—trajectories, transitions, and turning points—that are critical to life course scholarship. *Trajectories* are dynamic descriptors of health and well-being that typically describe a substantial period of the life span (Elder & Shanahan, 2006). For example, long-term patterns of an individual's behavior (e.g., physical activity and smoking) and health (e.g., depression and body mass index) can be described as trajectories. Importantly, each individual's life course is characterized by multiple, co-occurring trajectories (e.g., work, relationship, income, and health trajectories).

While trajectories typically capture the long-term picture of one's health and well-being, *transitions*—which are embedded within trajectories—usually take place within a relatively brief time frame. For example, the onset of parenthood or the aging of adolescents into adulthood may be described as transitions. A transition may also result in a *turning point*, defined as "a redirection of the life course through changes in situation, meaning, and/or behavior" (Elder, 2006, p. 2634). The transition to parenthood, for example, is associated with decreased alcohol consumption, at least in the short term (Wolfe, 2009).

FUNDAMENTAL CONCEPTS IN LIFE COURSE EPIDEMIOLOGY

Public health scholars have adopted a number of Elder's life course principles and concepts to advance a "life course epidemiology" or life course perspective on health. First and foremost, consistent with the *principle of life span development*, this perspective is premised on the idea that the body records all of our life experiences and, as a result, tells a story of one's past and that of the preceding generation (Kuh & Ben-Shlomo, 2004; Nguyen & Peschard, 2003). Thus, in order to understand present health and well-being, we must consider experiences and events that may have occurred years, decades, or even generations earlier. Second, life course epidemiology draws on

Elder's ideas that transitions, turning points, and durations embedded in social context have implications for health trajectories (Elder & Johnson, 2003), as well as the concept of cumulative dis/advantage (Dannefer, 1987; DiPrete & Eirich, 2006; O'Rand, 1996) to help explain the divergence of health trajectories (i.e., health disparities). What life course epidemiology adds to life course theory is a more clear delineation of the processes by which past experiences and events affect future health and development and, in doing so, a more nuanced explication of the *principle of timing* and the concepts of *trajectories*, *transitions*, and *turning points*. This task increases the utility of these principles and concepts for public health because it facilitates their operationalization in research, resulting in the collection of data that have the potential to help us identify the most appropriate timing and targets of strategies to improve health and reduce health disparities.

Toward this end, life course epidemiology posits that risk (and protective) factors may combine cross-sectionally and accumulate or interact with each other longitudinally to impact current, future, and intergenerational health (Kuh & Ben-Shlomo, 2004; Blane, 1999; Pollitt, Rose, & Kaufman, 2005), Thus, at least three life course models of health have been proposed: (1) a *latency*, "biological chains of risk," or critical/sensitive period model; (2) a *cumulative*, "accumulation of risk," or cumulative exposure model; and (3) a *pathway*, "social chains of risk," or social trajectory model (Berkman, 2009; Hertzman, 2004; Hertzman & Boyce, 2010; Kuh, Ben-Shlomo, Lynch, Hallqvist, & Power, 2003; Pollitt et al., 2005). As Figure 4–3 shows, a *latency* model suggests that early exposures are associated with later health risk, regardless of intervening exposures. A *cumulative* model posits that exposures across the life course combine to influence later health risk, producing a greater effect than would be produced by the same exposures at just one point in the life course. A *pathway* model is

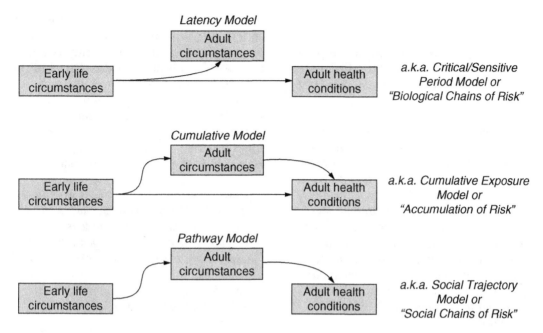

Figure 4–3 Three Life Course Models of Health

Source: Berkman, Lisa F. Social Epidemiology: Social Determinants of Health in the United States: Are We Losing Ground? Annual Review of Public Health 2009;30:2

one in which early experiences lead to a cascade of exposures and effects that eventually impact later health. It also suggests that changes (i.e., intervening exposures) in the trajectory at any point in time may modify the health effect (Hertzman, 2004; Pollitt et al., 2005).

These models are not mutually exclusive, but do have different implications for research and practice (Graham, 2002). In addition, although their visual depictions are gross oversimplifications of a more dynamic and complex set of intra- and inter-generational phenomena, the models are useful heuristics for considering mechanisms by which both beneficial and harmful exposures may affect the development *over time* of differential risk for adverse health outcomes across groups (e.g., racial/ethnic or socioeconomic groups). To date, however, limited evidence about which life course causal models underlie such group differences exists.

APPLICATIONS OF LIFE COURSE THEORY AND EPIDEMIOLOGY TO MCH

Historical Applications to MCH

Although the advent of life course epidemiology has been a key contributor to the widespread adoption of a life course perspective on MCH in recent years, its origins can be traced to at least 150 years ago when health reformers recognized the possibility that poor health could be transmitted from one generation to the next—a possibility that is consistent with the *principle of linked lives*. For example, it became clear to them that "if infant mortality was to be reduced, the health of all urban slum residents had to be improved" (Meckel, 1990, p. 22).

Similarly, it was nearly a century ago when MCH discourse began to include arguments consistent with the *principle of life span development*. For example, lack of knowledge about proper infant feeding and care among mothers was seen as the primary cause of infant mortality at the time, but this view did not supplant recognition of the potential impact of maternal health prior to pregnancy on birth outcomes. As Meckel (1990) observed:

> Even those infant welfare activists who evinced greatest faith in the power of advice had to admit that a mother's ability to carry and bear healthy infants could be seriously affected by a pre-gestative life of poor nutrition, debilitating physical activity, and exposure to infectious disease. Most physicians, for instance, were aware that childhood rickets, a common disease among the malnourished, often produced pelvic deformities that later complicated childbearing. (p. 170)

In the late 1940s, some of the first empirical evidence of this link came from a series of studies on adverse birth outcomes in Aberdeen, Scotland by Sir Dugald Baird and colleagues. They found that low birth weight and perinatal mortality were less common among taller women (who presumably enjoyed superior childhood nutrition) and those from higher social class origins. Moreover, a woman's social class during childhood predicted her likelihood of delivering a low birth weight infant *independent* of her current (adult) social class, suggesting that early life exposures may have an enduring effect on adult reproductive health (Baird, 1964). This suggestion is consistent with a *latency* or *critical/sensitive period* model.

Several decades later in the United States, Irvin Emanuel emerged as one of the earliest proponents of a life course perspective on reproductive health outcomes. For more than 3 decades, beginning in the early 1970s, Emanuel's research and review articles advanced an intergenerational model of reproductive health that emphasized how women's life course exposures—starting *in utero* and continuing into childhood and

beyond—influence the health of their offspring (e.g., Emanuel, 1986, 1993; Emanuel & Sever, 1973). Also noteworthy is Emanuel's early application of this model to the problem of racial disparities in birth outcomes (Emanuel 1986; Emanuel, Hale, & Berg, 1989). Commenting on the inability of prenatal care or genetic factors to account for these persistent disparities, Emanuel, Hale, and Berg (1989) observed that,

> It would be more fruitful to ask what it is about the lives of American black women which is apparently so hazardous to fetal and infant health, and we suggest that two aspects of their lives, the mothers' childhood environments and the environment in which their own pregnancies occur, merit additional study and attention. (p. 300)

Their conclusion that studying racial differentials in life course exposures, beginning *in utero*, is a more promising line of investigation than focusing on the prenatal period is an argument that reappeared 14 years later in Lu and Halfon's (2003) highly influential conceptual paper.

Other early examples of a life course perspective on MCH can be found in early theories and research linking infant and childhood exposures to a range of adult health outcomes. Interest in this topic dates back more than a century when there were growing concerns, in both the United States and Europe, about the physical degeneration of national populations. In particular, connections were made between the poor health of military recruits and early life health. During World War I, for example, 29% of American draftees were found to be physically unfit for military service, and the majority of their physical deficiencies could be traced to childhood illnesses, such as heart murmurs caused by scarlet fever or rickets-related physical deformities (Meckel, 1990).

One of the first empirical studies to link health across the full life span was published by Kermack, McKendrick, and McKinlay in 1934. Analyzing European data, they noted that the relative mortality rates of successive birth cohorts tended to track across the life course. In other words, cohorts that experienced lower infant and childhood mortality also experienced lower mortality across the full life span. This study, therefore, provides an early example of the *principle of historical time and place*.

Contemporary Applications to MCH

Now that there is renewed interest in adopting a life course perspective on MCH and a strong theoretical foundation on which to build, we have an opportunity to conduct even more nuanced life course MCH research. This potential is reflected in three important and illustrative areas of active MCH scholarship: (1) the role of *preconception* health and well-being on birth outcomes, (2) the long-term effects of adverse childhood experiences, and (3) the fetal origins of adult disease. In the paragraphs that follow, we review these areas of investigation, uncover their implicit life course theoretical underpinnings, and identify additional questions that life course theory compels us to ask.

1. Preconception Health and Well-Being

Studies of adverse birth outcomes have historically demonstrated a predominant focus on prenatal exposures—a practice that has limited our understanding of the factors that may precede pregnancy, or even the entire childbearing period, and be instrumental in precipitating preterm birth and low birth weight. As a result, many MCH scholars have grown interested in *preconception* health, viewing pregnancy as part of an integrated continuum or *trajectory* of health rather than a disconnected stage of development (Pies, Parthasarathy, Kotelchuck, & Lu, 2009). Consistent with the *principle of life span development*, therefore, the preconception health perspective argues that birth outcomes are affected not only by maternal exposures in the 9-month prenatal period, but also by maternal development across the life span prior to pregnancy.

For more than 2 decades, supporters of a preconception care agenda have promoted efforts to expand women's health care beyond the prenatal period to include preconceptional and interconceptional care (Moos, 2010). Despite these long-standing efforts, surprisingly little evidence exists on the relationship between prepregnancy maternal exposures and birth outcomes. To date, the most commonly studied exposures have been prepregnancy folic acid consumption, which has long been known to prevent neural tube defects (Wald, 1993), and prepregnancy obesity, which is associated with an increased risk of fetal death and macrosomic infant, prenatal and intrapartum complications (Arendas, Qiu, & Gruslin, 2008), and preterm delivery (Torloni et al., 2009). Emergent research suggests that daily consumption of vegetables prior to pregnancy (Weisman et al., 2011), preconception smoking and poor physical functioning (Haas et al., 2005), and prepregnancy depression (Gavin, Chae, Mustillo, & Kiefe, 2009) also may be associated with birth outcomes, although findings have been inconsistent across studies (e.g., Phillips, Wise, Rich-Edwards, Stampfer, & Rosenberg, 2010).

The focus on behavioral and psychosocial factors in the aforementioned studies reveals their bias toward factors that are amenable to healthcare intervention. Yet consistent with the principle of *human agency embedded in social context*, studies that focus on preconception (or early life) socioeconomic conditions also are important subjects for research on the contribution of preconception exposures to adverse birth outcomes. For example, a few studies have examined the effects of intergenerational changes or consistencies in individual-level and neighborhood-level socioeconomic status (i.e., early life versus contemporaneous socioeconomic status) on birth outcomes, independent of prenatal exposures (Colen, Geronimus, Bound, & James, 2006; Collins, David, Rankin, & Desireddi, 2009; Collins, Wambach, David, & Rankin, 2009; Love, David, Rankin, & Collins, 2010). Life course theory, however, makes clear that many important gaps in this body of literature remain to be filled. For example, these social mobility studies capture little of women's exposure histories prior to their pregnancies—e.g., exposures that intervene in the pathway between early life and adult factors (*principle of life span development*)—partially because they rely on data at only two time points. Nor do they examine the role of *duration, timing*, and *sequencing* to determine whether the effects of early life factors on later birth outcomes are lagged (*latency* or *critical/sensitive period model*), or when considered along with adult factors, interactive or *cumulative*.

Toward this end, one of the more active areas of investigation within the preconception health literature is concerned with the *weathering hypothesis*. This hypothesis, coined by Arline Geronimus (1992), refers to the potential cumulative negative impact of social environmental stressors on reproductive health and birth outcomes, and particularly the widening of black-white disparities in adverse birth outcomes with increasing maternal age (*principle of life span development* and *cumulative dis/advantage*). Among the stressors that she posits play roles in this process are socioeconomic challenges, residence in areas characterized by disadvantage and environmental hazards, and coping behaviors that are detrimental to health. In addition, she asserts that African American women may have limited access to health services and the informal social resources and institutions to which they have traditionally turned to offset the impact of these stressors, engaging instead in prolonged active or "high effort coping," which further damages health (Geronimus, 1992). In this way, the weathering hypothesis goes beyond cumulative dis/advantage by providing a more explicit description of the mechanisms

that lead to diverging trajectories of reproductive health decline (i.e., widening racial/ethnic disparities) as women age.

To date, evidence supporting the weathering hypothesis with respect to birth and other health outcomes remains incomplete. Although researchers have documented age patterns that are consistent with those that prompted the weathering hypothesis (e.g., Sastry & Hussey, 2003), the cumulative mechanisms posited by Geronimus to underlie racial differences in the rate of weathering have been underinvestigated. In most studies that purport to provide evidence of weathering, age serves merely as a proxy for those mechanisms. Another important limitation in this literature is that most studies have relied on cross-sectional data to evaluate a hypothesis that demands longitudinal data. Consequently, the majority of studies of the age-birth outcome relationship rest on the questionable assumption that contemporaneous circumstances reflect one's lifetime exposure history.

2. The Life Course Impact of Adverse Childhood Experiences

The long-term consequences of adverse childhood experiences, such as childhood maltreatment, are areas of MCH investigation that also reflect a life course perspective. Over the past 10–15 years, this topic has attracted increased attention due in large part to findings from the Adverse Childhood Experiences (ACE) Study, which has been following a cohort of adult Health Maintenance Organization (HMO) enrollees since the mid-1990s. In their initial paper, the ACE study team documented associations between adverse childhood experiences and a variety of adult health outcomes, including current smoking, severe obesity, depressed mood, attempted suicide, alcoholism, illicit drug use, sexual promiscuity, history of sexually transmitted infection, and chronic bronchitis or emphysema (Felitti et al., 1998). In subsequent papers, adverse childhood experiences have been linked to ischemic heart disease (Dong et al., 2004); anxiety, anger management, sleep disturbance, and memory impairment (Anda et al., 2006); mortality risk (Brown et al., 2009); and other outcomes.

Importantly, for most of these outcomes, the ACE study revealed evidence of a dose-response relationship: As the number of adverse childhood experiences increases so too do the odds of engaging in a health risk behavior or experiencing an adverse health outcome. Studies using other data sources have found a similar pattern. For example, in the 2001–2003 National Comorbidity Survey Replication involving a national probability sample of U.S. adults, a dose-response relationship between number of adverse childhood experiences (0–3) and multiple psychiatric outcomes was found among both women and men (Afifi et al., 2008). These findings are, therefore, consistent with a *cumulative* life course model.

Moreover, many fundamental principles and concepts of life course theory are implicit in this literature. Consistent with the *principle of life span development*, a key implication of the ACE study is that adult health and well-being can only be fully understood by considering early exposures along with more proximate influences. The *principle of linked lives* also is implicit in the study, as most of the adverse events experienced by children stem from the behaviors and experiences of people in their immediate social network. Many events, such as the incarceration of a parent or the change from a dual-parent to a single-parent household, also represent important *transitions* or *turning points* in a child's life.

Although these life course principles and concepts already permeate the literature on adverse childhood experiences, life course theory still has much more to offer this area of investigation. For example, our understanding of why experiences do not affect all individuals equally could benefit from greater attention to the life course *principle of timing*. Although existing research has devoted a great deal of attention to measuring the quantity of adverse childhood experiences, much remains to be learned about whether the timing (i.e., early vs. middle vs. late childhood), duration, or sequencing of exposures matters. The *principle of historical time and place* is also largely absent from this scholarship, leaving several other questions unanswered. For example, is it possible that the life course impact of a parental separation or divorce experienced in the 1940s, 1950s, or 1960s (when many ACE study participants were children) would differ from the same event experienced by the children of the 1980s, 1990s, or 2000s? Similarly, has the Great Recession of 2009 and its aftermath affected the quantity, frequency, duration, or severity of adverse childhood experiences?

3. Fetal Origins of Adult Disease

The fetal origins hypothesis, conceived by David Barker and associates, is one of the most prominent examples of a life course perspective on MCH. Consistent with the *principle of life span development* and a *latency (i.e., critical/sensitive period)* model, the hypothesis suggests that adult disease cannot be fully understood without considering early life exposures at critical or sensitive periods, beginning *in utero*, that may "program" the body's susceptibility to adult disease outcomes (Barker, 1998).

Much of the work on the fetal origins hypothesis has focused on fetal nutrition. Reflecting the life course *principle of linked lives*, fetal nutrition is a function of maternal nutrition (e.g., metabolism; pregnancy diet) and how well the placenta is able to transport nutrients from the mother to the fetus (Eriksson, Kajantie, Osmond, Thornburg, & Barker, 2010). Fetal undernutrition, it has been proposed, may produce permanent structural and functional changes that can increase one's risk for a variety of adult chronic diseases, including chronic kidney disease, hypertension, and diabetes. For example, in the presence of inadequate nutrition, the fetus may give priority to the brain and other vital organs over the kidneys (Eriksson et al., 2010), which in turn may reduce the number of nephrons, the basic functional units of the kidney. This reduction places greater stress on kidney function and ultimately damages the kidney (glomular sclerosis) and compromises its ability to regulate blood pressure (Barker, 1998). Hypertension, in turn, can further damage the kidney, potentially leading to a self-perpetuating process (Barker, 1998). Consistent with the life course *principle of timing*, the fetal origins hypothesis also suggests that fetal undernutrition in mid- to late gestation is most consequential for adult disease risk as this is the period when key developmental processes occur, such as those affecting the nephron count (Barker, 2006; Bateson et al., 2004) and glucose intolerance (Ravelli et al., 1998).

Support for these assertions comes from three strands of research: (1) experimental studies on rodents and other animals, (2) so-called "natural" experiments in humans (i.e., famines), and most commonly (3) large observational studies in human cohorts. First, evidence for fetal programming has been found in numerous animal studies, which have modeled the impact of a variety of maternal pregnancy exposures and conditions (e.g., caloric, protein, and micronutrient restriction; gestational diabetes) on offspring health. (For a review, see Fernandez-Twinn & Ozanne, 2010). Second, consistent with the life course *principle of historical time and place*, researchers have studied the adult disease outcomes of human birth cohorts exposed to famine—a natural experiment that allows us to study the long-term health impact of fetal undernutrition at different stages of pregnancy. For example, investigators have linked *in utero* exposure to the Dutch famine to a range of adult outcomes including obesity, schizophrenia, and a variety of metabolic and cardiovascular outcomes (Lumey et al., 2007; Stein et al., 2006).

The third and primary sources of evidence in fetal origins research have been large case-control and cohort studies on human populations. Since Wadsworth, Cripps, Midwinter, and Colley (1985) first reported a significant inverse association between birth weight and adult systolic blood pressure in the 1946 British birth cohort, well over 100 observational studies have been published on the association between birth weight and various adult health outcomes. One of the most consistent findings is a modest inverse association between birth weight and adult systolic blood pressure that generally ranges from −1.0 to −4.0 Hg/kg (Gamborg et al., 2007; Huxley, Shiell, & Law, 2000; Richardson et al., 2011). Recent meta-analyses also have reported an inverse relationship between birth weight and type 2 diabetes risk for birth weights less than approximately 4000 grams (Harder, Rodekamp, Schellong, Dudenhausen, & Plagemann, 2007; Whincup et al., 2008).

Although evidence to support the fetal origins hypothesis has been accumulating for more than 25 years, many important questions remain. How to measure fetal exposures continues to be a major challenge. Moreover, much remains to be learned about the mechanisms linking these exposures to future health. Therefore, based on the principles of *life span development, human agency embedded in social context*, and *timing*, we must ask, "What role do intervening exposures play in the link between birth weight and adult disease?" "What are the critical intervening exposures and periods?" Newer models, referred to as the "*developmental* origins of adult disease" (Adair & Dahly, 2005), are premised on emerging evidence about the role of postnatal exposures, such as childhood BMI (Hertzman & Boyce, 2010). Some scholars also acknowledge the need for research on intervening social and contextual factors (Avison, 2010). Genetic and epigenetic processes are also garnering increased attention.

IMPLICATIONS OF A LIFE COURSE PERSPECTIVE ON MCH POLICY AND PRACTICE

Traditional policy and practice responses to MCH (and other health) problems have rarely attempted to address them at multiple time points over the life course and simultaneously consider the social context in which they are embedded. The emphasis on prenatal care and neonatal care technologies to improve perinatal health outcomes in the United States, as well as the almost exclusive focus of U.S. health policy on health care, are just two examples of this neglect (Blane, 1999; Johnson, 2010b; Lu, 2010). Yet, adopting a life course perspective on MCH *research* will offer incomplete prospects for change if we do not also consider corresponding changes to *policy* and *practice*. In the sections that follow, we discuss these changes, and the challenges or barriers to implementing them. It should be noted that this discussion is biased heavily toward the U.S. policy and practice context, with which we are most familiar.

Implications for Timing of Policy Strategies to Improve MCH Outcomes

As we have discussed, the life course perspective on MCH and research stemming from it suggest that some of the key determinants of perinatal health outcomes precede conception (and perhaps even the entire childbearing period) and that the origins of many adult health problems can be traced to childhood. For many women, interventions initiated during pregnancy may provide "too little" and come "too late" to offset a lifetime of reproductive health-damaging exposures (Haas et al., 2005; Lu & Halfon, 2003; Moos, 2010). Thus, the first and most important change demanded by a life course perspective on MCH is to expand strategies for improving perinatal health beyond an exclusive focus on pregnancy

outcomes to a focus on the overall health of women, regardless of their childbearing history or plans (Halfon, DuPlessis, & Barrett, 2008; Hughes & Simpson, 1995; Misra, Grason, & Weisman, 2000). Focusing on early life health and development regardless of gender also seems warranted because, as life course research has shown, it holds the potential to improve population health during and beyond the transition into adulthood (Forrest & Riley, 2004; Lu, 2010), with a lighter burden on healthcare services than focusing on older-aged individuals (Blane, 1999).

Implications for Types/Targets of Policy Strategies to Improve MCH Outcomes

Not only does a life course perspective beg us to increase the time frame of interventions and policies that are introduced or developed to address MCH problems, but it also requires us to expand their range. By calling our attention to the embedding of human agency within social and larger contexts, life course theory suggests that we should intervene at multiple time points, and in multiple domains, to interrupt both downstream and upstream phenomena that contribute to MCH problems. This approach, however, requires that we expand our definition of health policy to include social policy (Blane, 1999; Woolf, 2009) because the health sector has little or no control over many of the upstream determinants of MCH (and other health) problems (Forrest & Riley, 2004). Social policies could influence population-wide exposures, such as adverse environmental conditions or income inequalities, thereby altering the multiple contexts in which individuals are embedded early enough to prevent the preconception or childhood precursors of adult health and disease (Forrest & Riley, 2004; Graham, 2004; Graham & Power 2004; Johnson, 2010b).

Challenges and Barriers to Policy and Practice Changes Derived from a Life Course Perspective

Several factors have the potential to complicate efforts to pursue the health and social policy changes we described previously. First, those changes make clear that policies stemming from a life course perspective on MCH will require collaboration between multiple entities involved in forming health and social policy. However, federal agencies that are playing a role (or can play a role) in MCH-relevant health and social policies are siloed and do not have a history of collaboration (Forrest & Riley, 2004). Future collaboration could be undermined by the lack of clarity about which agencies and policy makers would receive credit for MCH improvements resulting from policies that have not been viewed historically as health policies (Braveman & Barclay, 2009).

Second, if we begin to view social policy as health policy and shift our focus to childhood (or the preconception period more broadly) to improve perinatal health, we must change our expectations about the time frame needed to reap and evaluate the policy benefits (Braveman & Barclay, 2009; Forrest & Riley, 2004; Kawachi, Adler, & Dow, 2010). To date, the health impacts of social policies have not been evaluated or included in cost-benefit analyses (Dow, Schoeni, Adler, & Stewart, 2010; Forrest & Riley, 2004) likely because longer time frames for doing so, and probably a different set of monitoring and evaluation data, are needed.

Yet with the recent passage of the Patient Protection and Affordable Care Act of 2010, U.S. health policy continues to demonstrate a primary focus on health care. Thus, the inconsistencies between the proposed policy and practice changes and this act are obvious. First, although the Patient Protection and Affordable Care Act includes several provisions that have implications for MCH (Exhibit 4–A), it does not reflect the longitudinal, multilevel, and multifaceted nature of life course theory. Its sole focus on health care as a strategy for improving health distracts us from focusing on the preconception and childhood periods when the need for health care is presumably lower (Forrest & Riley, 2004). As a result, it also diverts our

---

- Ensures direct access to OB-GYNs without referral or preauthorization

- Creates a national home visiting program for high-risk families during pregnancy and the infant-toddler years

- Provides a new family planning coverage option in Medicaid

- Stipulates Medicaid coverage of tobacco cessation services for pregnant women

- Requires qualified health plans to provide minimum coverage for preventive care for infants, children, and adolescents, recommended immunizations, and additional preventive care and screening for women

- Maintains current Medicaid and Children's Health Insurance Plan (CHIP) eligibility for children until 2019

- Forbids preexisting condition exclusions for children

- Allows children to remain on their parent's individual/group health plans through age 26

- Prohibits sex-based discrimination

Exhibit 4–A Some MCH-Related Provisions of the 2010 Patient Protection and Affordable Care Act
Sources: Adapted from Johnson, 2010; Kaiser Family Foundation, 2010.

attention away from considering prevention policies, including social policies, that hold the potential for producing long-term population health improvements and reducing racial/ethnic disparities in health that have their origins in childhood (Forrest & Riley, 2004; Johnson, 2010b).

Implications for Practice

In addition to the broad policy implications of a life course perspective on MCH, it also has implications for public health and clinical practice. Specifically, it necessitates comprehensive healthcare services for women and their families over the entire life span, plus intensive services focused on critical or sensitive periods of development (Fine & Kotelchuck, 2010). To improve perinatal health, for example, it has been suggested that a continuum of care is needed—one that is "longitudinal (over time), vertical (within the health sector), and horizontal (across health and other sectors)" (Fine & Kotelchuck, 2010, p. 14). Toward this end, Halfon, Inkelas, and Hochstein (2000) have suggested creating life course health development organizations in the United States that would promote health by supplementing vertically integrated health management organizations with horizontal social services and longitudinal intervention programs.

Integration with community-based programs also may be necessary to reach women without access to the healthcare system who are often at highest risk (Misra & Grason, 2006). For example, individual communities throughout the United States have successfully developed MCH-specific life course organizations, including the Northern Manhattan Perinatal Partnership and the Contra Costa County Life Course Initiative, to meet the needs of women and children in their catchment areas. (See For Further Information for web addresses.) In developing countries, greater continuity of care could be achieved by integrating women's health and family planning services into programs to reduce infant and child mortality, and by further incorporating MCH programs into existing funding mechanisms for HIV/AIDS and infectious diseases (Horton, 2010).

In addition to continuity of care, a life course perspective on MCH implies that intensive services should be focused on specific points or periods in the life span, i.e., physiologically sensitive periods (such as childhood) or around socially defined transitions (such as the onset of the childbearing period), with emphasis on concurrence between the two (Halfon & Hochstein, 2002). Due to higher levels of developmental plasticity in young children and the effects of early life programming on adult outcomes, interventions at this time may be more cost-effective for improving health status in later life (Halfon et al., 2008). Programs implemented in children under age 5 have been shown to improve short- and long-term health outcomes (Guyer et al., 2009). Likewise, the increased emphasis on the preconception and interconception periods is expected to improve the timing of interventions surrounding this life stage (Atrash et al., 2008).

CONCLUSION

We have provided an introductory overview of the life course perspective and its applications to some of the most active areas of investigation in the MCH field. By tracing it to its roots in the social and behavioral sciences and linking it to historical and contemporary MCH scholarship, we demonstrated how the life course perspective offers a framework for understanding the factors and processes that contribute to our health and well-being over time and the immediate and larger historical, social, and temporal contexts in which health trajectories unfold. In doing so, we revealed the advantages of a life course approach over prevailing approaches to understanding and addressing MCH problems that focus primarily on contemporaneous and individual-level risk factors. We also showed how this approach can expand the range of questions asked and thereby produce information that has the potential to strengthen the evidence base for the life course-oriented policy and practice changes that have already begun to be proposed.

On both the global and domestic fronts, the challenges confronting the field of MCH are formidable, and new approaches to combat them are urgently needed. By expanding our focus and inspiring new questions, the life course perspective could be a much-needed catalyst for new strategies and solutions to the most intractable problems in MCH. Although elements of this perspective have been present in the field for at least 150 years, never before has it attracted as much attention and excitement as it has in the past decade. Consequently, opportunities for applying the life course perspective to MCH research, policy, and practice are burgeoning.

With these unprecedented opportunities come new responsibilities for all of us in the field of MCH. First, as we continue to refine the life course approach to MCH issues, it is critical that our work is informed by the best available theory, measurement, and evidence. Familiarity with life course theory and life course epidemiology is essential. Second, we must invest in cohort studies, which provide the best form of data for evaluating life course hypotheses. In the United States, ongoing cohort studies such as the National Longitudinal Study of Adolescent Health (Harris et al., 2009) provide unique opportunities to study life course influences on MCH outcomes (e.g., Richardson, 2009; Richardson et al., 2011). Third, as new life course-oriented MCH policies and practices are developed and implemented, we should insist that they are evidence-based and include monitoring and evaluation components. Although it is true that it may require years or even decades to detect the full impact of many life course initiatives, incorporating intermediate markers of progress should be possible. Fourth, until a more solid evidence base exists, we must exercise caution in pursuing the policy and practice changes implied by the life course paradigm. Although life course MCH evidence has been building for at least 75 years, our empirical foundation is still relatively thin and many key questions remain. Nevertheless, whether one views the life course perspective on MCH as a new paradigm or simply the revival of old ideas, most would agree that it has tremendous potential to impact MCH research, policy, and practice. By ensuring that life course policies and practices are based on the highest quality evidence and subjecting them to rigorous monitoring and evaluation, we can maximize the likelihood that this impact will be positive.

For Further Information

Online MCH Life Course Toolbox:
http://www.citymatch.org/lifecoursetoolbox/

MCHB Life Course Approach Resource Guide:
http://mchb.hrsa.gov/lifecourseapproach.html

MCH Life Course Research Network:
http://healthychild.ucla.edu/LCRN.asp

Northern Manhattan Perinatal Partnership:
http://www.sisterlink.com/

Contra Costa County Life Course Initiative:
http://cchealth.org/groups/lifecourse/

ACKNOWLEDGMENTS

Preparation of this chapter was supported by Award Numbers R01HD057073, R01HD058535, and T32-HD052468 from the Eunice Kennedy Shriver National Institute of Child Health & Human Development (NICHD). The content is solely the responsibility of the authors and does not necessarily represent the official views of the NICHD or the National Institutes of Health. The authors gratefully acknowledge Dr. Glen H. Elder, Jr., for his thoughtful comments on an earlier draft.

References

Adair, L., & Dahly, D. (2005). Developmental determinants of blood pressure in adults. *Annual Review of Nutrition, 25*, 407–434.

Afifi, T. O., Enns, M. W., Cox, B. J., Asmundson, G. J. G., Stein, M. B., & Sareen, J. (2008). Population attributable fractions of psychiatric disorders and suicide ideation and attempts associated with adverse childhood experiences. *American Journal of Public Health, 98*(5), 946–952.

Anda, R. F., Felitti, V. J., Bremner, J. D., Walker, J. D., Whitfield, C., Perry, B. D., Dube, S. R., & Giles, W. H. (2006). The enduring effects of abuse and related adverse experiences in childhood — A convergence of evidence from neurobiology and epidemiology. *European Archives of Psychiatry and Clinical Neuroscience, 256*(3), 174–186.

Arendas, K., Qiu, Q., & Gruslin, A. (2008). Obesity in pregnancy: Pre-conceptional to postpartum consequences. *Journal of Obstetrics and Gynaecology Canada, 30*(6), 477–488.

Atrash, H., Jack, B. W., Johnson, K., Coonrod, D. V., Moos, M. K., Stubblefield, P. G., Cefalo, R., Damus, K., & Reddy, U. M. (2008). Where is the "W"oman in MCH? *American Journal of Obstetrics and Gynecology, 199*(6 Suppl 2), S259–S265.

Avison, W. R. (2010). Incorporating children's lives into a life course perspective on stress and mental health. *Journal of Health and Social Behavior, 51*(4), 361–375.

Baird, D. (1964). Epidemiology of prematurity. *Journal of Pediatrics, 65*(6), 909–924.

Barker, D. J. P. (1998). In utero programming of chronic disease. *Clinical Science, 95*(2), 115–128.

Barker, D. J. P. (2006). Birth weight and hypertension. *Hypertension, 48*(3), 357–358.

Bateson, P., Barker, D., Clutton-Brock, T., Deb, D., D'Udine, B., Foley, R. A., Gluckman, P., Godfrey, K., Kirkwood, T., Lahr, M. M., McNamara, J., Metcalfe, N. B., Monaghan, P., Spencer, H. G., & Sultan, S. E. (2004). Developmental plasticity and human health. *Nature, 430*(6998), 419–421.

Berkman, L. F. (2009). Social epidemiology: Social determinants of health in the United States: Are we losing ground? *Annual Review of Public Health, 30*, 27–41.

Bhutta, Z. A., Chopra, M., Axelson, H., Berman, P., Boerma, T., Bryce, J., Bustreo, F., Cavagnero, E., Cometto, G., Daelmans, B., de Francisco, A., Fogstad, H., Gupta, N., Laski, L., Lawn, J., Maligi, B., Mason, E., Pitt, C., Requejo, J., Starrs, A.,

Victora, C. G., & Wardlaw, T. (2010). Countdown to 2015 decade report (2000–10): Taking stock of maternal, newborn, and child survival. *Lancet, 375*(9730), 2032–2044.

Blane, D. (1999). The life course, the social gradient, and health. In M. Marmot & R. G. Wilkinson (Eds.), *Social determinants of health* (pp. 64–80). Oxford: Oxford University Press.

Braveman, P., & Barclay, C. (2009). Health disparities beginning in childhood: A life-course perspective. *Pediatrics, 124*(Suppl. 3), S163–S175.

Brown, D. W., Anda, R. F., Tiemeier, H., Felitti, V. J., Edwards, V. J., Croft, J. B., & Giles, W. H. (2009). Adverse childhood experiences and the risk of premature mortality. *American Journal of Preventive Medicine, 37*(5), 389–396.

Cavanagh, S. E., & Huston, A. C. (2008). The timing of family instability and children's social development. *Journal of Marriage and the Family, 70*(5), 1258–1270.

Colen, C. G., Geronimus, A. T., Bound, J., & James, S. A. (2006). Maternal upward socioeconomic mobility and Black-White disparities in infant birthweight. *American Journal of Public Health, 96*(11), 2032–2039.

Collins, J. W., David, R. J., Rankin, K. M., & Desireddi, J. R. (2009). Transgenerational effect of neighborhood poverty on low birth weight among African Americans in Cook County, Illinois. *American Journal of Epidemiology, 169*(6), 712–717.

Collins, J. W., Wambach, J., David, R. J., & Rankin, K. M. (2009). Women's lifelong exposure to neighborhood poverty and low birth weight: A population-based study. *Maternal and Child Health Journal, 13*(3), 326–333.

Dannefer, D. (1987). Aging as intracohort differentiation: Accentuation, the Matthew Effect, and the life course. *Sociological Forum, 2*(2), 211–236.

DiPrete, T. A., & Eirich, G. M. (2006). Cumulative advantage as a mechanism for inequality: A review of theoretical and empirical developments. *Annual Review of Sociology, 32*, 271–297.

Dong, M. X., Giles, W. H., Felitti, V. J., Dube, S. R., Williams, J. E., Chapman, D. P., & Anda, R. F. (2004). Insights into causal pathways for ischemic heart disease — Adverse Childhood Experiences Study. *Circulation, 110*(13), 1761–1766.

Dow, W. H., Schoeni, R. F., Adler, N. E., & Stewart, J. (2010). Evaluating the evidence base: Policies and interventions to address socioeconomic status gradients in health. *Annals of the New York Academy of Sciences, 1186*, 240–251.

Elder, G. H., Jr. (1975). Age differentiation and the life course. *Annual Review of Sociology, 1*, 165–190.

Elder, G. H., Jr. (1979). Historical change in life patterns and personality. In P. B. Baltes & O. G. Brim (Eds.), *Life-span development and behavior* (pp. 117–159). New York: Academic Press.

Elder, G. H., Jr. (1994). Time, human agency, and social change: Perspectives on the life course. *Social Psychology Quarterly, 57*(1), 4–15.

Elder, G. H., Jr. (2006). Life course perspective. In G. Ritzer (Ed.), *The Blackwell Encyclopedia of Sociology* (pp. 2634–2639). Malden, MA: Blackwell.

Elder, G. H., Jr., & Johnson, M. K. (2003). The life course and aging: Challenges, lessons, and new directions. In R. A. Settersten (Ed.), *Invitation to the life course: Toward new understandings of later life* (pp. 49–84). Amityville, NY: Baywood Publishing Company, Inc.

Elder, G. H., Jr., Johnson, M. K., & Crosnoe, R. (2004). The emergence and development of life course theory. In J. T. Mortimer, & M. J. Shanahan (Eds.), *Handbook of the life course* (pp. 3–19). New York: Springer.

Elder, G. H., Jr., & Shanahan, M. J. (2006). The life course and human development. In R. E. Lerner (Ed.), *Handbook of child psychology. Vol. I: Theoretical models of human development* (6th ed., pp. 665–715). Hoboken, NJ: Wiley.

Emanuel, I. (1986). Maternal health during childhood and reproductive performance. *Annals of the New York Academy of Sciences, 477*, 27–39.

Emanuel, I. (1993). Intergenerational factors in pregnancy outcome. Implications for teratology? In H. Kalter (Ed.), *Issues and reviews in teratology* (pp. 47–84). New York: Plenum Press.

Emanuel, I., Hale, C. B., & Berg, C. J. (1989). Poor birth outcomes of American Black women: An alternative explanation. *Journal of Public Health Policy, 10*(3), 299–308.

Emanuel, I., & Sever, L. E. (1973). Questions concerning the possible association of potatoes and neural-tube defects, and an alternative hypothesis relating to maternal growth and development. *Teratology, 8*(3), 325–332.

Eriksson, J. G., Kajantie, E., Osmond, C., Thornburg, K., & Barker, D. J. P. (2010). Boys live dangerously in the womb. *American Journal of Human Biology, 22*(3), 330–335.

Feldacker, C., Emch, M., & Ennett, S. (2010). The who and where of HIV in rural Malawi: Exploring the effects of person and place on individual HIV status. *Health & Place, 16*(5), 996–1006.

Felitti, V. J., Anda, R. F., Nordenberg, D., Williamson, D. F., Spitz, A. M., Edwards, V., Koss, M. P., & Marks, J. S. (1998). Relationship of childhood abuse and household dysfunction to many of the leading causes of death in adults—the Adverse Childhood Experiences (ACE) Study. *American Journal of Preventive Medicine, 14*(4), 245–258.

Fernandez-Twinn, D. S., & Ozanne, S. E. (2010). Early life nutrition and metabolic programming. *Annals of the New York Academy of Sciences, 1212*, 78–96.

Fine, A., & Kotelchuck, M. (2010). *Rethinking MCH: The life course model as an organizing framework.* Washington, DC: U.S. Department of Health and Human Services, Health Resources and Services Administration, Maternal and Child Health Bureau. Retrieved on April 4, 2011 from http://www.hrsa.gov/ourstories/mchb75th/images/rethinkingmch.pdf.

Forrest, C. B., & Riley, A. W. (2004). Childhood origins of adult health: A basis for life-course health policy—A plea for policy attention to the way child health problems affect a person's entire lifespan. *Health Affairs, 23*(5), 155–164.

Gamborg, M., Byberg, L., Rasmussen, F., Andersen, P. K., Baker, J. L., Bengtsson, C., Canoy, D., Droyvold, W., Eriksson, J. G., Forsen, T., Gunnarsdottir, I., Jarvelin, M. R., Koupil, I., Lapidus, L., Nilsen, T. I., Olsen, S. F., Schack-Nielsen, L., Thorsdottir, I., Tuomainen, T. P., & Sorensen, T. I. (2007). Birth weight and systolic blood pressure in adolescence and adulthood: Meta-regression analysis of sex- and age-specific results from 20 Nordic studies. *American Journal of Epidemiology, 166*(6), 634–645.

Gavin, A. R., Chae, D. H., Mustillo, S., & Kiefe, C. I. (2009). Prepregnancy depressive mood and preterm birth in Black and White women: Findings from the CARDIA study. *Journal of Women's Health, 18*(6), 803–811.

Gennaro, S. (2005). Overview of current state of research on pregnancy outcomes in minority populations. *American Journal of Obstetrics and Gynecology, 192*(5, Suppl. 1), S3–S10.

Geronimus, A. T. (1992). The weathering hypothesis and the health of African-American women and infants: Evidence and speculations. *Ethnicity and Disease, 2*(3), 207–221.

Gershoff, E. T., Aber, J. L., Raver, C. C., & Lennon, M. C. (2007). Income is not enough: Incorporating material hardship into models of income associations with parenting and child development. *Child Development, 78*(1), 70–95.

Goldenberg, R. L., Culhane, J. F., Iams, J. D., & Romero, R. (2008). Epidemiology and causes of preterm birth. *Lancet, 371*(9606), 75–84.

Graham, H. (2004). Social determinants and their unequal distribution: Clarifying policy understandings. *Milbank Quarterly, 82*(1), 101–124.

Graham, H., & Power, C. (2004). Childhood disadvantage and health inequalities: A framework for policy based on lifecourse research. *Child Care Health and Development, 30*(6), 671–678.

Graham, H. (2002). Building an inter-disciplinary science of health inequalities: The example of lifecourse research. *Social Science and Medicine, 55*(11), 2005–2016.

Guyer, B., Ma, S., Grason, H., Frick, K. D., Perry, D. F., Sharkey, A., & McIntosh, J. (2009). Early childhood health promotion and its life course health consequences. *Academic Pediatrics, 9*(3), 142–149.

Haas, J. S., Fuentes-Afflick, E., Stewart, A. L., Jackson, R. A., Dean, M. L., Brawarsky, P., & Escobar, G. J. (2005). Prepregnancy health status and the risk of preterm delivery. *Archives of Pediatrics & Adolescent Medicine, 159*(1), 58–63.

Halfon, N., DuPlessis, H., & Barrett, E. (2008). Looking back at pediatrics to move forward in obstetrics. *Current Opinion in Obstetrics & Gynecology, 20*(6), 566–573.

Halfon, N., & Hochstein, M. (2002). Life course health development: An integrated framework for developing health, policy, and research. *The Milbank Quarterly, 80*(3), 433–479.

Halfon, N., Inkelas, M., & Hochstein, M. (2000). The health development organization: An organizational approach to achieving child health development. *The Milbank Quarterly, 78*(3), 447–497.

Hamilton, B. E., Martin, J. A., & Ventura, S. J. (2010). Births: Preliminary data for 2008. *National Vital Statistics Reports, 58*(16), 1–17.

Harder, T., Rodekamp, E., Schellong, K., Dudenhausen, J. W., & Plagemann, A. (2007). Birth weight and subsequent risk of Type 2 diabetes: A meta-analysis. *American Journal of Epidemiology, 165*(8), 849–857.

Harris, K. M., Halpern, C. T., Whitsel, E. A., Hussey, J., Tabor, J., Entzel, P., & Udry, J. R. (2009). *The National Longitudinal Study of Adolescent Health: Research design.* Retrieved on April 4, 2011 from http://www.cpc.unc.edu/projects/addhealth/design.

Hertzman, C. (2004). The life-course contribution to ethnic disparities in health. In N. B. Anderson,

R. A. Bulatao & B. Cohen (Eds.), *Critical perspectives on racial and ethnic differences in health in late life* (pp. 145–170). Washington, DC: The National Academies Press.

Hertzman, C., & Boyce, T. (2010). How experience gets under the skin to create gradients in developmental health. *Annual Review of Public Health, 31*, 329–347.

Hofferth, S. L., Reid, L., & Mott, F. L. (2001). The effects of early childbearing on schooling over time. *Family Planning Perspectives, 33*(6), 259–267.

Hogan, M. C., Foreman, K. J., Naghavi, M., Ahn, S. Y., Wang, M., Makela, S. M., Lopez, A. D., Lozano, R., & Murray, C. J. (2010). Maternal mortality for 181 countries, 1980–2008: A systematic analysis of progress towards Millennium Development Goal 5. *Lancet, 375*(9726), 1609–1623.

Horton, R. (2010). Maternal mortality: Surprise, hope, and urgent action. *Lancet, 375*(9726), 1581–1582.

Hughes, D., & Simpson, L. (1995). The role of social change in preventing low birth weight. *Future of Children, 5*(1), 87–102.

Hussey, J. M., Chang, J. J., & Kotch, J. B. (2006). Child maltreatment in the United States: Prevalence, risk factors, and adolescent health consequences. *Pediatrics, 118*(3), 933–942.

Huxley, R. R., Shiell, A. W., & Law, C. M. (2000). The role of size at birth and postnatal catch-up growth in determining systolic blood pressure: A systematic review of the literature. *Journal of Hypertension, 18*(7), 815–831.

Johnson, K. A. (2010a). Women's health and health reform: Implications of the Patient Protection and Affordable Care Act. *Current Opinion in Obstetrics & Gynecology, 22*(6), 492–497.

Johnson, R. C. (2010b). The place of race in health disparities: How family background and neighborhood conditions in childhood impact later-life health. In H. B. Newburger, E. L. Birch, & S. M. Wachter (Eds.), *Neighborhood and life chances: How place matters in modern America* (pp. 18–36). Philadelphia: University of Pennsylvania Press. Retrieved November 8, 2010 from http://socrates.berkeley.edu/~ruckerj/Johnson_UPENNBKChapter_neighborhoods.pdf.

Kaiser Family Foundation (2010). *Summary of new health reform law.* Retrieved on January 8, 2011 from http://www.kff.org/healthreform/8061.cfm.

Kawachi, I., Adler, N. E., & Dow, W. H. (2010). Money, schooling, and health: Mechanisms and causal evidence. *Annals of the New York Academy of Sciences, 1186*, 56–68.

Kermack, W. O., McKendrick, A. G., & McKinlay, P. L. (1934). Death-rates in Great Britain and Sweden: Some general regularities and their significance. *Lancet, 223*(5770), 698–703.

Kreager, D. A. (2007). Unnecessary roughness? School sports, peer networks, and male adolescent violence. *American Sociological Review, 72*(5), 705–724.

Kuh, D., Ben-Shlomo, Y., Lynch, J., Hallqvist, J., & Power, C. (2003). Life course epidemiology. *Journal of Epidemiology and Community Health, 57*(10), 778–783.

Kuh, D., & Ben-Schlomo, Y. (2004). Introduction. In D. Kuh, & Y. Ben-Schlomo (Eds.), *A life course approach to chronic disease epidemiology* (pp. 3–14). Oxford: Oxford University Press.

Langhoff-Roos, J., Kesmodel, U., Jacobsson, B., Rasmussen, S., & Vogel, I. (2006). Spontaneous preterm delivery in primiparous women at low risk in Denmark: Population based study. *British Medical Journal, 332*(7547), 937–939.

Love, C., David, R. J., Rankin, K. M., & Collins, J. W. (2010). Exploring weathering: Effects of lifelong economic environment and maternal age on low birth weight, small for gestational age, and preterm birth in African-American and White women. *American Journal of Epidemiology, 172*(2), 127–134.

Lu, M. C., & Halfon, N. (2003). Racial and ethnic disparities in birth outcomes: A life-course perspective. *Maternal and Child Health Journal, 7*(1), 13–30.

Lu, M. C. (2010). We can do better: Improving perinatal health in America. *Journal of Women's Health, 19*(3), 569–574.

Lumey, L. H., Stein, A. D., Kahn, H. S., van der Pal-de Bruin, K. M., Blauw, G. J., Zybert, P. A., & Susser, E. S. (2007). Cohort profile: The Dutch Hunger Winter Families Study. *International Journal of Epidemiology, 36*(6), 1196–1204.

Martin, J. A., Osterman, M. J. K., & Sutton, P. D. (2010). Are preterm births on the decline in the United States? Recent data from the national vital statistics system. *NCHS Data Brief, 39.*

Meckel, R. A. (1990). *Save the babies: American public health reform and the prevention of infant mortality, 1850–1929.* Baltimore: The Johns Hopkins University Press.

Merton, R. K. (1968). The Matthew Effect in science: The reward and communication systems of science are considered. *Science, 159*(3810), 56–63.

Merton, R. K. (1988). The Matthew Effect in science, II: Cumulative advantage and the symbolism of intellectual property. *Isis, 79*(4), 606–623.

Misra, D. P., & Grason, H. (2006). Achieving safe motherhood: Applying a life course and multiple determinants perinatal health framework in public health. *Women's Health Issues, 16*(4), 159–175.

Misra, D. P., Grason, H., & Weisman, C. (2000). An intersection of women's and perinatal health: The role of chronic conditions. *Women's Health Issues, 10*(5), 256–267.

Moos, M. K. (2010). From concept to practice: Reflections on the preconception health agenda. *Journal of Women's Health, 19*(3), 561–567.

Morken, N., Vogel, I., Kallen, K., Skjaerven, R., Langhoff-Roos, J., Kesmodel, U. S., & Jacobsson, B. (2008). Reference population for international comparisons and time trend surveillance of preterm delivery proportions in three countries. *BMC Women's Health, 8,* 16.

Morris, M., Kurth, A. E., Hamilton, D. T., Moody, J., & Wakefield, S. (2009). Concurrent partnerships and HIV prevalence disparities by race: Linking science and public health practice. *American Journal of Public Health, 99*(6), 1023–1031.

Nguyen, V., & Peschard, K. (2003). Anthropology, inequality, and disease: A review. *Annual Review of Anthropology, 32,* 447–474.

Organisation for Co-operation and Economic Development [OECD]. (2009). *Health at a glance 2009 - OECD indicators.* Paris, France: OECD Publishing. Retrieved June 26, 2010 from http://www.oecd-ilibrary.org/content/book/health_glance-2009-en.

O'Rand, A. M. (1996). The precious and the precocious: Understanding cumulative disadvantage and cumulative advantage over the life course. *The Gerontologist, 36*(2), 230–238.

Phillips, G. S., Wise, L. A., Rich-Edwards, J. W., Stampfer, M. J., & Rosenberg, L. (2010). Prepregnancy depressive symptoms and preterm birth in the Black Women's Health Study. *Annals of Epidemiology, 20*(1), 8–15.

Pies, C., Parthasarathy, P., Kotelchuck, M., & Lu, M. (2009). *Making a paradigm shift in maternal and child health: A report on the national MCH life course meeting.* Martinez, CA: Contra Costa Health Services. Retrieved on March 10, 2011 from http://cchealth.org/groups/lifecourse/pdf/2009_10_meeting_report_final.pdf.

Pollitt, R. A., Rose, K. M., & Kaufman, J. S. (2005). Evaluating the evidence for models of life course socioeconomic factors and cardiovascular outcomes: A systematic review. *BMC Public Health, 5,* 7.

Rajaratnam, J. K., Marcus, J. R., Flaxman, A. D., Wang, H., Levin-Rector, A., Dwyer, L., Costa, M., Lopez, A. D., & Murray, C. J. (2010). Neonatal, postneonatal, childhood, and under-5 mortality for 187 countries, 1970–2010: A systematic analysis of progress towards Millennium Development Goal 4. *Lancet, 375*(9730), 1988–2008.

Raphael, D. (2007). Public policies and the problematic USA population health profile. *Health Policy, 84*(1), 104–111.

Ravelli, A. C. J., van der Meulen, J. H. P., Michels, R. P. J., Osmond, C., Barker, D. J. P., Hales, C. N., & Bleker, O. P. (1998). Glucose tolerance in adults after prenatal exposure to famine. *Lancet, 351*(9097), 173–177.

Repetti, R. L., Taylor, S. E., & Seeman, T. E. (2002). Risky families: Family social environments and the mental and physical health of offspring. *Psychological Bulletin, 128*(2), 330–366.

Richardson, L. J. (2009). *The social structural context of pregnancy and adverse birth outcomes: The role of race, place, and time.* Doctoral dissertation, The University of North Carolina at Chapel Hill.

Richardson, L. J., Hussey, J. M., & Strutz, K. L. (2011). Origins of disparities in cardiovascular disease: Birth weight, body mass index, and young adult systolic blood pressure in the National Longitudinal Study of Adolescent Health. *Annals of Epidemiology, 21,* 598–607.

Sastry, N., & Hussey, J. M. (2003). An investigation of racial and ethnic disparities in birth weight in Chicago neighborhoods. *Demography, 40*(4), 701–725.

Schempf, A., Strobino, D., & O'Campo, P. (2009). Neighborhood effects on birthweight: An exploration of psychosocial and behavioral pathways in Baltimore, 1995–1996. *Social Science and Medicine, 68*(1), 100–110.

Shiono, P. H., Rauh, V. A., Park, M., Lederman, S. A., & Zuskar, D. (1997). Ethnic differences in birthweight: The role of lifestyle and other factors. *American Journal of Public Health, 87*(5), 787–793.

Stein, A. D., Zybert, P. A., Van der Pal-de Bruin, K., & Lumey, L. H. (2006). Exposure to famine during gestation, size at birth, and blood pressure at age 59 y: Evidence from the Dutch famine. *European Journal of Epidemiology, 21*(10), 759–765.

Swaroop, S., & Morenoff, J. D. (2006). Building community: The neighborhood context of social organization. *Social Forces, 84*(3), 1665–1695.

Torloni, M. R., Betran, A. P., Daher, S., Widmer, M., Dolan, S. M., Menon, R., Bergel, E., Allen, T., & Merialdi, M. (2009). Maternal BMI and preterm birth: A systematic review of the literature with meta-analysis. *Journal of Maternal-Fetal & Neonatal Medicine, 22*(11), 957–970.

U.S. Department of Health and Human Services [USDHHS]. (2000). *Healthy People 2010: Understanding and improving health and objectives for improving health. 2nd ed.* Washington, DC: U.S. Government Printing Office. Retrieved on April 1, 2011 from http://www.health.gov/healthypeople/2010/Publications/.

Van Dyck, P. C. *Moving from theory to practice: Life course, social determinants and health equity framework in maternal and child health.* Retrieved on April 4, 2011 from http://webcast.hrsa.gov/conferences/mchb/TitleV75/rams_transcripts/TheoryToPractice.pdf .

Wadsworth, M. E. J., Cripps, H. A., Midwinter, R. E., & Colley, J. R. T. (1985). Blood pressure in a national birth cohort at the age of 36 related to social and familial factors, smoking, and body mass. *British Medical Journal, 291*(6508), 1534–1538.

Wald, N. (1993). Folic acid and the prevention of neural tube defects. *Annals of the New York Academy of Sciences, 678,* 112–129.

Weisman, C. S., Misra, D. P., Hillemeier, M. M., Downs, D. S., Chuang, C. H., Camacho, F. T., & Dyer, A. M. (2011). Preconception predictors of birth outcomes: Prospective findings from the Central Pennsylvania Women's Health Study. *Maternal and Child Health Journal, 15,* 829–835.

Whincup, P. H., Kaye, S. J., Owen, C. G., Huxley, R., Cook, D. G., Anazawa, S., Barrett-Connor, E., Bhargava, S. K., Birgisdottir, B. E., Carlsson, S., de Rooij S. R., Dyck, R. F., Eriksson, J. G., Falkner, B., Fall, C., Forsen, T., Grill V., Gudnason, V., Hulman, S., Hypponen, E., Jeffreys, M., Lawlor, D. A., Leon, D. A., Minami, J., Mishra, G., Osmond, C., Power, C., Rich-Edwards, J. W., Roseboom, T. J., Sachdev, H. S., Syddall, H., Thorsdottir, I., Vanhala, M., Wadsworth, M., & Yarbrough, D. E. (2008). Birth weight and risk of Type 2 diabetes: A systematic review. *Journal of the American Medical Association, 300*(24), 2886–2897.

Willson, A. E., Shuey, K. M., & Elder, G. H., Jr. (2007). Cumulative advantage processes as mechanisms of inequality in life course health. *American Journal of Sociology, 112,* 1886–1924.

Wolfe, J. D. (2009). Age at first birth and alcohol use. *Journal of Health and Social Behavior, 50*(4), 395–409.

Woolf, S. H. (2009). Social policy as health policy. *Journal of the American Medical Association, 301*(11), 1166–1169.

World Health Organization [WHO]. (2009). *Women and health: Today's evidence, tomorrow's agenda.* Geneva: WHO Press.

DETERMINANTS OF HEALTH AND HEALTH SERVICES: THE DEVELOPMENTAL CYCLE

5

FAMILY PLANNING

Amy Tsui, Linda Piccinino, and C. Arden Miller

A sustainable U.S. is one where all Americans have access to family planning and reproductive health services...

(President's Council for Sustainable Development, 1996)

INTRODUCTION

This chapter begins with a discussion of family planning, organized programs to enable individual management of fertility. Family planning represents a key component of reproductive health services in the United States and elsewhere. Emphasis here features needs and programs in the United States.

Although contraceptive use has increased in the United States, so too has the percentage of births that are mistimed or unwanted. At the same time, in real dollars, public spending on contraceptive services through Title X of the Public Health Service Act declined by 58% between 1980 and 2000, whereas Medicaid has risen in prominence as the primary federal financing mechanism (Gold, Sonfield, Richards, & Frost, 2009; Poole & Hawkins, 1999). In real terms Title X funding began at $6 million in 1970 and grew to $160 million in 1980 and to $317 million in the fiscal year 2010 budget.

This chapter presents some of the history of family planning and reviews the status of family planning services in the United States in terms of their availability and barriers to their access. It also describes current and past levels and trends of contraceptive practice, the characteristics of users, the methods adopted, and sources of services. The likely future of family planning in the United States is discussed in terms of critical policy issues that prevent the population from achieving the status of an appropriately contracepting society. The chapter concludes with a call to reinforce commitment to the public financing of family planning services in the United States, even as the trend toward privatization of services continues and politicization over the services covered persists.

Clarification of terms is appropriate in this chapter. *Unintended* or *unplanned pregnancies* include those that are unwanted and those that are mistimed. *Unwanted pregnancies* and *unwanted childbearing* occur among women who report that they never intended to give birth or to continue childbearing. *Mistimed pregnancies* occur among women who report that at some time in the future they intended to bear one or more children but not at the time this pregnancy occurred. Data on these issues are based on surveys that in part require recall of intent, a procedure with a degree of uncertainty among some women and their partners (Tsui, McDonald-Mosley, & Burke, 2010).

As of 2005, the latest year for which national data are available, almost one half of women 15–44 years of age in the United States have experienced at least one unplanned pregnancy (Gold et al., 2009). Approximately one half of all pregnancies (3.1 million) in the United States are unintended. Half of these unintended pregnancies end in abortion. Approximately 35% of all live births are the result of unintended pregnancies. The proportion is higher among women in poverty, those unmarried, and those 18 to 24 years old. The consequences of these circumstances are dire for many women and children and underscore a pressing need for more effective programs of family planning (Gold et al., 2009; Kost & Forrest, 1995).

BACKGROUND

Efforts to control fertility date from earliest recorded history. Egyptian papyri recommend the insertion of a vaginal suppository containing crocodile's dung and honey mixed with sodium carbonate or the insertion of acacia tips. Soranos, a Greek physician writing in the second century, advised that for the prevention of conception, coitus should be avoided during critical times in the menstrual cycle. Other suggested methods included anointing the cervix with astringent materials or closing the *os uteri* with cotton (Major, 1954). The contraceptive effect of *coitus interruptus* has been known since antiquity. By an account in Genesis, Onan, required by tribal custom to sleep with his deceased brother's widow but not wishing

to establish a collateral family line, chose to spill his seed on the ground. Through history, various penile sheaths, often from strips of linen or animal membranes, have been tried as contraceptives.

The prevailing motivations for promoting access to contraception have changed from time to time. Concern for the well-being of unwanted children is one of them. Boswell (1988) estimated that from antiquity through the Renaissance, approximately one quarter of liveborn children were abandoned. Some of these children survived but many did not. Medieval chronicles report a harvest of infant corpses yielded by rivers such as the Nile and the Arno. Child abandonment was not a socially reprehensible method for coping with unwanted fertility. Rousseau, the noted 18th century French philosopher, wrote without apparent shame or regret that he abandoned all five of his children. It was a practice that not many theologians condemned, except for risk of committing the grave sin of incest by inadvertently having sexual relations with a previously abandoned daughter or son (Boswell, 1988).

Circumstances in the United States through the early decades of this century can be interpreted as evidence of socially sanctioned infanticide. Nearly every large city accommodated a foundling hospital, often with convenient provision for depositing unwanted infants. The mortality rates in those hospitals approached 90% (English, 1984). During the same period, upper-class French women boarded their unplanned infants with peasant families, a practice with a comparably high mortality rate (Klaus, 1993).

SUPPORTIVE RATIONALE

Some less stark considerations relate to unplanned childbearing. Infants and children have better survival rates, and survivors are healthier if they are born to mothers who are not at the extremes of the childbearing age span, if there is spacing of at least 2 years between births, and if family size is limited.

Unwanted childbearing poses health burdens beyond those that can be attributed to social and economic characteristics of the mother. For an unwanted pregnancy, the mother is less likely to seek prenatal care and is more likely to expose the fetus to harmful substances such as tobacco and alcohol. The child of an unwanted conception is more likely to be of low birth weight, to die in the first year of life, and to be abused. Kost, Landry, and Darroch (1998) studied more than 11,000 births from two 1988 national surveys in which the planned status of pregnancies was known and found a higher probability of negative outcomes, such as low birth weight or prematurity, early well-baby care and breastfeeding, for unintended than planned pregnancies. The risks and outcomes for a mistimed conception are of a similar nature but of lesser magnitude (Institute of Medicine, 1995). A systematic review by Shah and colleagues (Shah et al., 2011) finds increased odds of low birth weight and preterm birth associated with unintended, unwanted and mistimed pregnancies that end in a live birth. Concern about the effects of unwanted, mistimed, or excessive childbearing on the health of women has been conspicuous in the policy dynamics of family planning programs in this century. Childbearing and parenthood are low risk and rewarding experiences for people who want them. The risks and rewards become adverse for women at the extreme of childbearing years, women experiencing short interpregnancy intervals, women with health problems such as diabetes or hypertension, women with multiple pregnancies, and those women whose pregnancies are unwanted or mistimed. The adversities are biological, psychological (depression), economic, and social. Educational and career prospects for women are curtailed by unplanned childbearing. Women whose pregnancies are unwanted or mistimed are four times as likely as women with a planned pregnancy to be physically abused by their husband or partner (Gazmararian et al., 1995).

Maternal deaths from major complications of pregnancy (uncontrolled bleeding, blood clots to the lungs, and toxemia with high blood pressure and convulsions) are concentrated among fourth and higher order births and among very young women and those in the upper ranges of the childbearing years. These hazards are minimized among women given access to family planning.

When women have access to contraceptive services, they have reduced likelihood of resorting to dangerous illegal abortions for control of fertility. Under safe conditions, induced abortion is a low-risk procedure— with even fewer complications than childbearing. When access to abortion is limited, many women resort to unsafe procedures in order to avert pregnancy. Accurate data on illegal procedures are not readily available, but some estimates place the total number of illegal abortions the world over to be in the range of 22 million each year (Shah & Ahman, 2010). Associated deaths are estimated to number over 47,000, 13 % of the 358,000 maternal deaths that occur annually worldwide (World Health Organization, 2010).

During the early years of this century, Margaret Sanger worked as a public health nurse in the poorest sectors of New York City where she confronted appalling evidence of the plight of women caught in lives of excessive and unwanted fertility. She began promoting family planning, a cause that attracted many followers. Her work led to the formation of The Family Planning Federation, an organization that sponsored family planning clinics in nearly every community in the United States and in many other countries. It continues under the name of Planned Parenthood Federation of America as one of this country's largest organized providers of family planning services.

The eugenics theme has played a part in the promotion of family planning. In the early decades of this century, the view developed that society would be improved if only the "right" people were encouraged to propagate. This view today is greatly diminished but is not entirely absent. Voices from developing countries and from minority populations in the United States sometimes charge that the promotion of family planning is a covert expression of genocidal intent.

Concern about overpopulation has been a strong motivating force for family planning, especially in densely populated countries such as China, India, Indonesia, and Bangladesh. Malthus, in 1798, was one of the earliest analysts to point out that the growth of a population could outstrip the resources to support it. This consideration figured prominently in the United States during the 1970s when public programs to enable access to family planning, both domestically and internationally, were greatly expanded. As rational as the population theme may be in support of family planning, it is not now a strong influence in this country, Europe, or other countries that have passed through the fertility transition. The size of the population of the United States now changes largely in response to fluctuating migration patterns.

Historically, some countries have been more concerned about too little population than too much. Nationalistic rivalries in Europe during the late 19th and early 20th centuries caused many countries to adopt pronatalist policies, which offered strong inducements for childbearing, even among unmarried women (Klaus, 1993). These inducements and supportive services formed the basis for protections that contribute to favorable pregnancy outcomes and that persist to this day.

Feminists currently provide the strongest advocacy for abortion rights. Their concern is fortified by data on the health and well-being of women, but the cause is largely argued on the basis of human rights, an argument that the political process has thus far upheld even in a climate of increasing contention. Proponents maintain that women are entitled to sexual fulfillment that is free from the risk of unintended pregnancy. Denial of pregnancy prevention services is interpreted by some

voices as a form of social control over women by a male-dominated society. Advocacy for abortion services, for family planning, and for family planning services for poor women remains an urgent policy priority for workers in maternal and child health (MCH).

SOCIAL AND POLITICAL CONTEXT

Public health workers are apt to find the supportive rationale for family planning so compelling that countervailing forces are underestimated. These forces are considerable. In 1873, Anthony Comstock, secretary of the New York Society for the Suppression of Vice, induced Congress to pass an act prohibiting the use of the mails for obscene matter. Any content dealing with sex education or family planning was declared pornographic and was prohibited under provisions of the act. Comstockery (George Bernard Shaw's term) found even more stringent expression in various state laws. Margaret Sanger was arrested a number of times for lecturing and distributing pamphlets on family planning. As recently as the 1940s, an obstetrician in Connecticut was jailed for prescribing contraceptives for a married woman.

The tenets of nearly every organized religion are construed by some as supportive of family planning. Conversely, nearly every organized religion produces other voices that raise opposition. For many decades, the Catholic Church has been the strongest force in opposition. The official position of the church is supportive of family planning except by "unnatural" means. These include all currently available methods of contraception that are most effective. The "natural" methods approved by the church include periodic abstinence and breastfeeding, which tends to delay ovulation in some women. These methods have some effectiveness on a population-wide basis, but they are all high risk for individual couples who seek protection from unwanted childbearing. It is not surprising, as a consequence, that

Catholic women in the United States have a rate of abortion 22% higher than Protestant women (Jones, Darroch, & Henshaw, 2002b). Women of all ages, socioeconomic circumstances, religions, and races may find it necessary to have an abortion when faced with an unwanted pregnancy.

Withdrawal from intercourse before ejaculation is another "natural" method of attempted contraception. The annual failure rate for withdrawal is 22%, which means that 22 of 100 women will experience a pregnancy while using this method. Practicing this method over 3 years produces a cumulative failure rate of 52%. More than one half of such contraceptors will have an unwanted pregnancy.

The social reforms of the 1960s (e.g., Medicare, Medicaid, Head Start, the War on Poverty) included a prevailing attitude that family planning and population policy were appropriate matters for government action (Rosoff, 1988). Presidents Kennedy (the nation's only Catholic president) and Johnson spoke frequently in support of government-sponsored family planning programs. Support was bipartisan. President Nixon declared, "No American woman should be denied access to family planning assistance because of her economic conditions. I believe, therefore, that we should establish as a national goal the provision of family planning services... to all who want but cannot afford them" (Rosoff, 1988, p. 313). Former presidents Truman and Eisenhower served as honorary co-chairmen of Planned Parenthood Federation of America. As part of the War on Poverty, the MCH provisions of the Social Security Act were required to allocate to family planning a minimum of 6% of available funds and to offer services to "all appropriate cases." Congressman George H.W. Bush (R-TX) lent his support to a national program of government support for family planning clinics. Before his 1980 presidential campaign, he also supported the Supreme Court's decision of 1973, which protected a woman's constitutional right to abortion. Abortion remains a procedure not generally regarded as an appropriate method of family planning in the United States (unlike some countries in Eastern Europe) except as an alternative to be considered when contraception fails.

In 1970, Congress enacted Title X of the Public Health Service Act with broad bipartisan support, originally introduced by Senators Joseph Tydings (D-MD) and Charles Percy (R-IL) and Representatives James Scheuer (D-NY) and George H.W. Bush. Title X provided funds and implementation authority for a nationwide program of family planning clinics for poor women. Under this act, teenage women were generally eligible for services regardless of their parents' resources. The program expanded rapidly throughout the 1970s.

The political climate began to change toward the end of the decade. Beginning in 1976, under the Hyde Amendment, a rider attached to annual appropriations bills, Congress prohibited the use of Medicaid funds to pay for abortions. Aspirants to elective office began to reassess their positions supportive of family planning. Controversy over abortion grew as a conspicuous political issue. These changes were driven by the growing influence of a conservative political coalition given finance and voice by a Christian fundamentalist movement. The movement garnered support from a growing radio and television audience for charismatic media evangelists.

The election of Ronald Reagan to the presidency in 1980 marked a watershed in government policy. He omitted family planning funds from all of his budgets and spoke energetically in opposition to abortion. The "right to life," formulated around the abortion issue, became confusedly linked with negative attitudes toward family planning. As vice president, George H.W. Bush changed his position on both abortion and family planning.

During each year in the next decade and a half, a Democratic-majority Congress succeeded in restoring funds to Title X, holding them only to the 1981 funding level. After considering inflation, however, real financial support for the program has declined 58% by 2009. This decrease has been partially offset by increases in Medicaid funding for family planning services. Nationally, Medicaid provides 30% of all funding reported by family planning centers and Title X 24% (Fowler, Gable, & Wang, 2008). The election of a Republican Congress in 1994, strongly beholden to ultraconservative influences, brought new threats to the existence of public supported programs for family planning. The Republican administration under President George W. Bush showed little enthusiasm for family planning and actively promoted the practice of abstinence before marriage at the expense of education about family planning. The current Democratic administration of President Barack Obama has sought to raise Title X funding, but in a highly constrained budget environment success is uncertain.

The issue is not easily resolved. A strongly articulated view holds that easy access to contraception, especially for teenagers, has promoted irresponsible behavior, increasing early and extramarital sexual activity and, paradoxically, an increase in extramarital teenage childbearing. It is true that during the 1970s and 1980s more teenagers were engaging in sexual intercourse at earlier ages than in previous years (Alan Guttmacher Institute, 1994). It is also true that many difficult-to-measure influences other than access to contraception were brought to bear during those years. Ubiquitous media programming and advertising, often with provocative sexual content, and sexual maturation at younger ages are among the possible factors contributing to intercourse at earlier ages. However, since 1985, contraceptive use at first premarital sex among teenage females (ages 15 to 19) has risen to 84% in 2005–2008 (Mosher & Jones, 2010). Sexually active teen contraceptors favor use of condoms and pills.

An opposing view holds that access to contraception is not the problem but is in fact the solution. It is certainly true that during the 1980s programs to promote "just say no" and the abstinence-only programs of 2000–2008, both generously financed during Republican administrations, did not reverse trends in sexual behavior. It is also true that teenage fertility in this country had been at a stable level for many decades, increasing only slightly during the late 1980s, decreasing in the mid-1990s, and continuing to decline through the 2000s. The problem appears larger than it really may be because older women have reduced their fertility so much more than younger women, resulting in an increased proportion of newborns with teenage mothers.

Few good studies are available to resolve this controversy to everyone's satisfaction. Many public health workers are attracted by the findings of a controlled study by Zabin, Hirsch, Smith, Streett, and Hardy (1986) on the influence of a school-linked program of counseling and clinical services that included contraception. The onset of the age of first intercourse by participants in the study population was delayed by 13 months. More such studies are needed. This one suggests that when young people have information and related clinical services, their behavior becomes more responsible than without them. Experience from other industrialized nations is relevant. Many of them provide school-based sex education beginning at young ages and access to contraception when teenagers choose to become sexually active. Under these circumstances, the average age of first intercourse is no younger than in the United States, but teenage pregnancy and abortion rates are much lower (Santelli, Sandfort, & Orr, 2008). The U.S. experience with teenage pregnancy prevention programs includes relatively few judged to be effective (for a review, see Frost & Forrest, 1995; Kirby, 2002).

METHODS OF FAMILY PLANNING

Readers who are not thoroughly familiar with the physiology of sexual maturation, menstruation, and childbearing are urged to take time to study these processes with a standard text of physiology. Understanding the successes, failures, indications, and possible complications of various contraceptives is not possible without knowledge, for example, of the hormonal orchestration of reproduction. Some of the most widely used contraceptives manipulate female hormonal balances.

Successful family planning programs make available a variety of methods. No one of them is entirely satisfactory for all women or for all circumstances. Most women make use of different methods at different stages of their reproductive history. Condoms or diaphragms may be useful for relationships that are intermittent. A daily or quarterly contraceptive pill may be convenient for stable, continuing partnerships, and surgical sterilization may be chosen when plans for family formation are completed. Surgical sterilization, more often female than male, is the most commonly used method of contraception in the United States. Latex and polyurethane condoms and diaphragms are also useful for protection against sexually transmitted diseases (STDs).

Some methods rely on preventing the union of the ovum and sperm in normally ovulating women. Such methods include periodic abstinence (often identified as the rhythm method because it attempts to confine coitus to phases of the menstrual cycle when the woman is presumed not to be ovulating) and withdrawal, or onanism, when the male discontinues vaginal penetration before ejaculation. More effective methods of preventing union between ovum and sperm provide barriers such as the male and female condom, diaphragm, or cervical cap (the last infrequently used).

One of the most widely used contraceptive methods prevents ovulation by replacing the woman's normal hormonal cycle with an imposed one by means of a daily sequence of oral hormonal pills. The method is highly effective, but it requires diligence to remember to take the pills according to the prescribed schedule. Lapses reduce effectiveness; guidance on how to correct for lapses has no firm scientific basis. This problem is averted by adaptations of the hormonal method, such as the provision of the replacement hormones in a long-acting injection, effective for several months, or in subcutaneous implants, which can be effective for up to 5 years. If during this period a couple desires to conceive, the implants can be removed and fertility restored. In the last decade, contraceptive hormonal patches have become available that also are nonpermanent methods, but somewhat like the pill, these patches require that the user changes the patch on a weekly basis.

Various chemical agents can deactivate the sperm and hence prevent conception. These agents are prepared as vaginal foams, creams, gel strips, or jellies to be inserted into the vagina before intercourse or more commonly to be used in conjunction with other methods, such as the diaphragm or the condom.

The mode of action of some methods is not precisely known. For example, some models of the intrauterine device (IUD) may not actually prevent fertilization but act by disrupting implantation of the conceptum in the uterine wall. This matter has relevance to some people who take a microscopic view of a "right to life," charging that the device is not a contraceptive but an abortifacient. This view is contradicted when chemical agents, such as copper, are incorporated into the IUD. This is a highly effective method that acts by chemical, as well as by mechanical, means. IUDs currently available in the United States are contraceptives, not abortifacients (Sivin, 1989).

A postcoital "morning-after" regimen for taking certain oral contraceptive pills can also avert pregnancy. This method is widely used in Europe and already widespread in many other countries, available both by prescription and over the counter or "behind the counter" (i.e., requiring counseling at the point of purchase by a trained health professional). The morning-after pill is similarly available in the United States and its use, although still low, is increasing, particularly among young sexually active females. The contraceptive pill has been publicized as a means of "emergency contraception" for women having unprotected intercourse in the past 72 hours (Ellertson, 1996). Four fifths of family planning clinics offer emergency contraceptive pills (ECPs) on site (Guttmacher Institute, 2010). Jones, Darroch, and Henshaw, (2002a) estimated that ECP use prevented as many as 51,000 abortions in 2000. In view of the nearly 8 million women reporting condoms as their contraceptive method, emergency contraception presents an important and reassuring option (Trussell & Raymond, 2011).

Surgical sterilization by ligating the fallopian tubes or by severing the vas deferens is a choice elected by many individuals who have no further desire for family formation. The method is rarely ineffective, but it has the disadvantage of being almost irreversible if circumstances change and a couple desires a pregnancy.

The current and future focus of contraceptive research and development has expanded to include male methods (e.g., male pill and vas deferens clips, in addition to condoms and vasectomy). Although the nature of the male reproductive biology is often thought to limit contraceptive development for men, recent research on cellular and molecular events show some promising directions (Harrison & Rosenfield, 1996). At the behavioral level, much will be learned about the prevalence and the use of selected male methods with findings released from recent cycles of the National Survey of Family Growth.

Nearly 90% of women at risk of unintended pregnancy use a contraceptive at least some of the time. The methods they choose are shown in Table 5–1. The most

Table 5–1 Contraceptive Prevalence in the U.S.: 1982–2008 Prevalence and 2006–2008 Total Users

| Method | Contraceptive prevalence among women 15–44 | | | | 2006–2008 | |
	1982	1995	2002	2006–2008	Number of Users (in Thousands)	Percentage of Users
Sterilization	19.0	24.8	22.4	22.8	14,139	37.0
Tubal	12.9	17.8	16.7	16.7	10,356	27.1
Vasectomy	6.1	7.0	5.7	6.1	3,783	9.9
Pill	15.6	17.3	18.9	17.3	10,700	28.0
Implant	NA	0.8	0.8	0.7	420	1.1
Injectable	NA	1.9	3.3	2.0	1,223	3.2
Contraceptive ring	NA	NA	NA	1.5	917	2.4
IUD	4.0	0.5	1.3	3.4	2,120	5.5
Diaphragm	4.5	1.2	0.2	—	—	—
Condom	6.7	13.1	11.1	10.0	6,152	16.1
Periodic abstinence	2.2	1.5	0.9	0.6	420	1.1
Withdrawal	1.1	1.9	2.5	3.2	1,987	5.2
Other methods	2.7	1.1	0.6	0.2	153	0.4
Total	55.7	64.2	61.9	61.8	38,214	100.0

Definition of abbreviation: NA = not applicable.

Source: Piccinino LJ and Mosher WD, Trends in contraceptive use in the United States: 1982–1995, Family Planning Perspectives, 1998, 30(1):4–10 & 46.

frequently used methods (surgical sterilization and the pill) require a medical visit. (In many countries, the pill is available without a medical prescription.) Also, the use patterns change rapidly, particularly in response to concerns about sexually transmitted diseases (STDs). For people who are not in a stable monogamous relationship, the use of latex or polyurethane condoms is strongly recommended as the best protection next to abstinence to prevent venereal infection, including human immunodeficiency virus. Hormonal and other nonbarrier methods are not protective against STDs.

Use patterns also change rapidly in response to fear of complications. All of the methods described have greater health benefits than health risks, which are rare. Although in past years, a regime of higher dose hormonal pills than those now in use led some women to experience uncomfortable side effects, today's lower dose hormonal pills are equally effective. The IUD, recovering from the litigious aftermath of the Dalkon Shield distributed in the early 1970s, has undergone transformation with new systems releasing levonorgestrel, which reduce heavy bleeding. The earlier unpopularity of the IUD still can be seen in misinformation that prevails about the method among both users and providers.

Use patterns also respond to changes in contraceptive technology. Some of the most effective means of contraception have been available for only a few decades. Among female users between the survey years of 1982 and 1995, reliance on female and male sterilization increased from 34.1% to 38.6% and slipped back to 37.0% as of 2006–2008. The use of the hormonal pill has ranged from around 27.0% to 28.0%, whereas IUD use declined from 7.1% in 1982 to less than 1% in 1995, and has climbed up to 5.5% in 2006–2008. Reliance on periodic abstinence dropped during the same period from 3.9% to 1.1%. Among all users between 1982 and 2006–2008, use of the condom increased

from 12.0% to 16.1% (Mosher & Jones, 2010; Piccinino & Mosher, 1998). Further rapid change in use patterns is anticipated as a result of recent approved access to long-acting injectable and implanted hormonal contraceptives. The use of the condom since 1988 has risen also as a result of educational campaigns urging protection against STDs and acquired immunodeficiency syndrome (AIDS).

Malcolm Potts (1988) emphasized that women in the United States, compared with those in other developed countries, are inefficient contraceptors. Contributing factors include limitations in the United States on contraceptive information and services as well as restrictions on the methods available. The choices available to European women are greater and include easy access to postcoital contraceptives, a wider range of IUDs, and injectable or implanted contraceptives, only relatively recently approved for use in the United States. Santelli et al. (2008) have confirmed these disparities also exist for American teens compared to European teenagers.

The effectiveness of different family planning methods varies greatly. Failure rates for 1988 and circa 2002 of the most widely used methods are indicated in Table 5–2. Even for the most protective methods, the failure rates are substantial unless usage conforms perfectly to guidance. Failure rates are calculated only for the first year of use. As noted earlier, when failures are accumulated over multiple years of the reproductive life span, they are greatly increased. This circumstance is alarmingly confirmed by the finding that almost half of unintended pregnancies occur among women who are attempting some form of reversible contraception. This dismal record helps explain this country's high abortion rate. One in four pregnancies is terminated by induced abortion, nearly one in two among pregnant teenagers. Improving this record suggests the need for more effective contraception.

Table 5–2 First-Year (12-month) Contraceptive Failure Rates,* 1988 and 2002

Method	1988		2002	
	Perfect Use	**Typical Use**	**Perfect Use**	**Typical Use**
No method (chance)	85.0	85.0	85.0	85.0
Spermicides	3.0	30.0	18.0	28.0
Fertility awareness-based methods				
Standard days	NA	NA	5.0	NA
Two day method	NA	NA	4.0	NA
Ovulation method	NA	NA	3.0	NA
Symptothermal	NA	NA	0.4	NA
Sponge				
Parous women			20.0	24.0
Nulliparous women			9.0	12.0
Withdrawal	4.0	24.0	4.0	22.0
Periodic abstinence	9.0	19.0	20.2	25.0
Diaphragm	6.0	18.0	6.0	12.0
Condom (male)	2.0	16.0	2.0	18.0
Condom (female)	NA	NA	5.0	21.0
Combined pill	0.1	6.0	0.3	9.0
Patch (Evra)	NA	NA	0.3	9.0
IUD				
Copper T	0.8	4.0	0.6	0.8
Levonorgestrel (LNG)	NA	NA	0.2	0.2
Contraceptive ring	NA	NA	0.3	9.0
Injectables	0.3	0.4	0.3	6.0
Tubal sterilization	0.2	0.5	0.5	0.5
Vasectomy	0.1	0.2	0.1	0.15
Implants	0.04	0.05	0.05	0.05

*Estimated percentage of women experiencing an unintended pregnancy in the first year of use.

Definition of abbreviation: NA = not applicable.

Source: Trussell, J., & Raymond, E. G. (2011). Emergency contraception: A last chance to prevent unintended pregnancy. http://ec.princeton.edu/questions/ec-review.pdf [May 2011]. Hatcher, R. A., Trussell, J., Nelson, A. L., Cates, Jr., W., Stewart, F. H., Kowal, D. (Eds.). (2007). Contraceptive technology. 19th revised edition. New York, NY: Ardent Media, Inc. Alan Guttmacher Institute. (1993). Contraceptive use. Facts in brief. New York: Alan Guttmacher Institute (March 15, 1993).

FAMILY PLANNING PROVIDERS

Most users of reversible contraceptives obtain them from private physicians or managed-care organizations. Little is known about the scope or quality of those services. Approximately one user in three obtains services from a family planning clinic; the proportion is much higher for poor people, teenagers, and minority populations. A great deal is known about those clinics and their users. Accurate data are available on family planning agencies in the United States and their funding sources in 2009 (Guttmacher Institute, 2010). Studies show that:

- In FY2006 public expenditures for family planning services totaled $1.85 billion, of which Medicaid accounted for 71% and Title X 13%, with 12% from state appropriations.

- In 2006 8,199 family planning centers provided publicly funded family planning services, with 2,741 (33%) being health department clinics, 2,215 (27%) community or migrant health centers, 1,623 (29%) hospital or other clinics, and 868 (11%) Planned Parenthood Centers.

- Annually, more than 9 million women obtain contraceptive services from these providers, approximately 54% of those estimated to need publicly funded services.

- More than half (52%) of the agencies receive Title X funding for family planning services and account for two thirds of all family planning center clients.

- Some 2.3 million clients at family planning centers in 2006 were tested for chlamydia, 2.1 million for gonorrhea, 700,000 for syphilis and more than 650,000 for HIV, enabling early detection and treatment of STDs and prevention of subsequent infertility in young women.

- Eighty-five percent of counties in the United States had one or more publicly funded family planning clinics.

Most family planning clinics offer a great deal more than a range of contraceptives. A recent study (Gold et al., 2009) found that 9 in 10 agencies offer the pill, condom, and injectables, and 4 in 5 offer ECPs, up from 38% in 1995. A usual cluster of services would include pregnancy testing; screening for breast and cervical cancer; screening and treatment for STDs; screening for hypertension, anemia, and kidney disease; infertility and genetic counseling; abortion; and sometimes prenatal and postpartum care. This extensive array of services has led some analysts to suggest that family planning clinics should become comprehensive primary healthcare centers for women. In truth, family planning clinics are now the only or major source of health care for many women of reproductive age. The prospect of expanding the role of family planning clinics has some appeal, but it presents many problems. Among them is funding. Family planning is a low-cost service. As other more expensive services draw on the same resources, the family planning mission is diluted. A case can be made that the cause of family planning can best be served, as in many countries, by narrowly focused programs that strive for the widest possible participation of the population in need, leaving provision of other appropriate services to other providers.

The funding issue is central to consideration of the family planning mission. In 2006 federal and state governments spent an estimated $1.85 billion on family planning services, much of it through Medicaid (71%). The most important funding source for clinics dedicated to family planning services, however, is the federal Title X program, which contributes support to 52% of the agencies. Another important funding source for providers is MCH block grants from state and local governments. When considering all providers, not just the public clinics, the funding role of Medicaid and client fees increases appreciably. Other fee income and private contributions are minor sources of support, as is Social Services block grants (Finer, Darroch, & Frost, 2001).

More than seven million women received their most recent family planning services at a publicly subsidized clinic in 2006 (Guttmacher Institute, 2010). Title X clinics are especially important sources of care for low-income women, single and young women ages 15 to 24 years. One quarter of family planning clients at publicly funded centers were teenagers and nearly 2 million women under age 20 were served at these sites. Moreover, nationally funded family planning clinics helped their clients prevent 1.48 million unintended pregnancies (Gold et al., 2009).

Since the 1980s, family planning clinics have been caught in a squeeze between increased demand for more costly services and reduced funding. Some clinics have had to resort to increasing their fee income and withdrawing services from nonpaying clients. Financial challenges facing family planning centers include rising costs from providing multilingual, culturally sensitive and client-centered care, expanding STD and related diagnostic services, increased time allocated to high-quality patient counseling and education, and greater expenses on personnel salaries and a range of advanced contraceptive methods. Family planning clinics are also rapidly becoming the initial and main source of primary health care for many women.

NEEDS AND PROSPECTS

The fact that a high proportion of sexually active people practice contraception at least part of the time suggests that the need for it is widely known. The fact that such a high proportion of pregnancies is unintended and that the abortion rate is so high also suggest that the effective practice of contraception is poorly understood and that use of family planning services is insufficient. Use is especially low among women in households with incomes below 200% of poverty. For some women, access to family planning can be an expensive procedure, not always covered by health insurance, especially for young women and those of low income. Waiting times for

an appointment at family planning clinics have lengthened as clinic resources have shrunk. The need for a renewed national effort to enable planned childbearing is well established (Institute of Medicine, 2009).

Ever since the second Nixon administration in the early 1970s, a policy theme has gained strength to diminish the role of government, especially at the federal level, and to privatize as many public programs as possible. This theme has found expression, along with the political power to implement it, in the mid-1990s and most of the 2000s, with Congressional intent to make draconian cuts in the federal budget. In the early years of the 2010 decade, the Republican House of Representatives is seeking to eliminate Title X, or failing that, to fold it into Medicaid or MCH block grants. At the very best, this alternative would place public family planning at the uncertain discretion of different state governments. In many states, Planned Parenthood Federation affiliates, major providers of clinic services, would be shunted out of the funding stream. In other states, services in the public clinics would face serious political constraints. A consistent national policy and funding source for family planning would be lost. No strong private initiative shows promise of replacing it. What traditionally has been regarded as a public good, and one of the top 10 public health achievements of the 20th century in the United States (Centers for Disease Control, 1999) now becomes an individual burden.

Threats and uncertainties come from another direction. The Obama administration's Patient Protection and Affordable Care Act (ACA), passed in 2010, aims to expand health insurance coverage by 2014 to the millions presently uninsured, including many childless young adults. For this latter population, some have already gained coverage through their parents' insurance plans until they reach age 26. Starting in 2014, a large number of women and their partners will become eligible for Medicaid benefits that will cover their family planning needs. An almost similarly large group will be able to purchase private insurance through health exchanges established by the states beginning in 2014. Those who fall between 133% and 400% of the federal poverty level can receive subsidies toward their healthcare insurance premiums. Although Medicaid recipients will be able to access existing family planning and sexual and reproductive health services, the ACA intends that those covered through private health insurance will receive similar services standardized through a federally regulated essential health benefits package.

Plan enrollees increasingly are low-income individuals, often Medicaid recipients, who are locked into the system without resources to purchase services independent of the plan. There has been controversy over whether some providers (such as Catholic hospitals) may refuse to include family planning services under circumstances (such as "conscience clauses") when beneficiaries' choices of alternative providers are limited. Prospects for availability of family planning services through health insurance care plans should not be underestimated, however. Service priorities under the ACA will be driven by considerations of cost. Nearly all methods of averting unwanted childbearing, including abortion, are less costly than maternity care (Trussell et al., 1995). For this reason, insurance companies that do not explicitly cover the costs of abortion will sometimes do so if asked. Still, financing abortions is a less appealing prospect than preventing unplanned pregnancies.

The need for family planning clinics to continue functioning outside federally mandated health insurance plans, or under contract through Title X funding, is an ongoing concern. One study has found women reporting themselves as uninsured in order to continue to obtain family planning care from their preferred provider (Rosenbaum et al., 1994). No matter how the issue is resolved, there is room here for expert influence from public health. Sonfield and Gold (2011) identify three serious threats, the first being legal challenges to the ACA's requirement that all individuals have coverage. Second, Medicaid programs are under threat of drastic funding cutbacks, leaving millions of women of reproductive age uninsured. Third, the conservative agenda targets repeal of the ACA, and although likely to be blocked by a Democratic Senate, these efforts nevertheless place the act at risk and regulations regarding family planning care vulnerable to incremental changes at both the federal and state levels. A strong influence protective of user interests has not yet coalesced.

Standards for family planning, well established in Planned Parenthood clinics, need to be developed for healthcare reform plans. A pressing commitment for public health workers would be to define those standards, see to their incorporation into health exchange benefits packages and contracts, arrange to participate in quality review, develop data systems that enable accountability and outcome evaluations, train personnel capable of performing these tasks, and monitor the quality and outcome of services. The institutionalization of quality care standards for family planning under the ACA, drawing from the long experience of publicly funded clinics, is of utmost importance. Nothing in the history of this country suggests that the family planning needs of the population are likely to be met without the strongest possible advocacy.

References

Alan Guttmacher Institute. (1993, March 15). Contraceptive use. *Facts in brief*. New York: Alan Guttmacher Institute.

Alan Guttmacher Institute. (1994). The U.S. family planning program faces challenges and change. *Issues in brief*. Washington, DC: Alan Guttmacher Institute.

Boswell, J. (1988). *The kindness of strangers*. New York: Pantheon.

Centers for Disease Control and Prevention. (1999). Ten great public health achievements—U.S., 1900–1999. *Morbidity and Mortality Weekly Report, 48*, 241–243.

Ellertson, C. (1996). History and efficacy of emergency contraception: Beyond Coca-Cola. *Family Planning Perspectives, 28,* 44–48.

English, P. C. (1984). Pediatrics and the unwanted child in history: Foundling homes, disease and the origins of foster care in New York City, 1860 to 1920. *Pediatrics, 73,* 699–711.

Finer, L., Darroch, J. E., & Frost, J. J. (2001). U.S. agencies providing publicly funded contraceptive services in 1999. *Perspectives on Sexual and Reproductive Health, 34,* 15–24.

Fowler, C., Gable, J., & Wang, J. (2008). *Family planning annual report: 2006. National summary.* Research Triangle Park, NC: RTI International.

Frost, J. J., & Forrest, J. P. (1995). Understanding the impact of effective teenage pregnancy prevention programs. *Family Planning Perspectives, 27,* 188–195.

Gazmararian, J. A., Adams, M. A., Saltzman, L. E., Jonson, C. H., Bruce, F. C., Marks, M. S., & Zahniser, S. C. (1995). The relationship between pregnancy intendedness and physical violence in mothers of newborns. *Obstetrics and Gynecology, 85,* 1031–1038.

Gold, R., Sonfield, A., Richards, C., & Frost, J. (2009). *Next steps for America's family planning program: Leveraging the potential of Medicaid and Title X in an evolving health care system.* New York: Guttmacher Institute.

Guttmacher Institute. (2010). Facts on publicly funded contraceptive services in the U.S. *In Brief.* New York: Guttmacher, Institute.

Harrison, P., & Rosenfield, A. (Eds.). (1996). *Contraceptive research and development.* Washington, DC: National Academy Press.

Hatcher, R. A., Trussell, J., Nelson, A. L., Cates, W., Jr., Stewart, F. H., Kowal, D. (Eds.). (2007). *Contraceptive technology* (19th revised ed.). New York, NY: Ardent Media, Inc.

Institute of Medicine. (1995). *The best intentions: Unintended pregnancy and the well-being of children and families.* Washington, DC: National Academy Press.

Institute of Medicine. (2009). *A review of the HHS family planning program: Mission, management and measurement of results.* Washington, DC: National Academies Press.

Jones, R., Darroch, J. E., & Henshaw, S. K. (2002a). Contraceptive use among U.S. women having abortions in 2000–2001. *Perspectives in Sexual and Reproductive Health, 34,* 294–303.

Jones R., Darroch, J. E., & Henshaw, S. K. (2002b). Patterns in the socioeconomic characteristics of women obtaining abortions in 2000–2001. *Perspectives in Sexual and Reproductive Health, 34,* 226–235.

Kirby, D. (2002). Effective approaches to reducing adolescent unprotected sex, pregnancy and childbearing. *Journal of Sex Research, 39,* 51–57.

Klaus, A. (1993). *Every child a lion: The origins of maternal and infant health policy in the U.S. and France, 1890–1920.* Ithaca, NY: Cornell University Press.

Kost, K., & Forrest, J. D. (1995). Intention status of U.S. births in 1988: Differences by mothers' socioeconomic and demographic characteristics. *Family Planning Perspectives, 27,* 11–17.

Kost, K., Landry, D., & Darroch, J. (1998). The effects of pregnancy planning status on birth outcomes and infant care. *Family Planning Perspectives, 30,* 223–230.

Major, R. H. (1954). *A history of medicine* (Vol. 1). Springfield, IL: Charles C. Thomas.

Mosher, W. D., & Jones, J. (2010). *Use of contraception in the U.S.: 1982–2008. Vital Health Statistics, 23,* 1–44.

Piccinino, L., & Mosher, W. (1998). Trends in contraceptive use in the U.S.: 1982–1995. *Family Planning Perspectives, 30,* 4–10, 46.

Poole, V., & Hawkins, M. (1999). Pregnancy planning and unintended pregnancy. In, *Charting a course for the future of women's and perinatal health: Vol. II, Reviews of Key Issues* (pp. 81–102). Baltimore, MD: Women's and Children's Health Policy Center, Johns Hopkins School of Public Health and Maternal and Child Health Bureau, U.S. Department of Health and Human Services.

Potts, M. (1988). Birth control methods in the U.S. *Family Planning Perspectives, 20,* 288–296.

President's Council for Sustainable Development. (1996). *Sustainable America: A new consensus for the prosperity, opportunity and a healthy environment for the future.* Retrieved June 2011 from http://clinton2.nara.gov/PCSD/Publications/TF_Reports/amer-top.html. Rosenbaum, S., Shin, P., Mauskopf, A., Funk, K., Stern, G., & Zuvekus, A. (1994). *Beyond the freedom to choose: Medicaid, managed care and family planning.* Washington, DC: George Washington University Center for Health Policy Research.

Rosoff, J. (1988). The politics of birth control. *Family Planning Perspectives, 20,* 312–320.

Santelli, J., Sandfort, T., & Orr, M. (2008). Transnational comparisons of adolescent contraceptive use: What can we learn from these comparisons? *Archives of Pediatrics and Adolescent Medicine, 162*, 92–94.

Shah, I., & Ahman, E. (2010). Unsafe abortion in 2008: Global and regional levels and trends. *Reproductive Health Matters 18*, 90–101.

Shah, P., Balkhair, T., Ohlsson, A., Beyene, J., Scott, F., & Frick, C. (2011). Intention to become pregnant and low birth weight and preterm birth: A systematic review. *Maternal & Child Health Journal, 15*, 205–216.

Sivin, I. (1989). IUDs are contraceptives, not abortifacients: A comment on research and belief. *Studies in Family Planning, 20*, 355–359.

Sonfield, A., & Gold, R. (2011). Holding on to health reform and what we have gained for reproductive health. *Contraception*. DOI: 10.1016/j.contraception.2010.12.008.

Trussell, J., Leveque, J. A., Koenig, J. D., London, R., Borden, S., Henneberry, J., LaGuardia, K. D.,

Stewart, F., Wilson, T. G., Wysocki, S., & Strauss, M. (1995). The economic value of contraception: A comparison of 15 methods. *American Journal of Public Health, 85*, 494–503.

Trussell, J., & Raymond, E. G. (2011). Emergency contraception: A last chance to prevent unintended pregnancy. Retrieved May 2011 from http://ec.princeton.edu/questions/ec-review.pdf.

Tsui, A., McDonald-Mosley, R., & Burke, A. (2010). Family planning and the burden of unintended pregnancies. *Epidemiologic Reviews, 32*, 152–174.

World Health Organization (WHO). (2010). *Trends in maternal mortality: 1990 to 2008. Estimates developed by WHO, UNICEF, UNFPA and the World Bank*. Geneva: World Health Organization.

Zabin, L. S., Hirsch, M. B., Smith, E. A., Streett, R., & Hardy, J. B. (1986). Evaluation of a pregnancy prevention program for urban teenagers. *Family Planning Perspectives, 18*, 119–126.

6

MOTHERS AND INFANTS

Anjel Vahratian, Margaret Hicken,
Renee Schwalberg, and Milton Kotelchuck

At the present time medical schools do not prepare students for the work of preventing infant mortality . . . In short, preventive pediatrics must be taught. This becomes possible only when it is a required course based upon the present-day needs of the community. To be successful the preventive work in pediatrics must have a foundation in the knowledge that the faulty social structure is at the basis of many of the ills that are thrust upon infant flesh.

(Wile, 1910)

I am 37 years old and I am so worried and filled with perfect horror at the prospects ahead. So many of my neighbors die at giving birth to their children. I have a baby 11 months old in my keeping now, whose mother died. When I reached their cabin last Nov. it was 22 below zero, and I had to ride 7 miles horse back. She was nearly dead when I got there, and died after giving birth to a 14 lb. boy.

(Mrs. A-C-P, 1916)

INTRODUCTION

At the beginning of the 20th century, childbirth was still a life-threatening event for women in the United States. The risk of death to mothers and infants was substantial, and the available information and treatments were not adequate to assuage women's fears. Although the uneven distribution of risks has always placed disadvantaged groups in greatest jeopardy, the tragedy of a maternal or infant death elicits universal sympathy. Dr. Sara Josephine Baker, who became director of the New York City Bureau of Child Hygiene in 1908, coined the slogan "No Mother's Baby Is Safe Until Every Mother's Baby Is Safe" (Wertz & Wertz, 1982, p. 228). A pamphlet published by the U.S. Children's Bureau in 1913 proclaimed, "The infant death rate is the truest index of the welfare of any community" (Bremner, 1971, p. 966).

Infant deaths remain a widely used indicator of the general health and well-being of society. Infant mortality continues to plague developing countries at alarming rates, exacting significant social and economic costs and curtailing overall life expectancy. Although both maternal and infant mortality have been markedly reduced in this country, major racial and socioeconomic disparity persists as a gauge of social inequality. The relatively poor international ranking of the United States in infant mortality has been a source of national embarrassment. The last 3 decades have seen a great deal of effort targeted toward lowering the U.S. infant mortality rate, especially toward reducing the extremely high death rates of African American infants. The maternal and child health (MCH) community has focused on equalizing the life circumstances of mothers and the life chances of infants as a starting point toward greater social equity in the United States.

This chapter provides an overview of reproductive outcomes that are used as health indicators for mothers and infants. Definitions are provided, and epidemiologic trends and salient policy issues are briefly discussed. The notion of reproductive risk is explored and its usefulness examined in relationship to the defined outcomes. The chapter concludes with a review of current interventions in the field and some of the controversies that we face in setting program and policy priorities in the search for equity.

REPRODUCTIVE OUTCOMES

Infant Mortality

Definition

Formal efforts to study the health of populations began in Europe and the United States in the 1840s with the development of vital statistics systems in which the state, as opposed to the church, began to record births and deaths. The well-being of children has always been recognized as critical to a society's vitality and continuity, and the measurement of early death has been an important topic from the beginning of birth registration systems. In an era with no vaccinations or cures for infectious childhood diseases, the first efforts to examine the health of a state's youngest citizens focused on deaths of children under 5 years old. Childhood mortality, still calculated as a rate of such deaths per 1,000 children from birth to 5 years, is an important measure of a society's health. The World Health Organization (WHO) uses childhood mortality as part of a child survival index to make cross-national comparisons.

One can view the efforts of public health professionals over the past century as an effort to refine this broad health measure to assess infant health status better. As we have increasingly been able to affect the health of mothers and newborns, our ability to define and measure relevant components of infant health and morbidity has also improved. Measurement of MCH events is intended not only to enhance scientific understanding but also to facilitate effective interventions. By the 1870s, the present concept of infant mortality, the number of infant deaths per 1,000 live births, came into

use. The turn of the 20th century brought into focus the role of infectious diseases and poor nutrition, which took a heavy toll on infants throughout their first year. The MCH community began to divide infant mortality into neonatal mortality (deaths in the first 27 days of life per 1,000 live births) and postneonatal mortality (deaths from 28 to 364 days per 1,000 live births minus neonatal deaths). Neonatal deaths were generally attributed to biological birth complications and postneonatal deaths to environmental conditions and infectious diseases.

International comparisons are troubled by different historical and cultural perspectives on the meaning of infants' lives and deaths. In China, newborns are counted as being 1 year old at the time of birth. In some societies, an infant is not considered to be alive (and age is not calculated) until the time of christening, circumcision, or naming. A baby that dies before achieving the required status would not be enumerated as an infant death, and classification of neonatal and postneonatal deaths would be skewed by varying definitions.

Epidemiologic Trends

The reduction of the infant mortality rate in the United States from 150 deaths per 1,000 live births in 1900 to 6.86 per 1,000 in 2005 is one of the great public health success stories in the United States (Mathews & MacDorman, 2008). Over the last century, infant mortality has gone from being a common family tragedy to a relatively rare event. However, the overall rate has remained unchanged since 2000 and higher than the *Healthy People 2020* objective of 6.0 per 1,000.

With gains in technological control over environmental conditions and infectious diseases, the timing of infant mortality has gradually shifted toward early deaths, suggesting stronger biological determinants. Currently, most infant deaths occur in the neonatal period (4.54 deaths per 1,000 births in 2005) rather than the postneonatal period (2.32 deaths per 1,000 births in 2005) (Mathews &

MacDorman, 2008). In recent years, improvements in infant mortality have also been concentrated in the neonatal period, perhaps because of rapid gains in neonatology and enhanced regionalization of tertiary care. *Healthy People 2020* targets are 4.1 per 1,000 for neonatal deaths and 2.0 per 1,000 for postneonatal deaths.

Fifty-four percent of all infant deaths in 2005 were attributed to five causes: congenital malformations, disorders related to prematurity and low birth weight (LBW), sudden infant death syndrome (SIDS), newborn consequences of maternal pregnancy complications, and newborn consequences of cord complications (Mathews & MacDorman, 2008). The dramatic drop in SIDS deaths after the 1992 recommendation of the American Academy of Pediatrics to put infants to sleep on their backs or sides, rather than placing them on their stomachs, has continued at a slower pace.

Historically, there have been major disparities in infant mortality, which show no sign of diminishing. In 2005, infants of African American mothers were 2.3 times as likely to die in the first year as infants of white mothers (13.26 vs. 5.73 deaths per 1,000 live births) (Mathews & MacDorman, 2008). Racial comparisons in infant mortality usually focus on black/white differences because of the extreme gap in the outcomes for these groups. Overall mortality rates for Asian and Pacific Islander and Latino infants are similar or better than the white rate, although regional and subgroup variations belie the appearance of homogeneity. For example, in 2005, the Hispanic/Latino infant mortality rate in the United States as a whole was 5.62 deaths per 1,000 births but varied by ethnicity as follows: 4.42 for Cubans, 5.53 for Mexicans, and 8.3 for Puerto Ricans (Mathews & MacDorman, 2008).

Infant mortality rates in the United States tend to vary by geographic region and state. The highest rates tend to cluster among states in the South and Midwest. Both remote rural areas and metropolitan centers with large pockets of poverty and unemployment tend to have the highest rates. Variations by state also exist for race-specific rates. African Americans consistently fare worse, but the racial gap is more severe in some states than in others. For example, black:white infant mortality ratios in 2005 were as high as 3.16 in Wisconsin but were only 1.49 in Oregon (Mathews & MacDorman, 2008).

Low Birth Weight

Definition

Birth weight has been universally recognized as an important predictor of infant mortality and morbidity. Historically, all societies have known that tiny babies were more likely to die and that small infants who survived were developmentally vulnerable. In industrialized countries, the growth of specialized services for newborns and neonatal intensive care units in the 1950s and 1960s increased the focus on LBW and prematurity. Specific measures of newborn morbidity status arose in tandem with these developments. LBW can be thought of as having two possible causes, infants born too soon (prematurity) or infants born too small for their age (intrauterine growth restriction). Differential categorizations of small size that became popularized included definitions based on birth weight, gestational age or prematurity, and growth (birth weight levels corresponding to gestational age).

In 1948, WHO established 2,500 g. as the threshold for normal births. At first, LBW was the only criterion used to define infant size. With improved registration and the use of computerized databases, more detailed and sophisticated birth weight measures developed. Birth weight categories are generally defined as normal birth weight (NBW; 2,500 g. or more or at least 5 lb., 8.5 oz.), LBW (less than 2,500 g.), moderate LBW (1,500–2,499 g.), very LBW (VLBW; less than 1,500 g.), and extremely LBW (ELBW; less than 750 g). Births at less than 500 or 350 g.

are considered marginally viable and sometimes are excluded from live births. Infants
weighing 4,000 or 4,500 g. or greater are
sometimes considered separately as a high-
weight group with potential health risks.
Birth weight rates (more properly called
proportions) are defined as the percentages
of births in a weight category (i.e., number
of births in a given weight range per 100 live
births).

Epidemiologic Trends

LBW would appear to be an intransigent
problem in the United States. The lowest
recorded percentage of births below 2,500 g.
was 6.7% in 1984 (Martin et al., 2010), and
the rate slowly but steadily increased over
the next 2 decades. The percentage of LBW
births for the whole population rose from
7.0% in 1990 to 8.2% in 2008, whereas the
percentage of VLBW remained fairly stable
(1.27% in 1990 and 1.46% in 2008) (Martin
et al., 2010). These trends indicate that the
achievement of *Healthy People 2020* objectives (7.8% LBW and 1.4% VLBW) may be
unlikely.

Among white women, the increase in LBW
is primarily associated with a rise in multiple births caused by fertility drugs and other
assisted reproductive technologies, increased
inductions of labor, and cesarean deliveries.
LBW has also risen, although more modestly,
among singleton infants (Martin et al., 2010).
Rates of LBW (13.7%) and VLBW (3.0%)
among African Americans in 2008 remain
substantially elevated compared with the
rates for white infants (7.2% LBW and 1.2%
VLBW) (Martin et al., 2010). These persistent
problems have presented a frustrating challenge to the MCH community in its efforts to
improve birth outcomes and eliminate inequities. Buekens and Klebanoff (2001) have
observed that high rates of LBW and preterm
delivery may begin to seem inevitable to U.S.
observers because of public health failure,
and thus, innovative research and intervention strategies are more critically important
than ever.

Prematurity

Definition

Interest in the measurement of prematurity
is increasing with the recognition that most
infant deaths are due to low gestational age
and immaturity of the fetus, not size per se.
Prematurity has been defined somewhat
arbitrarily based on 40 weeks as the average length of pregnancy. Normal gestation is
defined as 37–41 weeks, although an early
term pregnancy is at 37–38 weeks gestation.
The criterion for premature gestation is
36 weeks or less, and for early or extremely
premature, it is 32 weeks or less. A late preterm birth is defined at 34–36 weeks gestation. Births at 42 or more weeks of gestation
are classified as postterm. Rates of prematurity are usually calculated as the percent of
premature births per 100 total live births.

Prematurity is more difficult to measure
accurately than birth weight. Gestational age
is usually defined as the difference between
the last menstrual period and the birth date,
minus 2 weeks; increasingly, ultrasonog-
raphy and newborn observational criteria,
such as the Dubowitz scoring system, are
also used to clinically estimate gestational
age. The completeness and accuracy of birth
certificate and medical record data on last
menstrual period vary according to mothers'
ability to recall menstrual information and
the accuracy of clinical judgment and record-
keeping.

Growth measures, which define intrauterine growth restriction or small for gestational
age (SGA), use percentages to rank infant
birth weights for a given gestational age
based on national norms (Alexander, Himes,
Kaufman, Mor, & Kogan, 1996). For example,
among all infants born at 39-weeks gestation
in the United States, 50% weigh more than
3,400 g. Babies are usually defined as SGA if
they rank in the lowest 10th percentile for a
given gestational age. The distinction between
prematurity and growth restriction has important implications for prevention efforts and
for subsequent morbidity and treatment of

the infant. Premature infants are more vulnerable to mortality, but if they survive, their life course may be quite normal. SGA infants have better survival rates but more subsequent developmental and health problems. Growth restriction often makes a greater contribution to LBW rates in developing countries compared with industrialized nations such as the United States. However, the utility of these growth measures is limited by the lack of international comparative norms as well as the need for fairly sophisticated data collection systems.

Epidemiologic Trends

The proportion of babies delivered prematurely (before 37 full weeks of gestation) has risen steadily in the United States, culminating in a 20% increase from 1990 to 2006. However, the preterm birth rate has been on the decline for the past 2 years. In 2008, the preterm birth rate was 12.3% (Martin et al., 2010). Despite the changing trend, this rate remains higher than the *Healthy People 2020* target of 11.4%. Racial and ethnic differences in preterm birth rates are of particular concern. The black:white prematurity ratio appears to be narrowing (from 2.2 to 1.6 between 1990 and 2008), as the preterm birth rate for both African American (17.5%) and white (11.1%) women has been decreasing.

There has been a major shift in the gestational age distributions of births in the United States over the past decade due to changes in obstetric practices, with postterm deliveries dropping precipitously and major increases in late preterm and early term births. The result is that the average length of pregnancy in the United States has dropped to 39 weeks (Martin et al., 2010). Although declines in preterm delivery would be desirable for the reduction of infant mortality, morbidity, and disability, improved prenatal screening and treatment sometimes contribute to iatrogenic prematurity when early intervention is judged to be beneficial. In other words, many obstetricians believe that medically induced prematurity may sometimes be preferable

to longer gestations in cases of maternal or fetal distress or a multiple pregnancy. Recent efforts by the March of Dimes, the American College of Obstetricians and Gynecologists, and others have been directed at changing these gestational age trends, emphasizing that all births if possible should be at 39 weeks gestation or longer.

Birth Weight-Specific Mortality

Definition

Public health analysts have attempted to capture the relationship between infant birth size and infant mortality by defining birth weight–specific mortality (BWSM), the number of infant deaths per 1,000 live births within a given weight category. For example, in the 2005 period linked birth/infant death data set in the United States, 57.4 infants died per every 1,000 born at LBW and 244.9 died for every 1,000 born at VLBW. These rates contrasted with only 2.3 deaths per 1,000 infants born at 2,500 g. or more (Mathews & MacDorman, 2008). BWSM is a very effective measure of a society's capacity to keep small infants alive.

Technically, the total infant mortality in society is the sum of all the infant mortality rates for each birth weight group. The infant mortality within each birth weight group is influenced by the frequency of births and the rate of survival of those births within that birth weight category. This definition is important because it suggests two approaches to improve infant mortality: reducing the number of small babies born through preventive public health interventions and improving the clinical neonatal health services to keep small babies alive. Both prevention and treatment approaches are critical to improving infant mortality rates in any society.

Epidemiologic Trends

Birth outcomes differ dramatically by birth weight. Thus, infant mortality trends are determined by changes in both the distribution of birth weights and the likelihood of death in each birth weight category. The majority of infants who are more likely to die are both very premature and VLBW. Newborns weighing 3,500–4,499 g. are least likely to die in the first year. Over two thirds (69%) of all infants who died in 2005 were LBW, and over half (54%) of infant deaths were VLBW. From 2000–2005, no significant declines were observed for infant mortality rates for infants weighing less than 2,000 g. (Mathews & MacDorman, 2008).

Infants of African American mothers died of causes associated with LBW at a rate four times the rate for white infants (Mathews & MacDorman, 2008). Although there is much debate over explanations for such differences, the BWSM survival rates of African Americans and whites of similar birth weight are not markedly different. The major source of the racial gap in infant mortality is differences in birth weight distributions, specifically the substantially greater rates of LBW, VLBW, and prematurity among African Americans.

Because of sophisticated neonatal intensive care technologies, the likelihood of survival is now approximately 95% at 1,250–1,499 g. compared with only 52% in 1960. Such dramatic improvements explain the overall decline in infant mortality over the last several decades, but technology may be reaching its limit in saving tiny newborns. Death rates for VLBW infants born less than 500 g. rose 1.3% between 2000 and 2005, and 86% of these infants died during this period (Mathews & MacDorman, 2008). The smallest survivors "are at much greater risk of experiencing lifetime disabilities such as blindness, developmental delays, and neurologic disorders, necessitating increased levels of medical and parental care" (Arias et al., 2003, p. 1224). The dissemination of high technology in neonatal and infant health services in the United States rivals any other country, but our population-based prevention efforts lag behind.

Perinatal Mortality

Definitions

The timing of the loss of a product of pregnancy is also important, and there are a number of opportunities for loss along the embryogenic timeline. It is not possible to estimate either the likelihood of fertilization or the rate of implantation of fertilized eggs. Once successful implantation of a fertilized egg is accomplished, research suggests that approximately 25% of implantations may fail before women are aware they are pregnant; spontaneous abortions or miscarriages then occur subsequently in approximately 15% of the clinically recognized pregnancies, although the measurement of any of these losses is imprecise. Thus, it appears that more than one third of all implanted pregnancies fail to result in a live birth. Spontaneous abortions frequently present a serious psychological loss for the mother and family. In spite of the high frequency of early pregnancy loss, general inattention to this important topic in women's health has hindered the development of any standardized measurements. The MCH field has a very limited understanding of the causes, risk factors, distribution or consequences of early pregnancy loss. Measuring early pregnancy loss remains a challenge for MCH research and an important topic for mothers and families.

Deaths after 20 weeks, but before birth, are defined as fetal deaths and are also rather poorly understood. Fetal mortality rates are approximately equal to neonatal mortality rates but are much less frequently studied (MacDorman & Kirmeyer, 2009). An arbitrary division is made between early (20–27 weeks) and late (28 + weeks) fetal deaths, often called stillbirths. Historically, these distinctions have become less clear with the increased potential for fetal surgery and life-saving interventions for infants born prematurely. In many European countries, the term perinatal mortality is used to refer to all deaths from 28 weeks gestation through 7 days of life (number of late fetal deaths plus early neonatal deaths per 1,000 live births). U.S. studies occasionally use this term but with varying definitions (MacDorman & Kirmeyer, 2009).

Epidemiologic Trends

From 1990–2003, the fetal mortality rate declined by an average of 1.4% per year (MacDorman & Kirmeyer, 2009). However, this trend has changed in recent years with no improvement. In 2005, the fetal mortality rate was 6.22 per 1,000 live births and fetal deaths, higher than the *Healthy People 2020* target of 5.6. The late fetal mortality rate has been on the decline over the past 25 years and was 3.03 per 1,000 live births and fetal deaths in 2005. The early fetal mortality rate is 3.13 in 2005. Similarly from 1990–2003, the perinatal mortality rate declined by 17% and then slowed through 2005 (6.64 deaths per 1,000 births 28 weeks gestation through 7 days of life). Fetal and perinatal mortality rates vary by race/ethnicity with substantially higher rates for non-Hispanic blacks as compared to non-Hispanic whites.

Maternal Mortality

Definition

As with indicators of infant health status, the definition of maternal outcomes has been evolving over time. Maternal mortality has traditionally been used as the sole women's health indicator, with measures estimating ratios of maternal deaths per 100,000 live births or women's average lifetime risks of dying from pregnancy-related causes. However, definitions and methods used for estimating maternal mortality have not been consistent. In the *International Classification of Diseases and Related Health Problems, Tenth Revision* (ICD-10), the World Health Organization defines maternal death as "the death of a woman while pregnant or within 42 days of termination of pregnancy, irrespective of the duration and site of the pregnancy, from any cause related to or aggravated by the pregnancy or its management but not from accidental or incidental causes" (World Health Organization, 2010, p. 4). From this definition, maternal deaths can be further classified as either direct or indirect in nature. Direct maternal deaths include those resulting from obstetric complications of the pregnant state (pregnancy, labor, and puerperium); from interventions, omissions, incorrect treatment; or from a chain of events resulting from any of these causes. Indirect maternal deaths include those resulting from preexisting disease or disease that developed during pregnancy, which was not due to direct obstetric causes but was aggravated by the physiologic effects of pregnancy. Deaths from unintentional or incidental causes presumed to be independent of childbearing are excluded, an omission that ensures conservative estimates of maternal mortality.

A limit of 42 days postpartum gives a narrow window for capturing fatalities related to the sequelae of pregnancy and childbearing. An important example is postpartum cardiomyopathy, a sometimes fatal condition that can manifest up to 6 months postpartum without previous signs. Studies that have extended the postpartum period to a full year have identified 6% to 11% additional deaths after 42 days (Atrash et al., 1988). To try to address this issue, late maternal death was included in the ICD-10 as an alternative concept of maternal death and as a means of capturing those deaths that occurred 6 to 52 weeks postpartum (WHO, 2010).

Epidemiologic Trends

An estimated 358,000 women worldwide die of maternal causes each year; 99% of these deaths occur in developing countries. Maternal mortality rates over 1,000 maternal deaths per 100,000 births still exist in some poor, underresourced countries. The United States had similarly high maternal mortality rates at the beginning of the 20th century.

The U.S. maternal mortality ratio[1] is estimated by the WHO (2010) at 24 deaths per 100,000 live births. However, maternal mortality is likely underestimated in all countries' registration systems, including that of the United States. For example, the official U.S. estimate for 2007 is 12.7 per 100,000 (Xu, Kochanek, Murphy, & Tejada-Vera, 2010). However, Horon (2005) showed that only 62% of maternal deaths in Maryland from 1993–2000 were identified from death certificates (Horon, 2005). The linkage of death certificates with medical examiner records for all women aged 10 to 50 who died between 1993 and 2000 and who had an undelivered or recent pregnancy helped to identify a more complete number of maternal deaths during this time period. Horon showed that the percentage of unreported deaths increased with the length of time between delivery and death. In the United States, substantial racial disparities in maternal mortality rates persist; Black non-Hispanic women die 3.3 times more often due to direct or indirect obstetric causes than white non-Hispanic women.

REPRODUCTIVE RISK

Extensive research has documented numerous factors, ranging from social to behavioral to biomedical, that are associated with poor birth outcomes such as infant mortality, LBW, and preterm birth. Here, we present approaches to the description of reproductive risk. As with other areas of health, the field of maternal and infant health is dominated by a biomedical approach to risk. However, there is growing interest in the longitudinal and social determinant factors that precede these more proximate risks. Therefore, along with a discussion of the approaches to risk description, we also discuss the approaches to the integration of the longitudinal, social, and biological determinants of poor birth outcomes.

Risk Factor Lists

The simplest and most common approach to the description of the risk of poor birth outcomes is the risk factor list. These lists are generated through the periodic reviews of the extant empirical literature. Risk factors are generally categorized in ways based on the strength of the evidence, attributable risk, social/behavioral versus biomedical, or those factors amenable to change. (For examples, see Berkowitz & Papiernik, 1993; Brown, 1985; Goldenberg, Culhane, Iams, & Romero, 2008; Kramer, 1987; Moore, 2003; Valero De Bernabe, et al., 2004.) Often authors focus on risk factors for either LBW or preterm birth as the outcome of interest.

In 1985, the Institute of Medicine (IOM) published a report on LBW that included a list of the "principal risk factors for low birthweight" (Brown, 1985). The risk factors in this list ranged from sociodemographic risks such as black race or low socioeconomic status (SES) to medical risks during pregnancy such as poor weight gain or hypertension. Others published a similar list on preterm birth, where the risk factors range from black race to gestational bleeding to in vitro fertilization pregnancy (Berkowitz & Papiernik, 1993).

More recently, authors have updated these risk factor lists, but in general, there have not been major changes in the risk factors that are associated with poor birth outcomes (Goldenberg & Culhane, 2007; Goldenberg et al., 2008; Muglia & Katz, 2010; Valero De Bernabe et al., 2004). The new or clarifying information that has been added to these lists is based on extensive research in the areas of infection, inflammation, genetics, and psychosocial stress (Goldenberg & Culhane, 2003; Harville, Hatch, & Zhang, 2005; Hobel & Culhane, 2003; Tsai et al., 2008). Although some new or more specific information has been added, fundamentally these risk factor lists have changed very little over the decades.

---

[1]Although the WHO calls it the maternal mortality ratio, the definition, maternal deaths per 100,000 live births, is the same as the U.S. definition of the maternal mortality rate.

The major advantage of the risk factor list approach is that it provides information for healthcare providers. For example, this information can be discussed with patients to facilitate behavior change both before and during the pregnancy (Kogan, 1995). In fact, some have narrowed these lists to those known factors theoretically amenable to intervention, such as chronic disease, cigarette smoking, and pregnancy planning (Moore, 2003). Furthermore, healthcare providers can use this information to develop obstetric plans for women at high risk for a poor birth outcome. With regard to preterm birth in particular, medical researchers support the development of risk factor lists to assist in the prediction of preterm birth within the current pregnancy (Goldenberg et al., 2008).

Although there may be some perceived benefit to the risk factor list approach, there are potential problems as well. First, all of the risk factors are given an equal weighting in these lists, when in reality only some are causal whereas others are markers for the actual causal factors. For example, black race, as a risk factor, is often seen as a proxy marker for social disadvantage and the risk exposure that accompanies that disadvantage (Blackmore et al., 1993). Most, if not all, of the risk factors are not independent but rather cluster (e.g., cigarette smoking, inadequate prenatal care, low socioeconomic status) or even interact (Cramer, 1987). Furthermore, there is no integration of social and biological determinants to better understand causal mechanisms.

Second, the focus on biomedical risk factors makes prevention of poor birth outcomes difficult or even impossible. Using intrauterine infection as an example, although it may present early in the pregnancy or even preconceptionally, it is generally not detectable until later in the pregnancy (Goldenberg, Hauth, & Andrews, 2000). Many other risk factors are health behaviors such as smoking, alcohol use, proper prepregnancy weight, and pregnancy weight gain. Although these risk factors may be attractive targets for risk reduction, according to Krieger's ecosocial framework health behaviors must be viewed within the context of the social and physical environment in which constraints are placed on the choices available for healthy behaviors (Krieger, 2001). Without an appreciation for the motivation for risky behaviors, behavior change will be a daunting task.

Third, although behavioral and biomedical risk factors may differ between LBW and preterm birth, the sociodemographic risk factors are the same. For example, black race, low SES, and unmarried marital status have been consistently associated with preterm birth, low birth weight, and infant mortality (Gortmaker & Wise, 1997; James, 1993; Wise & Pursley, 1992). The risk factor list approach obscures the important role of social determinants of poor birth outcomes.

Lastly, this approach leaves many poor birth outcomes unpredictable and unexplained. Many more outcomes are left unexplained when one considers that the strongest predictor of a LBW or preterm birth is a prior LBW or preterm birth, respectively (Mercer et al., 1999).

Multifactor Frameworks

In contrast, multifactor frameworks facilitate the integration and organization of risk factor lists into a theoretical causal story. Researchers have developed frameworks to address the complex nature of the causal mechanisms with regard to poor birth outcomes. These frameworks often integrate both models and theories (how and why, respectively) to describe the interconnected associations among risk factors and poor birth outcomes. The more complex frameworks provide temporal ordering to the risk factors, linking distal social factors such as race or socioeconomic status to health behaviors to biomedical risk factors to poor birth outcomes. (For example, see Lu & Halfon, 2003.) Some even broaden the notion of reproductive risk from health during current pregnancy to women's health over her life course. (For example, see Misra, Guyer, & Allston, 2003.)

Some frameworks focus solely on the biomedical complexities that precede a poor birth outcome. Figure 6–1 shows a framework linking preterm labor with preterm delivery (Lockwood & Kuczynski, 2001). Strictly biomedical frameworks such as this provide an outline for the causal flow of events that immediately precede poor birth outcomes, such as preterm delivery. However, they provide no information regarding the underlying causes of these outcomes and no guide for primary prevention.

Other frameworks describing poor birth outcomes actually do integrate social determinants with biological information. These contain the simplest approach to the integration of biological and social factors—what Diez Roux terms "social factors as antecedents to biologic processes" (Diez Roux, 2007, p. 569). For example, in Figure 6–2, the authors

outline their conceptual model for the role of the psychoneuroimmunologic (PNI) network of processes in the risk of preterm birth and low birth weight (Ruiz, Fullerton, & Dudley, 2003). The framework acknowledges some role for social determinants, but emphasizes the biomedical pathways.

Figure 6–3 shows a conceptual framework linking phenotypic race to very preterm (VPT) birth (Kramer & Hogue, 2009). The authors provide a complex framework based on both theory and a comprehensive review of the empirical literature. Note that the social risk marker of race is linked to very preterm birth through other distal determinants such as institutionalized racism and socioeconomic status (SES) and proximate biomedical determinants such as vascular dysfunction and inflammation.

Frameworks can facilitate hypothesis testing and further our understanding of causal mechanisms by providing the theorized and empirically supported, temporally ordered

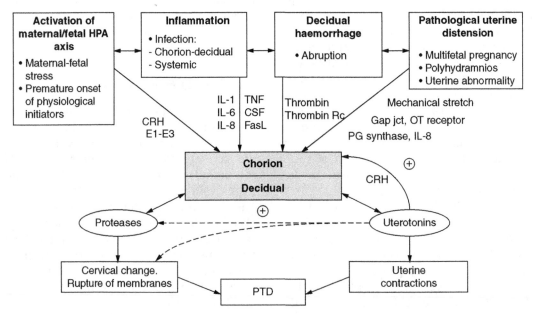

Figure 6–1 Pathways of Preterm Delivery Resulting from Preterm Premature Rupture of the Membranes and/or Preterm Labor

Source: Reprinted with permission from Lockwood, C. J., & Kuczynski, E. (2001). Risk stratification and pathological mechanisms in preterm delivery. *Paediatric and Perinatal Epidemiology, 15*(Suppl. 2), 78–89.

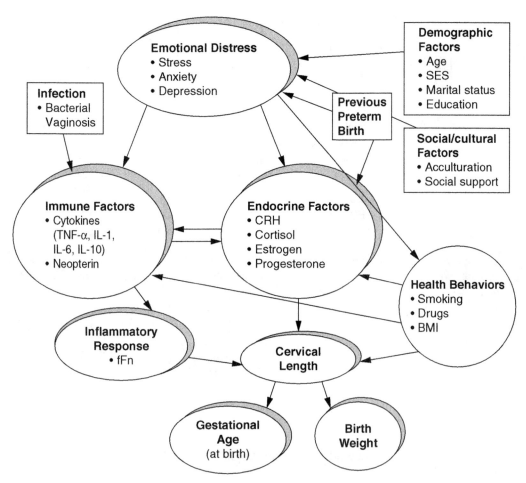

Figure 6–2 Depiction of the Psychoneuroimmunologic (PNI) Model in the Context of Preterm Birth. Numerous Factors Interact to Alter the Physiologic and Pathophysiologic Processes That Can Lead to Term and Preterm Labor

Source: Reprinted with permission from Ruiz, R. J., Fullerton, J., & Dudley, D. J. (2003). The interrelationship of maternal stress, endocrine factors and inflammation on gestational length. *Obstetrical & Gynecological Survey, 58*(6), 415–428.

mechanisms that link risk factors to poor birth outcomes. Furthermore, frameworks that integrate both social and biological information can also outline the theories regarding the consistent association between social factors such as race or SES and poor birth outcomes. These frameworks can help guide cost-effective and just policy and intervention development for the reduction of both absolute levels of poor birth outcomes but also social disparities in these outcomes.

Integrating Social and Biological Information

Of the research that integrates both social and biological mechanistic pathways that result in poor birth outcomes, the dominant approach is to view the social factors as antecedents to the biological events, as was mentioned previously. Although it is a step in the direction of a more holistic view of health, when depicting social factors merely as antecedents of biological processes, it becomes a

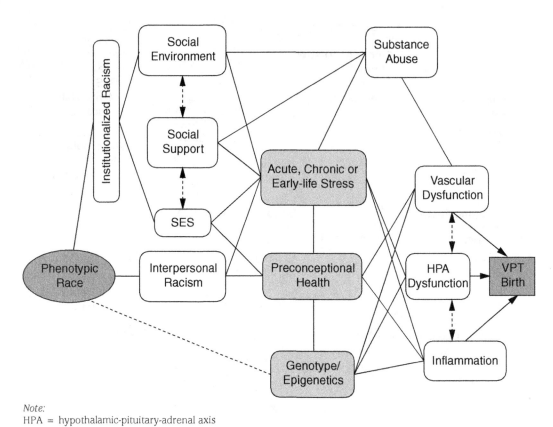

Note:
HPA = hypothalamic-pituitary-adrenal axis
SES = socioeconomic status.

Figure 6-3 Conceptual Framework for Understanding the Association of Race with Very Preterm (VPT) Birth

Source: Reprinted with permission from Kramer, M. R., & Hogue, C. R. (2009). What causes racial disparities in very preterm birth? A biosocial perspective. *Epidemiologic Reviews*, 31, 84–98.

major challenge to maintain the focus on the social factors.

As Diez Roux discusses, biomedical determinants dominate in current epidemiological frameworks, implying that it is possible to eliminate all social disparities in health outcomes if all of the proximate biomedical pathways are elucidated and addressed (Diez Roux, 2007). However, research indicates that a focus on these proximate pathways will not eliminate social disparities in poor birth outcomes. This is because the causes of poor birth outcomes are different from the causes of *social disparities* in poor birth outcomes (Link & Phelan, 1996; Rose, 2001).

For example, research has shown that social disparities in poor birth outcomes actually widen with the introduction of new technology meant to reduce these poor birth outcomes (Frisbie, Song, Powers, & Street, 2004; Gortmaker & Wise, 1997). Without addressing the social imbalance, those who are socially disadvantaged do not benefit from new technology compared to others.

Social factors such as race and SES determine exposure to behavioral, environmental, and biomedical risk for poor birth outcomes (Morello-Frosch & Shenassa, 2006). When proximate causes are addressed without regard for the fundamental social imbalances that created those proximate causes, new proximate causes will emerge to replace those that were addressed, ultimately leaving the health disparities in place (Link & Phelan, 1995; Link & Phelan, 1996).

Interactions among Risk Factors

The inability to reliably predict poor birth outcomes has led to the notion that certain risk factors may interact to result in different outcomes. For example, research shows that certain infections increase the risk for preterm birth (Goldenberg & Culhane, 2003; Ruiz, Fullerton, Brown, & Schoolfield, 2001). However, not all women who experience an infection experience a preterm birth. Researchers theorize that certain polymorphisms in important inflammatory pathway genes may explain these differential outcomes. For example, tumor necrosis factor-α (TNF-α), an inflammatory cytokine, appears to play an important role in the inflammatory pathway that links infection to preterm birth (Macones et al., 2004). The gene for the TNF-α gene (called TNFA) has been shown to have a moderating effect on the association between bacterial vaginosis and levels of TNF-α. With one polymorphism present, bacterial vaginosis results in high levels of TNF-α. With the other polymorphism present, bacterial vaginosis does not result in high levels of TNF-α (Genc, Vardhana, Delaney, Witkin, & Onderdonk, 2007).

Smoking has been linked to intrauterine growth retardation (Andres & Day, 2000; Horta, Victora, Menezes, Halpern, & Barros, 1997). However, research has also shown that it is linked to preterm birth in certain situations. Two genes, CYP1A1 and GSTT1, encode proteins involved in the metabolism of cigarette chemical byproducts. Researchers showed that smoking was associated with both low birth weight and preterm birth, but only for those women who carried a certain allele of either of these genes (Wang et al., 2002).

The research on interactions among risk factors for poor birth outcomes will likely provide further insight into the mechanisms that result in poor birth outcomes. However, most research on interactions deals with those among proximate risk factors, making the point of prevention difficult. More research is needed on the modifying effect of social factors on gene expression. For example, does social stress modify the gene expression of inflammatory processes? As with frameworks discussed previously, care must be taken to focus on social factors when examining the interactions among social and biological factors in order to focus resulting prevention attempts toward the social factors.

INTERVENTIONS

The manifestation of poor reproductive health outcomes is a function both of the maternal risks and any intervention that ameliorates those risks. Interventions to improve pregnancy outcomes for mothers and infants have probably existed since the earliest days of humanity, and folk traditions still abound. The histories of both public health and modern medicine are intimately tied to efforts to enhance the well-being of mothers and newborns. The dramatic reduction of both maternal and infant mortality in the 20th century testifies to the cumulative effects of multiple interventions.

Today a wide range of interventions aim to ensure healthy and successful pregnancies. Some of these interventions are tied directly to specific risk amelioration, whereas others are more closely associated with general health promotion. These interventions can be directed at the mother, the healthcare provider/healthcare system, or larger societal factors. For the purposes of this chapter, we divide interventions into five broad groups reflecting the developmental course of pregnancy and birth: (1) women's health care/life course, (2) preconception care, (3) antepartum or prenatal care, (4) intrapartum care, and (5) postpartum or interconception care.

Women's Health Care over the Life Course

The heart of MCH life course models is that the roots of reproductive health for both the newborn child and its mother are determined by the well-being of the mother over her life course. Optimal reproductive outcomes result from a continuous process of health promotion and disease prevention throughout the entire course of women's lives (Lu & Halfon, 2003). Infant health is intimately related to a mother's well-being from the time of her own conception, and the lifetime effects of childbearing are influenced by the totality of self-care and health care that mothers received.

Women's health care over the life course is the newest programmatic area for reproductive interventions. This focus has evolved historically from both the women's health and preconception health movements. The central issue for the MCH life course models has been to convert its innovative theoretical risk factor framework into practical longitudinal MCH programs and social determinant practices and policies that modify and enhance reproductive health.

This is a new area for intervention, and there are several distinct approaches being undertaken or conceptualized within this area. In practice, relatively few organized programs are directed over the life course to have a specific impact on reproductive health. There have been many innovative efforts, especially at the local level, to adapt MCH life course perspectives to MCH practice.

Most of the women's health care/life course health programs have focused on general health promotion, in particular health promotion for girls, as the means to enhance reproductive health in future pregnancies or more broadly as women's health/life course initiatives. These are either directly addressed to specific school-age girls or young teen participants (e.g., girls' clubs programs, chronic disease prevention programs, or obesity reduction or diabetes control programs) or more generally addressed through community-level health promotion, health education or behavioral change programs around diet, substance use, and/or physical activity for young women. All have an impact on both future reproductive health and women's own health; however, they are not directly organized as a specific "reproductive health" program.

A second type of women's health/life course interventions emphasizes community-level or place-based interventions, trying to enhance the community's overall health and reproductive health promoting capacity. Place-based practice and policy interventions/initiatives try to address the underlying social determinants of subsequent poor reproductive health. While the MCH field and its agencies in the United States are limited in their capacity to address fundamental social determinants such as poverty, housing, nutrition, etc., they can partner with other agencies to ensure that the community's overall capacity to foster more optimal women's and reproductive health are addressed. Specific creative examples in the United States include medical-legal partnerships, baby friendly hospitals, and children's environmental health assessment. The challenge is how to foster more far-reaching community-based strategies for infant mortality reduction that transcend the predominant medical paradigm.

Place-based collaboration, implicit in life course models of women's reproductive health, is rarely attempted in the United States. However, several local public health organizations are restructuring themselves as integrated life course and community empowering organizations (e.g., Alameda County, CA, the Northern Manhattan Perinatal Project, the Harlem Children's Zone). They are exploring these models for reproductive and life course health that try to simultaneously address women, family and community health, foster service integration, and utilize policy opportunities to have an impact on structural inequities (e.g., work, education, poverty, racism) (Lu et al., 2010).

Even if not so transformative, there are opportunities to develop longitudinal women's and reproductive health and health systems initiatives in every current MCH organization/program. Fine and Kotelchuck (2010) have emphasized the need for more vertical, horizontal, longitudinal, and holistic life course programmatic linkages. Vertical linkages refers to initiatives to improve handoffs/transitions within a health or public health-care organization, such as integrated primary to tertiary care, medical homes, and better compliance with referrals. Horizontal linkages refers to initiatives to foster better integration among various human service sectors, such as school-based health programs, Head Start dental screening programs, and prenatal care requirements for welfare benefits. Longitudinal integration refers to initiatives that deal with continuity over time, especially at critical transition points, such as new parenthood programs and improved care coordination for transitions such as from obstetrics to pediatrics and pediatrics to adult primary care. Women's health and reproductive care programs are especially susceptible to discontinuities over the life course, such as limited or no postpartum follow-up care for most women or the lack of reproductive health programs for sexually active teenagers. All programs would benefit from these kinds of formal restructuring, with a life course continuity orientation.

These new life course-inspired initiatives have yet to be evaluated for their impact on reproductive health. They reflect, however, the reappearance of social determinant programmatic content after decades of almost exclusively biomedical intervention models to improve birth outcomes and women's health in the United States. The majority of individual programmatic interventions for reproductive health, with a life course focus, derive primarily from expanding preconception health efforts to provide a broader time frame to improve women's health over the life course.

Preconception Health Care

Most reproductive health efforts have traditionally focused on women's health during pregnancy and thus, prenatal care. Preconception health care, as an ameliorative intervention and a formal preconception visit, derives from the innovative work of Cefalo and Moos (1995). They correctly argued that the critical stages of early fetal development are completed before many women enter prenatal care or even know with certainty that they are pregnant. "The period of greatest environmental sensitivity for [the] developing fetus is between 17 and 56 days after fertilization. Cell organization, cell differentiation, and organogenesis take place during this period, and any insult, whether nutritional, drug-related, or viral, can jeopardize fetal development . . . By the end of the eighth week after conception and certainly by the end of the first trimester, any major structural anomalies in the fetus have already developed" (Cefalo & Moos, 1995, pp. 2–3). Moreover, they argued that many of the major concerns of prenatal care could have been addressed prior to the beginning of the pregnancy, such as smoking cessation, achieving a healthy weight, and receiving needed vaccinations. They then created the first formal preconception care program in conjunction with family planning clinics in North Carolina, in an effort to shift medical care and counseling to an earlier period with a greater potential for primary prevention of early fetal loss, birth defects, and other adverse pregnancy outcomes. They stressed the importance of adequate information in ensuring full reproductive choice and counseled women on the extent to which they can increase their chance of healthy pregnancy and positive birth outcomes prior to conception. Preconception care was viewed as a form of primary care for women (Moos, 1989).

Around the same time, the Centers for Disease Control and Prevention (CDC) became interested in preconception care as part of its safe motherhood campaign and increased focus on the reproductive health of women. With the participation of all the major perinatal health groups in the United States, the CDC led an initiative to advance preconception health and health care in the United States. The goals of this initiative included improving the knowledge, attitudes, and behaviors of men and women related to preconception health, assuring that all women of childbearing age in the United States receive preconception care services that will enable them to enter pregnancy in optimal health, reducing risks indicated by a previous adverse pregnancy outcome through interventions during the interconception period, and reducing known disparities in adverse pregnancy outcomes. To achieve these four goals, CDC developed 10 strategic recommendations and specific action steps to achieve them. These recommendations are summarized in Table 6–1.

The CDC defined preconception care as "a set of interventions that aim to identify and modify biomedical, behavioral, and social risks to a woman's health or pregnancy outcome through prevention and management" (CDC, 2006, p. 3). At the individual level, components of preconception care include screening for risks, providing health education, and delivering effective interventions. Numerous maternal risk factors are identified by the CDC that can and should be addressed prior to conception, including chronic diseases, infectious diseases, reproductive concerns, genetic concerns, medication issues, personal behaviors, and exposures (CDC, 2006). Indeed, most of the risks identified on the previously presented risk factor lists are known and treatable before conception.

This work spawned special issues on preconception care in three professional journals: *Maternal and Child Health Journal* (2007), *American Journal of Obstetrics and Gynecology* (2008), and *Women's Health Issues* (2008). The CDC's efforts to implement preconception care represents a bold new

Table 6–1 CDC Recommendations to Improve Preconception Health and Health Care

1. Individual Responsibility Across the Lifespan
2. Consumer Awareness
3. Preventive Visits
4. Interventions for Identified Risks
5. Interconception Care
6. Prepregnancy Checkup
7. Health Insurance Coverage for Women with Low Incomes
8. Public Health Programs and Strategies
9. Research
10. Monitoring Improvements

Source: Centers for Disease Control and Prevention. (2006). Recommendations to improve preconception health and health care—United States: a report of the CDC/ATSDR Preconception Care Work Group and the Select Panel on Preconception Care. *MMWR, 55 (No. RR-6).* Retrieved May 16, 2011 from http://www.cdc.gov/mmwr/preview/mmwrhtml/rr5506a1.htm.

initiative to institute and transform the current reproductive health initiative prior to conception to enhance both women's health and pregnancy outcomes.

Unfortunately, there have been serious barriers to implementing preconception healthcare initiatives. Historically, these barriers have included limited insurance coverage for preconception visits and the reality that 50% of pregnancies are unplanned in the United States. If pregnancies are not planned, it is difficult to institute preconception care-specific interventions other than family planning. These have proven to be serious programmatic barriers to preconception care initiatives.

Since the extent of unplanned pregnancies may not readily change in the near future, preconception healthcare advocates have articulated a more general women's health/life course focus for preconception care. That is, they consider preconception care as basic primary care for women at any stage in her life. The proposed preconception interventions also ensure a healthy woman, whether or not she plans to become or becomes pregnant. Preconception care should serve as a bridge to more continuous services for women's general health needs. For this reason, Moos (2002) and others have advocated that one should offer preconception health care at every healthcare visit. "Rather than pursuing the 'add a category of service' mentality, what is needed is consolidation. Rather than further fragmenting care, we should reframe our existing array of services to look at the total woman first, and her reproductive status second. There is, in fact, little that could be recommended in routine preconception counseling that would not benefit the average woman's general health status, irrespective of eventual conceptions . . . Preconceptional wellness is women's wellness—healthy women are more likely to have healthy pregnancies and healthy offspring: It is that simple" (Moos, 2002, p. 72).

This attention to preconception care is evident in the *Healthy People 2020* objectives, which include four objectives specific to improving preconception health and behaviors.

Prenatal Care

The American College of Obstetricians and Gynecologists (ACOG) described four functions of prenatal care: (1) risk assessment, (2) serial surveillance, (3) health education, and (4) psychosocial support (Brann & Cefalo, 1992). The goals of risk assessment are to screen women in order to detect specific pregnancy risks for poor birth outcomes and to determine the most appropriate level of prenatal care, for example, to determine which women are medically at high risk needing specialized prenatal or obstetric care and which women have psychosocial needs requiring additional social services. The task of comprehensive prenatal care programs is

to provide treatment for women appropriate to their level of need.

Formal risk assessment is usually conducted at the first prenatal care visit. Unfortunately, risk screening tools have relatively low predictive value. At best, existing prenatal instruments can identify half of women who go on to experience perinatal deaths. Screening systems have inherent problems and limitations. Risk assessments are limited by our relatively weak understanding of mechanisms explaining poor pregnancy outcomes. Currently, the strongest predictors of adverse pregnancy outcomes are prior poor obstetric history, use of substances such as cigarettes, multiple gestations (i.e., twins, triplets, etc.), and vaginal infections. Predictions are much stronger for multiparous than for primiparous women.

Selwyn (1990) has outlined several dilemmas associated with risk assessment instruments based on the trade-off between sensitivity (detection of true positives) and specificity (detection of true negatives). The greater the chance of identifying women who are actually at risk (i.e., those who will have preterm birth), the lower the likelihood of accurately classifying low-risk women (i.e., those who go on to full-term deliveries). In other words, in selecting the cutoff points for measuring risks, providers must choose between overdiagnosis with unnecessary treatment of false positives as opposed to underdiagnosis and missed opportunities for preventive treatment of false negatives. Both of these possibilities carry the risk of medical complications and psychological distress. Repeated screening may be one way to improve the accuracy of risk assessment.

Serial surveillance is successive monitoring of the pregnant women and fetus to ensure that they are progressing properly through the normal developmental stages. The purpose of this screening is to detect deviations and then to make appropriate referrals or provide treatments for any identified problems of the pregnancy. For most women, this routine surveillance involves urinalysis, fundal (i.e., uterine) height measurement, weighing, and sometimes other tests such as alpha-fetoprotein screening and ultrasound to detect fetal abnormalities. Both ACOG and the U.S. Public Health Service (PHS) Expert Panel on the Content of Prenatal Care have developed detailed protocols for the timing and content of prenatal surveillance (Brann & Cefalo, 1992; PHS, 1989). Surprisingly, there has been no national meeting or consensus conference on the content of prenatal care despite major changes in content and practice over the last 10 years.

Health education is the provision of health information about the impact of pregnancy on women's health and physical changes, advice on behaviors to promote a healthy pregnancy and healthy infant (including nutrition, weight gain, exercise, and substance use), preparation for delivery, and knowledge of newborn care. Pregnancy provides a significant opportunity for instruction and advice to improve the health of the mother, her future offspring, and the entire family. Studies repeatedly show that pregnancy is a receptive period for health behavior change. Two thirds of women who have given birth have taken childbirth education classes, but disproportionately more white women (76%) than African American women (44%) receive this benefit (Lu et al., 2003).

Psychosocial support recognizes that pregnancy does not simply involve maternal physiological changes and embryological growth, but is embedded in a social, cultural, and emotional context. For many women, pregnancy is a time of great emotional flux. Clinical prenatal care providers as well as family and friends can provide needed support, both instrumental and psychological. Maternal depression, social isolation, exposure to violence, and substance use are some of the many psychosocial issues that may arise during and after pregnancy. Beyond clinical care settings, a variety of support programs have been developed to address prenatal psychosocial needs, including case management, pregnancy support groups,

centering pregnancy (group prenatal care), home visitation programs, and fatherhood involvement programs. Historically, a women's mental health during pregnancy was thought to influence the health of her fetus; this concept continues into the 21st century.

Currently in the United States, ACOG recommends 13 prenatal visits during pregnancy for a normal low-risk woman: the initial visit in the first 6 weeks, one visit per month until the 28th week, one visit every 2 weeks until the 36th week, and one visit per week thereafter. This standardized universal visit schedule was developed in the early part of the century in order to prevent maternal mortality, especially from eclampsia, a hypertensive disorder generally manifesting toward the end of pregnancy. It is important to note that this prenatal care schedule was developed primarily to improve maternal, not infant, health.

There have been some suggestions to change the visitation pattern. The USPHS report, *Caring for Our Future: The Content of Prenatal Care*, suggested fewer but more intensive prenatal care visits (PHS, 1989). According to the report, the timing of care should be shifted to increase visits toward the beginning of the pregnancy, including a preconception visit, in order to focus more on maternal health promotion activities. The PHS also recommended the establishment of different visitation schedules for primiparous and multiparous women. This and other proposals to modify the standard schedule have met with strong opposition from the professional obstetric community, even though the United States recommends more prenatal care visits than most European countries.

Prenatal care can be conceptualized very broadly or very narrowly. Narrowly defined, prenatal care represents only the ACOG recommended visits to a medical provider, that is, the provision of medical care during pregnancy. Broadly conceptualized, prenatal care comprises any intervention during pregnancy that enhances the health and well-being of mothers and their offspring.

A comprehensive definition of prenatal care would include nutrition counseling and food supplementation, childbirth preparation classes, mentoring and advice from a "resource mother," home visitation, and an array of other services.

In general, the MCH field takes a very broad view of prenatal care and encourages the inclusion of psychosocial, nutrition, health education, case management, and other services. Definitions of the scope of prenatal care reflect fundamental beliefs about what is truly needed to ensure a successful pregnancy. Surprisingly, inadequate evidence exists to assess conflicting beliefs about pregnancy care or to update guidelines for the content of prenatal care in the United States.

Prenatal care (PNC) utilization has improved steadily in the United States since 1988, with 74.6% of women in 2002 receiving at least adequate PNC. More recent data are unavailable because of revisions to the U.S. birth certificate. The gap in adequate use of prenatal care between racial/ethnic groups has also narrowed substantially (Rittenhouse, Braveman, & Marchi, 2003). Similar trends were noted by Alexander (Alexander et al., 2002).

There is widespread agreement that prenatal care is important and positive, but little research is available that documents the efficacy of prenatal care use or specific interventions to enhance birth outcomes and maternal health. The linkage between prenatal care and birth outcomes is actually quite difficult to study, as it involves complex definitional, methodological, design, and ethical issues. Randomized clinical trials (RCTs) assigning some women to a no-PNC group are not possible or desirable for ethical reasons, although RCTs of added new components of prenatal care are possible.

Kotelchuck (1994) and many others have shown that the impact of prenatal care on birth outcomes is a U-shaped function. Women with inadequate and those with intensive care have the poorest birth outcomes. Inadequate care is often a marker for psychosocial and socioeconomic difficulties that may result in medical conditions. A lack of preventive care or early treatment may exacerbate those problems. Women with intensive care are likely to have more severe medical needs and complications, although they may not necessarily be easily addressed by prenatal interventions. Their outcomes, although not optimal, would likely be worse without the intensive treatment they receive.

While comprehensive prenatal care is a strategy to address the nation's poor infant mortality rankings and continued disparities in the 1980s and 1990s (Institute of Medicine, 1985, 1988), the continued rising trends in poor birth outcomes and disparities in reproductive health in the United States have thrown further doubt on the efficacy of prenatal care to improve pregnancy outcomes. Moreover, most RCTs of enhanced or comprehensive PNC programs have not conclusively shown any impact on prematurity, LBW, or infant mortality. Various review articles have now concluded that PNC has, at best, only a limited impact on birth outcomes (e.g., Fiscella, 1995; Goldenberg & Rouse, 1998). These findings have cast doubt on the cost-effectiveness of comprehensive public PNC programs as interventions for improving pregnancy outcomes and have led in part to the growth in women's health/life course and preconception care initiatives.

Surprisingly, there have been relatively few efforts to examine the content of prenatal care, perhaps because of the inherent difficulty of examining the variety of ways the primary surveillance function of prenatal care is implemented, the absence of formal ACOG standards, and the recent lack of positive indications of prenatal care impact itself. Indeed, there has been no national meeting/consensus conference on the content of prenatal care over the past 20 years, despite major changes in content and practice of prenatal care, such as more and earlier clinical and genetic surveillance (e.g., the quad test for congenital markers of Down syndrome or spina bifida, more ultrasounds, HIV status determination), new psychosocial risk screening topics (e.g., intimate partner violence, maternal depression), more behavioral intervention programs to reduce smoking and increase physical exercise, and more use of electronic medical records and patient risk survey questionnaires.

Research findings suggest that the broad ACOG prenatal care recommendations, especially for risk assessment and health education, are not routinely followed (Peoples-Sheps, Hogan, & Ng'andu, 1996). Kogan et al. (1994) found that African American women were more likely than white women to have the recommended prenatal medical procedures performed, but less likely to receive advice about health behaviors. Findings from national survey data (Kogan, Alexander, Kotelchuck, Nagey, & Jack, 1994) indicate that receipt of health advice from PNC providers is an important contributor to LBW prevention.

Prenatal care is and will likely remain the principal mode of health service delivery during pregnancy, as it provides primary health care for mothers. The MCH field, in this era of healthcare reorganization and cost containment, is being challenged to demonstrate the effectiveness of specific components of prenatal care, especially the psychosocial and other nonmedical services. Along these lines there have been several recent efforts to change how prenatal care is delivered. Centering pregnancy is a national movement that supports the development of a group prenatal care model, in which small groups of women meet with a clinician in a setting that provides social support, empowerment, health education and health promotion/ health education in addition to clinical prenatal care surveillance. Advocates for this group prenatal care model believe that it helps women take more responsibility for their own prenatal care/surveillance and better balances the roles of the provider and the woman, who benefits from the collective power and wisdom of a community of women in the same stage of life. Research on group prenatal care has been favorable, showing both its popularity (Robertson et al., 2009) and its positive impact on birth outcomes in a randomized controlled trial (Ickovics et al., 2007). Similar group prenatal care and women's empowerment initiatives, with a more Afrocentric health education curriculum, are being used in the California Black Infant Health initiative, a community-based prenatal and postnatal program similar to Healthy Start.

The Healthy Start Program was designed to improve birth outcomes and reduce infant mortality rates in the nation's areas of highest need. An MCH Bureau-administered program, Healthy Start began as a pilot in 15 cities and rural areas in 1991 and has since expanded to include 96 sites in 37 cities and 2 territories (as of 2011). Healthy Start represents the ultimate programmatic expression of the 1980s/1990s efforts to address infant mortality with comprehensive prenatal care and enhanced services, plus increased community involvement and community-based initiatives. The program has three broad goals (Kotelchuck & Fine, 2000): (1) ensure access to/ use of high-quality comprehensive health services for all Healthy Start participants, including outreach, case management, and health education; (2) strengthen local health systems, including developing a local health systems action plan; and (3) bring a consumer/community voice to efforts to improve maternal and infant health, including utilizing a community consortium and consumer and provider councils to advise local grantee. The program is required to include five service components (outreach, case management, health education, depression screening, and interconception care) as well as four systems components (a consortium, a local health action plan, coordination and collaboration with Title V, and a sustainability plan). Healthy Start has been very flexible in adapting to newer, more current reproductive health initiatives, including father involvement and preconception care initiatives.

Healthy Start has also been systematically evaluated since its initial pilot in 1991. The evaluation of the 15 pilot sites found mixed results, with significant improvements in the initiation and consistent utilization of prenatal care, but no overall improvements in LBW rates, preterm deliveries, or infant mortality, though in a minority of sites birth outcome improvements were demonstrated (Devaney et al., 2000). Further studies showed that Healthy Start reached a higher risk population in its target areas and increased family planning usage (McCormick et al., 2001). A more recent evaluation has measured only "intermediate" outcomes to date, but reports that of the 96 sites currently in operation, nearly all have increased access to care and increased positive health behaviors among their participants, three quarters have increased the number of participants with a medical home, and a similar proportion have increased screening for perinatal depression among the providers in their communities (U.S. Department of Health and Human Services, 2008).

In many states and communities, home visiting programs provide prenatal support and educational services to pregnant women and parents of young children using registered nurses or paraprofessionals. Home visiting programs are designed to promote maternal, infant, and early childhood health, safety, and development, as well as strong parent-child relationships. High-quality, evidence-based home visiting programs can be seen as part of an early childhood system for promoting health and well-being for pregnant women and could provide an infrastructure for the provision of health education, psychosocial support, and case management services for high-risk pregnant women in their homes at the community level.

Historically, public health nurses conducted home visits to mothers with newborn children, a community-based program that disappeared as the locus of public health nursing shifted to the clinic. In the 1970s nurse and paraprofessional home visitation programs were reinstitutionalized but with a prenatal intervention focus. Today, many home visitation programs provide for prenatal to postnatal continuity. For European and other developed countries, home visitation remains an integral part of their universal reproductive health and infant care services.

Many home visiting programs begun in the 1970s were implemented and evaluated as randomized controlled experiments in specific communities to build a body of evidence of their effectiveness. These early trials found that women in the study sample showed reduced levels of smoking, reductions in preterm birth among smokers, reduction in pregnancy-associated hypertension, and increases in birth weight among infants born to adolescents, compared to the control populations (Kitzman et al., 1997; Olds, 2002). However like other comprehensive prenatal care programs, home visitation programs have not shown substantial impact on birth outcomes. To date, Olds' Nurse-Family Partnership model of home visiting has shown the greatest success based on evaluative randomized controlled trials (Kitzman et al., 2010; Olds et al., 2010; Rubin et al., 2011).

Men play a critical role in family formation and have important responsibilities in the preconception and prenatal periods, both in support of their partners and for their own development as partners and fathers. Unfortunately, men have not always felt welcome in MCH programs. In recent years, there have been more systematic, although still scattered, efforts to involve men (fathers) more actively in the preconception and prenatal care activities, as well as in delivery and parenthood initiatives (Frey et al., 2008). In part, these programs arose from a decline in marriage before childbearing and the differential absence of fathers in minority families with young children (Horn, 2000). The National Fatherhood Initiative (http://www.fatherhood.org), for example, has as its mission to improve the well-being of children by increasing the proportion of children growing up with involved, responsible, and committed fathers.

Healthy Start programs have actively embraced father involvement programs. For example, the San Mateo County Fatherhood Collaborative (Buckelew, Pierrie, & Chabra, 2006) joined together to (1) increase the community's awareness and support of fathers and men in the lives of children; (2) increase the health and well-being of children by increasing the strength and quality of their relationships with their fathers and male caregivers; and (3) improve the coordination of family services for fathers and encourage male responsibility in families. They creatively conducted a needs assessment of fathers in their county and identified their concerns in five areas: (1) personal development, (2) parenting skills, (3) family health, (4) employment and job training, and (5) legal assistance. Fatherhood programs that go beyond negative messages (i.e., don't do bad things to your partner) and include positive orientations to help men with their own developmental maturation as partners and fathers will be more effective in engaging them.

A final note on prenatal care: Although there has been a decreased emphasis in recent years on pregnancy-based prenatal care interventions as the principal means to ensure reproductive health, good birth outcomes, and reduced disparities, one can view the new women's health/MCH life course framework as once again giving emphasis to the need for good prenatal care (and a good prenatal care environment), not simply to focus on the immediate birth outcome, but to help ensure that both the mother and her newborn have a lifetime of good health and reproductive health outcomes.

Intrapartum Interventions

The delivery or intrapartum period is also an important time for interventions to improve birth outcomes for mothers and infants. Many of these interventions are pharmacological protocols and surgical procedures to augment the speed and safety of the birth process. Conflicting ideologies and values about childbirth have led to controversy about intercession in this period. Proponents of natural childbirth can cite evidence of the psychological and medical benefits of nonintervention, although most would recommend that women receive the highest quality of medical services at the first indication of need. In contrast, many clinical providers advocate for routine use of the latest medical technologies as an attempt to prevent any possible risk to the infant during delivery. Legal liability concerns, changing hospital practices, and trends in consumer demand influence the balance between these two orientations.

How should the MCH community balance the competing visions of birth as a natural process or as a risky event requiring the most advanced medical techniques available? Both views on the birth process capture a truth and express concern for the health of mothers and newborns. Women who have been historically excluded from high-quality health services may rightfully perceive an equal entitlement to technology. To some, natural childbirth is seen as the most psychologically and physically healthy manner to have a child; to others, it represents unnecessary endangerment of both mother and child. The debate is shaped by strong ideological views and personal experience, as well as strong professional identities and economic interests. How can we continue to reduce mortality and morbidity without disempowering women in the experience of pregnancy and birth?

There has been a major shift in the timing of births over the past 2 decades, due to substantial changes in obstetric practice. First, there has been a gradual rise in the percentage of labors that are induced (23.1% in 2008) in the United States. This rise in induced labor may be due in part because of changing trends in preterm delivery and cesarean section. However, it is unclear what proportion is medically indicated as opposed to elective.

A second change witnessed in the United States has been a 25% increase in the late preterm delivery rate (36–37 weeks gestation) from 1990–2006 (Martin et al., 2010). Although the delivery of an infant at 37–38 weeks may be safer than at 34 weeks or less, it is not without risk. Shapiro-Mendoza and colleagues (2008) showed that late preterm birth is an independent risk factor for newborn morbidity. In particular, they found a doubling of the newborn morbidity rate for each gestational week earlier than 38 weeks. If a mother experienced medical complications during pregnancy, a late preterm delivery of her child was associated with a higher risk for newborn morbidity compared to those who would be delivered at term (Shapiro-Mendoza et al., 2008). Similarly, infants delivered late preterm have a higher mortality rate compared to their term peers (Tomashek et al., 2007). It is unclear how much of the rise in late preterm births is due to (1) obstetricians' electively delivering babies early to prevent future harm, (2) changing cohort compositions (e.g., more multiple births due to assisted reproductive technologies and older mothers), (3) elective cesarean sections, or (4) a true rise in prematurity. This issue remains widely debated.

Another controversial change in obstetric practice in the United States has been the rise in cesarean section delivery. Cesarean section deliveries accounted for 32.3% of all births in 2008 (Martin et al., 2010). The rise in cesarean section deliveries is due to a rise in primary cesarean sections and a decline in vaginal birth after cesarean (VBAC). There is very strong evidence that cesarean section deliveries reduce maternal and infant mortality in specific delivery situations, such as obstructed labor and preeclamptic conditions. However, the optimal level of cesarean section deliveries is subject to much debate because they entail major surgery that introduces new risk to both mothers and infants (e.g., anesthesia complications, infection, iatrogenic prematurity). The national objective for *Healthy People 2020* is to reduce the cesarean delivery rate for first-time mothers to no more than 23.9 per 100 deliveries.

Besides the belief in the clinical safety and value of a cesarean section delivery, many financial, convenience, and legal incentives still make it a popular procedure for obstetricians. In 2007, the American College of Obstetricians and Gynecologists issued a committee opinion on cesarean delivery on maternal request. The committee concluded that cesarean delivery on maternal request is not recommended (1) before gestational age of 39 weeks, (2) based on the unavailability of effective pain management, or (3) for women desiring several children (ACOG, 2007). Although this is a popular argument, recent studies of elective cesarean delivery have shown very few women electing to have an elective cesarean delivery in the absence of cause (Declercq, Sakala, Corry, & Applebaum, 2007).

Controversy over the desirability of obstetric interventions and hospital competition has led both to more midwife-attended births and to marketing of more supportive, family-friendly birthing practices within hospitals, including the development of doula (labor support) programs. The vast majority of births (99%) take place in hospitals in the United States, and most deliveries are assisted by physicians (91.3%) (Martin et al., 2010). With increasing professionalization of the midwifery field, including the ability to obtain third-party reimbursement, there has been a steady increase to 8.0% in midwifery-assisted births over the past decade (7.5% by certified nurse midwives and 0.5% by other midwives) (Martin, 2010). Several European countries, including the Netherlands, have substantially more home births and more births assisted by midwives. Numerous studies have shown that birth outcomes for low-risk women attended by midwives are comparable, but with substantially fewer delivery complications (e.g., tears, C-section, anesthesia), to the outcomes of births attended by physicians.

Debate continues, however, about optimal settings, attendants, and modes of delivery. There has also been growth in the use of doulas (labor support coaches) to further enhance the birthing process for women. Studies show that they are well received and effective in reducing surgical obstetric interventions (McGrath & Kennell, 2008).

Postpartum or Interconception Care

A wide range of postpartum treatments can influence birth outcomes. The postpartum period, like the preconception period, is becoming a major focus for reproductive health initiatives. Traditionally, the postpartum period has addressed the quality of newborn services and access to neonatal medicine, public health infant mortality and morbidity prevention programs, infant transition to pediatric care and early intervention services if needed, and limited maternal postnatal follow-up. Today, a new focus is emerging on interconception care for maternal and infant health.

The postpartum period should be an important period for maternal intervention. Pregnancy is a major life event that can bring both joys and stresses to a woman's life. From a biological and social point of view, pregnancy and delivery are a stress test of life. Several critical postdelivery health risks may emerge that can have an impact on the woman's own subsequent health, her reproductive health in future pregnancies, and her capacity for optimal parenting. These include diabetes, hypertension, obesity, injuries, intimate partner violence and postpartum depression, as well as recovery from a cesarean delivery. Several other key health issues also emerge in this period, including subsequent family planning, breastfeeding, resumption of smoking or other substance use, and connectedness to primary care.

Traditionally, the 6-week postpartum follow-up visit is the only formal healthcare visit recommended to address maternal health. This visit focuses primarily on delivery follow-up care and family planning resumption, as too many mothers in the United States have no further contact with the healthcare system for themselves until their next pregnancy. Unfortunately, not all postpartum women attend this recommended medical visit. Recent data from the CDC show that only 89% of women attended a postpartum care visit 4 to 6 weeks after delivery (CDC, 2007). However, this prevalence was lower in some population subgroups, such as those who did not receive prenatal care (66%) and those who reported having 8 or fewer years of education (71%). As the 6-week postpartum visit is an opportune time to discuss postpartum family planning, it is apparent that the current system of care for postpartum women is inadequate for maternal health.

In the past decade, there has been a growth in the concept of interconception care, that is, in the development of an organized system for maternal (and infant) health care in the postpartum period. Much as preconception health care addresses women's health and reproductive health and health care before pregnancy, interconception care also addresses women's health but further along her life course. Interconception care can also be more narrowly viewed as preconception care for a subsequent pregnancy.

Interconception care recognizes the profound impact of pregnancy on women's health; it addresses the continuity of risk from one pregnancy to the next. However, this is still a relatively new and underappreciated topic in maternal and child health. Interconception care initiatives can be seen as a strategy to address women's health (postdelivery and longitudinally); as a strategy to enhance the health of the parent and caregiver, as a strategy to reduce subsequent infant mortality, and as a possible strategy to reduce racial disparities in birth outcomes.

As part of its new preconception health and healthcare initiative, the CDC has included interconception (postpartum) care as a key component of preconception care

(CDC, 2006), wherein care between two pregnancies is viewed, in part, as preconception care for the next pregnancy. The CDC is implicitly recommending both general preconception care for all women and specifically more intensive care for women with a poor birth outcome, because a prior poor birth outcome is the strongest risk factor predictor for a subsequent poor birth outcome.

The CDC's postpartum care recommendation initial steps include (1) monitoring the percent of women with postpartum visits; (2) developing interconception care and interconception care coordination models; (3) enhancing the content of postpartum visits to provide preconception care content; (4) using existing public health programs to link women to other postpartum services; and (5) using Title V and other existing public health programs to fund interconception care demonstration projects.

Interconception care should be easier than preconception care programs to implement, because virtually all births and mothers are known and easy to locate, and they are more operationally feasible using existing public health and clinical care programs. Most women stay engaged with the healthcare system for their children's pediatric care or for their own family planning. Interconception care programs do not depend on a planned pregnancy, and could build off of the existing 6-week postpartum visit. "We must conceptualize the six week postpartum visit not as the end of pregnancy, but as the beginning of a new women's longitudinal health initiative" (Kotelchuck, 2008).

New interconception care programs are being proposed (Lu et al., 2006). They recommend four postpartum visits, with the contents for each visit proposed. Many hospitals have already added a 2-week postpartum visit, especially for women who had cesarean section. Unfortunately, there are numerous barriers to such programs. Clinician supply of interconception care is low, as they have not traditionally provided it, and there are no clinical billing codes assigned for interconception care. Women have yet to demand it, since

traditionally there was no source of payment, little awareness of its value or availability, and more focus on their newborns' care.

Some disagree with the CDC recommendation that only women who had poor birth outcomes should have intensive interconception care; others believe that all women should have interconception care with special referral to a level of appropriate care for those with higher risk conditions (Kotelchuck, 2007).

Besides proposals for broader restructuring of interconception care programs, some very concrete maternal postpartum interventions are being proposed and implemented. One major set of clinical care initiatives involves increasing follow-up of high-risk women with chronic conditions, especially those that manifest in pregnancy, such as gestational diabetes or gestational hypertension. Virtually all major professional groups recommend follow-up screening for women with gestational diabetes, since it is a strong precursor of subsequent diabetes, and women would benefit from further dietary and clinical counseling (ACOG, 2009). Unfortunately, rates of follow-up testing for women with gestational diabetes are low. For example, a study in Philadelphia showed that only 20% of women with gestational diabetes received a documented order for postpartum diabetes mellitus screening by their obstetrician (Almario et al., 2008).

As with preconception care, existing public health programs have more readily embraced efforts to increase interconception care for both the mother and the infant. Healthy Start now requires each program site to offer as one of its core components interconception care (including case management, health education, and home visits) to all of its maternal and infant enrollees until the infant is 2 years of age. This is the first large national program to require postpartum care involvement. Healthy Start implementation is uneven, and sites report difficulty in client retention and balancing prenatal and postnatal activities (Brand et al., 2010), but they have learned large numbers of practical lessons/best practices in an interconception care learning collaborative (Badura et al., 2008).

The Centering Pregnancy program has expanded into Centering Parenting (postpartum group-based care) that allows for addressing women's postpartum health issues simultaneously with obtaining infant pediatric well baby visits. (See http://www.centeringhealthcare.org.) Its effectiveness has yet to be evaluated; but it does add a group empowerment component to an otherwise isolated and often nonexistent maternal health care. Pediatricians also offer some postpartum women's health care as part of their family care model, including assessing and counseling on maternal health issues such as smoking, intimate partner violence and abuse, and depression. Pediatric offices might be a good site for future interconception care programs, as women who bring their infants to pediatric offices have substantial morbidity (Kahn et al., 1999).

There has also been a new focus in the National Institute of Mental Health and the Maternal and Child Health Bureau on maternal depression and other mood disorders during and after pregnancy and their impact on subsequent women's and children's health and development. It is estimated that approximately 12 to 20% of women experience postpartum depression (CDC, 2008). Maternal depression is increasingly being viewed as a chronic illness, not solely as an episodic postpartum phenomenon. It has been linked to smoking, substance use, interpersonal violence, poor nutrition, and decreased access to and use of health care and family planning services. Several states, such as Illinois, now reimburse any provider for postpartum depression screening of Medicaid patients. New efforts in the Healthy Start initiative and other federal programs are addressing the identification, referral, and treatment of women with chronic depression around the time of pregnancy and early motherhood. These

initiatives include enhanced maternal depression screening and referral in pediatric care (a two-generation model of pediatric care) and in child development programs (including Early Head Start), as well as the development of community-based nonprofessional treatment programs and activities. The linkage of traditional MCH and reproductive clinical care with mental health services is a critical public health issue that deserves increased attention.

In sum, a series of postnatal public health and clinical programs exist that are directed toward both the mothers' and infants' health, but they are scattered programs without a coherent and comprehensive maternal health legacy. There are many more opportunities to develop programs that could assess, treat, and better ensure maternal postpartum health over the life course. For example, very few prevention programs focus on resumption of maternal smoking in the postpartum period, despite the fact that half of women who stop smoking cigarettes during pregnancy resume smoking after delivery. The postpartum period is also extremely important as the initiation into parenthood for new mothers, their partners, and their families. For routine uncomplicated deliveries, the postpartum hospitalization should offer opportunities for physical recovery and stabilization of the mother and newborn, psychological adaptation, maternal education, and observation of both the mother's and infant's health status. Current insurance and hospital policies allow little time for any of these functions, and the duration of hospitalization for delivery has become a major public health and policy issue. The average length of stay for a hospital delivery is approximately 2 days for a vaginal birth and 4 days for a C-section, much shorter than the time required for manifestation of many problems that require medical care and advice. Often women are discharged even more quickly. Initially, early discharge programs were offered only to low-risk women in order to free hospital beds and to meet consumer demand for a less medicalized birth experience. In such programs in the 1970s, women were carefully screened for participation and received extensive in-home follow-up services. As cost-containment pressures have become more dominant, early discharge has become routine and involuntary for almost all women without serious medical complications.

Margolis, Kotelchuck, and Chang (1997) showed that women discharged early are actually more likely to be those with risk characteristics, such as teenagers and women lacking private health insurance. The consequences of this fiscally driven policy for MCH are unknown. By the late 1990s, the U.S. Congress and 43 states had passed legislation mandating insurers to cover postpartum hospital stays for a minimum of 48 hours after vaginal deliveries and 96 hours after C-sections. The impact of that legislation has generally been favorable, with decreases in rehospitalization for neonatal jaundice and fewer subsequent emergency department visits, especially for those newborns with early home follow-up visits (Meara, Kotagal, Atherton, & Lieu, 2004).

Access to regionalized neonatal intensive care units for high-risk infants and improvements in neonatal medicine have dramatically improved infant survival (BWSM rates) over the last half century. Recent advancements in intrapartum antibiotics, high-frequency ventilation, and surfactant, an agent that enhances the elasticity of the fetal lung surface, have dramatically improved birth outcomes and the quality of life for premature VLBW newborns. Surfactant has had a major impact on premature infants with RDS; it is estimated that 50% of the decrease in the U.S. infant mortality rates in the 1990s was due to the introduction and use of this agent. There have been no new breakthrough neonatal interventions in the past decade, which is reflected in the relative stability of BWSM rates (Mathews & MacDorman, 2008) and the lack of significant improvement in infant mortality rates in the 21st century. There is some concern that the increasing frequency of VLBW infant survival may be associated with an increase in the incidence of cerebral palsy.

One of the most successful recent public health programs directed at infant mortality is the American Academy of Pediatrics' "Back to Sleep" campaign. This campaign, begun in 1992, encourages parents to place infants to sleep on their backs or sides, rather than placing them on their stomachs, in order to reduce the incidence of Sudden Infant Death Syndrome (SIDS), the leading cause of postneonatal death in the United States. Deaths associated with SIDS have dropped dramatically (over 50%) since 1992 as infants sleeping in the supine position increased from only 13% in 1992 to 74% in 2009 (National Infant Sleep Position Study, 2011). The decline in SIDS deaths has continued at a slower pace in recent years.

CONTINUED IMPROVEMENTS IN REPRODUCTIVE HEALTH INTO THE 21ST CENTURY

Major improvements in reproductive health were one of the great achievements of public health in the 20th century. Reductions in infant mortality (from 150 to 7 infant deaths per 1,000 births) and maternal mortality (from 750 to 10 maternal deaths per 100,000 births) have dramatically changed the lives and expectations of mothers, children, and families. These achievements were accomplished through a broad array of public health activities and struggles. There have been substantial changes in our understanding of the causes of poor birth outcomes, in clinical and public health practices to address reproductive health, in opportunities for women, and in the overall public health of our communities, as well as changes in the role and responsibility of government for the health of our newest citizens and their parents.

Political and professional challenges remain to further improving reproductive health in the United States and abroad. Our scientific and epidemiologic knowledge base about reproductive outcomes remains inadequate. We need to strengthen women's health/life course programs, preconception care, prenatal care, delivery services, postpartum, and interconception care intervention programs. The success of European experiences with comprehensive health and social benefits for mothers and families suggests that birth outcomes are not impervious to public health interventions. Finally, and perhaps most important, we must improve our reproductive health policies and funding support in order to implement necessary and successful public health and social welfare programs. The continued existence of severe disparities remains an unacceptable burden on the African American community, a stark reminder of societal inequities and injustice, and a compelling challenge to the MCH field. The new MCH life course perspective can provide us with new insights and humility about our future endeavors. The political and professional legacy of our MCH foremothers and forefathers should be a challenge, and an inspiration, to improve reproductive health care further for mothers and infants in the 21st century.

References

Alexander, G. R., Himes, J. H., Kaufman, R. B., Mor, J., & Kogan, M. (1996). A United States national reference for fetal growth. *Obstetrics & Gynecology, 87*, 163–168.

Alexander, G. R., Kogan, M. D., & Nabukera, S. (2002). Racial differences in prenatal care use in the United States: are disparities decreasing? *American Journal of Public Health, 92*, 1970–1975.

Almario, C. V., Ecker, T., Moroz, L. A., Bucovetsky, L., Berghella, V., & Baxter, J. K. (2008). Obstetricians seldom provide postpartum diabetes screening for women with gestational diabetes. *American Journal of Obstetrics and Gynecology, 198*, 528.e1–528.e5.

American College of Obstetricians and Gynecologists, Committee on Obstetric Practice. (2007). ACOG Committee Opinion: Cesarean delivery on maternal request. *Obstetrics and Gynecology, 110*, 1501–1504.

American College of Obstetricians and Gynecologists, Committee on Obstetric Practice (2009). ACOG Committee Opinion: Postpartum screening for abnormal glucose tolerance in women who had gestational diabetes. *Obstetrics and Gynecology, 113*, 1419–1421.

Andres, R. L., & Day, M.-C. (2000). Perinatal complications associated with maternal tobacco use. *Seminars in Neonatology, 5*(3), 231–241.

Arias, E., MacDorman, M. F., Strobino, D. M., & Guyer, B. (2003). Annual summary of vital statistics: 2002. *Pediatrics, 112*, 1215–1230.

Atrash, H. K., Koonin, L. M., Lawson, H. W., Franks, A. L., & Smith, J. C. (1990). Maternal mortality in the United States, 1979–1986. *American Journal of Obstetrics and Gynecology, 76*, 1055–1060.

Badura, M., Johnson, K., Hench, K., & Reyes, M. (2008). Healthy Start lessons learned on interconception care. *Women's Health Issues, 18*, S61–S66.

Berkowitz, G. S., & Papiernik, E. (1993). Epidemiology of preterm birth. *Epidemiologic Reviews, 15*, 414–443.

Blackmore, C. A., Ferre, C. D., Rowley, D. L., Hogue, C. J., Gaiter, J., & Atrash, H. (1993). Is race a risk factor or a risk marker for preterm delivery? *Ethnicity & Disease, 3*(4), 372–377.

Brand, A., Walker, D. K., Hargreaves, M., & Rosenbach, M. (2010). Intermediate outcomes, strategies, and challenges of eight healthy start projects. *Maternal and Child Health Journal, 14*, 654–665.

Brann, A. W., & Cefalo, R. C. (Eds.). (1992). *Guidelines for perinatal care* (3rd ed.). Evanston, IL, Washington, DC: American Academy of Pediatrics and American College of Obstetricians and Gynecologists.

Bremner, R. H. (Ed.). (1971). *Children and youth in America: A documentary history* (Vol. 2, Pt. 8). Cambridge, MA: Harvard University Press.

Brown, S. S. (1985). Can low birth weight be prevented? *Family Planning Perspectives, 17*(3), 112–118.

Buckelew, S. M., Pierrie, H., & Chabra, A. (2006). What fathers need: a county-wide assessment of fathers of young children. *Maternal and Child Health Journal, 10*, 285–291; Epub 2005 Oct. 18.

Buekens, P., & Klebanoff, M. (2001). Preterm birth research: From disillusion to the search for new mechanisms. *Pediatric and Perinatal Epidemiology, 15*(Suppl. 2), 159–161.

Cefalo, R. C., & Moos, M. K. (1995). *Preconceptional health care: A practical guide* (2nd ed.). St. Louis, MO: Mosby.

Centers for Disease Control and Prevention. (2006). Recommendations to improve preconception health and health care—United States: a report of the CDC/ATSDR Preconception Care Work Group and the Select Panel on Preconception Care. *MMWR, 55* (No. RR-6).

Centers for Disease Control and Prevention. (2007). Postpartum care visits—11 states and New York City, 2004. *MMWR, 56,* 1312–1316.

Centers for Disease Control and Prevention. (2008). Prevalence of Self-Reported Postpartum Depressive Symptoms—17 States, 2004–2005. *MMWR, 57,* 361–366.

Cramer, J. C. (1987). Social factors and infant mortality: identifying high-risk groups and proximate causes. *Demography, 24,* 299–322.

Declercq, E. R., Sakala, C., Corry, M. P., & Applebaum, S. (2007). Listening to mothers II: Report of the second national U.S. survey of women's childbearing experiences: conducted January-February 2006 for childbirth connection by Harris Interactive® in partnership with Lamaze International. *Journal of Perinatal Education, 16,* 9–14.

Devaney, B., Howell, E. M., McCormick, M., & Moreno, L. (2000). *Reducing infant mortality: Lessons learned from Healthy Start.* Final report. Princeton, NJ: Mathematica Policy Research.

Diez Roux, A. V. (2007). Integrating social and biologic factors in health research: A systems view. *Ann Epidemiol, 17*(7), 569–574.

Fine, A., & Kotelchuck, M. (2010). Rethinking MCH: The Life Course Model as an organizing framework. Concept paper to the Maternal and Child Health Bureau, Retrieved October 2, 2001 from http://www.aucd.org/docs/lend/hrsa_kotelchuck _lifecourse2010.pdf.

Fiscella, K. (1995). Does prenatal care improve birth outcomes? A critical review. *Obstetrics and Gynecology, 85,* 468–479.

Frey, K. A., Navarro, S. M., Kotelchuck, M., & Lu, M. C. (2008). The clinical content of preconception care: preconception care for men. *American Journal of Obstetrics and Gynecology, 199,* S389–S395.

Frisbie, W. P., Song, S. E., Powers, D. A.,& Street, J. A. (2004). The increasing racial disparity in infant mortality: Respiratory distress syndrome and other causes. *Demography,* 41(4), 773–800.

Genc, M. R., Vardhana, S., Delaney, M. L., Witkin, S. S., & Onderdonk, A. B. (2007). TNFA-308G > A polymorphism influences the TNF-alpha response to altered vaginal flora. *Eur J Obstet Gynecol Reprod Biol, 134*(2), 188–191.

Goldenberg, R. L., & Culhane, J. F. (2003). Infection as a cause of preterm birth. *Clinics in Perinatology, 30*(4), 677–700.

Goldenberg, R. L., & Culhane, J. F. (2007). Low birth weight in the United States. *American Journal of Clinical Nutrition, 85*(2), 584S–590S.

Goldenberg, R. L., & Rouse, D. J. (1998). Prevention of premature birth. *New England Journal of Medicine, 339,* 313–320.

Goldenberg, R. L., Culhane, J. F., Iams, J. D., & Romero, R. (2008). Epidemiology and causes of preterm birth. *Lancet, 371,* 75–84.

Goldenberg, R. L., Hauth, J. C., & Andrews, W. W. (2000). Intrauterine infection and preterm delivery. *New England Journal of Medicine, 342*(20), 1500–1507.

Gortmaker, S. L., & Wise, P. H. (1997). The first injustice: socioeconomic disparities, health services technology, and infant mortality. *Annu Rev Sociol, 23,* 147–170.

Harville, E. W., Hatch, M. C., & Zhang, J. (2005). Perceived life stress and bacterial vaginosis. *Journal of Women's Health (Larchmont), 14*(7), 627–633.

Hobel, C., & Culhane, J. (2003). Role of psychosocial and nutritional stress on poor pregnancy outcome. *Journal of Nutrition, 133,* 1709–1717.

Horn, W. F. (2000). Fathering infants. In J. D. Osofsky, & H. E. Fitzgerald, (Eds). *Handbook of infant mental health.* New York: Wiley and Sons, Inc.

Horon, I. L. (2005). Underreporting of maternal deaths on death certificates and the magnitude of the problem of maternal mortality. *American Journal of Public Health, 95,* 478–482.

Horta, B. L., Victora, C. G., Menezes, A. M., Halpern, R., & Barros, F. C. (1997). Low birthweight, preterm births and intrauterine growth retardation in relation to maternal smoking. *Paediatric and perinatal epidemiology, 11*(2), 140.

Ickovics, J. R., Kershaw, T. S., Westdahl, C., Magriples, U., Massey, Z., & Reynolds, H. (2007). Rising SS. Group prenatal care and perinatal outcomes: A randomized control trial. *Obstetrics & Gynecology, 110,* 330–339.

Institute of Medicine, Committee to Study the Prevention of Low Birthweight. (1985). Preventing low birthweight. Washington, DC: National Academy Press.

Institute of Medicine. (1988). Prenatal care: Reaching mothers, reaching infants. Washington, DC: National Academy Press.

James, S. A. (1993). Racial and ethnic differences in infant mortality and low birth weight. A psychosocial critique. *Annals of Epidemiology, 3*(2), 130–136.

Kahn, R. S., Wise, P. H., Finkelstein, J. A., Bernstein, H. H., Lowe, J. A., & Homer, C. J. (1999). The scope of unmet maternal needs in pediatric settings. *Pediatrics, 103*(3), 576–581.

Kitzman, H. J., Olds, D. J., Cole, R. E., Hanks, C. A., Anson, E. A., Arcoleo, K. J., Luckey, D. W., Knudtson, M. D., Henderson, Jr., C. R., & Holmberg, J. R. (2010). Enduring effects of prenatal and infancy home visiting by nurses and children: Follow-up of a randomized trial among children at age 12 years. *Archives of Pediatrics and Adolescent Medicine, 164*, 412–418.

Kitzman, H., Olds, D. L., Henderson, Jr., C. R., Hanks, C., Cole, R., Tatelbaum, R., McConnochie, K. M., Sidora, K., Luckey, D. W., Shaver, D., Engelhardt, K., James, D., & Barnard, K. (1997). Effect of prenatal and infancy home visitation by nurses on pregnancy outcomes, childhood injuries, and repeated childbearing: a randomized controlled trial. *JAMA, 278*, 644–652.

Kogan, M. D., Alexander, G. R., Kotelchuck, M., Nagey, D. A., & Jack, B. W. (1994). Comparing mothers' reports on the content of prenatal care received with recommended national guidelines for care. *Public Health Reports, 109*, 637–646.

Kogan, M. D. (1995). Social causes of low birth weight. *Journal of the Royal Society of Medicine, 88*(11), 611–615.

Korenbrot, C. C. (2002). Preconception care: A systematic review. *Maternal and Child Health Journal, 6*, 75–88.

Kotelchuck, M. (1994). The adequacy of prenatal care utilization index: Its US distribution and association with low birthweight. *American Journal of Public Health, 74*, 1086–1092.

Kotelchuck, M. (2008). *Women's health and preconceptional care between pregnancies: Development of internatal care programs.* Delaware Summit on Maternal and Child Health, Dover, DE.

Kotelchuck, M., & Fine, A. (2000). *The Healthy Start Initiative: Strategic assessment and policy options.* Washington, DC: U.S. Department of Health and Human Services, Health Resources and Service Administration.

Kramer, M. S. (1987). Determinants of low birth weight: methodological assessment and meta-analysis. *Bulletin of the World Health Organization, 65*, 663–737.

Kramer, M. R., & Hogue, C. R. (2009). What causes racial disparities in very preterm birth? A biosocial perspective. *Epidemiologic Reviews, 31*, 84–98.

Krieger, N. (2001). The ostrich, the albatross, and public health: An ecosocial perspective—or why an explicit focus on health consequences of discrimination and deprivation is vital for good science and public health practice. *Public Health Reports, 116*, 419–423.

Link, B. G., & Phelan, J. (1995). Social conditions as fundamental causes of disease. *J Health Soc Behav, Spec No*, 80–94.

Link, B. G., & Phelan, J. C. (1996). Understanding sociodemographic differences in health—the role of fundamental social causes. *Am J Public Health, 86*(4), 471–473.

Lockwood, C. J., & Kuczynski, E. (2001). Risk stratification and pathological mechanisms in preterm delivery. *Paediatric and Perinatal Epidemiology, 15*(Suppl. 2), 78–89.

Lu, M. C., & Halfon, N. (2003). Racial and ethnic disparities in birth outcomes: A life-course perspective. *Maternal and Child Health Journal, 7*, 13–30.

Lu, M. C., Prentice, J., Yu, S. M., Inkelas, M., Lange, L. O., & Halfon, N. (2003). Childbirth education classes: Sociodemographic disparities in attendance and the association of attendance with breastfeeding initiation. *Maternal and Child Health Journal, 7*, 87–94.

Lu, M. C., Kotelchuck, M., Culhane, J. F., Hobel, C. J., Klerman, L. V., & Thorp, Jr., J. M. (2006). Preconception care between pregnancies: The content of internatal care. *Maternal and Child Health Journal, 10*, S107–S122.

Lu, M. C., Kotelchuck, M., Hogan, V., Jones, L., Wright, K., Halfon, N. (2010). Closing the Black-White gap in birth outcomes: a life-course approach. *Ethnicity and Disease, 20*, S2-62-76.

MacDorman, M. F., & Kirmeyer, S. (2009). Fetal and perinatal mortality, United States, 2005. *National Vital Statistics Reports, 57*(8). Hyattsville, MD: National Center for Health Statistics.

Macones, G. A., Parry, S., Elkousy, M., Clothier, B., Ural, S. H., & Strauss, J. F. (2004). A polymorphism in the promoter region of TNF and bacterial vaginosis: preliminary evidence of gene-environment interaction in the etiology of spontaneous preterm birth. *American Journal of Obstetrics and Gynecology, 190*(6), 1504–1508.

Margolis, L. H., Kotelchuck, M., & Chang, H-Y. (1997). Factors associated with early maternal postpartum discharge from the hospital. *Archives of Pediatrics & Adolescent Medicine, 151,* 466–472.

Martin, J. A., Hamilton, B. E., Sutton, P. D., Ventura, S. J., Mathews, T. J., & Osterman, M. J. K. (2010). Births: Final data for 2008: *National Vital Statistics Reports, 59*(1), Hyattsville, MD: National Center for Health Statistics.

Mathews, T. J., & MacDorman, M. F. (2008). Infant mortality statistics from the 2005 period linked birth/infant death data set: *National Vital Statistics Reports, 57*(2), Hyattsville, MD: National Center for Health Statistics.

McCormick, M. C., Deal, L. W., Devaney, B. L., Chu, D., Moreno, L., & Raykovich, K. T. (2001). The impact on clients of a community-based infant mortality reduction program: the national healthy start program survey of postpartum women. *American Journal of Public Health, 91,* 1975–1977.

McGrath, S. K., & Kennell, J. H. (2008). A randomized controlled trial of continuous labor support for middle-class couples: effect on cesarean delivery rates. *Birth, 35,* 92–97.

Meara, E., Kotagal, U. R., Atherton, H. D., & Lieu, T. A. (2004). Impact of early newborn discharge legislation and early follow-up visits on infant outcomes in a state Medicaid population. *Pediatrics, 113,* 1619–1627.

Mercer, B. M., Goldenberg, R. L., Moawad, A. H., Meis, P. J., Iams, J. D., Das, A. F., et al. (1999). The preterm prediction study: effect of gestational age and cause of preterm birth on subsequent obstetric outcome. National Institute of Child Health and Human Development Maternal-Fetal Medicine Units Network. *American Journal of Obstetrics and Gynecology, 181*(5, Pt 1), 1216–1221.

Misra, D. P., Guyer, B., & Allston, A. (2003). Integrated perinatal health framework. A multiple determinants model with a life span approach. *American Journal of Preventive Medicine, 25,* 65–75.

Moore, M. L. (2003). Preterm labor and birth: what have we learned in the past two decades? *Journal of Obstetric, Gynecologic, and Neonatal Nursing, 32*(5), 638–649.

Moos, M.-K. (1989). Preconceptional health promotion: a health education opportunity for all women. *Women Health 1989, 5*(3), 55–67.

Moos, M.-K. (2002). Preconceptional health promotion: Opportunities abound. *Maternal and Child Health Journal, 6,* 71–74.

Morello-Frosch, R., & Shenassa, E. D. (2006). The environmental "riskscape" and social inequality: implications for explaining maternal and child health disparities. *Environ Health Perspect, 114*(8), 1150–1153.

Mrs. A-C-P to Julia Lathrop, Chief of the US Children's Bureau (1971, June 24). October 19, 1916, folder 634, Ethel S. Dummer Papers. Schlesinger Library, Radcliffe College. In R. H. Bremner (Ed.), *Children and youth in America: A documentary history* (p. 1071). Cambridge, MA: Harvard University Press.

Muglia, L. J., & Katz, M. (2010). The enigma of spontaneous preterm birth. *New England Journal of Medicine, 362*(6), 529–535.

National Infant Sleep Position Study. Retrieved March 23, 2011 from http://dcc2.bumc.bu.edu/Chimenisp/Tables_in_PDF/NISP%201992-2009%20The%20usual%20sleep%20position.pdf.

Olds, D. L. (2002). Prenatal and infancy home visiting by nurses: from randomized trials to community replication. *Prevention Science, 3,* 153–172.

Olds, D. L., Kitzman, H. J., Cole, R. E., Hanks, C. A., Arcoleo, K. J., Anson, E. A., Luckey, D. W., Knudtson, M. D., Henderson, Jr., C. R., Bondy, J., & Stevenson, A. J. (2010). Enduring effects of prenatal and infancy home visiting by nurses on maternal life course and government spending: Follow-up of a randomized trial among children age 12 years. *Archives of Pediatrics and Adolescent Medicine, 164,* 419–424.

Peoples-Sheps, M. D., Hogan, V. K., & Ng'andu, N. (1996). Content of prenatal care during the initial work-up. *American Journal of Obstetrics and Gynecology, 174,* 220–226.

Public Health Service Expert Panel on the Content of Prenatal Care. (1989). *Caring for our future: The content of prenatal care.* Washington, DC: U.S. Public Health Service.

Rittenhouse, D. R., Braveman, P., & Marchi, K. (2003). Improvements in prenatal insurance coverage and utilization of care in California: An unsung public health victory. *Maternal and Child Health Journal, 7,* 75–86.

Robertson, B., Aycock, D., & Darnell, L. (2009). Comparison of centering pregnancy to traditional care in Hispanic mothers. *Maternal and Child Health Journal, 13,* 407–414.

Rochat, R., Koonin, L. M., Atrash, H. K., & Jewett, J. F. (1988). Maternal mortality in the United States: Report from the Maternal Mortality Collaborative. *Obstetrics and Gynecology, 72*, 91–97.

Rubin, D. M., O'Reilly, A. L. R., Luan, X., Dai, D., Russel Localio, A., & Christian, C. W. (2011). Variation in pregnancy outcomes following statewide implementation of a prenatal home visitation program. *Archives of Pediatric and Adolescent Medicine, 165*, 198–204.

Ruiz, R. J., Fullerton, J., Brown, C. E. L., & Schoolfield, J. (2001). Relationships of cortisol, perceived stress, genitourinary infections, and fetal fibronectin to gestational age at birth. *Biological Research for Nursing, 3*, 39–48.

Ruiz, R. J., Fullerton, J., & Dudley, D. J. (2003). The interrelationship of maternal stress, endocrine factors and inflammation on gestational length. *Obstetrical & Gynecological Survey, 58*(6), 415–428.

Selwyn, B. J. (1990). The accuracy of obstetric risk assessment instruments for predicting mortality, low birth weight, and preterm birth. In I. R. Merkatz & J. E. Thompson (Eds.), *New perspectives on prenatal care*. New York: Elsevier.

Shapiro-Mendoza, C. K., Tomashek, K. M., Kotelchuck, M., Barfield, W., Nannini, A., Weiss, J., & Declercq, E. (2008). Effect of late-preterm birth and maternal medical conditions on newborn morbidity risk. *Pediatrics, 121*, e223–e232.

Tomashek, K. M., Shapiro-Mendoza, C. K., Davidoff, M. J., & Petrini, J. R. (2007). Differences in mortality between late-preterm and term singleton infants in the United States, 1995–2002. *Journal of Pediatrics, 151*, 450–456.

Tsai, H. J., Liu, X., Mestan, K., Yu, Y., Zhang, S., Fang, Y., et al. (2008). Maternal cigarette smoking, metabolic gene polymorphisms, and preterm delivery: new insights on GxE interactions and pathogenic pathways. *Human Genetics, 123*(4), 359–369.

U.S. Department of Health and Human Services, Health Resources and Services Administration, Maternal and Child Health Bureau. (2008). *A profile of Healthy Start: Findings from Phase I of the Evaluation 2006*. Rockville, MD: Author.

Valero De Bernabe, J., Soriano, T., Albaladejo, R., Juarranz, M., Calle, M. E., Martinez, D., et al. (2004). Risk factors for low birth weight: a review. *European Journal of Obstetrics & Gynecology and Reproductive Biology, 116*(1), 3–15.

Wang, X., Zuckerman, B., Pearson, C., Kaufman, G., Chen, C., Wang, G., et al. (2002). Maternal cigarette smoking, metabolic gene polymorphism, and infant birth weight. *Jama, 287*(2), 195–202.

Wertz, R. W., & Wertz, D. C. (1982). *Lying-in: A history of childbirth in America*. New York: Schocken Books.

Wile, I. S. (1910). Do medical schools adequately train students for the prevention of infant mortality? Transactions of the American Association for Study and Prevention of Infant Mortality. In R. H. Bremner (Ed.), *Children and youth in America: A documentary history* (Vol. 2, Pt. 8, p. 965). Cambridge, MA: Harvard University Press.

Wise, P. H., & Pursley, D. M. (1992). Infant mortality as a social mirror. *New England Journal of Medicine, 326*(23), 1558–1560.

World Health Organization. (2010). *Trends in maternal mortality: 1990 to 2008*. Geneva: World Health Organization.

Xu, J. Q., Kochanek, K. D., Murphy, S. L., & Tejada-Vera, B. (2010). Deaths: Final data for 2007. *National vital statistics report, s58*(19). Hyattsville, MD: National Center for Health Statistics. 2010.

7

THE CHILD FROM ONE TO FOUR: THE TODDLER AND PRESCHOOL YEARS

J. Kerr, D. Steffen, and J.B. Kotch

The importance of early childhood for future health cannot be overstated. During this period, the children, born totally helpless and dependent, gain the cognitive intelligence (IQ[1]) and social-emotional intelligence/executive functions (EQ[2]) necessary for successful school entry. Their physical growth accelerates at a rate only rivaled by that of adolescence. It is, however, their emotional and social growth that determines their school readiness. Of particular concern recently has been the lack of the child's development of emotional self-regulation, ability to shift attention successfully, exhibit inhibitory control, and develop working memory- the components of executive functioning.

(Shonkoff, Boyce, & McEwen, 2009)

INTRODUCTION

In recognition of the importance of this developmental phase, the *Healthy People 2020 Health Objectives for the Nation* have added an emphasis on the life course approach to health and have established an early and middle childhood stage. Its first objective is to "increase the proportion of children who are ready for school in all five domains of healthy development: physical development, social-emotional development, approaches to learning, language, and cognitive development" (USDHHS, n.d.).

Children are born ready to learn and grow and have feelings that are affected positively by nurturing relationships. Like seeds, their growth will occur if the seed's biological makeup is sound (nature) and they enjoy safe, secure, and loving relationships (nurture). To grow a seed requires the proper climate (child and family policies), soil (physical and social environments), and water (nurturing relationships).[3] The extent to which these factors combine determines how much resilience and strength the seed-child needs to weather the inevitable life stressors s/he will face. If appropriate support is not given, early childhood can be a period of great risk. Inadequate nutrition and inadequate health care can predispose the preschool child to potential health problems that compromise future growth and development. Inadequate parenting or insufficient social and cognitive stimulation can

---

[1]Intelligence Quotient
[2]Emotional intelligence Quotient
[3]See Figure 2: The Social-Ecological Model, in Middlebrooks, J. S., & Audage, N. C. (2008). *The Effects of Childhood Stress on Health across the Lifespan*. Atlanta, GA: Centers for Disease Control and Prevention, National Center for Injury Prevention and Control, p. 11. The seed, water, soil and climate correspond with individual, relationship, community and society levels of the model.

jeopardize the successful transition to school and lead to subsequent academic and social problems (Farel & Kotch, 2005).

THE PRESCHOOL CHILD

Children at 1 to 4 years of age develop language, locomotion, social relationships, and the knowledge and skills that make successful school entry possible (Farel & Kotch, 2005). They begin to interact with the world outside their home through communication and play. They develop a sense of identity and initiative and can follow directions and stories. They learn how to dress, toilet, wash hands, and brush teeth. Their imaginations explode with creativity and vision as they differentiate fantasy from reality.

According to Erikson (1950), the preschool child's developmental tasks are to achieve a sense of autonomy and to experience individual initiative. The successful completion of these tasks is a necessary prerequisite of the individuality and purposeful activity that will be called on when the child enters school. The interpersonal relationships that the child develops during this period will be long lasting, as in the case of family relationships, and will also be models for future relationships. The American Academy of Pediatrics (2011) lists the following language, cognitive, and social and emotional milestones a child should reach by age 4 to 5 years:

Language

- Recalls part of a story
- Speaks sentences of more than five words
- Uses future tense
- Tells longer stories
- Says name and address

Cognitive

- Can count 10 or more objects
- Correctly names at least four colors

- Better understands the concept of time
- Knows about things used every day in the home (money, food, appliances)

Social and emotional

- Wants to please friends
- Wants to be like her friends
- More likely to agree to rules
- Likes to sing, dance, and act
- Shows more independence and may even visit a next-door neighbor by herself
- Aware of sexuality
- Able to distinguish fantasy from reality
- Sometimes demanding, sometimes eagerly cooperative

Successful early childhood development that sets the stage for successful school entry, and advancement is possible if we value and nurture the innate potential of the child. In order to successfully achieve this goal, we must know more about both the nature and nurture factors that both contribute to the overall health of the preschool child. In the next sections we discuss who are the preschool population of children, their health-related issues and their contributing and protective factors, the policies and programs that can ameliorate their issues and bring out the child's potential, and finally, the issues and opportunities that face the preschool child and their advocates in the future.

DEMOGRAPHICS

U.S. births increased 3% between 2005 and 2006 (Martin, et al., 2008). Children currently 4 years old were part of that cohort, which had the largest increase in births since 1961. Births and birth rates increased in all race groups. Hispanic births comprised 24% of all births in 2006 compared with 15% in 1990, and the actual number of births to Hispanic women was more than 1 million for the first time (Martin, et al., 2008).

As of 2008 there were 21 million children under the age of 5 in the United States, comprising 6.9% of the U.S. population (Martin, et. al, 2008). There were slightly more boys born than girls, but because boys have a higher mortality rate, females become the majority by the age of 30 years. The majority (56%) of children are non-Hispanic white. Demographic trends indicate that the ethnic composition of the preschool population, and consequently of all children in the United States, is shifting toward nonwhite. The sex and race distribution of children less than 5 years old in the United States as of 2008 is shown in Table 7–1.

The percentage of children who are Hispanic increased more than 50% between 1980 and 2009. These children are projected to comprise almost 30% of the child population by 2021. In contrast, the percentage of black, non-Hispanic children has remained at approximately 15% since 1980 and is expected to decline slightly to 14% by 2021. Asian-only children made up 4% of the U.S. child population in 2009 and are expected to increase to 5% of the child population in that same time frame. The percentage of non-Hispanic white children fell from 61% to 56% in 2009 and is expected to decline further to 51% by 2021 (Child Trends Data Bank, 2010).

Teen childbearing rose in 2006, the first increase after 14 years of steady decline. Childbearing by unmarried women reached an historic high at 38.5% of all births. This is 20% higher than in 2002 when the upturn began (Martin, et al., 2008).

Poverty

Poverty is one of the most powerful determinants of a young child's health. From birth through infancy and childhood, poverty is associated with higher mortality and morbidity for a wide range of conditions, including behavioral and emotional disorders, spanning virtually every sphere of a child's life. Approximately one in five U.S. children (and one in four minority children) lives in poverty—the highest child poverty rate in the world among developed countries.

Poverty is a contributor to preventable illness in the United States and is associated with many risks for poor health among young children. In 1913, the Children's Bureau conducted a landmark study of infant deaths. Adverse pregnancy outcomes among poor women include a greater likelihood of low birth weight and postnatal complications. Poor children are more likely to have inadequate or inappropriate nutrition. Malnutrition is associated with both undernutrition and obesity. Both have short- and long-term health effects. They are both associated with iron deficiency anemia and can have vague symptoms like fatigue and weakness. More serious symptoms include growth retardation and poor cognitive and social development related to social deprivation (Armstrong, Dorosty, Reilly, & Emmett, 2003).

Definition of Poverty

The federal definition of poverty has thresholds based on the number of people in a family and its pretax income. Different assistance programs use different thresholds as eligibility criteria. A child living in extreme poverty is defined as a child living in a family with income less than 50% of the poverty threshold. Below poverty, but above extreme poverty, is defined as 50–99% of the poverty threshold. Low income is defined as 100–199% of the poverty threshold. Medium income is defined as 200–399% of the poverty threshold. High income is defined as being at or above 400% of the poverty threshold.

For example, a family with one child where one parent works a minimum wage job of $7.25 at 40 hours each week for 52 weeks ($15,090 annually) is considered low income. With two children, however, the family falls below the poverty line (Forum on Child and Family Statistics, 2010). In the United States 51% of children are at or below 250% of poverty. Twenty-three percent of

Table 7–1 Resident Population, by Race, Hispanic Origin, and Single Years of Age: 2008 (U.S. Census Bureau, 2010) [in thousands]

| | Total | Race | | | | | | Hispanic origin \1 | Not-Hispanic White alone |
		White alone	Black or African American alone	American Indian, Alaska Native alone	Asian alone	Native Hawaiian and Other Pacific Islander alone	Two or more races		
Total	**304,060**	**242,639**	**39,059**	**3,083**	**13,549**	**562**	**5,167**	**46,944**	**199,491**
Under 5 years old	21,006	15,771	3,150	286	931	51	817	5,288	11,065
Under 1 year old	4,313	3,220	660	61	189	10	173	1,108	2,237
1 year old	4,276	3,187	660	60	189	10	169	1,109	2,204
2 years old	4,171	3,130	627	57	185	10	163	1,060	2,191
3 years old	4,122	3,104	610	55	185	10	157	1,023	2,196
4 years old	4,124	3,130	593	53	183	10	154	988	2,238

Source: U.S. Census Bureau, "Monthly Resident Population Estimates by Age, Sex, Race, and Hispanic Origin for the United States: April 1, 2000 to July 1, 2008" (released May 14, 2009).

\1 Persons of Hispanic origin may be any race.
U.S. Census Bureau. 2010. The 2010 Statistical Abstract. Table 10. Retrieved June 26, 2011 from http://www.census.gov/compendia/statab/2010/cats/population.html.

1- to 4-year-olds are at 100% poverty (Annie E. Casey Foundation, 2010). Several national trends over the past 40 years have contributed to the rise in poverty. Major adjustments in the economy, such as the replacement of skilled, unionized manufacturing jobs with lower paid, lesser skilled, nonunionized service sector jobs, coupled with increasing proportions of children living with one parent, usually the mother, and failure of social welfare programs to keep pace with inflation, conspire to keep approximately one in five children (and one in four minority children) in poverty (Farel & Kotch, 2005). The decreased real value of wages earned by workers with less education, reductions in real value of income transfer programs, and adverse interactions between these factors and social and emotional problems of families (such as domestic violence) are integral factors in child poverty. Domestic violence significantly reduces the annual number of work hours of the victim (Tolman & Wang, 2005). Regardless of whether the mother works, the low-income level of mother-headed families is made worse by the persistent failure of fathers to meet child support obligations.

Housing

Approximately half of families that are poor live in neighborhoods with concentrated poverty (Annie E. Casey Foundation, 2010). Poor communities suffer from a lack of public resources, economic investment, and political power, all of which exacerbate the disadvantages of poverty (Knitzer, 2002). Leventhal and Brooks-Gunn (2004) demonstrated that achievement scores of male students who moved to low-poverty neighborhoods were higher than their counterparts in high-poverty neighborhoods.

Poor communities offer few safe places for children to congregate and play. Consequently, children who live in neighborhoods that are poor are less likely to participate in sports or after-school activities. Economic, social, health, and other factors thus converge to stunt the intellectual, emotional, and physical development of poor children.

Cohabiting

Kennedy and Bumpass (2008) did extensive analysis of cohabitation and children's living arrangements based on the National Survey of Family Growth 1997–2001 (Table 7–2).

Table 7–2 Mother's Union Status at Birth, Children Born 1997–2001 and 1990–1994

	Point Estimates[a]		Bounds on Imputed Data, 1997-2001[b]	
	1990–94	1997–01	Assign to Marriage 1997–01	Assign to Single 1997–01
Marital births	73	66	68	65
All nonmarital births	27	34	32	35
Single mother	16	16	14	17
Cohab mother	11	18	18	18
TOTAL	3825	2678	2678	2678

[a]Point estimates are calculated using imputed values for date of marital separation.
[b]In 2002, because of the large amount of missing marital separation dates, parent's marital status at birth could not be determined with certainty for 5% of children in 2002. Bounds were created by assuming that (1) all of these children were born to married parents, and (2) all were born after the marriage dissolved.

Source: Data from Table 7 in "Cohabitation and Children's Living Arrangements: New Estimates from the United States," by S. Kennedy and L.L. Bumpass, 2008, *Demographic Research, 19*, p. 1679.

There was both an increase of prevalence and duration of unmarried cohabitation from 1990–1994 to 1997–2001. They concluded that two-fifths of all children spend some time in a cohabiting family by age 12, a highly influential factor in poorer outcomes than those of the children of married parents, such as poor academic performance, emotional problems, depression, behavioral problems and delinquency. Lower income is among a number of factors making U.S. cohabiting unions potentially disadvantageous environments for raising children.

Child poverty also increases the need for special education services because it affects children's health, behavior, and as a consequence, cognitive development and academic achievement. One-third of mothers of poor children with individualized education plans (IEPs) did not finish high school compared with 7% of mothers whose children with IEPs are not in poverty, reinforcing the conclusion that parental education is the best predictor of poverty. Poverty alone had a negative effect on teacher ratings of approaches to learning (U.S. Department of Education, 2001).

Poverty and the low educational level of the household combine to form an almost insurmountable culture of deprivation, which is difficult to overcome. In 2008 36% of heads of household with a child had an associate degree or higher. Forty-eight percent had a high-school diploma or GED. Sixteen percent of American homes with children were headed by a parent without a high school education (Annie E. Casey Foundation, 2010).

HISTORICAL CHANGES IN THE HEALTH STATUS OF PRESCHOOL CHILDREN

The improvement in the health status of preschool-age children in the United States in the 20th century is the greatest of any infant or child age bracket. Using fatality as a proxy measure of health status, it may be said that preschool children in the United States are healthier now than ever before. Fatalities among 1- to 4-year-olds fell 98% from 1900 to 1998 (Guyer, Freedman, Strobino, & Sondik, 2000), and it continues to fall. The death rate for children aged 1–4 years old in 2005 was 8% lower than in 2000 (Martin, et al., 2008).

Indisputably, the story behind this modern public health miracle is the control of infectious diseases. Of the 97% decline in mortality that occurred between 1900 and 1985, 93% occurred before 1950, approximately the time of the introduction of antibiotics to the general public (Fingerhut, 1989). Therefore, the lives saved and morbidities prevented are attributable almost entirely to improved public health services such as sanitation, immunization, food safety, and the promotion of personal hygiene by public health workers on the one hand and to improved living standards resulting in reductions in family size, improved nutrition, improved housing conditions, and decreased crowding on the other. There is no credible basis for the claim that personal medical care made anything more than a marginal contribution to this "spectacular" (Guyer, et al., 2000, p. 1313) improvement in health and life expectancy enjoyed by U.S. children.

In her autobiography, Dr. Sara Josephine Baker (1873 to 1945), the first woman to receive a doctorate in public health and founder of New York City's Division of Child Hygiene, the first government-sponsored agency in the world dedicated to child health, described the activities contributing to the improvement of the health of children in her jurisdiction. These included training 30 public health nurses to teach recent immigrants preventive health practices such as proper ventilation, bathing, breastfeeding, and clothing for infants and young children. Baker's Division of Child Hygiene offered health education and advice, screening and referral, and pure milk in the "baby hygiene stations" that she set up. She trained midwives, introduced hygiene into New York

City classrooms, isolated children with infectious diseases by keeping them out of school, and placed orphaned children from hospitals with loving foster mothers. By the time of her retirement in 1923, New York's child death rate was the lowest of any city in the United States or Europe (Grolier Library of North American Biographies, 1994).

In her comprehensive review of trends in childhood mortality in the United States, Fingerhut (1989) documented the precipitous drop in death rates for the 1- to 4-year-old age group, from 1,980 per 100,000 in 1900 (based on death registration states that included 26% of the U.S. population) to 50 per 100,000 in 1985. By 2005, this rate had declined still further to 32 per 100,000 (Martin, et al., 2008). At the same time, preschool children in the United States experience higher mortality rates than their peers in other Western countries, primarily because of excessive injury deaths. The success in reducing the death rate in this age group represents primarily the success in reducing natural causes of death. In 1900, natural causes accounted for the death of 93% of all 1- to 4-year-olds in the United States. Diphtheria, diarrhea, enteritis, and pneumonia together caused the deaths of 10% of all 1- to 4-year-olds. By 1985, however, all natural causes (including but not limited to infectious diseases) accounted for 55% of the deaths of all 1- to 4-year-olds (Fingerhut, 1989). By 2005, the leading causes of death in this age group, in order, had become unintentional injury, congenital anomalies, malignant neoplasms, homicide, heart disease, and (finally) influenza and pneumonia, reflecting the relatively greater success in preventing natural causes of death compared with external causes (Bloom & Cohen, 2007). The rate of every one of them decreased with the single exception of homicide. The 1- to 4-year homicide rate increased from 0.6 per 100,000 in 1950 to 2.9 in 1995, after which it resumed its decline, to 2.2 per 100,000 in 2005 (Bloom & Cohen, 2007).

EPIDEMIOLOGY OF MAJOR HEALTH PROBLEMS

Poor health habits initiated during this period of life can lead to obesity, diabetes, and cardiovascular disease (Maffeis & Tato, 2001). Recent investigation has connected early childhood health to adult health. Poor childhood health increases more than three times the odds of having self-reported poor adult health. This association is independent of health risk factors and socioeconomic status (Haas, 2007).

In the 2007 National Survey of Children's Health, 86.7% of parents with children 1 to 4 years old ranked their children's health as excellent or very good. Only 68% of parents with household income at or below poverty level, however, felt that way (Bloom, Cohen, & Freeman, 2009).

Whereas preventive health services, exemplified by immunizations, play a prominent role at this age period, it is also true that, as children approach school age, the greatest threat to their lives becomes intentional and unintentional injury, which at best can only modestly be affected by personal health care. Similarly, many of the leading causes of morbidity in this period either seem resistant to medical intervention or are increasing in prevalence as a result of advances in medical technology and treatment. All of these circumstances suggest the need to consider better integrated, community-based prevention strategies and social policy as interventions of choice in this age group. In this chapter, we describe the demographics, history, and health status of 1- to 4-year-olds in the United States, their access to health services, and programs and policies relevant to this age group.

Chronic Conditions

Trends over the past 30 years demonstrate that the incidence of serious acute illness in children has fallen. In its place now are chronic conditions (Wise, 2007). The vast majority (78%) of children 1 to 4 years old do not have chronic conditions. For those with chronic conditions 14% have only one, and 8% have two or more. The more prevalent chronic condition is asthma, followed by learning disabilities, attention deficit hyperactivity disorder, speech, and conduct disorder (Kogan & Newacheck, 2007). Chronic conditions are responsible for > 90% of all childhood medical causes of death and contribute to the social disparities in child health (Wise, 2007). Even though relatively few children have chronic conditions, their care accounts for a large portion of child health care expenditures (Wise, 2007).

Each year there are about 60,000 infants (1.5% of newborns) who are born at less than 30 weeks' gestation and have a birth weight of less than 1500 grams. Bronchopulmonary dysplasia develops in approximately 20% of them (Baraldi & Filippone, 2007). It is the most common respiratory disease of infants and is associated with high use of health services and costs (Baraldi & Filippone, 2007). Bronchopulmonary dysplasia is a multisystem disorder, which "may be associated with a number of other conditions, including growth retardation, pulmonary hypertension, neurodevelopmental delay, hearing defects, and retinopathy of prematurity. Consequently, interdisciplinary follow-up is often required" (Baraldi & Filippone, p. 1946).

Premature babies, some of them now surviving at 23 weeks' gestation, have complex, chronic health issues and disabilities. Their parents must learn how to feed and take care of them, and they require multiple specialists to care for them—pediatric ophthalmologists, neurologists, orthopedists, gastroenterologists, psychiatrists. Many need physical therapy, occupational therapy, and speech therapy. These same services are needed for children with congenital anomalies, Down Syndrome and heart defects (Lantos, 2010). Parents and the health care and educational systems are not always prepared to care for these special needs infants and children.

Neonatal intensive care units (NICUs) are profitable, but follow-up clinics lose money (Lantos, 2010). Medicaid is the primary payer in NICU follow-up clinics, and reimbursement is considered to be poor. These special needs babies and children need a plethora of services, which are rarely well coordinated or integrated. According to Lantos (2010), in the case of one academic medical center's dilemma (which is "emblematic of those that play out in every academic medical center in the country, day in and day out"), "saving premature babies is better business than helping them thrive" (p. 2114).

Disabilities

The prevalence of disabilities in young children is difficult to quantify. The rate may vary from 0.22% to 44% depending on what definition of disability is used (van der Lee, Mokkink, Grootenhuis, Heymans, & Offringa, 2007). Young children with disabilities are significantly more likely to live in poverty than children without disabilities, and low-income families are burdened more by expenses than higher income families (Newacheck, Inkelas, & Kim, 2004).

Mental retardation is a broad classification, including conditions for which the etiologies are numerous and diverse. Legislative and social initiatives can reduce the incidence of some conditions associated with mental retardation such as preterm births and alcohol consumption during pregnancy, but most cases of mental retardation have no known cause. In addition to mental retardation, neuromuscular disorders such as muscular dystrophy, sensory impairments such as blindness and deafness, learning disabilities, and conditions such as epilepsy and autism all fall under the developmental disabilities classification (Farel & Kotch, 2005).

In the 1960s, intelligence tests were used to identify children with mental retardation, and services were offered primarily in special schools or residential institutions. The current practice of mainstreaming children with mental retardation grew out of concern that the segregated environment of special classes or institutions deprived children with mental retardation of experiences necessary for effective socialization. The widespread use of IQ testing as the criterion for decisions about services was also criticized for having stigmatizing consequences that were difficult to overcome. Although there is not a consistent viewpoint about classifying children with mild mental retardation, severe mental retardation (defined as IQ < 50) is usually recognizable before children reach school age. The prevalence of preschool-age children with severe mental retardation ranges from 3 to 5 per 1,000 children. However, the definition of severe mental retardation as an IQ of less than 50 is problematic because IQ alone does not describe individual differences in adaptive skills or the presence of other conditions that may impede effective coping by a child whose IQ is above this cutoff.

Accurate prevalence rates for developmental disabilities are not available. The Federal Interagency Forum on Child and Family Statistics (2010) estimated that 60% of young children have no risk of developmental disability. Fourteen percent have low risk, 16% moderate risk, and 10% high risk. Children in poverty have higher rates of developmental disabilities than children from higher income families. Developmental disabilities stem from poor birth outcomes, which are partly related to the poor health status of their mother, illness of infancy, and the environment in which the child grows. Low socioeconomic status is associated with poor language skills and learning ability (Herring, et al., 2006). It contributes to chaotic homes and lifestyles, which in turn decrease the child's ability to self-regulate executive functioning. Without a stable foundation from which to grow, the young child has difficulty achieving developmental milestones. These milestones are the building blocks upon which preschoolers construct their early educational framework.

Children with developmental disabilities, by definition, have functional limitations in at least three of the following seven areas: self-care, receptive or expressive language, learning, mobility, self-direction, capacity for independent living, and economic self-sufficiency (Herring, et al., 2006). Parents' observations, perceptions, concerns, and action are what bring the young child to the attention of medical providers. The PEDS (Parents' Evaluation of Developmental Status) eight-question survey can help predict risk of developmental issues based on the age of the child (Glascoe, 2003).

Surveillance of developmental disabilities is difficult because case definitions often rely on clinical judgment, and there are no standard national or state-specific definitions for developmental disabilities. Furthermore, developmental disabilities may not be manifest at the age of 1 year and become apparent only as the child matures. Recent mandates to provide preschool special education services may generate useful data about children under 4 years with developmental disabilities (Farel & Kotch, 2005).

Asthma

Asthma, a chronic inflammatory disorder of the airways, is the most common chronic disease of childhood, affecting about 7.1 million children. Its prevalence ranges from 5.2% in South Dakota and Idaho to 14.4% in Delaware (American Lung Association, 2010). The proportion of children with asthma and its severity vary by race, ethnicity, and income. The prevalence of asthma in low-income children is higher than in children above 100% of poverty, and obesity increases the odds of having asthma. Black children have a 1.3 times higher chance of having asthma than white children (Saha, Riner, & Liu, 2005).

Asthma is one of the primary causes of school and preschool absence and in 2008 was attributed to 14.4 million lost days of education. The prevalence of asthma in school-aged children has been reported by the International Study of Asthma and Allergies in Children but has not been studied in preschoolers. This is partly due to the difficulty of diagnosis and treatment (Bisgaard & Szezler, 2007; Bush, 2007; Øestergaard & Prahl, 2007; Pedersen, 2007).

Eliciting a detailed history requires skill. Most preschool children have no physical signs of asthma. The differential diagnosis for coughs is complicated by a history of prematurity or a recent viral infection (Pedersen, 2007). There is not consensus when to use a nebulizer or a spacer. Young children are not able to use peak flow meters, devices that help with differentiation in older children (Bush, 2007). In short, there is need for more evidence-based research in this age group.

Obesity

Childhood obesity continues to be a leading public health concern. Children who are obese in preschool have a greater chance of being obese later in life (Sharma, et al., 2009). Childhood obesity is associated with a range of complications that affect a child's risk for poor physical and mental health. Obese children are more likely to develop type II diabetes, cardiovascular disease, orthopedic problems, hypertension, and many other medical and psychological conditions including social rejection and low self-esteem (Strauss, 2000). Although certain individuals may have a greater genetic predisposition to obesity, the prevalence of obesity has occurred far too rapidly for increased prevalence of these genes to account for the epidemic.

The Pediatric Nutrition Surveillance System (PedNSS) monitors the nutritional status of low-income children who participate in federal maternal and child health programs for routine care, nutrition education, and supplemental food. The 2002 PedNSS, which summarized 2001 data, reported that the prevalence of overweight was 13.5% for children aged birth to 5 years old and 14.3% for children 2 to 5 years old. The highest rates were among American Indian or Alaska Native (17.7%) and Hispanic (19.0%) children, and the lowest rates were among black and white children (11.8%) (Polhamus, et al., 2004).

In 2008 the Centers for Disease Control and Prevention (CDC) looked at trends and obesity prevalence in obesity using PedNSS data from 1998–2008 and found similar results. The results indicated that obesity prevalence among low-income, preschool-aged children increased steadily from 12.4% in 1998 to 14.5% in 2003, but subsequently remained essentially the same, with a 14.6% prevalence in 2008 (Sharma, et al., 2009). Overweight has increased among all racial and ethnic groups, with the greatest increase occurring among white children. An increase was seen in all racial and ethnic groups except American Indian and Alaska Native children, for whom the prevalence, consistently higher than all other groups, has remained stable. Findings from PedNSS are consistent with trends found for the increase of overweight among children in the U.S. population as a whole (Polhamus, et al., 2004).

Early recognition and prevention are essential for addressing obesity. Research into conditions that precipitate early childhood obesity has focused on several issues. For example, studies among infants of the role of breastfeeding and the early introduction of solid foods concluded that an infant's dietary patterns alone do not explain the development of overweight in early childhood (Parsons, Power, Logan, & Summerbell, 1999). Other studies have investigated feeding practices among mothers of children 2 to 5 years of age. Baughcum, et al. (2001) argued that a mother's feeding practices and her beliefs about a child's desirable weight affect the growing child's ability to regulate his or her own appetite. Although there was not a specific style of feeding that was associated with obesity in young children, low-income mothers had significantly different feeding behaviors from high-income mothers, as measured by the Preschooler Feeding Questionnaire.

The impact of having a television in the bedroom on a child's risk of obesity was examined in children between 1 and 5 years of age. Based on a survey conducted among families enrolled in one of New York State's Women, Infants, and Children (WIC) programs (n = 52,761) and specific information about the child's height, weight, and body mass index, a television in the child's bedroom was a strong marker of increased risk for being overweight (Dennison, Erb, & Jenkins, 2002). Another survey of participants in the New York City Neighborhood WIC Program was attached to demographic information collected as part of certification for WIC. Nelson, Chiasson, and Ford (2004) concluded that 40% of the children 2 to 4 years of age were or were at risk for overweight.

Oral Health

The oral health of preschool children is a growing public health problem in the United States. Caries, or cavities, represent tooth decay, which is a severe problem among low-income, minority preschool children. Dental care is associated with fewer decayed teeth and more filled teeth (Sohn, Ismail, Amaya, & Lepkowski, 2007).

In the National Survey of Children's Health 2007, 77.9% of parents of children ages 1 to 5 years old reported that overall their children's teeth were in excellent or very good condition. The condition of children's teeth, however, was different by income category. Of children with household incomes below 100% poverty (see demographics section for illustration of poverty levels), only half (49.8%) of parents reported that the condition of their children's teeth was excellent or very good. As income rose, so did parents' perception of their children's dental health. Between 100–199% of poverty 61.3% reported excellent or very good condition; 76% at 200–399%, and 84.8% above 400% of poverty (Dietrich, Culler, Garcia, & Henshaw, 2008).

Access to dental insurance is one barrier to dental care. Children with private dental insurance have four times greater chance of seeing a dental provider than children without insurance. Having Medicaid increases the odds one and a half times higher than for noninsured children (Sohn, Ismail, Amaya, & Lepkowski, 2007).

Medicaid covers dental care for children, but adult dental insurance is expensive. One study found only 27% of mothers of Medicaid children had a dental provider (Grembowski, Spiekerman, & Milgrom, 2007). Not surprisingly, higher educational achievement and income are associated with better dental care for young children. Parents who visit the dentist for preventive care are five times more likely to take their children to the dentist (Sohn, Ismail, Amaya, & Lepkowski, 2007).

A study of Medicaid enrolled children in North Carolina found that preschool-aged children who had early dental visits were more likely to continue with dental care (Savage, Lee, Kotch, & Vann, 2004). Children who are Women, Infants and Children Food Supplement Program recipients (see section on WIC later in the chapter for more information) are more likely to have dental care than nonrecipients. This may be related to health care referrals which are a deliberate programmatic component of WIC (Lee, Rozier, Kotch, Norton, & Vann, 2004; Lee, Rozier, Norton, Kotch, & Vann, 2004).

Mental Health

Attention to the prevalence and distribution of mental health disorders among preschool-aged children is relatively new (Knitzer & Cooper, 2006; Perry, Kaufmann, & Knitzer, 2007). Despite a popular belief to the contrary, young children can grapple with mental health problems. Bricker, Davis, and Squires (2004) asserted that the prevalence of young children with evidence of mental health problems is rising, reporting that recent surveys suggest that 10% to 25% of young children have mild to serious disorders. Grupp-Phelan, Harman, and Kelleher (2007) examined National Hospital Ambulatory Medical Care Survey data from 1995–2001 and found that mental health-related emergency department visits were growing at a faster rate and higher intensity than visits for chronic illnesses. Davis (2010) documented that mental health visits of children with deployed parents increased 11% between 2006 and 2007. Their visits for behavioral disorders jumped 19% and stress disorders 18%.

There is no consensus on the definition of psychiatric problems or criteria in young children (Egger & Angold, 2006). Early childhood mental health research sometimes has ambiguous findings (Essex, et al., 2006). It is difficult to differentiate normative individual variations in temperament, behavior and emotions in this age group (Egger & Angold, 2006). Mental health conditions in young children may have different presentations than in older children or adults, making them difficult to distinguish from early childhood behaviors. Commonly identified problems include hyperactivity, restlessness, attention seeking, difficult-to-control behavior, bedwetting, daytime wetting, food fads, difficulty settling down at bedtime, and night waking. These problems are most frequently associated with maternal depression, poor family relationships, and marital disharmony.

Mental health services include individual or family counseling, medications, or specialized therapies. However, many of these services are not accessible due to lack of insurance coverage or not enough providers, particularly for children under the age of 5. Among children aged 2 to 5 years who had an ongoing emotional, developmental, or behavioral problem that required treatment or counseling, only 42.2% accessed treatment or counseling (National Survey of Children's Health, 2007).

Bricker, Davis, & Squires (2004) described five barriers to early identification that still remain in 2011:

1. The development of mental health screening programs is impeded by the intrinsic variability of behavior among young children.
2. Physicians and other providers are often not as attuned to mental health evaluation as they are to other health indicators.
3. Poor recognition of mental health problems by providers may be confounded by uneasiness at labeling a child as well as awareness that many insurance plans provide only limited coverage.
4. Family members or other caregivers may not be sensitive to possible disturbances in a child's development. Guidelines for the identification of early mental health and behavior problems in 3- to 5-year-old children under the Individuals with Disabilities Education Act (IDEA) are limited. Vague eligibility guidelines under IDEA, in addition to limited community-based options for screening, diagnosing, and evaluating children in this age group, reduce opportunities for treating problems.
5. There are few low-cost, easily administered instruments for screening young children.

Early identification of mental health problems is critical. Children whose conditions are identified early benefit from earlier preventive intervention. Without such intervention, mental health problems in young children may limit the formation of strong and constructive relationships with peers and adults and impair the acquisition of adaptive, cognitive, and language skills necessary for early school preparedness (Farel & Kotch, 2005).

Maternal depression is associated with loss of financial support and household food insecurity. Low-income single female parents have two to four times the rate of clinical depression as that found in the general population (Lennon, Blome, & English, 2001). Domestic violence then magnifies the effect of maternal depression and has a negative impact on school functioning (Silverstein, Augustyn, Cabral, & Zuckerman, 2006). Casey and colleagues found that maternal depression was associated with decrease or loss of public assistance, household food insecurity, child health rating of fair or poor, and history of child hospitalization since birth. Depressed mothers report poorer child health status in infants and toddlers (Casey, et al., 2004). Maternal depression is inextricably connected to a child's general health and has been associated with conduct disorder and emotional problems (Leschied, Chiodo, Whitehead, & Hurley, 2005).

The U.S. Preventive Services Task Force recommends depression screening for adults (O'Connor, Whitlock, Beil, & Gaynes, 2009; U.S. Preventive Services Task Force, 2009). Screening mothers of young children is of particular importance because of the impact of maternal depression on children. Although prevalence rates vary, one study found consistency between screening (16.9%) and at 1 year follow-up (18.5%) and that 46.3% of women with elevated initial symptoms continued to have elevated symptoms at follow-up (McCue, Horwitz, Briggs-Gowan, Storfer-Isser, & Carter, 2007). They concluded this indicates the lack of diagnosis and treatment of maternal depression. This is further confirmed by a national survey of 888 randomly selected primary care pediatricians, which found that 57% felt responsible for recognizing maternal depression, but 64% did not believe they had adequate training to diagnose or counsel (Olson, et al., 2002). This does not bode well for mothers needing help or for their children. Addressing maternal needs is critical to the health and development of young children.

External Causes

Injuries are the single leading cause of death among all children over the age of 6 months. In the 1- to 4-year-old age group, intentional and unintentional injuries combined account for over 43% of all deaths (Xu, Kochanek, Murphy, & Tejada-Vera, 2010). Among 1- to 4-year-olds in the United States drowning was the leading cause of unintentional injury death (accounting for 29%), followed by motor vehicle traffic injuries (27%), fires or burns (13%), suffocation (9%), and pedestrian injuries (USDHHS/HRSA/MCHB, 2010). Whereas the death rate for unintentional injury declined between 2007 and 2008, the rate of death due to homicide increased slightly (Xu, et al., 2010).

Among these increasing homicides, perhaps the most tragic is child abuse, defined here as physical harm deliberately inflicted by a caretaker. Although many parents whose use of corporal punishment may have led to the death of a child might not have "intended" to kill the child, the result is the same. The difference between the intention to teach the child a lesson by hurting him or her and deliberately intending to harm him or her is merely semantic. Unfortunately, many cases of child abuse fail to achieve the medical examiner's threshold for diagnosing child maltreatment as the cause of death, resulting in underreporting of the incidence of fatal child abuse (Herman-Giddens, 1991; Kotch, Chalmers, Fanslow, Marshall, & Langley, 1993). Despite the fact that child maltreatment reports appear to be declining in the United States, estimated child maltreatment fatalities are going up (USDHHS/ACF/ACYF, 2010). The proliferation of child fatality teams in the United States is evidence of the recognition that fatal child abuse is preventable if, by more accurate identification, we can learn who is at risk and when to intervene.

It is impossible to know the true incidence of child maltreatment in the U.S. Official statistics reflect the activities of public agencies in response to reported cases, and child protection teams do not even investigate a third of referrals that come to their attention (USDHHS/ACF/ACYF, 2010). The most recent National Incidence Study (Sedlack, et al., 2010), a survey within a sample of counties in the United States to enumerate cases both known to child protective services (CPS) and known to other agencies and organizations, was last conducted in 2005–2006.

Far more injuries are nonfatal than fatal, but the causes and incidence of nonfatal injury are less well documented than those of fatal injury. The top 10 leading causes of hospitalizations for injury (all unintentional) in this age group include falls, poisoning, foreign bodies, struck by or against an object, burns, bites and stings, motor vehicle injury, and near drowning (CDC, 2011). Although less serious medically, nonfatal injuries, the leading cause of disability after congenital and perinatal causes, actually cost the United States more in indirect costs than fatal injuries, given that the present value of total lost productivity caused by nonfatal injuries is greater than that caused by fatal injuries. In fact, of the over $4 billion lifetime cost of injury in the 0- to 4-year-old age group in 1985, 33% is the indirect cost of injury morbidity compared with 23% for injury mortality (Rice, MacKenzie, & Associates, 1989).

ACCESS TO CARE

Access to care has several meanings but primarily indicates being able to see a health care provider (overall access). Part of access is related to insurance coverage, and there are disparities. Only 6% of whites are uninsured as compared with 7% of African Americans, 17% of Native American, and 21% of Hispanics (Selden & Hudson, 2006). Medical insurance coverage for children has improved tremendously over the past 15 to 20 years because Medicaid expansion and the Children's Health Insurance Programs (CHIP) have afforded children health care coverage.

In 2005, however, 62% of uninsured children (5.5 million) were not enrolled (Selden & Hudson, 2006). Part of the reason for this is income ineligibility (parents' incomes are above the cutoff), and part is parents not making application. If a family's experience with public welfare has not been positive or

if information about Medicaid rules under welfare reform are not adequately communicated, families may not know that their children are eligible for public sources of health insurance. Cumbersome enrollment procedures, stigma associated with public programs, language barriers, and misunderstanding about the value of insurance all undermine enrollment.

Having insurance coverage is one factor in access to care. Actually using the services is another component of access. The Medical Expenditure Panel Survey, an annual household survey sponsored by the Agency for Healthcare Research and Quality, provides data for evaluating trends in health insurance status that include estimates of health care use, expenditures, sources of payment, quality, and insurance coverage. According to a recent report, between 2000 and 2002 only 43.7% of children 0 to 18 years old had a well-child visit during a 12-month period of time, and 39.4% had none over a 2-year period (Selden, 2006). Well-child visit participation was higher with infants and children with special health needs, children whose parents were college educated and whose incomes were more than four times above the poverty level. Uninsured children had the lowest levels of well-child visits at 35% (Selden, 2006).

Access is also related to having a medical home or usual source of care. The concept is that with continuity of care comes improved health. Not having a usual source of medical care can be related to not having providers in the area who accept the child's coverage, transportation to the provider, cultural and language barriers, and perceptions of when it is appropriate to see a provider. One study found an association between not having insurance for 1 to 4 months and not having a medical home (Cummings, Laverrada, Rice, & Brown, 2009). Ninety percent of whites have medical homes, followed by 87% of Asians, 77% of blacks, 68% of Latinos, and 61% of Native Americans (Flores & Tomany-Korman, 2008).

Access to care can also mean being able to see a specialist. This is particularly important with severe health issues common. Many children with special health care needs do not access health services because their parents do not recognize the need for those services (Porterfield & McBride, 2007.)

Access is also related to how easy it is to contact a provider (contact accessibility), how long to get an appointment (appointment accessibility), and how easy it is to get to the provider (geographic accessibility) (Hall, Lemak, Steingraber, & Shaffer, 2008). In a Florida study interviewers posed as Medicaid recipients trying to make appointments. They found that, although 87% of providers were accepting new patients, only 68% were taking new Medicaid patients. The study showed that it is sometimes hard to reach a provider and make an appointment. Twenty-two percent of first calls were not answered. Only one-third of the providers had weekend or evening appointments (Hall, et al., 2008). Simply providing insurance coverage to low-income children will not expand access to care and reduce unmet need without also developing a delivery system that will serve them (Rosenbach, et al., 1999).

PROGRAMS AFFECTING PRESCHOOLERS

Immunizations

A large part of the precipitous drop in child deaths is related to immunization. Immunizations are the *sine qua non* of a personal preventive health intervention. Immunizations exemplify disease prevention, the delivery of a direct service to individuals for the purpose of preventing a specific disease. Immunizations have been proven to be cost beneficial and are the basis for the routine schedule of health maintenance services recommended for preschool children by the American Academy of Pediatrics and others. The Healthy People 2010 immunization goal of 80% coverage of 19- to 35-month-olds has been met

(Sondik, Huang, Klein, & Satcher, 2010). The Healthy People 2020 goal is 90%.

Up-to-date immunization of 36- to 48-month-olds in the United States includes three vaccines for the prevention of polio (IPV); four diphtheria/tetanus/acellular pertussis (DTaP); one measles, mumps and rubella (MMR); at least one Haemophilus influenzae type B; three hepatitis B; and one varicella (Centers for Disease Control, 2010a). Up-to-date immunizations are required of children in licensed child care settings. For kindergarten entry after the fourth birthday, the child must receive a fifth DTaP, fourth IPV, and second MMR (Centers for Disease Control, 2010a).

Early Care and Education

Increasing numbers of preschool children are being cared for outside the home. In 2009, 85% of children from birth through 6 years of age (not yet in kindergarten) whose mothers worked outside the home 35 hours or more each work spent time in child care on a regular basis with persons other than their parents (Forum on Child and Family Statistics, 2010). Children from birth through the age of 2 years were more likely to be in home-based care, either with a relative or nonrelative, than to be in center-based care. Children ages 3 to 6 years who were not yet in kindergarten were more likely to be in a center-based child care arrangement. Center-based care includes child care centers, preschools, Head Start programs, nursery school, prekindergartens, and early childhood education programs.

There is no conclusive research that child care is better or worse than care by a parent, but the classic work, *From Neurons to Neighborhoods*, demonstrates consistently that high-quality, age and developmentally appropriate child care benefits children's cognitive, language, and social development than low quality care (Shonkoff & Phillips, 2000). The Task Force on Community Preventive Services is an independent, nonfederal, volunteer body of public health and prevention experts, whose members are appointed by the director of the CDC. The group considers results from the literature and makes recommendations that inform policy and practice. The Task Force recommends that low-income 3- to 5-year-olds participate in publicly funded, center-based, comprehensive early childhood development programs. This is based on evidence that participation helps to prevent delays in cognitive development, promotes school readiness and decreases placement in special education (Centers for Disease Control, 2010b). Low-income children who receive high-quality early education have greater academic achievement, higher graduation rates, and less need for special education services (Dearing, McCartney, & Taylor, 2009; McCartney, Dearing, Taylor, & Bub, 2007).

The use of child care and preschool is not without risk. Child care centers and preschool settings that meet the American Academy of Pediatrics and American Public Health Association standards (AAP/APHA, 1992) account for only half of the centers in the United States (Rigby, Ryan, & Brooks-Gunn, 2007). Strong evidence shows that group child care increases the frequency of infectious disease among young children. Most of the illnesses that children are exposed to in group child care are annoying but benign. However, the same mode of transmission that increases the risk of diarrhea also increases the risk of hepatitis A. The same mode of transmission that increases the risk of upper respiratory infection also increases the risk of otitis media and meningitis.

The means to prevent the most common form of meningitis in preschoolers, H. influenza meningitis, is straightforward—immunization. Diarrhea, however, may be caused by any of a number of parasites, viruses, and bacteria. Lyman et al. (2009) concluded that viruses are major causes of acute gastroenteritis in child care centers, and there is an immunization for rotavirus, the most common viral cause of diarrhea

in young children. However, there are no immunizations for the diarrheas caused by the many remaining pathogens. Most prevention strategies rely on scrupulous hand washing and environmental sanitation and hygiene, but utilizing diapering, hand washing, and food preparation equipment specifically designed to decrease contagion significantly decreased diarrheal illness and absences in staff and children in child care centers even more (Kotch, et al., 2007).

The picture with respect to injuries among children in out-of-home care is not clear, given the absence of any U.S. studies based on community-wide samples of children. However, Schwebel, Brezausek, & Belsky (2006) found that, among the 1,225 children they studied, those who spent more time in nonparental child care environments were at slightly reduced risk for unintentional injury. The authors believe that not only were the centers safe because of regulations; the adults in the child care settings may be teaching safety to the children. The United Kingdom Millennium Study, however, cautioned that a lack of access to high-quality child care can lead to a widening of inequalities in injury (Pearce, Ferguson, Abbas, Graham, & Law, 2010). The challenge is to make child care even safer. Adult supervision, safer playground equipment and impact-absorbing playground surfaces, scheduled activities, barriers to exposure to household hazards such as poisonous cleaning substances and medications, and less time spent in the car all contribute to reduced injury risk for children in organized child care centers.

Head Start

The federal Head Start program was launched in 1965 as part of President Johnson's War on Poverty. The program was a response to sobering statistics about the number of young children who were very poor. The Head Start program was a national initiative to help improve the odds that poor young children would succeed in life. From the beginning, Head Start was envisioned as a comprehensive program that would provide child care and parent education, evaluate enrolled children's health systematically, monitor children's nutritional and emotional status, screen for hearing and vision, and provide a climate that would nurture social and behavioral competence among enrolled children to ensure that they enter school with a foundation similar to that of their more economically advantaged peers.

Access to health services was a fundamental theme in Head Start programming. These services include (1) a comprehensive health services program that encompasses a broad range of medical, dental, nutrition, and mental health services; (2) preventive health services and early intervention; and (3) service coordination to link the child's family to an ongoing health care system to ensure that the child continues to receive comprehensive health care even after leaving Head Start (USDHHS/ACF/ACYF, 2000). Ten percent of Head Start enrollment is reserved for children with disabilities, most of whom have hearing or speech/language impairments. Children with low-incidence, severe disabilities such as blindness, deafness, and mental retardation are enrolled in the Head Start population in approximately the same proportion as in the IDEA, Part B program for 3- and 4-year-olds. Head Start also enrolls children with feeding tubes and children served by full-time aides. For low-income areas and neighborhoods, Head Start is often the only program serving families who have children with severe disabilities (USDHHS/ACF/ACYF, 2000).

The importance of starting positive child development experiences at birth was reinforced by a new component included in the reauthorization of the Head Start Act in 1994, Early Head Start. The concept for Early Head Start was similar to that of the initial Head Start program, but support and education for the parents of these very young children were reinforced. By 2000, 6% of the overall Head Start enrollment was served in Early Head Start (USDHHS/ACF/ACYF, 2000).

As many low-income parents with young children shifted from public assistance to regular employment and hours away from home increased, the need for the unique family supports provided by Head Start programs grew. However, the parent involvement component, with the goal of engaging parents as classroom volunteers or as recipients of home visits, cannot be effective when parents are expected to be employed full time or enrolled in job training. Changes in the economic and political environment will continue to have a powerful effect on the demand for Head Start programs.

Challenges for Head Start include the demand for expanding the program and ensuring the quality of Head Start services, particularly teacher training. The low wages typically paid to Head Start staff precipitate turnover and jeopardize program quality. Economic uncertainty and the vulnerability of young children form the crucible within which child development services are designed. These services consequently are heavily weighted toward ameliorating existing situations rather than improving outcomes in the long term. Nevertheless, evaluations of Head Start emphasize the positive outcomes for most of the children and families who have been enrolled in these services. Not surprisingly, Head Start programs enjoy bipartisan support.

Individuals with Disabilities Education Act

The Individuals with Disabilities Education Act (IDEA) provides early intervention services for young children (from birth through age 2) and special education services for children ages 3 to 5. By intervening early, developmental delays and learning disabilities are addressed to improve children's educational framework. Early intervention includes physical, occupational, and speech therapy and special education.

Which services children receive depends on individual needs. Some children receive all services, others only one. According to

Bloom, Cohen, and Freeman (2009), the 2008 National Health Interview Survey indicated that 2.8% of children from age 1 to less than 3 years receive early intervention services, whereas 5.4% of children aged 3 to less than 6 years received special education services. Children in poverty are more likely to receive early intervention services (4.2%), in contrast with 3.2% of those with household incomes between 200% and 399% of poverty and 1.9% percent of those in highest income categories.

Part B Preschool Grants Programs

Compelling evidence over the past 50 years has affirmed that special interventions for young children with disabilities and their families during the preschool years increase the child's developmental and educational gains. In 1986, the federal government reinforced the importance of preschool services for children with developmental delays or disabilities by establishing the Preschool Grants Program (Section 619 of Part B) under amendments to the Education of the Handicapped Act, referred to as the IDEA since 1990. This legislation expanded earlier incentives to encourage states to entitle all 3- through 5-year-old children with disabilities to a free and appropriate public education. By 1993, every state and jurisdiction assured free and appropriate public education for all preschoolers with disabilities. The Preschool Grants Program is the only federal program exclusively serving preschool-age children with disabilities. State education agencies are awarded formula grants from the U.S. Department of Education to implement the program through local education agencies and other community service agencies. The Preschool Grants Program is the second largest federal program focusing on 3- to 5-year-old children.

Services provided under Part B may include, but are not limited to, assistive technology devices and services, audiology, counseling services, early identification and assessment, medical services for diagnosis or evaluation, occupational therapy, parent counseling and training, physical therapy, psychological services, recreation, rehabilitation counseling services, school health services, social work services in schools, special education, speech pathology, and transportation. All children who are eligible for services under Part B must have an individual education plan (IEP) developed by parents and providers to develop goals for a child's program of services and to determine which special education and related services are necessary to reach these goals and the setting(s) in which these services will be provided. Related services are provided when they are necessary to assist a child with benefiting from special education.

Innovations and increased interagency collaboration have promoted services that are comprehensive and cost effective. However, some difficult issues persist. Translating the vision of inclusion is difficult in many communities where, historically, children with disabilities may have been placed in more segregated, distinct settings. Although local school systems may be integrating older children into the public school classrooms, child care settings have traditionally been more autonomous. This situation is compounded by the dearth of preschool or child care resources, particularly in rural areas. Furthermore, providing services for children with more rare conditions requires establishing channels of communication among diverse providers, resources in the public and private sector, and families. Communities in which child care rather than preschool services is the norm require special collaborative initiatives between health care and educational providers.

Part C Infant and Toddler Program

Part C, the infant/toddler section of IDEA, is a mechanism for developing systems of family-centered services for infants and toddlers, with or at risk for disabilities, and their families. The 1986 legislation required states that chose to participate in the Part C (previously,

Part H) program to develop state and local infrastructures to respond to the requirement for service delivery systems. Over the course of the 5-year planning period, states were required to apply for continued funding from the U.S. Department of Education and to document their progress in developing the different elements of the system required by the legislation. At the end of the 5-year program implementation process, it was expected that all eligible infants, toddlers, and their families would be entitled to a gamut of comprehensive, coordinated services. By 1992, the complicated process of developing appropriate policies, including interagency agreements, at the state and local levels slowed progress toward full implementation of the law. Furthermore, budget constraints experienced by many federal and state programs forced states to narrow their conceptualization of appropriate populations to serve. In fact, only nine states and jurisdictions opted ultimately to serve infants and toddlers "at risk" for developmental problems (Shackelford, 2004).

All states are required to address 16 minimum requirements in their state plans. States are required to identify a "lead agency" for the Part C program. In more than half of the states, the health department is the lead agency. An Individualized Family Service Plan (IFSP) for each eligible child must be developed with families in order to ensure its responsiveness to families' unique concerns, priorities, and needs. Extensive regulations direct state early intervention programs to improve community awareness and identification of children with or at risk for developmental disabilities. For example, under IDEA, the Child Find system requires each state to ensure that all children with disabilities or suspected of having disabilities are located, identified, and evaluated. The Child Find system must be coordinated with all other Child Find initiatives, including Supplemental Security Income (SSI), Title V, and Early and Periodic Screening, Diagnosis, and Treatment (EPSDT). Explicit regulations for

community outreach, participation of diverse early childhood personnel, and development and monitoring of IFSP have shaped the implementation and evaluation of early intervention programs.

The IFSP has several components related to health care. For example, the IFSP must describe the child's physical development, including vision and hearing. Health care services and nursing services that would enable the child to benefit from other early intervention services must be provided. Medical services, in so far as they are necessary for diagnostic and assessment purposes, are also included in early intervention services. Other services that the child needs such as well-child care or surgery must also be documented in the IFSP, although not paid for by Part C. Such information helps provide a more complete picture of the child and family's needs for services and for tracking a child's health status, particularly when the child does not have a primary care physician.

Early Intervention

Early intervention refers to the provision of services to young children between birth and school age with or at risk for developmental disabilities and their families. Educational, health care, supportive, social, and therapeutic services are among those provided. Early intervention services can be delivered in a center or the child's home. Teams of specialized professionals (teachers, social workers, allied health therapists) as well as community workers, who may provide very personal support even if they lack formal training or education, staff early intervention programs.

The health care system historically has been the first point of professional contact for families with young children with developmental problems. Assessing a child's needs and resources in the context of the family shifted the orientation of the relationship between caregivers and interventionists and fostered the development of more refined identification and assessment procedures for infants and preschool children and emphasizes the importance of the family. Families and children develop unique mechanisms to compensate for the child's special needs. Consequently, the family must be the context where assessment and intervention take place.

Under federal law, states are given considerable discretion in establishing eligibility criteria for early intervention services among the following three groups: infants with established conditions that are likely to lead to delay, infants with developmental delay, or infants who are at risk for developmental delay. However, identifying accurate, culturally sensitive risk factors has been difficult. Precursors of developmental delay have been identified more accurately by including the impact of multiple family risk factors, such as stressful life events, mother's educational level, mother's mental health status, and father's presence in the home. The child's relationships within the larger context of family and community are central to understanding the likelihood of success in school.

There is considerable evidence that properly designed programs with well-defined goals can affect parenting behavior that, in turn, can facilitate favorable outcomes. By this means, children with developmental disabilities and socioeconomic disruption are given the greatest opportunity to pursue a life course in which the consequences of these risk factors are kept to a minimum.

Special Supplemental Nutrition Program for Women, Infants, and Children

The Special Supplemental Food Program for Women, Infants, and Children (WIC) (renamed The Special Supplemental Nutrition Program for Women, Infants, and Children in 1994) began as a demonstration in 1972. The goal was to improve the health of pregnant and lactating women, infants, and children by combining nutrition supplements, nutrition education, and access to health services. From its inception, WIC was conceived of as a food and nutrition program with a mandated connection to health care. Congress deliberately chose to avoid any stigma associated with welfare programs by administratively placing WIC in the Food and Nutrition Service of the U.S. Department of Agriculture (USDA). As Senator Hubert H. Humphrey (1972), one of the architects of the new program, said at the time, such placement would ensure that the program would "not be mismanaged in terms of some other programs."

Since 1972, thanks in part to a series of lawsuits to overcome the Nixon administration's deliberate impounding of WIC funds, the program has expanded rapidly. Today it serves nearly 8 million clients in an average month, including nearly 60% of poor children under the age of 4, at an annual cost of $5 billion (USDA, 2011). A beneficiary of the combined forces of agricultural interests, retail stores, child health and nutrition advocates, and drug companies that produce infant formula, WIC has survived major policy challenges, including threats of budget cuts in 1995. The success of WIC is undoubtedly attributable also to the fact that it is the most evaluated program of all federal social programs, and most of those evaluations have demonstrated the health benefits and the cost effectiveness of WIC.

The overwhelming majority of these evaluations have focused on pregnancy outcome. During pregnancy, WIC services include vouchers for milk, cheese, eggs, fruit juice, dried peas, beans or peanut butter, and iron-fortified grain products. Recently, regulatory changes have been introduced to increase the initiation and duration of breastfeeding. In addition, WIC services are offered as an adjunct to health care, and thus, pregnant women attracted by free food also receive prenatal care, as well as group and individual nutrition education. The evaluations of WIC have not attempted to disaggregate the separate contributions of health care, nutrition supplements, and nutrition education, but as a package, WIC has been shown to increase the mean birth weight and mean gestational age of newborns (Foster, Jiang, & Gibson-Davis, 2010). Prenatal WIC participation is associated with significant improvements in black infant mortality rates and reduced racial disparities in infant mortality between blacks and whites (Khanani, Elam, Hearn, Jones, & Maseru, 2010). WIC also has been shown to reduce Medicaid expenses for newborns in the first year of life (Swann, 2010), hence the assertion that, in addition to providing a net health benefit, WIC also saves money.

There is less evidence about the benefits of WIC for the preschool child. As with the pregnant woman, an eligible child who has a nutritional risk and who is income eligible (185% of the Federal Poverty Income Guidelines in most states) is entitled to food vouchers for milk and milk products, eggs, peanut butter, iron-fortified cereals, and vitamin C–rich juices. In addition, the parent or guardian (and in some cases the child) participates in nutrition education, and the child must have access to medical care. One early study showed that WIC participation improved immunization rates (Kotch & Whiteman, 1982).

More recent studies of WIC have documented its positive effect on the nutrition intake and access to health care of preschool children. Buescher et al. (2003) used linked birth, Medicaid, and WIC records to show that WIC children used more health services, both preventive and curative, than matched children on Medicaid but not on WIC. Lee, Rozier, Kotch, Norton, and Vann (2004) used the same data set to look specifically at the use of dental services. Not only did WIC increase the use of preventive and restorative dental care for children 0 to 5 years old compared with Medicaid children not on WIC, those on WIC also used fewer emergency dental care services. Finally, Richards, Merrill, Baksh, and McGerry (2010) demonstrated that WIC increased access to medical care.

Home Visiting

Over the past 15 years, home visiting programs, funded by private and public sources, have flourished. An estimated 3,000 or more home visiting projects are under way across the United States, operating through local initiative or under the more than 70 state-based efforts in progress in 2009 (Johnson, 2011). Once a strategy for addressing the special needs of immigrant populations, current models build on evidence about the critical early years in a child's life and positive reports from specific home visiting models. All home visiting programs emphasize the delivery of services to young children and their families in their homes and parents' vital role in guiding their child's development. The overarching home visiting model asserts that by seeing the young child in the environment in which the family lives, the home visitor can tailor services to meet the unique needs of the family. In addition, the personal relationship between parents and home visitors bridges the loneliness and isolation between families and their communities. Similar to early intervention programs, home visiting describes a strategy for delivering services rather than a homogeneous or unalterable program (Farel & Kotch, 2005).

The implementation of home visiting programs varies widely. For example, most programs attempt to prevent child abuse and neglect by improving parenting skills and promoting healthy child development. Some programs also work to improve mothers' lives by supporting their efforts to return to school, to postpone subsequent pregnancies, and to earn a living. Some programs begin during pregnancy, whereas others begin when a child is born or even later. The length of most programs is 2 to 4 years. The background for home visitors ranges from individuals with bachelor's, master's, or nursing degrees to paraprofessionals who live in the communities being served (Johnson, 2011).

Almost unique among evaluation protocols implemented in the field, several home visiting programs have attempted to provide evidence for a causal connection between their programs and outcomes by using experimental designs that randomly assign families either to receive home visiting services or to be in control groups that receive other services or no services beyond periodic screenings. In a review of the effect of home visiting on child maltreatment, Duggan et al. (2007) concluded that the results were mixed. Furthermore, even evaluations showing a positive effect indicate that improvement is modest. Program evaluators used an array of approaches to assess whether parents' knowledge of child development and parents' perceptions of their effectiveness changed. In some cases, parent self-report scales and observations of mother–children interaction were used. Program evaluations document some change in parents' attitudes as a result of the home visiting program, but not necessarily in their behaviors (Wasik, Bryant, Lyons, Sparling, & Ramey, 1997).

Similarly, despite promoting the importance of prenatal care and the use of preventive health visits, none of the six evaluation studies found improvements in immunization rates or number of well-child visits. Results for assessments of children's development and behavior similarly suggested only modest, if any, improvement. The Nurse Home Visitation Program (Olds, et al., 2007, 2010), however, has documented reduction of women's rates of subsequent births, longer spacing between first and second births, improved relationship stability, and children's improved adjustment to elementary school. A mother's ability to assume responsibilities associated with a steady job and to postpone a second pregnancy may make it possible for her to emerge from poverty and focus her efforts on her child (Farel & Kotch, 2005).

As currently practiced, most home visiting programs exemplify secondary prevention, addressing risks factors and early indicators of parenting problems rather than targeting the general population of young families. All home visiting programs focus on changing parenting behaviors rather than addressing the underlying social, cultural, and economic threats to healthy child growth and development. The results from evaluations of home visiting programs to date demonstrate that expectations for home visiting programs can be only modest at best and, most important, that home visiting cannot be the only strategy for serving families with young children at risk for health and developmental outcomes (Farel & Kotch, 2005).

As of this writing the Patient Protection and Affordable Care Act of 2010 (Public Law 111-148) is supporting a new federal Maternal, Infant, and Early Childhood Home Visiting Program by funding state-based home visiting programs throughout the United States. By law, the U.S. Department of Health and Human Services will grant money to states that have "evidence-based" home visiting programs. To qualify as "evidence based," programs must have models that demonstrate a positive impact through randomized controlled trials or quasi-experimental research designs (Johnson, 2011). What level of evidence will be required for approving states' home visiting programs remains to be determined.

OUTSTANDING ISSUES

Child Abuse and Neglect

Public involvement in child protection in the United States can be traced to the 1874 case of Mary Ellen, a beaten, emaciated New York City child who was found chained to a bed in her tenement apartment. The New York Society for the Prevention of Cruelty to Animals, in the absence of any analogous agency, public or private, dedicated to the prevention of cruelty to children, took the case to court and won. Subsequently, the New York Society for the Prevention of Cruelty to Children emerged, later becoming the

American Humane Association (American Humane Association, n.d.). Child protection remained primarily a responsibility of voluntary agencies until the outcry, prompted by the publication of Kempe's seminal article, "The Battered Child Syndrome," resulted in local and state social service involvement (Kempe, Silverman, Steele, Droegemueller, & Silver, 1962).

The federal government has been directly involved in child abuse and neglect services since 1973, when model Child Abuse and Neglect legislation was first passed (U.S. Congress, 1973). Because social services are under state jurisdiction, the federal government is limited to providing child maltreatment services through grants-in-aid. In the model legislation, the Congress provided funds for state Child Protective Services (CPS), which defined child maltreatment more or less the same way that the model legislation does and included mandatory reporting in state legislation. As a result, every state now has a mandatory reporting law, and federal support for child maltreatment services is channeled to states through the social services block grant (Title XX of the Social Security Act).

Overworked and understaffed CPS agencies are constrained to investigate every legitimate report and provide services to the substantiated cases (approximately 30% of all reports), leaving little time, money, or energy for prevention. Public health has been in the forefront of prevention services for families at risk of abuse and neglect (Barber-Madden, Cohn, & Schloesser, 1988), but identifying such families remains a crude science at best. Although there is some evidence that home visiting services can reduce reporting rates among at-risk families, there is no evidence that, short of removing the child from the home, CPS interventions actually reduce the risk of subsequent abuse. Approximately one-third of CPS cases are re-reported. Because ethical considerations preclude a randomized, controlled trial of CPS interventions, there is no way of knowing if this recidivism rate is higher or lower

than would be the case without CPS. The National Study of Child and Adolescent Well-being (NSCAW), a longitudinal study of a representative sample of CPS cases funded by the Administration for Children and Families under congressional mandate that is following a representative sample of CPS cases, included only children and families who had had experience in the child welfare system (USDHHS/ACF/OPRE, n.d.).

Autism Spectrum Disorder

Autism Spectrum Disorder (ASD) is a range of diagnoses including autism, Pervasive Developmental Disorder (PDD), and Asperger's Syndrome. Autism affects children's language development, communication, and social skills. Children with Asperger's disorder have normal speech and language but impaired social skills. They focus intensely on one thing and perseverate. PDD has severe language and communication delays in addition to poor social skills (Kogan & Newacheck, 2007).

The prevalence varies, depending on whether Asperger's Syndrome and PDD children are included. The 2007 National Survey of Children's Health (sample size 78,037) used parent report that a doctor had told them their child had autism. Autism is more prevalent in boys than girls, and non-Hispanic black children are less likely than whites to have the disorder. The point-prevalence was 110 per 10,000, around 673,000 children, which is higher than previous estimates in the United States (Kogan & Newacheck, 2007).

There are many possible reasons for this increase. The diagnosis of autism was changed in 1994 to include children with typical intellectual abilities as well as those with more limited skills. At that time there was evidence that early, intensive behavioral treatment could make a difference for autistic children. In response, the federal government changed the educational definition of disabilities to include autism, which meant children could access services. This in turn resulted in a major public education campaign to alert parents to the importance of identifying autism as early as possible. These campaigns have resulted with increasing numbers of children being diagnosed and families receiving appropriate support.

According to Helt, et al., 2008, 3–25% of children with ASD improve fully in that they no longer meet the criteria for autism, but they may continue to have other problems with development or behavior. Early identification of developmental disorders, meaning between birth and 3 years old, is essential to young children's well being. Screening tests should be done at 9, 18, and 24 months, and children identified with special needs should receive early intervention (Allison, et al., 2007).

It is extremely frustrating for families not to know what caused their child's autism. Many environmental factors influence the development of autism, but nothing is conclusively associated with it. It is logical for parents to want answers, so in 1998 when Wakefield postulated that the MMR vaccine and the preservative thimerosal caused autism, there was a parental backlash against immunizations. Twenty epidemiologic studies— retrospective, observational studies, ecological studies, and prospective observational studies with substantial statistical power— proved that MMR and thimerosal do not cause autism (de los Reyes, 2010; Gerber & Offit, 2009). *Lancet*, which published the 1998 study, withdrew it and subsequently accused Dr. Wakefield of outright fraud (Deer, 2011). Nevertheless, many parents and advocacy groups continue to believe there is a causative link with immunization. The AAP strongly supports immunizing children on time as well as pursuing investigation by the Centers for Disease Control and Prevention and National Institutes of Health to determine what factors in our modern environment may be contributing to autism (AAP, 2010).

Attention Deficit Disorder (ADD)/ Attention Deficit Hyperactivity Disorder (ADHD)

During the preschool period children develop what is called executive function (EF). This EF is what enables a child to control his or her impulses and actions, to focus and problem solve (Garon, Bryson, & Smith, 2008). This developmental milestone forms an extremely important foundation, from which cognition processes develop from childhood through adulthood.

Attention Deficit Disorder/Attention Deficit Hyperactivity Disorder (ADD/ADHD) is a disorder that is characterized by impaired executive function (Thorell & Wåhlstedt, 2006). Children with ADD are chronically inattentive and unable to focus on tasks. Children with ADHD also demonstrate impulsive hyperactivity to the extent that it interferes with daily functioning. ADHD has been characterized as a neurobehavioral, psychiatric disease that sometimes manifests as conduct disorder and aggression. The symptoms interfere with their social development (Hay, Hudson, & Liang, 2010).

ADHD worldwide-pooled prevalence is 5.29% (Polanczyk, de Lima, Horta, Biederman, & Rohde, 2007). In the United States, 2.4 million children, or 8.7% of children 8 to 15 years old, meet the *DSM-IV* criteria for ADHD. It is more commonly seen in boys than girls. ADHD affects rich and poor children alike. Poor children, however, are more likely than higher income children to meet the criteria for ADHD but are less likely to receive medication (Froehlich, et al., 2007).

The cause of ADHD is unknown, and it is difficult to diagnose in preschoolers (Smith & Corkum, 2007). There is some evidence of sleep disorder in children with ADHD (Hiscock, Caterford, Ukommunne, & Wake, 2007; Sung, Hiscock, Sciberras, & Efron, 2008; Taylor, 2009). Most likely "the behavior and symptoms of ADHD result from the interplay of individual predispositions and the surroundings. The symptoms at a particular time in life will vary and be influenced by factors having positive or negative effects on symptoms" (Sagvolden, Johansen, Aase, & Russell, 2005, p. 397).

There is controversy in the treatment of ADD and ADHD. Counterintuitively, stimulants like Methylphenidate, commonly known as Ritalin™, and Dextroamphetamine (Adderall™) are prescribed for school-age children and older with ADD or ADHD. Their safety and efficacy in children under the age of 5 has not been widely studied; understandably parents of preschoolers are reluctant to give these medications to their children (Staller, 2007).

Children with ADHD have difficulty with academic achievement. Given the epidemiology of this condition, this has large economic implications. "The severity of the problems associated with ADHD and the pervasiveness of its symptoms suggest that efforts to find better ways to teach the relatively small number of children diagnosed with ADHD could have a large payoff in terms of improving the academic outcomes of many children with milder symptoms" (Currie & Stabile, 2006, p.1115).

CONCLUSION

A social problem becomes a part of a nation's policy agenda when a particular issue catches the public's attention or when a group with a special interest advocates for its own particular cause. We do not have a national agenda with a child health focus in the United States. Rather than being an end in itself, child health is more often considered a means to some other end, such as life expectancy or productivity, and expenditures for child health services must be justified in terms of cost benefit in addition to health benefit. An alternative approach, grounded in the Universal Declaration of Human Rights, would make the child entitled to special care and assistance simply by virtue of his or her being a child. As it says in the UN Convention on the Rights of the Child (Article 3.1),

"In all actions concerning children, whether undertaken by public or private social welfare institutions, courts of law, administrative authorities or legislative bodies, the best interests of the child shall be a primary consideration" (United Nations, 1990).

Despite rhetoric to the contrary, the United States, alone among developed countries, has not committed the resources necessary to ensure access to an appropriate level of health services nor committed resources sufficient to achieving optimal health status for its youngest citizens. Rather, it has chosen a categorical approach to child health, ignoring opportunities to address the underlying causes of suboptimal child health on a population-wide basis. The current legislative process, through U.S. House and Senate committee structures, perpetuates the practice of responding to the fragmented perspectives of the many disease-specific special interests. As a result, health and developmental outcomes occurring at the furthest ends of the chain of causality get attention and funding, while the underlying social problems that determine children's health and well-being are ignored. The broad array of public programs supported by the federal government is symptomatic of our cultural preference for throwing life preservers to drowning children rather than preventing them from falling into the water in the first place. Although healthier than ever, the health status of subpopulations of preschool children in the United States has been deteriorating relative to that observed in other developed countries. The current generation of children in the United States may be the first in history to be less healthy than its parents.

Were the United States to make a national commitment to its children, ready and waiting to grow and develop to their optimal potential, then as a society it would acknowledge its responsibility to provide the best possible climate for the expression of that potential (child and family-friendly policies). It would prepare the soil in which its children could sink their roots (healthy communities and families), apply fertilizer to enhance their full potential growth (education and recreation), provide stakes and string to guide their development (guidance and discipline), and protect them from weeds and harmful bugs (safe social and physical environments and promotion of healthy behaviors). Given these supports the next generation will grow into a beautiful garden. The alternative, increasing disparities, increasing low birth weight, increasing obesity, increasing ADD/ADHD, increasing autism and other social, emotional and mental health disorders, is bleak. One will reap what one sows. The cultivation of strong child advocates ready to lead will be needed to succeed in growing healthy toddlers and preschoolers.

References

Allison, C., Williams, J., Scott, F., Stott, C., Bolton, P., Baron-Cohen, S., & Brayne, C. (2007). The Childhood Asperger Syndrome Test (CAST). *Autism, 11*(2), 173.

American Academy of Pediatrics. (2010). Children's health topics. Retrieved May 26, 2011 from http://www.healthychildren.org/English/health-issues/conditions/chronic/Pages/Sound-Advice-on-Autism.aspx.

American Academy of Pediatrics. (2011). Developmental milestones: 4 to 5 year olds. Retrieved July 15, 2011 from http://www.healthychildren.org/English/ages-stages/preschool/pages/Developmental-Milestones-4-to-5-Year-Olds.aspx.

American Academy of Pediatrics & American Public Health Association. (1992). *Caring for our children: National health and safety standards; Guidelines for out-of-home child care programs.* Oak Grove Village, IL and Washington, DC: Authors.

American Humane Association. (n.d.). Mary Ellen Wilson. Retrieved July 14, 2011 from http://www.americanhumane.org/about-us/who-we-are/history/mary-ellen-wilson.html.

American Lung Association. (2010). Asthma and children fact sheet. Retrieved December 11, 2010 from http://www.lungusa.org/lung-disease/asthma/resources/facts-and-figures/asthma-children-fact-sheet.html.

Annie E. Casey Foundation. (2010). *Kids count data book 2010: State profiles of child well-being.* Baltimore, MD: Annie E. Casey Foundation. Retrieved June 11, 2010 from http://datacenter.kidscount.org/data/acrossstates/Rankings.aspx?ind=102.

Armstrong, J., Dorosty, A., Reilly, J., & Emmett, P. (2003). Coexistence of social inequalities in undernutrition and obesity in preschool children: Population based cross sectional study. *Archives of Disease in Childhood, 88*(8), 671.

Baraldi, E., & Filippone, M. (2007). Chronic lung disease after premature birth. *New England Journal of Medicine, 357*(19), 1946–1955.

Barber-Madden, R., Cohn, A., & Schloesser, P. (1988). Prevention of child abuse: A public health agenda. *Journal of Public Health Policy, 9,* 167–176.

Baughcum, A. E., Powers, S. W., Johnson, S. B., Chamberlin, L. A., Deeks, C. M., Jain, A., & Whitaker, R. C. (2001). Maternal feeding practices and beliefs and their relationships to overweight in early childhood. *Journal of Developmental & Behavioral Pediatrics, 22*(6), 391–408.

Bisgaard, H., & Szefler, S. (2007). Prevalence of asthma-like symptoms in young children. *Pediatric Pulmonology, 42*(8), 723–728.

Bloom, B., & Cohen, R. A. (2007). Summary health statistics for U.S. children: National health interview survey, 2006. *Vital and Health Statistics. Data from the National Health Survey, (10)*234, 1–79.

Bloom, B., Cohen, R. A., & Freeman, G. (2009). Summary health statistics for U.S. children: National health interview survey, 2008. *Vital and Health Statistics. Data from the National Health Survey, 244*(10), 1–81.

Bricker, D., Davis, M. S., & Squires, J. (2004). Mental health screening in young children. *Infants and Young Children, 17,* 129–144.

Buescher, P. A., Horton, S. J., Devaney, B. L., Roholt, S. J., Lenihan, A. J., Whitmire, J. T., & Kotch, J. B. (2003). Child participation in WIC: Medicaid costs and use of health care services. *American Journal of Public Health, 93*(1), 145–150.

Bush, A. (2007). Diagnosis of asthma in children under five. *Primary Care Respiratory Journal, 16*(1), 7–15.

Casey, P., Goolsby, S., Berkowitz, C., Frank, D., Cook, J., Cutts, D., Black, M. M., Zaldivar, N., Levenson, S., & Heeren, T. (2004). Maternal depression, changing public assistance, food security, and child health status. *Pediatrics, 113*(2), 298–304.

Centers for Disease Control and Prevention. (2010a). Recommendations and guideline. Retrieved May 14, 2011 from http://www.cdc.gov/vaccines/recs/default.htm.

Centers for Disease Control and Prevention. (2010b). The community guide—early childhood development programs: Comprehensive, center-based programs for children of low-income families. Retrieved May 14, 2011 from: http://www.thecommunityguide.org/social/centerbasedprograms.html.

Centers for Disease Control and Prevention. (2011). WISQARS: Leading causes of nonfatal injury reports. Retrieved June 26, 2011, from http://webappa.cdc.gov/sasweb/ncipc/nfilead2001.html.

Child Trends Data Bank. (2010). Racial and ethnic composition of the child population. Retrieved May 14, 2011 from http://www.childtrendsdatabank.org/?q = node/234.

Cummings, J. R., Lavarreda, S. A., Rice, T., & Brown, E. R. (2009). The effects of varying periods of uninsurance on children's access to health care. *Pediatrics, 123*(3), e411.

Currie, J., & Stabile, M. (2006). Child mental health and human capital accumulation: The case of ADHD. *Journal of Health Economics, 25*(6), 1094–1118.

Davis, C. B. E. (2010). Parental wartime deployment and the use of mental health services among young military children. *Pediatrics, 126*(6), 1209–1210.

de los Reyes, E. C. (2010). Autism and immunizations: Separating fact from fiction. *Archives of Neurology, 67*(4), 490–492.

Dearing, E., McCartney, K., & Taylor, B. A. (2009). Does higher quality early child care promote low-income children's math and reading achievement in middle childhood? *Child Development, 80*(5), 1329–1349.

Deer, B. (2011). How the case against the MMR vaccine was fixed. *British Medical Journal, 342*, c5347, doi: 10.1136/bmj.c5347, (doi: 10.1136/bmj.c5347).

Dennison, B. A., Erb, T. A., & Jenkins, P. L. (2002). Television viewing and television in bedroom associated with overweight risk among low-income preschool children. *Pediatrics, 109*, 1028–1035.

Dietrich, T., Culler C., Garcia, R. I., & Henshaw, M. M. (2008). Racial and ethnic disparities in oral health: The National Survey of Children's Health. *Journal of the American Dental Association, 139*(11), 1507–1517.

Duggan, A., Caldera, D., Rodriguez, K., Burrell, L., Rohde, C., & Crowne, S. S. (2007). Impact of a statewide home visiting program to prevent child abuse. *Child Abuse & Neglect, 31*(8), 801–827.

Egger, H. L., & Angold, A. (2006). Common emotional and behavioral disorders in preschool children: Presentation, nosology, and epidemiology. *Journal of Child Psychology and Psychiatry, 47*(3–4), 313–337.

Erikson, E. H. (1950). *Childhood and society* (2nd ed.). New York: W.W. Norton and Co.

Essex, M. J., Kraemer, H. C., Armstrong, J. M., Boyce, W. T., Goldsmith, H. H., Klein, M. H., Woodward, H., & Kupfer, D. J. (2006). Exploring risk factors for the emergence of children's mental health problems. *Archives of General Psychiatry, 63*(11), 1246–1256, (doi: 10.1001/archpsyc.63.11.1246).

Farel, A., & Kotch, J. (2005). The child from 1 to 4: the toddler and preschool years. In J. B. Kotch (Ed.), *Maternal and child health: Programs, problems, and policy in public health* (2nd ed.). Sudbury, MA: Jones and Bartlett Publishers.

Fingerhut, L. A. (1989). Trends and current status in childhood mortality, United States, 1900–1985. *Vital and Health Statistics* (Series 3, No. 26. DHHS Pub. No. [PHS] 89-1410). Washington, DC: U.S. Department of Health and Human Services, Public Health Service, Centers for Disease Control, National Center for Health Statistics.

Flores, G., & Tomany-Korman, S. C. (2008). Racial and ethnic disparities in medical and dental health, access to care, and use of services in US children. *Pediatrics, 121*(2), e286.

Federal Interagency Forum on Child and Family Statistics. *America's Children: Key National Indicators of Well-Being, 2010.* Washington, DC: U.S. Government Printing Office.

Foster, E. M., Jiang, M., & Gibson-Davis, C. M. (2010). The effect of the WIC program on the health of newborns. *Health Services Research, 45*(4), 1083–1104.

Froehlich, T. E., Lanphear, B. P., Epstein, J. N., Barbaresi, W. J., Katusic, S. K., & Kahn, R. S. (2007). Prevalence, recognition, and treatment of attention-deficit/hyperactivity disorder in a national sample of US children. *Archives of Pediatrics and Adolescent Medicine, 161*(9), 857–864.

Garon, N., Bryson, S. E., & Smith, I. M. (2008). Executive function in preschoolers: A review using an integrative framework. *Psychological Bulletin, 134*(1), 31–60.

Gerber, J. S., & Offit, P. A. (2009). Vaccines and autism: A tale of shifting hypotheses. *Clinical Infectious Diseases, 48*(4), 456–461. (doi:10.1086/596476).

Glascoe, F. P. (2003). Parents' evaluation of developmental status: How well do parents' concerns identify children with behavioral and emotional problems? *Clinical Pediatrics, 42*(2), 133–138.

Grembowski, D., Spiekerman, C., & Milgrom, P. (2007). Disparities in regular source of dental care among mothers of Medicaid-enrolled preschool children. *Journal of Health Care for the Poor and Underserved, 18*(4), 789–813.

Grolier Library of North American Biographies. (1994). Activists (Vol. 1, pp. 15–16). Danbury, CT: Grolier Educational Corporation.

Grupp-Phelan, J., Harman, J. S., & Kelleher, K. J. (2007). Trends in mental health and chronic condition visits by children presenting for care at US emergency departments. *Public Health Reports, 122*(1), 55–61.

Guyer, B., Freedman, M. A., Strobino, D. M., & Sondik, E. J. (2000). Annual summary of vital statistics: Trends in the health of Americans during the 20th century. *Pediatrics, 106,* 1307–1317.

Haas, S. A. (2007). The long-term effects of poor childhood health: An assessment and application of retrospective reports. *Demography, 44*(1), 113–135.

Hall, A. G., Lemak, C. H., Steingraber, H., & Schaffer, S. (2008). Expanding the definition of access: It isn't just about health insurance. *Journal of Health Care for the Poor and Underserved, 19*(2), 625–638.

Hay, D., Hudson, K., & Liang, W. (2010) Links between preschool children's prosocial skills and aggressive conduct problems: The contribution of ADHD symptoms. *Early Childhood Research Quarterly, 25*(4), 493–501.

Helt, M., Kelley, E., Kinsbourne, M., Pandey, J., Boorstein, H., Herbert, M., & Fein, D. (2008) Can children with autism recover? If so, how? *Neuropsychology Review, 18*(4), 339–366.

Herman-Giddens, M. E. (1991). Underreporting of child abuse and neglect fatalities in North Carolina. *North Carolina Medical Journal, 52,* 634–639.

Herring, S., Gray, K., Taffe, J., Tonge, B., Sweeney, D., & Einfeld, S. (2006). Behaviour and emotional problems in toddlers with pervasive developmental disorders and developmental delay: Associations with parental mental health and family functioning. *Journal of Intellectual Disability Research, 50*(12), 874–882.

Hiscock, H., Canterford, L., Ukoumunne, O. C., & Wake, M. (2007). Adverse associations of sleep problems in Australian preschoolers: National population study. *Pediatrics, 119*(1), 86–93.

Humphrey, H. H. (1972, August 16). *Congressional Record.* U.S. Congress, 92d Congress, 2d Session, S28588. Washington, DC: Government Printing Office.

Johnson, K. (2011). New evidence on program impact can guide implementation of federal home visiting program. *Archives of Pediatrics and Adolescent Medicine, 165*(3), 198–204.

Kempe, C. H., Silverman, F. N., Steele, B. F., Droegemueller, W., & Silver, H. K. (1962). The battered child syndrome. *Journal of the American Medical Association,* 181, 17–24.

Kennedy, S., & Bumpass, L. (2008). Cohabitation and children's living arrangements: New estimates from the United States. *Demographic Research, 19,* 1663–1692. (doi: 10.4054/DemRes.2008.19.47).

Khanani, I., Elam, J., Hearn, R., Jones, C., & Maseru, N. (2010). The impact of prenatal WIC participation on infant mortality and racial disparities. *American Journal of Public Health, 100*(S1), S204–S209.

Knitzer, J. (2002). *Promoting resilience: Helping young children and parents affected by substance abuse, domestic violence, and depression in the context of welfare reform* (Children and welfare reform Issue Brief 8). New York: National Center for Children in Poverty, Columbia University.

Knitzer, J., & Cooper, J. (2006). Beyond integration: Challenges for children's mental health. *Health Affairs, 25*(3), 670–679. (doi:10.1377/hlthaff.25.3.670).

Kogan, M. D., & Newacheck, P. W. (2007). Introduction to the volume on articles from the national survey of children's health. *Pediatrics, 119*(Suppl.), S1–S3. (doi: 10.1542/peds.2006-2089B).

Kotch, J. B. (Ed.). (2005). *Maternal and child health: Programs, problems, and policy in public health* (2nd ed.). Sudbury, MA: Jones and Bartlett Publishers.

Kotch, J. B., & Whiteman, D. (1982). Effect of a WIC program on children's clinic activity in a local health department. *Medical Care, 20,* 691–698.

Kotch, J. B., Chalmers, D. J., Fanslow, J. L., Marshall, S., & Langley, J. D. (1993). Morbidity and death due to child abuse in New Zealand. *Child Abuse and Neglect, 17,* 233–247.

Kotch, J. B., Isbell, P., Weber, D. J., Nguyen, V., Savage, E., Gunn, E., Skinner, M., Fowlkes, S., Virk, J., & Allen, J. (2007). Hand-washing and diapering equipment reduces disease among children in out-of-home child care centers. *Pediatrics, 120*(1), e29–e36.

Lantos, J. (2010). Cruel calculus: Why saving premature babies is better business than helping them thrive. *Health Affairs, 29*(11), 2114–2117.

Lee, J. Y., Rozier, R. G., Kotch, J. B., Norton, E. C., & Vann, W. F., Jr. (2004). The effects of child WIC participation on use of oral health services. *American Journal of Public Health, 94*(5), 772–777.

Lee, J. Y., Rozier, R. G., Norton, E. C., Kotch, J. B., & Vann, W. F., Jr. (2004). The effects of the Women, Infants, and Children's Supplemental Food Program on dentally related Medicaid expenditures. *Journal of Public Health Dentistry, 64*(2), 76–81.

Lennon, M. C., Blome, J., & English, K. (Eds.). (2001). *Depression and low-income women: Challenges for TANF and welfare-to-work policies and programs.* New York: National Center for Poverty, Columbia University.

Leschied, A. W., Chiodo, D., Whitehead, P. C., & Hurley, D. (2005). The relationship between maternal depression and child outcomes in a child welfare sample: Implications for treatment and policy. *Child & Family Social Work, 10*(4), 281–291.

Leventhal, T., & Brooks-Gunn, J. (2004). A randomized study of neighborhood effects on low-income children's educational outcomes. *Developmental Psychology, 40*(4), 488.

Lyman, W. H., Walsh, J. F., Kotch, J. B., Weber, D. J., Gunn, E., & Vinjé, J. (2009). Prospective study of etiologic agents of acute gastroenteritis outbreaks in child care centers. *Journal of Pediatrics, 154*(2), 253–257.

Maffeis, C., & Tato, L. (2000). Long-term effects of childhood obesity on morbidity and mortality. *Hormone Research, 55*(1), 42–45.

Martin, J. A., Kung, H. C., Mathews, T., Hoyert, D. L., Strobino, D. M., Guyer, B., & Sutton, S. R. (2008). Annual summary of vital statistics: 2006. *Pediatrics, 121*(4), 788–801.

McCartney, K., Dearing, E., Taylor, B. A., & Bub, K. L. (2007). Quality child care supports the achievement of low-income children: Direct and indirect pathways through caregiving and the home environment. *Journal of Applied Developmental Psychology, 28*(5-6), 411–426.

McCue-Horwitz, S., Briggs-Gowan, M. J., Storfer-Isser, A., & Carter, A. S. (2007). Prevalence, correlates, and persistence of maternal depression. *Journal of Women's Health, 16*(5), 678–691.

National Survey of Children's Health. (2007). *The mental and emotional well-being of children. A portrait of states and the Nation, 2007.* Retrieved November 13, 2011, from http://www.mchb. hrsa.gov/nsch/07emohealth/national/mhs/ pages/3ccebdc.html

Nelson, J. A., Chiasson, M. A., & Ford, V. (2004). Childhood overweight in a New York City WIC population. *American Journal of Public Health, 94*, 458–462.

Newacheck, P. W., Inkelas, M., & Kim, S. E. (2004). Health services use and health care expenditures for children with disabilities. *Pediatrics, 114*(1), 79–85. (doi:10.1542/peds.114.1.79).

O'Connor, E. A., Whitlock, E. P., Beil, T. L., & Gaynes, B. N. (2009). Screening for depression in adult patients in primary care settings: A systematic evidence review. *Annals of Internal Medicine, 151*(11), 793–803.

Olds, D. L., Kitzman, H. J., Cole, R. E., Hanks, C. A., Arcoleo, K. J., Anson, E. A., Luckey, D. W., Knudtson, M. D., Henderson, C. R., Jr., & Bondy, J. (2010). Enduring effects of prenatal and infancy home visiting by nurses on maternal life course and government spending: Follow-up of a randomized trial among children at age 12 years. *Archives of Pediatrics and Adolescent Medicine, 164*(5), 419–424.

Olds, D. L., Kitzman, H., Hanks, C., Cole, R., Anson, E., Sidora-Arcoleo, K., Luckey, D. W., Henderson Jr., C. R., Holmberg, J., & Tutt, R. A. (2007). Effects of nurse home visiting on maternal and child functioning: Age-9 follow-up of a randomized trial. *Pediatrics, 120*(4), e832–e845.

Olson, A. L., Kemper, K. J., Kelleher, K. J., Hammond, C. S., Zuckerman, B. S., & Dietrich, A. J. (2002). Primary care pediatricians' roles and perceived responsibilities in the identification and management of maternal depression. *Pediatrics, 110*(6), 1169–1176.

Østergaard, M. S., & Prahl, P. (2007). Diagnosis of preschool asthma: Parents' comments and typical phrases may ease history-taking. *Primary Care Respiratory Journal: Journal of the General Practice Airways Group, 16*(3), 194–195. (doi:10.3132/ pcrj.2007.00035).

Parsons, T. J., Power, C., Logan, S., & Summerbell, C. D. (1999). Childhood predictors of adult obesity: A systematic review. *International Journal of Obesity Related Metabolism Disorders, 23*(Suppl. 8), S1–S107.

Pearce, A., Li, L., Abbas, J., Ferguson, B., Graham, H., & Law, C. (2010). Does childcare influence socioeconomic inequalities in unintentional injury? Findings from the UK millennium cohort study. *Journal of Epidemiology and Community Health, 64*(2), 161–166. (doi:10.1136/jech.2009.092643).

Pedersen, S. (2007). Preschool asthma—not so easy to diagnose. *Primary Care Respiratory Journal: Journal of the General Practice Airways Group, 16*(1), 4–6. (doi:10.3132/pcrj.2007.00011).

Perry, D. F., Kaufmann, R. K., & Knitzer, J. (2007). *Social and emotional health in early childhood.* Baltimore, MD: Paul H. Brookes Publishing Company.

Polanczyk, G., de Lima, M. S., Horta, B. L., Biederman, J., & Rohde, L. A. (2007). The worldwide prevalence of ADHD: A systematic review and metaregression analysis. *American Journal of Psychiatry, 164*(6), 942–948.

Polhamus, B., Dalenius, K., Thompson, D., Scanlon, K., Borland, E., Smith, B., & Grummer-Strawn, L. (2004). *Pediatric nutrition surveillance 2002 report.* Atlanta, GA: U.S. Department of Health and Human Services, Centers for Disease Control and Prevention.

Porterfield, S. L., & McBride, T. D. (2007). The effect of poverty and caregiver education on perceived need and access to health services among children with special health care needs. *American Journal of Public Health, 97*(2), 323–329. (doi: 10.2105/AJPH.2004.055921).

Rice, D. P., MacKenzie, E. J., & Associates. (1989). *Cost of injury in the United States: A report to Congress.* San Francisco, CA: University of California, Institute for Health and Aging, and Baltimore, MD: The Johns Hopkins University, Injury Prevention Center.

Richards, R., Merrill, R. M., Baksh, L., & McGarry, J. (2010). Maternal health behaviors and infant health outcomes among homeless mothers: U.S. Special Supplemental Nutrition Program for Women, Infants, and Children (WIC) 2000–2007. *Preventive Medicine, 52*(1), 87–94.

Rigby, E., Ryan, R. M., & Brooks-Gunn, J. (2007). Child care quality in different state policy contexts. *Journal of Policy Analysis and Management, 26*(4), 887–908.

Rosenbach, M. L., Irvin, C., & Coulam, R. F. (1999). Access for low-income children: Is health insurance enough? *Pediatrics, 103,* 1167–1174.

Sagvolden, T., Johansen, E. B., Aase, H., & Russell, V. A. (2005). A dynamic developmental theory of attention-deficit/hyperactivity disorder (ADHD) predominantly hyperactive/impulsive and combined subtypes. *Behavioral and Brain Sciences, 28*(3), 397–419.

Saha, C., Riner, M. E., & Liu, G. (2005). Individual and neighborhood-level factors in predicting asthma. *Archives of Pediatrics and Adolescent Medicine, 159*(8), 759–763.

Savage, M. F., Lee, J. Y., Kotch, J. B., & Vann, W. F., Jr., (2004). Early preventive dental visits: Effects on subsequent utilization and costs. *Pediatrics, 114*(4), e418–e423.

Schwebel, D. C., Brezausek, C. M., & Belsky, J. (2006). Does time spent in child care influence risk for unintentional injury? *Journal of Pediatric Psychology, 31*(2), 184–193.

Sedlak, A. J., Mettenburg, J., Basena, M., Petta, I., McPherson, K., Greene, A., & Li, S. (2010). *Fourth National Incidence Study of Child Abuse and Neglect (NIS-4): Report to Congress, Executive Summary.* Washington, DC: U.S. Department of Health and Human Services, Administration for Children and Families.

Selden, T. M. (2006). Compliance with well-child visit recommendations: Evidence from the medical expenditure panel survey, 2000–2002. *Pediatrics, 118*(6), e1766–e1778.

Selden, T. M., & Hudson, J. (2006). Access to care and utilization among children: estimating the effects of public and private coverage. *Medical Care, 44*(5), I-19–I-26. (doi: 10.1097/01.mlr.0000208137.46917.3b).

Shackelford, J. (2004). *State and jurisdictional eligibility definitions for infants and toddlers with disabilities under IDEA* (NECTAC Notes No. 14). Chapel Hill, NC: The University of North Carolina at Chapel Hill, FPG Child Development Institute, National Early Childhood Technical Assistance Center.

Sharma, A., Grummer-Strawn, L., Dalenius, K., Galuska, D., Anandappa, M., Borland, E., Mackintosh, H., & Smith, R. (2009). Obesity prevalence among low-income, preschool-aged children—United States, 1998–2008. *Morbidity and Mortality Weekly Report, 58*(28), 769–770.

Shonkoff, J. P., & Phillips, D. (Eds.). (2000). *From neurons to neighborhoods.* Washington, DC: National Academies Press.

Shonkoff, J. P., Boyce, W. T., & McEwen, B. S. (2009). Neuroscience, molecular biology, and the childhood roots of health disparities: Building a new framework for health promotion and disease prevention. *Journal of the*

American Medical Association, 301(21), 2252–2259. (doi:10.1001/jama.2009.754).

Silverstein, M., Augustyn, M., Cabral, H., & Zuckerman, B. (2006). Maternal depression and violence exposure: Double jeopardy for child school functioning. *Pediatrics, 118*(3), e792–e800.

Smith, K. N. G., & Corkum, P. (2007). Systematic review of measures used to diagnose attention-deficit/hyperactivity disorder in research on preschool children. *Topics in Early Childhood Special Education, 27*(3), 164–173.

Sohn, W., Ismail, A., Amaya, A., & Lepkowski, J. (2007). Determinants of dental care visits among low-income African-American children. *Journal of the American Dental Association, 138*(3), 309–318.

Sondik, E. J., Huang, D. T., Klein, R. J., & Satcher, D. (2010). Progress toward the Healthy People 2010 goals and objectives. *Annual Review of Public Health, 31*, 271–281.

Staller, J. A. (2007). Psychopharmacologic treatment of aggressive preschoolers: A chart review. *Progress in Neuro-Psychopharmacology and Biological Psychiatry, 31*(1), 131–135.

Strauss, R. S. (2000). Childhood obesity and self-esteem. *Pediatrics, 105*(1), e15.

Sung, V., Hiscock, H., Sciberras, E., & Efron, D. (2008). Sleep problems in children with attention-deficit/hyperactivity disorder: Prevalence and the effect on the child and family. *Archives of Pediatrics and Adolescent Medicine, 162*(4), 336–342.

Swann, C. A. (2010). WIC eligibility and participation: The roles of changing policies, economic conditions, and demographics. *The BE Journal of Economic Analysis & Policy, 10*(1), 1–30.

Taylor, E. (2009). Sleep and tics: Problems associated with ADHD. *Journal of the American Academy of Child & Adolescent Psychiatry, 48*(9), 877–878.

Thorell, L. B., & Wåhlstedt, C. (2006). Executive functioning deficits in relation to symptoms of ADHD and/or ODD in preschool children. *Infant and Child Development, 15*(5), 503–518.

Tolman, R. M., & Wang, H. C. (2005). Domestic violence and women's employment: Fixed effects models of three waves of women's employment study data. *American Journal of Community Psychology, 36*(1), 147–158.

United Nations. (1990). Convention on the rights of the child. Retrieved July 15, 2011 from http://www2.ohchr.org/english/law/pdf/crc.pdf.

U.S. Congress. (1973). Child Abuse Prevention and Treatment Act, PL 93-247.

U.S. Department of Agriculture, Food and Nutrition Service. (2011). WIC Program: Average monthly benefit per person FY (Data as of June 30, 2011). Retrieved May 30, 2011 from http://www.fns.usda.gov/pd/25wifyavgfd$.htm.

U.S. Department of Education. (2001). *24th annual report to Congress on the implementation of the Individuals with Disabilities Education Act.* Washington, DC: US Government Printing Office.

U.S. Department of Health and Human Services. (n.d.). Healthy People 2020 summary of objectives. Early and middle childhood. Retrieved May 14, 2011 from http://www.healthypeople.gov/2020/topicsobjectives2020/pdfs/Childhood.pdf.

U.S. Department of Health and Human Services, Administration for Children and Families, Administration on Children, Youth and Families, Children's Bureau (USDHHS/ACF/ACYF). (2010). *Child maltreatment 2009.* Retrieved July 15, 2011 from http://www.acf.hhs.gov/programs/cb/pubs/cm09/index.htm.

U.S. Department of Health and Human Services, Administration for Children and Families, Administration on Children, Youth and Families, Head Start Bureau (USDHHS). (2000). *Head Start performance standards.* Washington, DC: Author.

U.S. Department of Health and Human Services, Health Resources and Services Administration, Maternal and Child Health Bureau (USDHHS/HRSA/MCHB). (2010). *Child health USA 2010.* Rockville, MD: U.S. Department of Health and Human Services, 2010. Retrieved June 26, 2011 from http://www.mchb.hrsa.gov/publications/pdfs/childhealth2010.pdf.

U.S. Department of Health and Human Services, Administration on Children and Families, Office of Planning, Research and Evaluation (USDHHS/ACF/OPRE). (n.d.). National Survey of Child and Adolescent Well-Being (NSCAW), 1997–2010 Retrieved July 14, 2011 from http://www.acf.hhs.gov/programs/opre/abuse_neglect/nscaw/

U.S. Preventive Services Task Force. (2009). Screening for depression in adults: U.S. Preventive Services Task Force recommendation statement. *Annals of Internal Medicine, 151*(11), 784–792.

van der Lee, J. H., Mokkink, L. B., Grootenhuis, M. A., Heymans, H. S., & Offringa, M. (2007). Definitions and measurement of chronic health conditions in childhood: A Systematic review.

Journal of the American Medical Association,
297(24), 2741–2751.

Wasik, B. H., Bryant, D., Lyons, C., Sparling, J. J.,
& Ramey, C. T. (1997). Home Visiting. In R. T.
Cross, D. Spyker, &C. W. Haynes (Eds.). *Help-*
ing low birthweight premature babies: The Infant
Health and Development Program (pp. 27–41).
Stanford, CA: Stanford University Press.

Wise, P. H. (2007). The future pediatrician: The
challenge of chronic illness. *Journal of Pediatrics,*
151(5), S6–S10.

Xu, J. Q., Kochanek, K. D., Murphy, S. L., & Tejada-
Vera, B. (2010). Deaths: Final data for 2007.
National Vital Statistics Reports, 58(19). Hyatts-
ville, MD: National Center for Health Statistics.

8

THE SCHOOL-AGE CHILD

Jonathan B. Kotch and Paula Hudson Collins

"When I was born in 1920, if you wanted to visit your family on Sundays you . . . went to the graveyard . . . My brother and sister died when I was seven. Half of my family was gone! Tell me, dear children, how many of your friends died while you were growing up?"
"None," said Rodney at last.
"None! You hear that? . . . Six of my best friends died by the time I was ten!"

(Bradbury, 1994, pp. 133, 135)

INTRODUCTION

The transition to school for any child, whether reared primarily at home or with significant experience in out-of-home care, is the most profound transition for most children until the transition to work or residential college. Upon school entry, the child becomes a worker, responsible for "producing things" (Erikson, 1950, p. 259). Although success in making this transition does not guarantee future health and happiness, in the developed world these days it is a rare individual who can become a healthy and productive adult after a failed career in school. Indeed, years of completed education are a powerful predictor of health status. Applying regression techniques to data from the National Vital Statistics System, the National Longitudinal Mortality Study, and the Area Resource File, Singh and Yu (1996) concluded, "The lower the level of educational attainment and the greater the poverty, the higher the childhood mortality rates" (p. 512).

The child entering the realm of formal education moves from a learning style based mostly on personal contacts to one based on symbols. The child's world expands from the familiar, circumscribed environment of direct experience to one whose history extends back over centuries and forward infinitely in time and space (Dewey, 1956). As his or her physical and intellectual worlds expand, so do physical risks. It is in the early school years that injury becomes the cause of nearly half (46%) of all childhood deaths (Anderson & Smith, 2003). In this chapter, we review the demography, health status, health services, and health programs affecting U.S. children who are 5 to 9 years of age.

DEMOGRAPHICS

Currently, children who are 5 to 9 years old constitute 6.6% of the American population (Howden & Meyer, 2011). According to the 2010 Census, U.S. children 5 to 9 years old numbered approximately 20,348,657, a 1%

decrease since the 2000 Census. There were 10,389,638 boys and 9,959,019 girls (Howden & Meyer, 2011). Detailed data on age by race and Hispanic origin from the 2010 Census are not yet published as of this writing. The Census Bureau's American FactFinder online (U.S. Census, n.d.) permits one to query census data from the American Community Survey (ACS) from as recently as 2008. In that year the racial composition of the U.S. population of 5- to 9-year-olds was estimated to be as follows: 13,755,579 white only children, 2,788,378 African American only children, 185,184 American Indian and Alaska Native only children, 824,883 Asian only children, and 28,651 Native Hawaiian and other Pacific Islander children. These figures do not include children of more than one race. Among all U.S. children 5 to 9 years old in 2008, 4,353,113 were Hispanic or Latino (U.S. Census Bureau, n.d.).

FAMILY STRUCTURE

According to the ACS (U.S. Census Bureau, n.d.), there were an estimated 113,101,329 households in the United States in 2008, of which 75,030,551 were family households (i.e., two or more household residents were related by blood or marriage). Of these, 34,727,021 included related children under the age of 18, and only 20.2% of the 34,727,021 were family households with children of school age (6 to 17 years). Put another way, only 6.2% of all of the households in the United States in 2008 were family households living with their school-age children. The implications of this very small number on future prospects for public funding of children's services should be a major concern of child advocates.

In 2005, the number of single householder families with own children under 18 was approximately 11 million, of which 77% were maintained by a female householder. By 2008 the total was slightly less, as was the total female-headed single households with children under 18, but the total male-headed single households with children under 18 had increased slightly (U.S. Census Bureau, n.d.). The percentage of all families within each racial group maintained by a single-parent (male or female) varies greatly, with 10.1% for white, non-Hispanic families, 33.3% for African Americans, 6.1% for Asians, and 19.6% for Hispanics of any race (Kreider & Elliot, 2009).

CHILDREN AND POVERTY

In 2009, 42% of school-age children 6 to 11 years of age, or 10.3 million children, lived in low-income families (< 200% of poverty). Of those, nearly half (5 million) lived in poverty. Both the number and the percentage of school-age children living in poverty have been on the rise since 2000. These figures are somewhat better than those for children under 6, but worse than those of children 12 to 17. Race and ethnicity are strong predictors of low income. (See Table 8–1.)

Parental education, employment, and marital status are strong predictors of poverty. For example, 30% of children 6 to 11 in married couple families were low income compared to 69% of children in single-parent families. Only 28% (even that is too high) of children 6 to 11 living in a family where at least one parent worked full time were low income, compared with 91% of children in families where no adult worked. Finally,

Table 8–1 Number and Percentage of Low-Income Children by Race and Ethnicity, U.S., 2009

	Number (millions)	Percent
White	3.8	28
African American	2.1	64
Asian	0.3	30
American Indian	0.1	64
Other race	0.3	43
Hispanic	3.6	64

Source: Courtesy of the National Center for Children in Poverty, Mailman School of Public Health, Columbia University.

87% of children lived with parents who have less than a high school diploma, compared with 63% with parents with no more than a high school diploma and 27% with at least one parent with at least some college (Chau, Thampi, & Wight, 2010). Not surprisingly, only 17% of poor children have private health insurance, but poor children are more likely to be insured by either a private or a public source than children in families at 100–200% of poverty thanks to Medicaid, which covers 66% of poor children 6–11 years old (Chau, Thampi, & Wight, 2010).

HEALTH STATUS

The years from 5 to 9 are the healthiest of any age bracket in the United States (Miniño, Xu, Kochanek, & Tejada-Vera, 2009) if judged by the mortality rate, 13.7 per 100,000 in 2007 (a decrease from 15.8 per 100,000 in 2000) (Centers for Disease Control, National Center for Health Statistics, 2010). Major concerns in child health shifted during the 20th century from "natural causes" (infectious diseases primarily) to so-called new morbidities (injury-related mortality and morbidity; psychological, emotional, and learning disorders; and chronic physical and developmental conditions) (USDHHS/HRSA/MCHB, 1991). Improved living standards, community-based health promotion and disease prevention, and effective immunization against infectious diseases have all made major contributions in reducing childhood mortality and morbidity in the 20th century. Nevertheless, the United States is still behind other industrialized nations in childhood mortality, primarily because of excess deaths attributable to injury (Williams & Kotch, 1990). The majority of unintentional injury deaths among children 5 to 14 years old resulted from motor vehicle traffic crashes (USDHHS/HRSA/MCHB, 2010). Although seat belt use and other safety measures (such as child-proof safety caps, smoke detectors, bicycle helmets, and flame-retardant clothing) have reduced mortality rates caused by

unintentional injury, rates of death because of violence rose among children until about 1991 in the case of homicide (Fox & Zawitz, 2003) and 1994 in the case of suicide (Snyder & Swahn, 2003). Both homicide and suicide have generally declined for this age group between 1999 and 2007.

EPIDEMIOLOGY OF MAJOR HEALTH PROBLEMS

Natural Causes

Death rates in the 5- to 9-year-old age group declined 66% from 1900 to 1933, 62.5% between 1933 and 1950, 33.3% from 1950 to 1970, and 50% from 1970 to 1985 (Fingerhut, 1989). That 50% decline was the highest of any age bracket among all people in the United States. Deaths among U.S. 5- to 9-year-old children declined another 19.2% between 1985 and 1998 (Centers for Disease Control, National Center for Health Statistics, 2003) and another 18.9% between 1999 and 2007 (Centers for Disease Control, National Center for Health Statistics, 2010). Over the course of the 20th century, from 1900 and 1998, the death rate for 5- to 9-year-olds in the United States declined 96%. Because natural causes were declining faster than external causes (e.g., 69% between 1933 and 1950 for natural causes compared with 35% for external causes) (Fingerhut, 1989), the proportion of all deaths attributable to external causes has been increasing. In 1900, an estimated 89.9% of child deaths were due to natural causes. Sometime between 1970 and 1971, natural causes resulted in fewer than 50% of deaths among U.S. 5- to 9-year-old children for the first time in history (Fingerhut, 1989).

Infectious Diseases

In 1900, diphtheria alone caused 10% of all deaths in U.S. school-aged children (Fingerhut, 1989). By 1992, there was no infectious disease among the top five killers of such children (Guyer, Freedman, Strobino, & Sondik, 2000). On the other hand, infectious disease is the leading cause of visits to the doctor for sick care (Hardy, 1991) and one of the top five causes of hospitalization in this age group (USDHHS/HRSA/MCHB, 2010).

The 1988 Child Health Supplement to the National Health Interview Survey (NHIS-CHS) (Adams & Hardy, 1989) asked respondents about nine of the most common childhood infectious diseases. Using a 7-year age bracket (5 to 11), the survey discovered that repeated ear infections were the most common complaint in the past year (8.8%), followed by repeated tonsillitis (5.5%). Half of school-age children who had either condition had to limit their activity. Pneumonia was the leading infectious disease cause of hospitalization, but children with mononucleosis were hospitalized longer. Children in the 5- to 11-year-old bracket were the most likely to have surgery for repeated tonsillitis or repeated ear infections, to lose the most school days and spend more time in bed because of mononucleosis, and to see the doctor for repeated tonsillitis and bladder or urinary infections (Hardy, 1991).

Chronic Illness

In 1998, the Maternal and Child Health Bureau defined children with special health needs or chronic conditions as "those who have or are at increased risk for a chronic physical, developmental, behavioral, or emotional condition and who also require health and related services of a type or amount beyond that required by children generally" (McPherson, et al., 1998, p. 138). According to the 2005–2006 National Survey of Children with Special Health Care Needs, approximately 13.7 million children under 18 have special health care needs such as allergies, asthma, attention deficit/attention deficit/hyperactivity disorder (ADD/ADHD), depression/anxiety/emotional problems, migraine/frequent headaches, and mental retardation. These and other conditions are responsible for functional difficulties such as respiratory problems, learning problems, behavior problems, speech and language

problems, social problems, and chronic pain (Data Resource Center, n.d.). Expenditures for children with special health care needs (CSHCN) account for 70–80% of all medical expenditures for all children (Institute of Medicine, 1988). The most recent prevalence reports from the 2005–2006 national survey of CSHCN indicate that, for children 6 to 11 years old with a special health care need, the most prevalent conditions (not unduplicated) include allergies (55.7%), asthma (41.4%), ADD/ADHD (34.0%), learning difficulties (45.4%), speech–language difficulties (23.4%), migraine or frequent headaches (14.1%), mental retardation (11.3%), and depression/anxiety/eating disorder/other emotional problem (20.6%) (National Survey of Children with Special Health Care Needs, n.d.). The prevalence of CSHCN does not vary significantly by income, but it does by race/ethnicity. The prevalence of special health care needs varies by the race/ethnicity of the child. The prevalence is highest among multiracial children (18.0%), followed by non-Hispanic white (15.5%), non-Hispanic Black (15.0%), American Indian/Alaska Native (14.5%), and Native Hawaiian/Pacific Islander children (11.5%). The prevalence of special health care needs is lowest among Hispanic children (8.3%) and Asian children (6.3%) (USDHHS/HRSA/MCHB, 2008).

The absolute numbers of children with chronic illness are not expected to change dramatically in the coming decades (Newacheck & Taylor, 1992). Although more children with chronic conditions will survive because of improvements in medical technology and practice, these increases will be offset by demographic trends leading to fewer births (National Center for Health Statistics, 1995). Nonetheless, the prevalence of children with chronic conditions continues to increase. Growing populations of children with special health care needs include those who are dependent on advanced medical technology such as ventilators, gastrostomies, and tracheostomies (Palfrey, et al., 1991). Comparing National Health Interview

Survey data from 2005 (Bloom, Dey, & Freeman, 2006) to 2009 (Bloom, Cohen, & Freeman, 2010) suggests that conditions such as asthma, allergies and learning disabilities are inching up. However, improvements in diagnosis may account for some of the increase (Richardson, 1989; Schidlow & Fiel, 1990).

Mental Health

For many decades, emotional and behavioral problems among children were treated because they were seen as precursors of adult disorders. As the 20th century drew to a close, these problems have come to be seen as also important in their own right (Drotar & Bush, 1985). The President's New Freedom Commission on Mental Health reports that between 5% and 9% of school-age children suffer from serious emotional disorders, manifesting in impairments that range from behavioral problems to depression. Findings from the 1992 to 1994 National Health Interview Survey on Disability (NHIS-D) and related studies suggest that between 17% to 22% of children from birth to 17 years old suffer from some form of diagnosable mental illness, indicating that the use of psychological assistance for children had increased by more than 7% to 12% since results of the 1988 NHIS-CHS results were published (Halfon & Newacheck, 1998).

Data from the 1988 NHIS-CHS indicate that the cumulative proportion of children who have ever had emotional or behavioral problems should increase fairly steadily with age. The proportion of children who had ever had an emotional or behavioral problem rose from 5.3% at the age of 3 to 5 years, to 12.7% at ages 6 to 11 years, to 18.5% at ages 12–17 years. This is consistent with the results of the National Survey of Children's Health (NSCH), which reported that 8.4% parents of 6- to 11-year-olds indicated that their children consistently demonstrated problematic behavior, compared with 9.3% of parents of 12- to 17-year-olds (NSCH, 2007). Increases in childhood psychological disorders have been attributed to the growing proportions of children who experience parental divorce, were born outside of marriage, or are raised in conflict-filled families or low-income, low-education, single-parent households (Zill & Schoenborn, 1990).

NHIS-CHS data also indicate that the prevalence of childhood emotional and behavioral problems showed significant variation across family income groups, with children from less advantaged backgrounds standing a somewhat greater chance of exhibiting such problems (Zill & Schoenborn, 1990). Similarly, the NSCH revealed that children with these conditions are more likely to have low family incomes than children without them: of children with at least one emotional, behavioral, or developmental condition, 24.8% had family incomes below the federal poverty level, compared to 17.1% of children without one of these conditions (USDHHS/HRSA/MCHB, 2009).

Although mental health problems are relatively common among children, especially among those with health problems (Drotar, 1981; Goldberg et al., 1979), most cases are mild and resolve without treatment. Nonetheless, there is a core of persistent, disabling disorders—notably conduct disorder, multiple disorders, autism, and child schizophrenia—that require focused and sustained treatment. Data from the 1988 NHIS-CHS indicate that the overall prevalence of emotional or behavioral problems was 13.4% of all children 3 to 17 years old. By 1996, the 6-month prevalence of any mental or addictive disorders among 9- to 17-year-olds was reported by the Surgeon General to be 20% (USDHHS, 1999). Yet, of children whose parents reported that they needed mental health treatment, 40% did not receive mental health care or counseling (USDHHS/HRSA/MCHB, 2010). This fact should be of great concern to maternal and child health practitioners in that (1) the etiology of most childhood emotional and behavioral problems is not well understood, (2) many providers have not been adequately trained to recognize and deal with these types of problems, and (3) procedures for referring children for psychological diagnosis and treatment are not standardized. Thus, there is believed to be a substantial group of young people with developmental or behavioral disorders whose problems go untreated and perhaps even unrecognized (Silverman & Koretz, 1989). Because of the significant life stresses faced by children with emotional and behavioral difficulties, untreated mental health problems can often lead to further difficulties in adolescence and adulthood. There is growing recognition that prevention and early intervention work to reduce the prevalence of, or the consequences of, mental health problems in children (USDHHS, 1999).

Developmental Disabilities

In 1984, the Developmental Disabilities Act (PL 98-527) referred to a developmental disability as a "severe, chronic condition attributable to a mental or physical impairment, manifest before the age of 22 and likely to continue indefinitely." More recently, the Developmental Disabilities Assistance and Bill of Rights Act Amendments of 1999 define the concept of developmental concerns of young children "to include both substantial developmental delays or specific congenital or acquired conditions that will likely result in substantial functional limitations in three or more major life activities, including self-care, receptive and expressive language, learning, mobility, self-direction, capacity for independent living, and economic self-sufficiency if services are not provided." Developmental concerns experienced by children can challenge typical development in the key domains: cognition, social and emotional growth, language and communication, and physical growth and skill (Hogan, Rogers, & Msall, 2000). These concerns may be due to inherited genetic influences or environmental influences (or a combination of genetic and environmental factors) and may have their genesis during the prenatal, perinatal, or postnatal periods. Examples of genetically based concerns include Down syndrome, Fragile X syndrome, phenylketonuria, and Tay-Sachs disease. Environmentally based concerns may include the consequences of encephalitis, meningitis, rubella (German measles), fetal alcohol syndrome, lead poisoning, poor nutrition, unintentional injury, and child abuse. A host of individual and cultural–familial factors is associated with environmentally based concerns such as parental educational level, family history, and patterns of parent–child interaction. The prevalence estimate data from the 2007 National Survey of Children's Health indicate that 3.2% of U.S. children 17 years old and less have had a delay in their development (USDHHS/HRSA/MCHB, 2009), rising to 4.1% for children 6–11 (NSCH, 2007). As with mental health problems, the rate of treatment for these problems should be of concern to MCH practitioners.

Learning Disabilities

The proportion of children whose parents reported in 2009 that they were told that they had a learning disability (including ADD/ADHD) was 8% (Bloom, Cohen, & Freeman, 2010), higher than the 6.5% reported in the 1988 NHIS-CHS (Zill & Schoenborn, 1990). Furthermore, in contrast to developmental delays, most learning disabilities (LDs) are not fully apparent until the child gets to school and starts trying to read, write, and calculate. Therefore, there is a substantial rise in the prevalence of LDs as children reach school age. The proportion of children with LDs jumped from 1% at 3 to 5 years old to 11% among 12- to 17-year-olds (Child Trends Data Bank, 2003).

The prevalence of LDs also varied by family structure, income, and gender. Low income, single mother as parent, and male gender are all associated with an increased prevalence of LD (NSCH, 2007). The situation for race/ethnicity is more complicated, however. Hispanic children 2 to 17 years are less likely to have a diagnosis of ADD than white non-Hispanics but more likely to have learning disabilities, whereas black non-Hispanic children are less likely to have ADD but more likely to have learning disabilities than

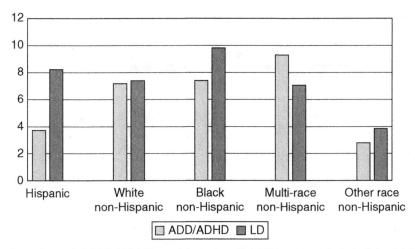

Figure 8–1 Prevalence of ADD/ADHD and learning disabilities by race/ethnicity, children 2–17 years, U.S. 2007.

Source: Data from: National Survey of Children's Health, 2007.

multiracial non-Hispanic children (NSCH, 2007). (See Figure 8–1.)

Moreover, Zill and Schoenborn (1990) pointed out that there is evidence that LDs were underidentified in populations of different race in 1988. The reason for this is that blacks and Hispanics have higher rates than whites of the risk factors for LDs—low parental education and income levels, low birth weight, single parenthood, etc. However, it is important to keep in mind the different cultural perceptions and mores of whites and persons of different race regarding what constitutes a learning deficiency (how it is both perceived and defined) and how much and what type of information should be shared with strangers (Jackson, 1981; Jones & Roberts, 1994; Nettles, 1994; Telfair & Nash, 1996). As well, private health insurance coverage is associated with a higher prevalence of ADD only (Pastor & Reuben, 2002). Given more limited access to medical care, black children may be less likely to have had a LD diagnosed as such than white children.

Finally, in the 1988 NHIS-CHS, approximately 5% of all children 3 to 17 years old, or more than three-quarters of those with LDs, had received treatment or counseling for their disabilities, and most of these children (three-fifths) had received treatment or counseling in the previous 12 months (Zill & Schoenborn, 1990).

External Causes

External causes (including both intentional and unintentional injury) are the leading causes of death of children 1 to 14 years old. Unintentional injury causes the most deaths between ages 5 and 14 years. Homicide was the fourth leading cause of death for 5- to 9-year-olds and third for 10- to 14-year-olds, whereas suicide, not a top 10 leading cause of death for 5 to 9, was the fourth leading cause of death in 10- to 14-year-olds (Centers for Disease Control [CDC], National Center for Injury Prevention and Control, 2007). Injury disproportionately affects males and children of different races. Among children 5 to 14 years old, American Indian/Alaska Native males had the highest death rates in 2007, followed in order by African American males and white males. African American females had the highest injury death rate among all females, albeit lower than white

Table 8–2 All Injury Deaths and Rates per 100,000 All Races, Both Sexes, Ages 5 to 14, United States, 2007

Race	Sex	Number of Deaths	Population	Crude Rate	Age-Adjusted Rate**
White	Males	1,218	16,061,751	7.58	7.58
	Females	766	15,260,544	5.02	5.02
		1,984	**31,322,295**	**6.33**	-
Black	Males	415	3,315,181	12.52	12.46
	Females	237	3,211,294	7.38	7.36
		652	**6,526,475**	**9.99**	-
Am Indian/AK Native	Males	39	282,808	13.79	13.83
	Females	19*	273,735	6.94*	6.95
		58	**556,543**	**10.42**	-
Asian/Pac Islander	Males	47	999,356	4.70	4.76
	Females	33	968,630	3.41	3.44
		80	1,967,986	4.07	-
Total		**2,774**	**40,373,299**	**6.87**	-

Source: Centers for Disease Control and Prevention, National Center for Injury Prevention and Control. WISQARS. (2007). United States All Injury Deaths and Rates per 100,000. Retrieved July 16, 2011 from http://webappa.cdc.gov/sasweb/ncipc/leadcaus10.html.

males, followed by American Indian/Alaska Native females and finally white females. Asian/Pacific Islander males and females had the lowest injury death rates of all (CDC, National Center for Injury Prevention and Control, 2007). (See Table 8–2.)

Community-based strategies to prevent injury have largely been successful in reducing death rates. Examples of such successes include seat belt use and other safety measures that have lowered traffic fatalities, smoke detectors to reduce deaths caused by house fires, childproof caps on medications, and bicycle helmets (Singh & Yu, 1996). Rates of death caused by homicide rose among children 5 to 14 years old by a factor of two to three between the mid-1980s and the mid-1990s, after which date homicide rates have been decreasing (Fox & Zawitz, 2003).

Injuries more often are not fatal. In the 5- to 9- and 10- to 14-year-old age groups, injury is the third leading cause of hospitalization, resulting in 91,000 hospital discharges in 2007 (USDHHS/HRSA/MCHB, 2010). Unfortunately, not all of these children are discharged well. Injury is the leading cause of acquired disability among school-aged children. In addition to hospitalization, injury may result in an emergency room or doctor visit, activity limitation, days lost from school, bed-disability days, etc.

HEALTH CARE ACCESS AND UTILIZATION

The use of health services by children is qualitatively different from that of adults. Children use proportionately more ambulatory and preventive care and less hospital care than adults (Keane, Lave, Ricci, & LaVallee, 1999). As a direct result, annual health care costs for children (excluding infants) are less than those of adults, even of adults less than 65 years old. For the majority of children 5 to 17 years old (85%), average medical care expenditures totaled $1,663, compared with $2,974 of adults 18 to 44 and $5,843 for older adults less than 65 (Agency for Healthcare Research and Quality, 2008). Nevertheless, 29% of that expense was paid out of pocket, compared with 21% for 18- to 44-year-olds and 17% for 45- to 64-year-olds (Agency for Healthcare Research and Quality [AHRQ], 2011). This compares with 21% out-of-pocket costs for children 6 to 17 that was paid out during the period 1996–1998 (McCormick, et al., 2001).

The need for immunizations and indeed for routine well-child visits in general declines in the school years. This explains why school-age children (6 to 17 years old) were more likely to have had no doctor visit, and less likely to have had four or more visits, than children under 6 during the years of 1997 to 2009 (CDC, 2010a). Another reason for lack of a doctor visit for routine medical care or for not having a regular source of routine health care in the first place is uninsuredness (Kenney, Dubay, & Haley, 2000; Newacheck, Hughes, Hung, Wong, & Stoddard, 2000; Schoen & Dezroches, 2000). Children constitute a significant proportion of the growing uninsured population. In 2009, 8.3 million children under 18 years of age lacked health insurance (Holahan, 2011). In actual numbers, this corresponded to a decrease of nearly 1 million over the levels of uninsured children reported for the year 2000. That uninsuredness declined for children during the Great Recession is entirely due to Medicaid and the Child Health Insurance Program (CHIP), which covered 4 million more children in 2009 compared with 2007, whereas employer-based coverage declined by 2.5 million children in the same period (Holahan, 2011). Not surprisingly, privately

insured children 6 to 17 were least likely to have had no doctor visit in 2008–2009 (9.5%), compared with children on Medicaid (12.5%) and with the uninsured (39.8%) (CDC, 2010b).

This inequity seems to characterize the nation's approach to children's health care needs in general. Although private insurance coverage increases with increasing child age, the drop in public health insurance coverage (primarily Medicaid and CHIP) from under 4 to ages 13 to 17 is steep, resulting in increasing uninsuredness with age (AHRQ, 2011). At the same time, private health insurance coverage of all children less than 18 years old, both employer-based health coverage and private nongroup coverage, is decreasing steadily (Holahan, 2011). Although Medicaid and other public health insurance have been able to compensate thus far, policy initiatives at the national level to cut Medicaid funding and eliminate federal entitlements to Medicaid are ominous.

The Medicaid and CHIP programs are associated with substantial improvement in access to and use of health care services for low-income children. However, 17.2% of children in poverty remain uninsured (Kaiser Family Foundation, 2010). Numerous barriers to Medicaid enrollment have prevented many eligible children from enrolling in the program. This problem has been further exacerbated by welfare reform (welfare-to-work initiatives), which dismantled previous policies that automatically conferred Medicaid eligibility to children in families receiving Aid to Families with Dependent Children or welfare (Garrett & Holahan, 2000; Sochalski & Villarruel, 1999). Sochalski and Villarruel (1999) reported that many children in families leaving welfare are still eligible for Medicaid based on income eligibility criteria. However, several reasons are given for many of these children becoming uninsured. First, welfare administrators fail to inform families of their continuing eligibility. Second, families may not understand the eligibility rules. Third, a stigma is frequently attached to receiving Medicaid, and finally, many administrative challenges exist for states and families (Garrett & Holahan, 2000; Sochalski & Villarruel, 1999).

The fate of children who are eligible for Medicaid but who remain unenrolled mirrors that of children who are uninsured. Davidoff, et al. (2000) pooled Medicaid-eligible children from the 1994 and 1995 National Health Interview Survey and classified them according to insurance status (Medicaid enrollee; eligible but unenrolled and without insurance; and eligible but unenrolled with private insurance). Comparative analyses were completed examining measures of access (having a particular physician at a usual source of care, clinic waiting time, having an unmet health need) and use of healthcare services (adequacy of immunizations, having visited a doctor's office in the past 2 weeks, amount of money spent on medical care). Uninsured Medicaid-eligible children fared least well on all the access to care indicators studied. With respect to use, uninsured Medicaid-eligible children had the lowest levels of immunization adequacy and tended to be less likely to have visited the doctor's office in the past 2 weeks. They were more likely to have used nonhospital outpatient, hospital outpatient, and the hospital emergency room than Medicaid enrollees. Although privately insured Medicaid-eligible children generally had better health care access and use profiles than Medicaid enrollees, they were significantly more likely to spend more than $500 per year for out-of-pocket healthcare expenses.

In view of the evidence that having some form of insurance, whether private or public, improves access to health care for children, attempts to provide health insurance coverage to other uninsured low-income non-Medicaid eligible children are warranted. The Children's Health Insurance Program was created in response to the growing problem of these uninsured children. The program was enacted as Title XXI of the Social Security Act and appropriates funds through the Balanced Budget Act of 1997 for states to provide health insurance to children from birth through 18 years old (Halfon, et al., 1999; Sochalski & Villarruel, 1999). The program, funded for 10 years, was reauthorized in 2009. States have the option to use the funds to expand their Medicaid programs, to establish new or expand existing child health insurance programs apart from the Medicaid program, or to use a combination plan with Medicaid expansion and a state plan available. Although not an entitlement like Medicaid, the Children's Health Insurance Program offers tremendous potential for improving access to care for children in the target population.

The aggregate numbers for health insurance coverage mask differences in health insurance and access to health care by child or family characteristics. For example, Hispanic children are less likely to have health insurance than white, non-Hispanic, or black children (Kaiser Family Foundation, 2010). Uninsured children are much more likely to have no usual source of care than are children who have health insurance. For example, 29% of children who were not insured had no usual source of health care. This was more than 11 times the percentage of children with private health insurance who had no usual source of health care (Federal Interagency Forum, 2010). Finally, merely having health insurance does not tell the whole story. Twenty-three and a half percent of parents of children with insurance reported that insurance was inadequate in terms of one or more of the following criteria: (1) out-of-pocket costs were not reasonable, (2) insurance usually did not provide necessary benefits or services, or (3) insurance usually did not allow the child to see the family's preferred provider (USDHHS/HRSA/MCHB, 2010).

SCHOOL HEALTH

"No knowledge is more crucial than knowledge about health. Without it, no other life goal can be successfully achieved."

(Ernest L. Boyer, 1983, p. 304)

School health activities were one of the earliest public health interventions targeted specifically at children. Leading the way were Dr. Sarah Josephine Baker and Lillian Wald, who, based in New York's Henry Street Settlement, organized in 1893 the first visiting nurse service and subsequently the first school health nursing program in the country. These early efforts both used the school setting to shortcut infectious disease surveillance strategies in an effort to identify and quarantine children who were a threat to others and directed health education, screening, and disease prevention activities for the benefit of the children served and their families.

Public school entry is the first time since birth that essentially all children in the United States are within the purview of an institutional setting. This creates an opportunity for proactive health intervention that has only partly been taken advantage of in this country. Traditional school health activities, such as screening tests and routine medical history and examination, were considered of "low effectiveness" (p. 112) and "limited value" (p. 123), respectively (American Academy of Pediatrics, 1981). On the other hand, a comprehensive and coordinated school health program cannot only promote a child's achievement of health literacy, "the capacity to obtain, interpret, and understand basic health information and services and the competence to use such information and services in ways which enhance health" (Joint Committee on National Health Education Standards, 1995, p. 5). It can also make a direct contribution to the general education of the child. According to J. Michael McGinnis, former Director of Disease Prevention and Health Promotion of the U.S. Public Health Service, a child who is not healthy will not "profit optimally from the educational process" (American School Health Association, 1994).

"Efforts to improve school performance that ignore health are ill-conceived, as are health improvement efforts that ignore education" (National Commission on the Role of the School and the Community in Improving Adolescent Health, 1990, p. 9). Comprehensive school health education is defined

as classroom instruction that addresses the physical, mental, emotional, and social dimensions of health; develops health knowledge, attitudes and skills; and is tailored to each age level. School health education is designed to motivate and assist students to maintain and improve their health, prevent disease, and reduce health-related risk behaviors (Marx & Wooley, 1998, p. 43). Often, education professionals define school health as health knowledge, health instruction, health education, and health literacy, whereas their public health counterparts tend to define school health as school health services. However, the Centers for Disease Control and Prevention (CDC) have promoted a coordinated approach to school health since the mid-1980s. This framework is referred to as Coordinated School Health Programs and is extensively described by Marx and Wooley (1998) in *Health Is Academic*.

The goals of a coordinated school health program are to promote health, prevent injury and disease, prevent high-risk behavior, intervene to help children in need or at risk, help those with special needs, and promote positive health and safety behaviors. The program has eight separate components. The eight components of a Coordinated School Health Program (CSHP) include the following: (1) comprehensive school health education; (2) physical education; (3) school nutrition services; (4) school health services; (5) a healthy school environment; (6) school counseling, psychological and social services; (7) school-site health promotion for staff; and (8) family and community involvement. Although the Coordinated School Health Model (CSH) promotes the eight components of a healthy school, the key to "coordinating" the program lies with the successful collaboration of school and health professionals routinely working together to address school health issues.

As discussed previously, *comprehensive school health education* focuses on the health information, strategies, and skills taught to students. Health education is to be integrated into the academic curriculum and to result in changes in students' knowledge, attitudes, behaviors, and skills (American School Health Association, 1994). This classroom-based instruction provides age-appropriate information in a proper scope and sequence of health topics, skills, and behaviors. It is designed to motivate and assist students to maintain and improve their health, prevent disease, and reduce health-related risk behaviors by helping the children develop appropriate health knowledge, attitudes, and skills. Typically, elementary students receive health instruction taught by their regular classroom teachers in lessons often integrated into other subjects such as reading a book about an unhealthy rabbit in language arts or plotting a graph during math showing the number of fruits and vegetables eaten by the student each day for a week. Time for health instruction competes with other equally important and tested subjects during the elementary students' school day.

Physical education is planned, sequential instruction that promotes lifelong physical activity. It is designed to develop basic motor skills, sports skills, and physical fitness as well as to enhance students' mental, physical, social, and emotional abilities. Physical education classes should devote at least 50% of course time to instruction that can translate into a lifetime program of health-related physical activity. Physical education and physical activity, although linked, cannot accurately be described as interchangeable. They represent two very different philosophies. *Physical education* involves teaching students the skills, knowledge, and confidence they need to lead physically active lives. It should be taught by a licensed physical education specialist and/or a health and physical education teacher. On the other hand, *physical activity* is actual bodily movement that may be practiced as part of a physical education curriculum. The CDC recommends that children receive a minimum of 60 minutes of moderate to vigorous physical activity each day for optimal health. In support of this recommendation, several states

have adopted policies promoting and/or requiring physical activity. For example, in North Carolina, K-8 students receive 30 minutes of physical activity during the school day as required by the North Carolina State Board of Education's Healthy Active Children Policy (HSP-S-000) adopted in 2003. Creative teaching methods and materials such as "Energizers," which are classroom-based physical activities for elementary and middle school students, have been developed and are available at no charge to teachers and may be accessed at www.nchealthyschools.org. In Texas, many of the public schools have adopted the CATCH program (Coordinated Approach to Child Health) to advance a coordinated school health model and increase physical activity for students and staff members.

School nutrition services focuses on the integration of nutritious, affordable, and appealing meals; nutrition education; and the creation of an environment that promotes healthy eating behaviors for all children. The school meals program is designed to maximize each child's education and health potential. School food service and nutrition include both nutritionally appropriate meals at a reasonable price and education in making responsible, healthy food choices. Good nutrition along with physical activity are essential to preventing chronic disease and obesity among not only our nation's youth but worldwide. The obesity epidemic and efforts to address it are currently receiving a great deal of media attention.

The *school environment* addresses not only children's safety from injury and toxic exposures but a supportive psychosocial environment as well. The healthy school environment addresses the physical, emotional, and social climate of the school. It is designed to provide a safe physical facility, as well as a healthy and supportive social environment that fosters learning. For example, many school administrators and public health professionals recognize that fostering a safer school environment requires a more vigorous approach to stopping bullying in schools.

School counseling, psychological services, and *social services* include activities that focus on the cognitive, emotional, behavioral, and social needs of individuals, groups, and families. Counseling, guidance, and mental health address direct services to students with psychosocial needs, in conjunction with other community-based resources. These services are designed to prevent and address problems, facilitate positive learning, and enhance the development of healthy behaviors.

School-site health promotion for staff or *worksite health promotion* is directed at school district employees and includes assessment, education, and fitness activities for school faculty and staff. Its purpose is to maintain and improve the health and well-being of school faculty and staff who serve as role models for the students and their families.

Family and community involvement in schools creates partnerships among schools, families, community-based groups and health care providers, and individuals. This involvement maximizes the resources and expertise available in addressing the healthy development of children, youth, and their families. Integration of school and community-based health activities seeks to maximize health and health-related services for school-age children through coordination, integration, and communication with parents and existing health resources (American School Health Association, 1994).

Many states have adopted the use of School Health Advisory Councils (SHACs), also known as School Health Councils (SHCs), to assist schools in organizing health-related action plans and strategies within the CSH framework. These councils are minimally composed of representatives from each of the previously described eight components of the coordinated school health program plus a student, a school administrator, and a public health partner.

Health services in school are a special case. School health services include preventive services, health education, emergency care, as well as management and referral of acute and chronic health conditions. These services are designed to identify and prevent health problems and injuries as well as to provide health care for students. These may vary from the minimum required by law (such as dental, hearing, vision and spinal screening, and sports physicals) to the delivery of hands-on personal health services on school grounds. School-based and school-linked health centers, totaling approximately 30 in the early 1980s (U.S. General Accounting Office, 1994), now number 1,909 as of 2007–2008, according to the National Assembly on School-Based Health Care (NASBHC, 2007–2008). Although most common in high schools (33.3%), school-based health centers are not unknown at the elementary and middle school levels. Approximately 9.6% of all school-based and school-linked health centers are based in elementary schools, and 7.8% are based in middle schools. Another 6.8% serve elementary and middle school combinations, and the remainder serve other grade-level combinations (NASBHC, 2007–2008).

Many different school-based and school-linked health center models exist. They may be staffed by school district employees or local health department employees, may be available to a specific subpopulation of the student body or to all (with parental consent), may be limited to screening and referral for initial complaints, or may provide comprehensive primary and preventive care. In most cases, midlevel providers, primarily nurse practitioners and physician assistants, provide the bulk of the services. The most controversial issue that has to be confronted in establishing a school-based health center at the secondary school level, the provision of reproductive health services, is less of an issue at the elementary school level. Financing, staffing, third-party reimbursement, and responding to dental and mental health needs are continuing problems. Nevertheless, the school-based health centers are low cost, convenient, and "can improve children's access to health care . . . especially those who are poor or uninsured" (U.S. General Accounting Office, 1994, p. 5).

There are often three markers—poverty, poor educational attainment, and poor health—of obstacles to succeeding in school (Collins & Lee, 2008). However, schools can best teach, encourage, and promote healthy behaviors among students by being model environments for these behaviors and by providing evidence-based curricula in a safe and healthy learning environment (Atkinson & Collins, 2010). Just imagine a school of the future focused on academics as well as the overall well-being of each student and staff member. In this school, students would have water bottles at their desks to help them stay hydrated throughout the day. The school cafeteria would serve only healthy *à la carte* foods and beverages and ample fresh fruits and vegetables. More students would select meals offered through the school meals program, meeting national guidelines and other nutritional requirements. Candy and unhealthy treats such as those that are high in fat and sugar would not be used for fundraisers or for rewards for students. Teachers would model healthy eating. Physical fitness would be encouraged by allowing more students to participate in sports and physical activities through intramural activities, clubs, and special interest groups. Positive exercise habits would be modeled by teachers who take the opportunity to enjoy physical activity alongside their students during their daily recess or physical education classes. Physical education for students would focus on activities that are fun and engaging in adequate facilities and with proper equipment. The teachers' lounge would be stocked with healthy alternatives to the usual vending machine fare, and there would be onsite wellness programs to help teachers focus on their own health needs. Staff wellness programs would include activities to promote

reaching and maintaining a healthy weight, stress management, and smoking cessation. The school facility would be connected to the community by sidewalks or bike pathways to enable more students to walk safely to school. The outdoor campus of the school would be pleasant and inviting. Gardens on the school grounds would provide seasonal flowers, wildlife habitat, and even fruits or vegetables for consumption. These gardens would be tended by students, parents, or faculty volunteers and would meet the various local, state and federal guidelines insuring food safety. This vision represents the ideal! Parts of this vision already exist in our schools; other parts remain dreams for the future. By implementing the eight essential components of the Coordinated School Health Model, schools can partner with broader community efforts to improve the health status of our young people (Collins & Lee, 2008).

OUTSTANDING ISSUES

Child Abuse and Neglect

Child maltreatment victimization declines with age, such that school-age children are less likely to be reported than preschool children, and preschool children are less likely to be reported and substantiated than infants and toddlers (USDHHS/ACF/ACYF/CB, 2010). However, the proportion of type of maltreatment changes with age. Younger children are more likely to be victims of neglect, whereas older children are more likely to be victims of physical and sexual abuse (USDHHS/HRSA/MCHB, 2010). Neglect prior to age 2 years can have greater impact on children's behavioral outcomes than either neglect between ages 2 and 4, or physical abuse anytime between birth and age 4 (Kotch, et al., 2008).

After declining in the 1990s, official reports of child abuse and neglect went up somewhat in 2000 from 1.18% to 1.22% of all U.S. children (USDHHS/ACF/ACYF/CB, 2002). The increase does not only reflect an increased awareness and willingness to report (National Center for Health Statistics, 1995). In her reanalysis of the 1986 national incidence study, Sedlak (1991) concluded that the increased incidence of child maltreatment between 1980 and 1986 "reflected increases in the incidence of occurrence of moderate injury cases" (Sedlak, 1991, p. 3–15). Subsequent to Sedlak's analysis, a Gallup poll reported that a survey of parents revealed a rate of abuse 16 times that estimated by official statistics (Lewin, 1995).

We are now witnessing another period of decline in official child maltreatment rates. There has been a decrease in the number of reports and the number of substantiations in the five years between 2005 and 2009. The unique number of children who were investigated by child protective services (CPS) agencies across the United States fell to a low of 3 million (40.3 per 1,000), and the victimization to 693,174 children (9.3 per 1,000). However, there are reasons to take this apparent decline with a grain of salt. The total number of "dispositions" (when CPS assigns a finding to a case) has not declined in the same 5 years. This may be a consequence of the fact that the proportion of all allegations that are considered for an investigation (now 62%) has been declining, and an increasing number of cases accepted for an investigation are referred for an alternative response before substantiation is determined.

A telling statistic that makes one skeptical of claims that maltreatment is diminishing is the child fatality rate. Child maltreatment fatalities have continued to increase during the same period that official child maltreatment rates were reportedly declining. In 2009, child maltreatment fatalities reached 1,770 victims, or 2.34 per 100,000, a 5-year high. Neglect is the most common type of maltreatment associated with child death. Analyzing the children by mutually exclusive types of maltreatment reveals that 36.7% of all child fatalities suffered from multiple maltreatment types, among which neglect associated with multiple types was more common than physical abuse associated with multiple types. Among deaths associated with mutually exclusive types of maltreatment, 35.8% of child fatalities died exclusively from neglect, and 23.2% died exclusively from physical abuse (USDHHS/ACF/ACYF/CB, 2010).

Children who have experienced abuse and neglect are at increased risk for experiencing adverse health effects and behaviors as adults, including smoking, alcoholism, drug abuse, physical inactivity, severe obesity, depression, suicide, sexual promiscuity, and certain chronic diseases (USDHHS/ACF/ACYF/CB, 2002). The role of the CPS agency is to respond to the needs of children who are alleged to have been maltreated and to ensure that they remain safe. This has become increasingly problematic as fewer allegations are investigated and fewer investigations lead to substantiations, which disposition would require that services be provided.

Different patterns of maltreatment among school-age children are reported by the Fourth National Incidence Study (NIS-4) than are described in official reports. The NIS-4 (Sedlak et al., 2010) relies on community sentinels rather than CPS agencies for its data, and report two levels of risk, a Harm Standard and an Endangerment Standard. In fact, school-age children 6 to 8 years old have the highest rates of neglect (Endangerment Standard) compared to either 16- and 17-year-olds or younger children. On the other hand, disproportionate increases in types of maltreatment (Harm Standard sexual abuse and Endangerment Standard overall maltreatment, neglect, and emotional neglect). The authors (Sedlak, et al., 2010) suggest that these changes since the NIS-3 evidence "broad vulnerability across the age spectrum" (p. 9).

In order to qualify for federal CPS funding, states must implement child abuse and neglect legislation that mandates reporting, conforms with federal definitions of abuse and neglect, and provides prevention and treatment services within the guidelines of the law (U.S. Congress, 1973). Unfortunately, CPS agencies as currently constituted are inadequate to the task. Problems include underfunding; inadequate and inadequately trained staff; lack of coordination among the legal, criminal justice, health, social service, and education communities; inadequate or conflicting laws and policies; and a lack of responsibility among the general public (U.S. Advisory Board, 1995). Most cases reported to CPS and accepted for investigation are not substantiated, and according to McCurdy and Daro (1992), hundreds of thousands of substantiated cases do not even receive basic services.

The answer to child maltreatment is prevention. Successful home visiting programs, such as the Nurse Family Partnership, have demonstrated reduced rates of maltreatment reports among a select population of high risk families (Olds, et al., 2007), but primary prevention at the community level requires knowing maltreatment's underlying causes. As yet, few resources have been expended to understand the etiology of abuse and neglect. Not only are the funds not available for causal research into child abuse and neglect inadequate, but the very agency designated by Congress to lead the national effort to investigate the phenomenon of child maltreatment, the National Center on Child Abuse and Neglect, was abolished by the welfare reform legislation that emerged from the 1996 Congress and replaced by a lower level Office on Child Abuse and Neglect. Nevertheless, it is clear that child abuse and neglect cannot be overcome without attention to social and economic conditions (poverty, substandard housing, inadequate education, broken families, unwanted pregnancy, unemployment, substance abuse, and low-quality child care) that put children and families at risk of a myriad of health problems. In addition, stressful life events and lack of social support have been shown to contribute to the risk of reported abuse and neglect (Kotch, et al., 1995).

HIV/AIDS

Pediatric acquired immunodeficiency syndrome (AIDS) is defined as clinical AIDS in children less than 13 years of age. AIDS was not recognized in children until well after its initial description in adults (Work Group on HIV/AIDS, 1988). Initially, it was difficult to distinguish AIDS from other rare congenital immunodeficiency diseases in children, but several researchers convincingly demonstrated that the human immunodeficiency virus (HIV) affects the pediatric as well as the adult population (Work Group on HIV/AIDS, 1988).

The face of pediatric AIDS has changed. When first recognized in children, HIV infections were seen primarily among hemophiliacs and neonatal intensive care unit graduates, as these were children who had multiple exposures to blood products. Effective screening and processing of the blood supply have largely eliminated this vector of transmission (Stuber, 1989). It is now well understood that HIV in children is transmitted by three routes: (1) from mothers to infants during the perinatal period, (2) through parenteral exposure to infected body fluids, primarily blood, and (3) through sexual contact (Rogers, 1987). Perinatal transmission remains the primary form of transmission of HIV in children. Evidence suggests that HIV is transmitted from infected mothers to their infants in utero by transplacental passage of the virus, during labor and delivery through exposure to infected maternal blood and/or vaginal secretions, and postnatally through non-exclusive breastfeeding.

New HIV infections among newborns have dropped significantly since the introduction of AZT-based regimens in 1995. Perinatal transmission continues to occur because of HIV-positive pregnant women who have not received appropriate care. With proper maternal treatment, the risk of passing HIV from mother to child is 1.5% compared with over 20% without treatment (National Institute of Allergy and Infectious Disease, 2002).

Thanks to antiretroviral therapy before, during and after pregnancy, the number of new cases of HIV in children has plummeted from 894 in 1992 to only 41 in 2008 (USDHHS/HRSA/MCHB, 2010).

The pediatric AIDS crisis is one small part of the overall crisis of AIDS, and it is also distinct from it. Today, most children with AIDS were born with HIV infection—born into families often living in poverty in which one or both parents may be HIV infected and drug dependent (Oleske, 1989). Minority children, many of whom face urban poverty, poor health, a lack of access to adequate health care, and educational disadvantages, comprise the majority of pediatric AIDS cases. Non-Hispanic black children represented 65% of pediatric HIV cases in the United States in 2008, although they are only 15% of the U.S. population in this age group (USDHHS/HRSA/MCHB, 2010).

Pediatric HIV disease, including AIDS, differs from the disease in adults in a variety of ways. Children with AIDS often develop severe bacterial infections, and a large proportion has mental or motor retardation (National Institute of Allergy and Infectious Diseases, 2002). The natural history of the disease is not only different in children; it is less well understood than in adults. Moreover, AIDS progresses very differently in different children. Most of the children reported with perinatally acquired AIDS (87%) had met the Centers for Disease Control case definition for AIDS before their third birthday, whereas 3% were diagnosed after their sixth birthday. HIV-infected children frequently are slow to reach milestones in motor skills and mental development such as crawling, walking, and speaking. As the disease progresses, many children develop neurologic problems such as difficulty walking, poor school performance, seizures, and other symptoms of HIV (National Institute of Allergy and Infectious Disease, 2000). Children with AIDS become sicker and die faster than do adults. Like adults with HIV infection, children with HIV develop life-threatening opportunistic infections. Serious bacterial infections occur in children more frequently than adults, and they are more likely to suffer from chronic diarrhea. Pneumocystis carinii pneumonias the leading cause of death in HIV-infected children with AIDS. In addition, a lung disease called lymphocytic interstitial pneumonitis, rarely seen in adults, occurs more frequently in HIV-infected children. This condition, like Pneumocystis carinii pneumonia, can make breathing more progressively difficult and often results in hospitalization (National Institute of Allergy and Infectious Disease, 2000). Infected infants and children who receive comprehensive health care have markedly fewer hospitalizations and experience an improved quality of life. However, this care comes at a price. Oleske (1989), Osterholm and MacDonald (1987), and Boland et al. (1992) pointed out that on average the lengths of hospital stay for children with AIDS are longer and their bills are higher than comparable children with acute or other chronic conditions.

Families raising children with HIV/AIDS differ from families living with other chronic illnesses in important ways. Mothers, and sometimes fathers and siblings, also may be infected. Thus, several family members may require medical treatment, and the family may have experienced the death of one or more of its members. Moreover, HIV/AIDS is a stigmatizing condition that can isolate individuals or families from usual supports, which is often compounded by stigma associated with drug use, poverty, and minority ethnic status (Rehm & Franck, 2000).

MCH practitioners should keep in mind that children with AIDS have a particular dependency—in many cases, virtually total dependency—on the community and on government. This unique dependency arises from the complexity of their health-care needs and the high costs of treatment, the stigma that they often face, the fragility of their families, and the poverty into which they are so often born. Furthermore, as paraphrased from Osterholm and MacDonald

(1987), MCH practitioners must first realize in a straightforward but compassionate manner that the great weight of pediatric AIDS will continue to fall on our communities of color, particularly in the inner city. It will be important for those working with these communities and the communities themselves to take ownership in developing creative solutions to addressing the complex problems associated with pediatric HIV/AIDS. In other words, individuals, communities, public health agencies, MCH practitioners, and government all need to respond.

Migrant and Immigrant Children

A subgroup of the school-aged population that has grown exponentially over the last decade is the offspring of immigrants to the United States. Children of immigrants are expected to account for more than half of the growth in the school-aged population between 1990 and 2010 (Nord & Griffin, 2000). Overall, the percentage of all children living in the United States with at least one foreign-born parent rose from 15% in 1994 to 23% in 2010 (Federal Interagency Forum, 2010). It is estimated that most of the population growth over the next 30 years will occur through immigration and births to immigrants and their children. The majority of children in immigrant families are of Hispanic or Asian origin (Hernandez, 2000). The proportion of children in the United States who are non-Hispanic whites is projected to drop from 54% in 2010 to only 38% in 2050 (Federal Interagency Forum, 2010).

Limited research is available on the health, development, and access to health care of the children of immigrants, who experience overwhelming issues involved with growing up in an environment dramatically different from that of their agemates. Several factors are believed to elevate a child's risk for negative health, developmental, and educational outcomes. A foreign-born child living with at least one foreign-born parent is more likely to be living with a parent without a high school degree or equivalent and to be living in poverty than a native-born child with a foreign-born parent, and that child is more likely to be living with a parent without a high school degree and in poverty than a native-born child with no foreign-born parent (Federal Interagency Forum, 2010). Finally, in 2009, 63% of school-age Asian children and 66% of school-age Hispanic children spoke a language other than English at home, compared with 6% of both white, non-Hispanic and black, non-Hispanic school-age children, and 16% of both school-age Asian and school-age Hispanic children spoke another language at home and had difficulty with English (Federal Interagency Forum, 2010).

The health of immigrant children is confounded by their disproportionate representation among migrant farmworker families. In their randomized study of 300 migrant farmworker families in eastern North Carolina, Weathers, Minkovitz, O'Campo, & Diener-West (2003) found over 99% of caregivers to be foreign born, as were 69% of their children. As a result, the vast majority of the children were uninsured. Despite resource and sociodemographic barriers to care, caregivers managed to obtain needed health services for their children. Nevertheless, 53% of caregivers reported unmet health care needs among their children. The authors point out a paradox, however. Caregivers of migrant children report 87% of the time that their children's health status is excellent or very good, compared with only 73% of Hispanic children in the United States overall. This suggests a possible "healthy migrant effect" (Weathers, Minkovitz, O'Campo, & Diener-West, 2004), that parents deliberately choose their healthier children to accompany them to the fields. If this were true, Weathers et al. predict that the proportion of foreign-born children among migrant farmworker families would increase with age, and in fact, this was the case.

CONCLUSION

Although on average school-age children may be the healthiest population group in the United States, they are also among the most vulnerable. Although benefiting at an unprecedented extent from public health advances in the areas of infectious disease and other natural causes of morbidity and mortality, school-age children are threatened by injuries, both intentional and unintentional. Chronic and handicapping conditions, behavioral morbidities including social and emotional problems, LDs, and social problems such as abuse and neglect, demand attention. Nevertheless, it is during the school-age years that enormous potential exists for reaching vast numbers of children with services and health-promoting strategies; it is in this age group, for the first time since birth, that children in the United States are nearly universally accessible through a helping institution. Using the schools to enforce immunization requirements demonstrates how reaching children and their families at this stage of their development can be successful. Recognizing this, Freedman, Klepper, Duncan, and Bell (1988) proposed that public schools be used to define insurable groups for the purpose of obtaining health care coverage for uninsured and underinsured children and their families. Initiatives such as school-based health centers and coordinated school health programs could be expanded to include setting the stage for healthier adolescence and adulthood by emphasizing injury prevention, physical activity, oral health, good nutrition, and healthful, prosocial interpersonal relationships. Teachers and others in schools see children every day and would be appropriate sources for early referral for health, developmental, social, and emotional problems, if resources were available to respond. Inadequate funding and preoccupation with so-called family rights has prevented the United States from maximizing the potential of generations of children.

References

Adams, P. F., & Hardy, A. M. (1989). Current estimates from the national health interview survey: United States, 1988. National Center for Health Statistics. *Vital and Health Statistics, 10*(173).

Agency for Healthcare Research and Quality. (2008). Total health services—mean and median expenses per person with expense and distribution of expenses by source of payment: United States, 2008. Medical Expenditure Panel Survey Household Component Data. Generated interactively. Retrieved July 17, 2011 from http://www.meps.ahrq.gov/mepsweb/data_stats/quick_tables_results.jsp?component = 1&subcomponent = 0&tableSeries = 1&year = -1&SearchMethod = 1&Action = Search.

Agency for Healthcare Research and Quality. (2011). Medical Expenditure Panel Survey. Complete Set of Health Insurance Coverage Series in PDF Format, first half of 2010. Table 1. Health insurance coverage of the civilian noninstitutionalized population: Percent by type of coverage and selected population characteristics, United States, first half of 2010. Retrieved July 17, 2011, from http://www.meps.ahrq.gov/mepsweb/data_stats/summ_tables/hc/hlth_insr/2010/alltables.pdf.

American Academy of Pediatrics. (1981). *School health: A guide for health professionals*. Evanston, IL: Author.

American School Health Association. (1994). *Guidelines for comprehensive school health programs* (2nd ed., ASHA publication #G011). Kent, OH: American School Health Association.

Anderson, R. N., & Smith, B. L. (2003). Deaths: Leading causes for 2001. National Vital Statistics Reports (Vol. 52, No. 9). Hyattsville, MD: National Center for Health Statistics.

Atkinson, J., & Collins, P. H. (2010). The role of schools in prevention. *North Carolina Medical Journal, 71*(1), 75–78

Bloom, B., & Tonthat, L. (2002). Summary statistics for U.S. children: National Health Interview Survey, 1997. *Vital and Health Statistics, 10*(203).

Bloom, B., Cohen, R. A., & Freeman, G. (2010). Summary health statistics for U.S. children: National

Health Interview Survey, 2009. National Center for Health Statistics. *Vital and Health Statistics, 10*(247).

Bloom, B., Dey, A. N., & Freeman, G. (2006). Summary health statistics for U.S. children: National Health Interview Survey, 2005. National Center for Health Statistics. *Vital and Health Statistics, 10*(231).

Boland, M., Conviser, R., Kelly, M., Connor, E., Rapkin, R., & Oleske, J. (1992). Care needs of HIV-infected children at New Jersey Children's Hospital. *AIDS & Public Policy Journal, 7*, 7–17.

Boyer, E. L. (1983). *High School: A Report on Secondary Education in America.* New York: Harper & Row, Inc.

Bradbury, R. (1994). No news, or what killed the dog? *American Way, 27*, 133, 135.

Centers for Disease Control and Prevention. (2001). U.S. HIV and AIDS cases reported through June 2001. *HIV/AIDS Surveillance Report. Midyear edition, 13*(1). Atlanta, GA: U.S. Department of Health and Human Services.

Centers for Disease Control and Prevention. (2002). Cases of HIV infection and AIDS in the United States, 2002. *HIV/AIDS Surveillance Report, 14*, 1–40.

Centers for Disease Control and Prevention. (2008). Healthy youth! Alcohol and drug use. Retrieved October 12, 2011 from http://www.cdc.gov/healthyyouth/alcoholdrug/.

Centers for Disease Control and Prevention. (2010a). Health USA 2010. Child and adolescent health. Access and utilization of health care. Table 79 (page 1 of 3). Health care visits to doctor offices, emergency departments, and home visits within the past 12 months, by selected characteristics: U.S., selected years 1997–2009. Retrieved October 12, 2011 from http://www.cdc.gov/nchs/data/hus/hus10.pdf#079.

Centers for Disease Control and Prevention. (2010b). Health USA 2010. Child and adolescent health. Access and utilization of health care. Table 78 (page 1 of 2). No health care visits to an office or clinic within the past 12 months among children under 18 years of age, by selected characteristics: U.S., average annual, selected years 1997–1998 through 2008–2009. Retrieved October 12, 2011 from http://www.cdc.gov/nchs/data/hus/2010/078 .pdf.

Centers for Disease Control and Prevention, National Center for Health Statistics (CDC/NCHS). (2003). Compressed mortality file 1979–1998. CDC WONDER online database, compiled from Compressed Mortality File CMF 1968–1988, Series 20,

No. 2A, 2000 and CMF 1989–1998, Series 20, No. 2E, 2003. Retrieved October 12, 2011 from http:// wonder.cdc.gov/cmf-icd9.html.

Centers for Disease Control and Prevention, National Center for Health Statistics (CDC/NCHS). (2010). Compressed mortality file 1999–2007. CDC WONDER online database, compiled from Compressed Mortality File 1999–2007 Series 20 No. 2M, 2010. Retrieved October 12, 2011 from http://wonder.cdc.gov/cmf-icd10.html.

Centers for Disease Control and Prevention, National Center for Injury Prevention and Control. (2007). WISQARS™. 10 leading causes of death, US, all races, both sexes 2007. Retrieved July 16, 2011 from http://webappa.cdc.gov/sasweb/ncipc/leadcaus10.html.

Centers for Disease Control and Prevention, National Center for Injury Prevention and Control. (2011). Injury prevention & control: Data & statistics (WISQARS™). Fatal injury data. Retrieved July 16, 2011 from http://www.cdc.gov/injury/wisqars/fatal .html.

Chau, M., Thampi, K., & Wight, V. R. (2010). *Basic facts about low-income children, 2009: Children aged 6 through 11.* New York: Columbia University, National Center for Children in Poverty.

Child Trends Data Bank. (2003). Learning disabilities. Retrieved October 12, 2011 from http://www .childtrendsdatabank.org/archivepgs/65.htm.

Collins, P. H. (2006). Coordinating school efforts to help address the obesity epidemic in North Carolina. *North Carolina Medical Journal, 67*(4), 293–295.

Collins, P. H., & Lee, H. N. (2008). School health policy in North Carolina. *North Carolina Medical Journal, 69*(6), 461–465.

Data Resource Center for Child and Adolescent Health. (n.d.). Who are children with special health care needs? Child and Adolescent Health Measurement Initiative, Oregon Health & Science University. Retrieved October 12, 2011 from http://childhealthdata.org/docs/nsch-docs/whoarecshcn _revised_07b-pdf.pdf.

Davidoff, A. J., Garrett, A. B., Makuc, D. M., & Schirmer, M. (2000). Medicaid-eligible children who don't enroll: health status, access to care, and implications for Medicaid enrollment. *Inquiry, 37*(2), 203–218.

Dewey, J. (1956). *The child and the curriculum.* Chicago: University of Chicago Press.

Drotar, D. (1981). Psychological perspectives in chronic childhood illness. *Journal of Pediatric Psychology, 6*, 211–228.

Drotar, D., & Bush, M. (1985). Mental health issues and services. In N. Hobbs & J. M. Perrin (Eds.), *Issues in the care of children with chronic illness*. San Francisco: Jossey-Bass.

Erikson, E. H. (1950). *Childhood and society* (2nd ed.). New York: W.W. Norton and Co.

Federal Interagency Forum on Child and Family Statistics. (2010). *America's children in brief: Key national indicators of well-being, 2010*. Washington, DC: U.S. Government Printing Office.

Fingerhut, L. A. (1989). Trends and current status in childhood mortality, United States, 1900–1985. *Vital and Health Statistics* (Series 3, No. 26. DHHS Pub. No. [PHS] 89-1410). Washington, DC: U.S. Department of Health and Human Services, Public Health Service, Centers for Disease Control, National Center for Health Statistics.

Fox, J. A., & Zawitz, M. W. (2003, January). *Homicide trends in the US: 2000 update*. NCJ 197471. BJS Crime Data Brief, Washington, DC: U.S. Department of Justice, Office of Justice Programs, Bureau of Justice Statistics.

Freedman, S. A., Klepper, B. R., Duncan, R. P., & Bell, S. P., Jr. (1988). Coverage of the uninsured and underinsured: A proposal for school enrollment-based family health insurance. *New England Journal of Medicine, 318*, 843–847.

Garrett, B., & Holahan, J. (2000). *Welfare leavers, Medicaid coverage, and private health insurance*. Assessing the New Federalism Brief B-13. Washington, DC: The Urban Institute.

Goldberg, R. T., Isralsky, M., & Shwachman, H. (1979). Vocational development and adjustment of adolescent with cystic fibrosis. *Archives of Physical Medicine and Rehabilitation, 60*, 369–374.

Guyer, B., Freedman, M. A., Strobino, D. M., & Sondik, E. J. (2000). Annual summary of vital statistics: Trends in the health of Americans during the 20th century. *Pediatrics, 106*, 1307–1317.

Halfon, N., & Newacheck, P. W. (1998). Prevalence and impact of parent reported disabling mental health conditions among U.S. children. *Child & Adolescent Psychiatry, 38*, 600–609.

Halfon, N., Inkelas, M., & Newacheck, P. W. (1999). Enrollment in the State Child Health Insurance Program: A conceptual framework for evaluation and continuous quality improvement. *Milbank Quarterly, 77*(2):181–204, 173.

Hardy, A. M. (1991). Incidence and impact of selected infectious diseases in childhood. *Vital and Health Statistics, 10*(180), (DHHS Pub. No. [PHS] 91–1508).

Hernandez, D. (Ed.). (1999). *Children of immigrants: Health, adjustment and public assistance*. Washington, DC: National Academy Press. Retrieved October 12, 2011 from http://www.nap.edu/openbook/0309065453/html.

Hogan, D. P., Rogers, M. L., & Msall, M. E. (2000). Functional limitation and key indicators of well-being in children with disability. *Archives of Pediatric and Adolescent Medicine, 154*, 1042–1048.

Holahan, J. (2011). The 2007–09 recession and health insurance coverage. *Health Affairs, 30*(1), 145–152.

Howden, L. M., & Meyer, J. A. (2011). *Age and sex composition*. 2010 Census Briefs. Washington, DC: U.S. Department of Commerce, Economics and Statistics Administration, U.S. Census Bureau.

Institute of Medicine. (1988). *The future of public health*. Washington, DC: National Academy Press.

Jackson, J. J. (1981). Urban black Americans. In A. Harwood (Ed.), *Ethnicity and medical care*. Cambridge, MA: Harvard University Press.

Joint Committee on National Health Education Standards. (1995). *National health education standards: Achieving health literacy*. New York: American Cancer Society.

Jones, D. J., & Roberts, V. A. (1994). Black children: Growth, development, and health. In L. Livingston (Ed.), *Handbook of black American health: The mosaic of conditions, issues, policies, and prospects*. Westport, CT: Greenwood Press.

Kaiser Family Foundation. (2010). The uninsured. A primer. Supplementary Data Tables. Table 2. Health Insurance Coverage of Children, 2009. Retrieved July 17, 2011 from http://www.kff.org/uninsured/upload/7451-06_Data_Tables.pdf.

Keane, C. R., Lave, J. R., Ricci, E. M., & LaVallee, C. P. (1999). The impact of a children's health insurance program by age. *Pediatrics, 104*, 1051–1058.

Kenney, G., Dubay, L., & Haley, J. (2000). Health insurance, access, and health status of children: Findings from the nation survey of America's families, in Urban Institute, SNAPSHOTS of America's Families II (1–8), Washington, DC: Urban Institute.

Kotch, J. B., Browne, D., Ringwalt, C. L., Stewart, P. W., Ruina, E., Holt, K., Lowman, B., & Jung, J.-W. (1995). Risk of child abuse or neglect among a cohort of low income infants. *Child Abuse and Neglect, 19*, 1115–1130.

Kotch, J. B., Lewis, T., Hussey, J. M., English, D., Thompson, R., Litrownik, A., et al. (2008). The importance of early neglect for childhood aggression. *Pediatrics, 121*, 725–731.

Kreider, R. M., & Elliott, D. B. (2009). *America's families and living arrangements: 2007*. Current Population Reports, P20-561. Washington, DC: U.S. Census Bureau.

Lewin, T. (1995, December 7). Parents poll finds child abuse to be more common. *The New York Times*.

Marx, E., & Wooley, S. (1998). *Health is academic, A guide to coordinated school health programs*. New York: Teachers College Press.

McCormick, M. C., Weinick, R. M, Elixhauser, A., Stagnitti, M. N., Thompson, J., & Simpson, L. (2001). Annual report on access to and utilization of health care for children and youth in the United States: 2000. *Ambulatory Pediatrics, 1, 3–15*.

McCurdy, K., & Daro, D. (1992). *Current trends in child abuse reporting and fatalities: The results of the 1991 annual fifty state survey*. Chicago: National Center on Child Abuse Prevention Research.

McPherson, M., Arango, P., Fox, H., Lauver, C., McManus, M., Newacheck, P. W., Perrin, J. M., Shonkoff, J. P., & Strickland, B. (1998). A new definition of children with special health care needs. *Pediatrics, 102*, 137–140.

Miniño, A. M., Xu, J., Kochanek, K. D., & Tejada-Vera, B. (2009). *Death in the United States, 2007*. NCHS data brief, no 26. Hyattsville, MD: National Center for Health Statistics.

National Assembly on School-Based Health Care. (2007–2008). *School-based health centers: National census, School year 2007–2008*. Washington, DC: Author. Retrieved October 12, 2011 from http://ww2 .nasbhc.org/NASBHCCensusReport07-08.pdf.

National Center for Health Statistics. (1995). *Health, United States, 1994*. Hyattsville, MD: U.S. Public Health Service.

National Center for Health Statistics. (1994). National Health Interview Survey-Disability Supplement. Rockville, MD: National Center for Health Statistics.

National Commission on the Role of the School and the Community in Improving Adolescent Health, (1990). Code blue: Uniting for healthier youth. Arlington, VA: National Association of State Boards of Education and the American Medical Association.

National Institute of Allergy and Infectious Disease. (2002). Mother-to-infant HIV transmission rate less than 2% in Phase III perinatal trial (PACTG 316). Bethesda, MD: Author.

National Survey of Children with Special Health Care Needs. (n.d.). Data Resource Center for Child and Adolescent Health. Retrieved October 12, 2011 from http://childhealthdata.org/learn/NS-CSHCN.

National Survey of Children's Health (NSCH). (2007). Child and Adolescent Health Measurement Initiative, Data Resource Center for Child and Adolescent Health website. Retrieved October 12, 2011 from http://childhealthdata .org/learn/NSCH.

Nettles, A. (1994). Scholastic performance of children with sickle cell disease. *Journal of Health and Social Policy, 5*, 123–140.

Newacheck, P. W., & Taylor, W. R. (1992). Childhood chronic illness: Prevalence, severity, and impact. *American Journal of Public Health, 82*, 364–370.

Newacheck, P. W., Hughes, D. C., Hung, Y., Wong, S., & Stoddard, J. J. (2000). The unmet needs of America's children. *Pediatrics, 105*, 989–997.

Nord, C. W., & Griffin, J. A. (1999). Educational profile of 3 to 8 year old children of immigrants. In D. Hernandez (Ed.), *Children of immigrants: Health, adjustment, and public assistance* (pp. 348–409). Washington, DC: National Academy Press. Retrieved October 12, 2011 from http:// www.nap.edu/openbook/0309065453/html.

North Carolina State Center for Health Statistics. Retrieved October 12, 2011 from http://www.epi .state.nc.us/SCHS/.

North Carolina Department of Public Instruction and Department of Health and Human Services. (2007). NC Youth Risk Behavior Surveillance Survey, Retrieved October 12, 2011 from http://www .nchealthy schools.org/data/yrbs/.

Olds, D. L., Kitzman, H., Hanks, C., Cole, R., Anson, E., Sidora-Arcoleo, K., Luckey, D. W., Henderson, C. R., Jr., Holmberg, J., Tutt, R. A., Stevenson, A. J., & Bondy, J. (2007). Effects of nurse home visiting on maternal and child functioning: Age-9 follow-up of a randomized trial. *Pediatrics, 120*, e832. DOI: 10.1542/peds.2006-2111.

Oleske, J. M. (1989). Children with HIV infection: Dilemmas in management. *Caring, 8,* 32–35.

Osterholm, M. T., & MacDonald, K. L. (1987). Facing the complex issues of pediatric AIDS: A public health perspective. *Journal of the American Medical Association, 258*, 2736–2737.

Palfrey, J. S., Walker, D. K., Haynie, H., Singer, J. D., Porter, S., Bushey, B., & Cooperman, P. (1991). Technology's children: Report of a statewide census of children dependent on medical supports. *Pediatrics, 87,* 611–618.

Pastor, P. N., & Reuben, C. A. (2002). Attention deficit disorder and learning disability: United States, 1997–98. National Center for Health Statistics. *Vital and Health Statistics, 10*(206).

Rehm, R. S., & Franck, L. S. (2000). Long-term goals and normalization strategies of children and families affected by HIV/AIDS. *Advances in Nursing Science, 23*, 69–82.

Richardson, S. A. (1989). Transition to adulthood. In R. E. K. Stein (Ed.), *Caring for children with chronic illness: Issues and strategies.* New York: Springer Publishing Company.

Rogers, M. F. (1987). Transmission of human immunodeficiency virus infection in the United States. In B. K. Silverman & A. Waddell (Eds.), *Report of the Surgeon General's workshop on children with HIV infection and their families* (pp. 17–19). Rockville, MD: U.S. Department of Health and Human Services, Public Health Service, Health Resources and Services Administration, Bureau of Health Care Delivery and Assistance, Division of Maternal and Child Health.

Schidlow, D., & Fiel, S. (1990). Life beyond pediatrics: transition of chronically ill adolescents from pediatric to adult care systems. *Medical Clinics of North America, 74,* 1113.

Schoen, C., & Dezroches, C. (2000). Uninsured and unstably insured: The importance of continuous insurance coverage. *Health Services Research, 35*, 187–206.

Sedlak, A. J., Mettenburg, J., Basena, M., Petta, I., McPherson, K., Greene, A., and Li, S. (2010). *Fourth National Incidence Study of Child Abuse and Neglect (NIS–4): Report to Congress, Executive Summary.* Washington, DC: U.S. Department of Health and Human Services, Administration for Children and Families.

Sedlak, A. (1991, September 5). *National incidence and prevalence of child abuse and neglect: 1988* (rev. report). Rockville, MD: Westat.

Silverman, M. M., & Koretz, D. S. (1989). Preventing mental health problems. In R. E. K. Stein (Ed.). *Caring for children with chronic illness, issues, and strategies* (pp. 213–229). New York: Springer Publishing Co.

Simpson, G. (1993, Winter). *Determining childhood disability and special needs children in the 1994–95 NHIS on disability.* Paper presented at the American Statistical Association annual meeting.

Singh, G. K., & Yu, S. M. (1996). US childhood mortality, 1950–1993: Trends and socioeconomic differentials. *American Journal of Public Health, 86,* 505–512.

Snyder, H. N., & Swahn, M. H. (2003, March). *Juvenile suicides, 1981–1998.* Youth Violence Research Bulletin. Washington, DC: U.S. Department of Justice, Office of Justice Programs, Office of Juvenile Justice and Delinquency Prevention.

Sochalski, J. A., & Villarruel, A. M. (1999). Improving access to healthcare for children. *Journal of the Society of Pediatric Nursing, 4,* 147–154.

Stuber, M. L. (1989). Coordination of care for pediatric AIDS: The development of a maternal-child HIV task force. *Developmental and Behavioral Pediatrics, 10,* 201–204.

Telfair, J., & Nash, K. B. (1996). Delivery of genetic services to African Americans. In N. L. Fisher (Ed.), *Ethnic and cultural diversity and its impact on the delivery of genetic services.* Baltimore, MD: The Johns Hopkins University Press.

U.S. Advisory Board on Child Abuse and Neglect. (1995). *A nation's shame: Fatal child abuse and neglect in the United States.* Executive Summary. Washington, DC: US Advisory Board on Child Abuse and Neglect.

U.S. Census Bureau (n.d.). American FactFinder. Retrieved July 17, 2011 from: http://factfinder.census.gov/home/saff/main.html?_lang = en&_ts = .

U.S. Congress. (1973). Child Abuse Prevention and Treatment Act, PL 93-247.

U.S. Department of Health and Human Services (USDHHS). (1999). Children and mental health. In *Mental health: A report of the Surgeon General.* Rockville, MD: U.S. Department of Health and Human Services, Substance Abuse and Mental Health Services Administration, Center for Mental Health Services, National Institutes of Health, National Institute of Mental Health. Retrieved April 25, 2004 from http://www.surgeongeneral.gov/library/mentalhealth/chapter3/sec1.html

U.S. Department of Health and Human Services, Administration for Children and Families, Administration on Children, Youth and Families, Children's Bureau (USDHHS/ACF/ACYF/CB). (2002). *Child maltreatment, 2000.* Washington, DC: Author. Retrieved October 12, 2011 from http://www.acf.hhs.gov/programs/cb/pubs/cm00/cm2000.pdf.

U.S. Department of Health and Human Services, Administration for Children and Families, Administration on Children, Youth and Families, Children's Bureau (USDHHS/ACF/ACYF/CB). (2010). *Child maltreatment 2009.* Washington, DC: Author. Retrieved October 12, 2011 from http://www.acf.hhs.gov/programs/cb/pubs/cm09/cm09.pdf.

U.S. Department of Health and Human Services, Health Resources and Services Administration, Maternal and Child Health Bureau (USDHHS/HRSA/

MCHB). (1991). *Healthy children 2000* (DHHS Pub. No. HRSA-MCH-91-2). Washington, DC: U.S. Government Printing Office.

U.S. Department of Health and Human Services, Health Resources and Services Administration, Maternal and Child Health Bureau (USDHHS/HRSA/MCHB). (2008). *The National Survey of Children with Special Health Care Needs Chartbook 2005–2006*. Rockville, MD: U.S. Department of Health and Human Services.

U.S. Department of Health and Human Services, Health Resources and Services Administration, Maternal and Child Health Bureau (USDHHS/HRSA/MCHB). (2009). *The National Survey of Children's Health 2007*. Rockville, MD: U.S. Department of Health and Human Services. Retrieved October 12, 2011 from http://mchb.hrsa.gov/nsch/07main/.

U.S. Department of Health and Human Services, Health Resources and Services Administration, Maternal and Child Health Bureau (USDHHS/HRSA/MCHB). (2010). *Child health USA 2010*. Rockville, MD: U.S. Department of Health and Human Services.

U.S. General Accounting Office. (1994). *Health care reform: School-based health centers can promote access to care* (GAO/HEHS-94-166). Washington, DC: Author.

Weathers, A., Minkovitz, C., O'Campo, P., & Diener-West, M. (2003). Health services use by children of migratory agricultural workers: Exploring the role of need for care. *Pediatrics, 111*(5), 956–963.

Weathers, A., Minkovitz, C., O'Campo, P., & Diener-West, M. (2004). Factors associated with unmet need for medical care access to care for children of migratory agricultural workers. *Pediatrics, 113*, e276.

Williams, B., & Kotch, J. B. (1990). Excess injury mortality among children in the US: Comparison of recent international statistics. *Pediatrics, 86*(Suppl.), 1067–1073.

Work Group on HIV/AIDS. (1988). Pediatric AIDS. *Public Health Reports, 103*(Suppl. 1), 94–98.

Zill, N., & Schoenborn, C.A. (1990). *Developmental, learning, and emotional problems: Health of our nation's children, US, 1988. Advance data from vital and health statistics* (No. 190). Hyattsville, MD: National Center for Health Statistics.

9

IMPROVING ADOLESCENT HEALTH IN THE 21ST CENTURY

Sara Buckelew and David Knopf

I would there were no age between ten and three-and-twenty, or that youth would sleep out the rest; for there is nothing in between but getting wenches with child, wronging the ancientry, stealing, fighting.

(Shakespeare, 1925)

Adolescence is a new birth, for the higher and completely human traits are now born. . . . These years are the best decade of life. No age is so responsive to all the best and wisest adult endeavor.

(Hall, 1904, pp. xiii and xviii)

INTRODUCTION

No age group is more maligned or idealized than adolescence. This cultural ambivalence has profound implications for the health of adolescents, resulting in sometimes dismissing adolescent problems as inevitable, sometimes minimizing adolescent concerns and issues as trivial, and sometimes developing anxiety-driven, ideologically based policies. Adolescent health is often injected into the core political-cultural debates regarding justice and the range and role of government in such areas as abortion, sexuality, family values, poverty, and social opportunity. Clearly, adolescents have significant problems as a population, and these problems have significant repercussions for young people and society now and in the future. Public health professionals and advocates have long sought to improve the health of adolescents, increase concern for their needs, and apply public health principles to efforts to improve their health, both now and in the future.

Compared with other age groups, adolescents are generally healthy, but they should be of high public health concern for several reasons. Certain populations of adolescents have poor health status, and many of these are in the direct care of public agencies, such as the incarcerated, those in foster care, and Native Americans. Many of the major health problems of adolescents are psychosocially based and thus should be amenable to prevention efforts. Because many health-related behaviors that cause significant adult morbidity and mortality begin in adolescence and may be less well embedded in younger people, changes in these behaviors during adolescence may pay long dividends for the public's health (Burt, 2002). Another important reason to attend closely to adolescent health is that adolescents are the immediate next pool of parents, workers, and citizens, and thus, their health will very soon affect the health of succeeding generations, the economy, and the body politic. Adolescent problems such as juvenile crime, motor vehicle injuries, pregnancy, and sexually transmitted diseases often affect other generations directly. Finally, just as parents feel some urgency to complete the unfinished business of socialization as the opportunity to influence the development of their offspring draws to a close in adolescence (Smetana, 1989), so too should society.

This chapter considers the importance, nature, and context of adolescent development. The epidemiology of adolescent health illustrates the pervasiveness of psychosocial factors in understanding adolescent health status. Considering these issues leads us to the identification of several cross-cutting themes that guide public health efforts for youth. The themes of (1) addressing risk behavior; (2) enhancing adolescent development; (3) increasing access to broadly conceived, comprehensive, youth-oriented services; and (4) establishing evidence-based interventions can guide federal, state, and community efforts. Several public health tools will be considered in exploring efforts to establish and monitor national health objectives, to increase access to high-quality services, to reduce motor vehicle and suicidal fatalities, to decrease unintended adolescent pregnancy, and to enhance adolescent fitness.

First, who are adolescents? Some use biological markers such as the beginning and completion of puberty. Others would use social definitions such as leaving the family of origin, becoming economically independent, or becoming a legally responsible adult (usually at 18 years old). Some would even combine in the adolescent group both teenagers and youth and thus include those up to their mid-20s, reflecting the continued developmental issues and lack of true independence of many in their mid-20s. For public health purposes, age-based definitions, although crude, are easiest to apply, but even age definitions vary. Some resources such as the Centers for Disease Control and Prevention (CDC) typically report health data in varying age blocks such as less than 18, 5 to 14, 15 to 24, or even 15 to 64, thus confusing and obscuring much data with issues of other ages. For the purposes

of this chapter, adolescence usually refers to those who are in the second decade of life.

ADOLESCENCE IN THE 21ST CENTURY

"It wasn't always this way...or was it?"

Some have argued that adolescence is a recent invention (Kett, 1993), but historical reviews illustrate a long awareness of unique issues in the second decade of life and some important differences over time. The term adolescent was not in common use until G. Stanley Hall's (1904) publication of a two-volume text, *Adolescence: Its Psychology, and Its Relations to Anthropology, Sex, Crime, Religion, and Education*. Before this time, the age group was more often referred to as "youth," which had a connotation of semi-independent participation in economic activities and typically ranged from age 12 to the early to mid-20s (Modell & Goodman, 1990). Before the industrial revolution, the transition by youth to full adulthood often included fostering out to apprenticeships for working class youth and to boarding school for the elite, both of which were seen as semiautonomous phases still monitored by adults.

Industrialization changed the ways youth become adults, and this distressed many. With industrialization, urbanization, and the expansion of the middle class in the late 19th century, the semi-independent status faded, and youth became increasingly dependent on their families and marginalized economically. Age-segregated training became the norm for the second decade of life, and the mixed social class American public high school emerged as the uniquely American means to foster upward social mobility for the working and middle classes. Hall's publication became an important part of the movement that focused on the character development of an age group, which was seen as vulnerable and malleable. When working class youth did not respond to these bourgeois reformers' attempts, they were again seen as troublesome, and the label of juvenile delinquent developed. Hall believed adolescents should be protected from precocity—adult experiences and responsibilities that come too early. This view fit well with the changing needs of the economy for fewer unskilled laborers and the changing view of the family as less an economic unit and more an emotional refuge to protect children. In contrast to the popular imagination, protected child development, family stability, and multigenerational relationships have become possible norms only within the last century. This changing view of adolescence as a protected transition time may not be universally accepted and may be particularly difficult for non-European immigrants, who come from different historical, economic, and cultural traditions.

Demographics of Adolescence

In the last 2 decades, the total adolescent population between 10 and 19 years increased from 34 million in 1990 to nearly 42 million in 2009. The adolescent population will become increasingly heterogeneous, with the percentage of those who do not consider their heritage primarily European increasing from 18.5% in 1980 to 45% by 2025 according to Census Bureau projections (National Adolescent Health Information Center [NAHIC], 2003). This change may result in adolescents being regarded as even more alien and becoming more marginalized. Hispanic youth are expected to be 22% of the total in 2025, African American 14%, and Asian/Pacific Islander 8%. Although two-thirds of all young people younger than 18 years lived with two parents in 2000, this percentage is down considerably since 1970, when 87.1% lived with two parents. In 2009, nearly one in five adolescents lived in poverty, a rise since the low in 2002. There continue to be large racial differences, with 46% of African American adolescents living with two parents (NAHIC, 2003), and more than half of all African American youth living in low income or poverty in 2008 (Douglas-Hall & Chua, 2009). Most adolescents now live in suburbs (54%) rather than central cities

(27%) or rural areas (19%), and more live in the South than any other region.

The Context of Adolescent Development

Part of the difficulty in approaching adolescence has been in understanding the nature of adolescence. Many still think of adolescents not as people but as monstrosities to be avoided at best and endured and controlled at worst. Population-based studies do not confirm this negative view of normal adolescence. Most adolescents do not describe extreme moodiness but rather describe positive relationships with their parents. Most parents describe their own adolescents in mostly positive terms. Numerous studies find that approximately 80% of adolescents are growing up and becoming responsible adults without major difficulty (Offer & Schonert-Reichl, 1992). The consequence of the view that adolescence is inevitably a time of "storm and stress" for most youth is that problems may be dismissed as inherent to adolescence rather than seen as signs of significant psychological or social problems that can be modified. A more rounded view has developed in the social psychological literature of adolescence as a time of transitions with occasional perturbation (Steinberg, 2000) needing a "prolonged supportive environment with graded steps toward autonomy" (Irwin, 1987, p. 2). Indeed, some research suggests adolescence is more problematic for parents than for teenagers because of the parent's own developmental and relationship issues (Steinberg, 2000).

Biological Development

Biological changes, particularly the development of the reproductive and endocrine systems, are often considered the engine for the train of many issues related to adolescent development. For females, pubertal changes may begin as early as age 8 years with the first stages of breast development. Height spurts commonly occur between the ages of 9.5 to 14.5 years and menarche between 10.5 and 15.5 years of age. Males typically develop a little later, with testicular enlargement between 10.5 and 13.5 years of age and rapid growth in height and other dimensions approximately a year after that (U.S. Congress, 1991b). Although the pubertal process takes a predictable course, there is much variation in timing between individuals such that normal puberty may be considered anywhere from years 8 to 18.

There are also significant historical and environmental variations in the timing of puberty. At the beginning of the 20th century, age of menarche averaged 14.5 years in the United States, and thus puberty was often not completed until near the end of high school. Currently, the average age of menarche is 12.5 years, and thus the process is now often completed before high school. Data also demonstrate that there are racial differences in the timing of puberty. The exact causes of these changes are unknown but are usually attributed to reductions in infectious disease and changes in nutrition, including the increase in obesity.

Most people would agree that adolescents' thought processes are different from those of children and of adults. Recent research has focused on neuroimaging (including magnetic resonance imaging [MRI]) as a means to better understand pubertal and biological changes in the adolescent brain. Changes in the brain during adolescence are complex, with maturation and increase in associated cognitive activity, different systems (cognitive and emotional) maturing at different rates and selective elimination or pruning of the nervous system occurring throughout adolescence (Giedd, 2008).

Psychological Development and Social Health

Because so much of public health work regarding adolescence is focused on the behavioral changes of adolescents, it is necessary for public health workers to have an understanding of adolescent psychological

and social development. Although the growth and development of the reproductive system are widely recognized, few appreciate the increasing complexity of mental operations made possible by neurologic and cognitive maturation in adolescence and young adulthood, a process that facilitates the transformations in identity, personal relationships, and social roles. Until the last 2 decades, most thinking about young people's cognitive ability has followed Piaget's developmental stage theories of a necessary and inevitable sequence from concrete thinking through simple abstractions, cognitive comparisons, perspective taking, and empathy to formal operations and synthesis using self-awareness, experience, judgment about the thinking process, and multiple strategies for making logical inferences. It is now recognized that the processes are much more environmentally supported or hindered than previously thought, more specific to content areas of interest, and take much longer than commonly assumed. "Rampant relativism," questioning everything, intolerance of inconsistency, literalism, and difficulty with understanding inferences and consequences, all common to earlier adolescents, may be seen as expected signs of incomplete neurocognitive maturity that may continue to develop into the 20s. Those attempting to influence adolescent risky behavior will need to take particular notice of adolescent cognitive development and perceptions of risk and vulnerability (Keating & Halpern-Felsher, 2008; Millstein & Halpern-Felsher, 2002).

Much psychological research and theorizing have described normal adolescence during three phases. In the early adolescence phase, the central tasks are described as coming to terms with physical changes, the accompanying need for a changing body image, and increased cognitive abilities. Ego development is described as frequently impulsive and self-focused (Sayer et al., 1995). In the middle adolescence phase, the central tasks are developing independent relationships with peers and establishing a sexual identity while balancing continuing relationships with family. Ego development is now described as conformist because it is usually group and peer centered and thus externally imposed. The late adolescence phase is often described as having the central tasks of completing the establishment of autonomy by determining vocational orientations and planning to exit the family of origin. The ego in late adolescence is described as postconformist in that there is increased internal control, greater reliance on internalized principles, appreciation of more subtle differences in motivation, and awareness of multiple causation. Some developmental psychologists have noted that the drive toward autonomy does not preclude maintaining healthy connections to the family of origin and that most young adults in their 20s continue to receive significant support from their families.

An important part of psychological and social development that too often is isolated from these topics is sexuality development. Developmental challenges related to the sexual unfolding of adolescents have been defined as (1) developing positive feelings about one's body, (2) learning to manage feelings of sexual arousal and desire, (3) developing new forms of autonomy and intimacy, and (4) developing skills to control the consequences of sexual behavior (Brooks-Gunn & Paikoff, 1993). Adolescents are exposed to considerable sexually oriented advertisements and entertainment; nevertheless, adolescents receive inconsistent messages from adults about the acceptability of sexual expression. This American cultural contradiction between a sexualized environment and the unacceptability of sexual behavior places youth in a double bind, tends to drive sexual decision making away from adult influence, and makes accessing contraceptives psychologically difficult for many. One example of these contradictions is shown in a 5-year longitudinal study of those who pledged virginity until marriage. The pledgers had similar sexual behavior as

matched nonpledgers, but were less likely to use birth control or condoms (Rosenbaum, 2009a). Increasingly, researchers and public health advocates are considering how to view adolescent sexual behavior in the context of healthy life course development (Halpern, 2010) as the federal government moves away from supporting abstinence-only prevention programming.

National studies on the sexuality development of adolescents have tended to assume that all adolescent respondents are heterosexual. A significant number of youth are nonheterosexual based on sexual orientation, attraction, identity, and/or behavior but may not consider themselves homosexual (Savin-Williams & Ream, 2007). A large survey of high school students in Minnesota found that 4.5% considered themselves "predominantly homosexual," and 10.7% "weren't sure" of their sexual orientation (Remafedi, Resnick, Blum, & Harris, 1992). The concept of normal, healthy homosexual behavior is rarely discussed, but a few attempts have noted issues in parallel with those of heterosexuals, including coming to terms with one's self-identity, being able to achieve intimacy, and planning for the consequences of sexual activity. The massive stigmatization, alienation from supportive adults, and violence toward those with different sexual orientations result in greater difficulty achieving a healthy sexual identity. Family rejection has been associated with poor health outcomes and higher risk behavior including a suicide rate more than 8 times that of more accepting families (Huebner, Diaz, & Sanchez, 2009). Some have noted that loss of traditional support rituals normally available to teens has led to distinctive subcultures offering different forms of community supports (Remafedi, 1989).

Social relationships also go through changes in adolescence. Families continue to be important, and as noted previously here, relationships are generally positive; however, significant changes still exist. Boundaries become more permeable, such that adolescents and their families often have to find ways to accommodate new relationships. Conflict increases somewhat during early adolescence, particularly between mothers and daughters, usually about household chores. The adolescent defines the conflict as about issues of personal choice, but parents perceive the conflict as about issues of social propriety. Parent–adolescent conflict usually subsides by middle adolescence and is seldom threatening to family cohesion (Smetana, 1995). A substantial amount of research has attempted to define parenting correlates of adolescent competency, usually defined in terms of school achievement, psychological health, and healthy behavior (Baumrind, 1987; Steinberg, Blatt-Eisengart, & Cauffman, 2006). Using both longitudinal convenience samples and large-scale, population-based school samples, these studies analyzed parenting on two dimensions, amount of control or demandingness and amount of nurturance or warmth as perceived by the teenager. This approach identified four basic types of parenting: (1) authoritative (sometimes called democratic) parents who are demanding but warm and nurturing; (2) authoritarian families who may be demanding but are not seen by the adolescent as warm or nurturing; (3) permissive parents who are nurturing but not demanding; and (4) neglectful or inattentive parents who are neither demanding nor warm toward the adolescent. Adolescents with authoritarian or authoritative parents generally achieve better than the other two groups, but young people with authoritative parents score higher on measures of psychological health and healthy behavior. The youth who fared the worst were those with neglectful parents. The degree of effect in most studies is rather low, and the distinctions between types somewhat imprecise, as most parents fall toward the middle on the two dimensions. This has been replicated among other cultural groups with similar results, but the positive impact of authoritative parenting is even more modest among African American families (Steinberg, Mounts, Lamborn, & Dornbusch, 1991).

Environmental Context of Adolescent Health and Development

The context of adolescents' lives is also affected by the larger society. Legal structures, schools, neighborhoods, the economy, and the media all have influence on the health and well-being of young people.

Legal structure The legal structure affects adolescent development by establishing a series of regulatory steps designed to reduce risky behavior until the young person is deemed, by virtue of age, to be capable. Statutes related to tobacco, alcohol, driving, sexual consent, medical consent, and financial responsibility are all based on judgments about adolescent developmental abilities and needs for protection. Although states differ, generally, beginning about age 12 years, adolescents begin to have more legal rights (such as the ability to get confidential treatment for sexually transmitted diseases), and they progress in the direction of increasing legal autonomy in the areas of driving privileges (usually 16 to 18 years), consent for medical treatment (14 to 18 years), sexual consent (13 to 18 years), confidentiality (14 to 18 years), contracts (18 years), purchase of controlled substances such tobacco (18 years), and the last legal right in most states, buying alcohol (21 years). On the surface, such variation seems inconsistent, which can be quite irritating to some youth, but such inconsistency reflects attempts at accommodation between the reality of increasing adolescent autonomy and the need for continued adult involvement and responsibility.

Most important, state laws do recognize the need for minors to be able to consent, thus having confidentiality regarding sexual health issues, in order to encourage treatment of sexually transmitted infections and to allow access to contraception (English & Kenney, 2003). Although until recently the trend in the law has been to increase legal rights for young people, legal access to medical treatment, especially regarding sexuality and abortion, continues to be highly controversial (English, 2002). Failure to ensure confidential care has meant that many youth who engaged in risky health behavior have not received needed health care (Lehrer et al., 2007), and restrictions on abortion consent by requiring waiting periods, parental consent, and/or parent notification, have resulted in increased unintended pregnancy, particularly among poor youth and among African American youth. (Coles et al., 2010). Confidentiality issues are discussed further in this chapter in the context of adolescent access to health care. The important issue of legal obligation to pay for services and the ability of minors to qualify for state-funded health care also vary widely. Some states allow minors to become eligible for Medicaid for reproductive healthcare services ("sensitive services") based on their own income and assets rather than their family's income. Without such eligibility, confidentiality provisions are rather hollow because the medical bill may be sent home.

Although most adolescents progress from being legally dependent on parents, many have different legal paths to adulthood, which often makes them of particular concern to public health. In 2008, approximately 81,000 young people were in juvenile justice facilities, and another half million were on court-ordered supervision (Sickmund, 2010). Of the 423,773 in foster care on September 30, 2009, 48% were in the second decade of their life (U.S. Department of Health and Human Services, Administration for Children and Families, 2010a). Homeless and runaway youth have also been a particular focus of public health efforts due to the high incidence of health and mental health problems. This group of minors living without adults includes often overlapping groups of runaways, "throwaways" who have been expelled by their parents, street youth, and systems youth. Little data exist on the size of these populations, although population studies have estimated that between 1.6 million to 2.8 million youth run away from home each year (Toro, Dworsky, & Fowler, 2007).

Schools American high schools are the dominant social institution in adolescents' lives. The schools struggle to implement three competing overarching goals: preparing students for employment, preparing students for college, and creating responsible citizens. Since schools have such a major influence on adolescent health and development, they are often a major site for public health interventions. Poor school adaptation as shown through dropping out, grade retention, and a lack of participation in school activities has been associated with pregnancy, delinquency, substance use, unemployment, and reduced earnings (U.S. Congress, 1991b), and poor engagement in school has been associated with high-risk behavior (Resnick et al., 1997). The link between school disengagement and health problems suggests that problems such as dropping out of school should be seen as public health problems requiring multiple systems interventions (Freudenberg & Ruglis, 2007). Although the problems of poor school adaptation may be most related to poverty and social class issues, some factors of school structure and environment have been associated with poorer adaptation and engagement such as large overall size, high teacher-student ratio, and high concentrations of poverty. Efforts to increase academic standards by using standardized testing, requiring more rigorous academic courses, and tracking by ability have increased academic performance for a few and increased the numbers of students taking advanced mathematics and sciences. These efforts have also increased grade retention, school dropout, and alienation among more marginal students without improving overall test scores (Balfanz, 2009). Other attempts at school reform that affect adolescent health have been efforts to integrate social and emotional learning throughout the school experience (Greenberg et al., 2003).

Disparities based on ethnic and racial identity continue to plague schools. Most students still attend schools that are functionally segregated. Forty percent of white students attend schools that are 90% white, and 30%

of minority students attend schools in which 90% of all students are African American, Hispanic, or Native American. Only one-fifth of all schools could be considered racially balanced (Balfanz, 2009). Seldom recognized has been the significant improvement in educational performance of minorities from 1971 until 1996 (Ferguson, 2001). This improvement may reflect the tremendous discrepancy between whites and blacks under mostly officially segregated conditions until the 1970s, changes in family structure, and improvement in parental education (Grissmer, Kirby, Berends, & Williamson, 1995). Nevertheless, the gap in performance continues with little change in the last decade (National Center for Education Statistics, 2010).

Neighborhood and community

Neighborhood and community effects on adolescent development are most studied in terms of the consequences of concentrations of poverty in urban environments. Less often studied are rural/urban differences. Poor urban neighborhoods have more single mothers, more unemployed men, more substance abuse, and fewer positive role models (National Research Council, 1993). The consequences for adolescents of living in a neighborhood with a high concentration of poverty include more risky behavior, poorer educational achievement, and high rates of pregnancy, delinquency, and violent crime. The effects are particularly strong on males (Katz, King, & Liebman, 2001). The negative effects have been attributed to (1) a lack of institutional resources, (2) impaired relationships and social connections, and (3) neighborhood norms that do not encourage collective efficacy and do not support social control over inappropriate behavior (Browning et al., 2008). The concentration of poverty in neighborhoods, which had been increasing for decades, declined substantially in the 1990s (Jargowsky, 2003).

Neighborhoods vary by more than poverty concentration. A study of small cities in the Midwest found important differences between communities independent of poverty.

Community assets may be defined as policies and practices that support families, facilitate positive interactions with and between youth, and endorse more prosocial values (Blyth, 1993). Communities that had more of these assets tended to have adolescents who had lower frequency of risk behaviors, substance abuse, pregnancy, antisocial behavior, depression, and vandalism.

Economic influences

Economic influences on adolescent health and development are poorly understood because researchers seldom obtain income data directly and instead use proxy measures such as parental education or race. Nevertheless, the influence on health and development is considerable. The poorer the adolescent, the more likely the youth will be disabled, have a chronic condition, have emotional or behavioral problems, lack health insurance, not see a healthcare provider, not see a dentist, or have unmet medical needs (Newacheck, Hung, Park, Brindis, & Irwin, 2003a). Poorer adolescents have long been known to have more school problems, get pregnant earlier, and be arrested more often than nonpoor adolescents (U.S. Congress, 1991c).

Economic changes affect family behavior. Because of declining wage structure, and increasing single parenthood, more family caretakers need to be employed outside of the home. Children living with only one of their parents have increased from 10% of the population in 1965 to 26.3% in 2008, a percentage that has not changed since 1994 (Grall, 2009). Adolescents at home without adult supervision are engaged in more risk behavior, regardless of economic status (Richardson, Radziszewska, Dent, & Flay, 1993). Economic problems also affect parenting behavior. Longitudinal studies of middle-class Iowa families who had major decreases in income found increased parental depression and hostility, particularly among the men, which resulted in greater negativity by the father toward the adolescent children in the family, which in turn was associated with more antisocial behavior and depression among the adolescents (Elder, Conger, Foster, & Ardelt, 1992). This research group has also found that exposure to poverty specifically in adolescence resulted in earlier parenthood by these adolescents, whose toddlers exhibited more externalizing behaviors (Scaramella et al., 2008). Other studies have associated poverty with fewer positive role models for adolescents, restricted geographic mobility resulting in exposure to riskier neighborhoods, greater disengagement from society (particularly among African American males), and greater difficulty with becoming employed (Sum & Fogg, 1991). Although poverty increases the risks of poor transitions, it should be recognized that two-thirds of poor adolescents are not poor as adults (Edelman & Ladner, 1991).

It can be expected that the economic recession of 2008–2010 will have significant impact on adolescent's lives. Commentators have noticed increased youth unemployment and more difficulties for young adults establishing economic independence. Whether or not the economic difficulties will reverse the generally positive trends in adolescent health status (to be discussed later) remains to be seen.

The media and technology   The media are often seen as a major influence on adolescent development, usually in terms of stimulating desire, fostering violence, socializing adolescents into the market economy, and supporting passivity. Over the last decade, media have changed dramatically, with teens now spending time on the Internet including social networking sites and on their mobile phones including texting. With advances in technology, such as the advent of "smart phones," media are constantly at the fingertips of young people, with teens and tweens always plugged in and available to their friends. Young people spend an average of 7.5 hours per day consuming media, including television, Internet, music, and video games (Rideout, Foehr, & Roberts, 2010). Often they are using multiple forms of media at once, packing in an average of over

10.5 hours in that 7.5 hours. Television is still the most popular form of media used by teens, and potential negative health impacts include effects of television on academic performance, weight, and increased risk behavior, including substance use and earlier sexual activity (Villani, 2001). Others have linked increases in gender stereotyping, consumerism, and aggressiveness to television watching (Strasburger, 2004). Texting has increased in popularity, with 75% of teens owning cellphones and over 50% of teens texting daily. Of those, 50% text over 50 times per day (Lenhart, Ling, Campbell, & Purcell, 2010). Texting and driving has been a major public health concern for teens. Adolescents are also increasingly using social networking sites, with 73% of online teens now using these sites (Lenhart, Purcell, Smith, & Zickuhr, 2010). Concerns about these sites include teens posting sexual content or content related to substance use, which may affect future employment. Another concern is that teens will contact strangers, resulting in a threat to their safety, although research has shown that the majority of teens connect with people they already know on social networking sites, rather than contacting strangers.

ADOLESCENT HEALTH STATUS

Although adolescents are generally healthy, there are important exceptions, disparities, and unhealthy patterns. Adolescent mortality increased during the mid-1990s but is now at an all-time low. The causes of death have changed over the decades from mostly infectious disease-related causes in 1950 to mostly injury, both intentional and unintentional, today. Epidemiologic analysis of adolescent health problems indicates the pervasiveness of behavioral factors in the morbidity and mortality of adolescents, and many of these same behaviors initiated during adolescence contribute to the morbidities and mortalities experienced in adulthood. This section includes discussion of the sources of data regarding adolescent health, a consideration of data related to well-being, and an overview of the current status of adolescent health, ill health, and related behaviors.

Data Sources for Adolescent Health

Data about adolescent health have increased over the last decade. The most widely used assessment of adolescent health behaviors has been the CDC's Youth Risk Behavior Surveillance System. The YRBSS uses national, state, and local samples of high school students throughout the United States to measure the incidence and prevalence of the specific behaviors among adolescents that lead to their most important health problems. The YRBSS is also used by schools, communities, and states to assess health risk status and to target interventions. An important limitation of the YRBSS has been that it does not include higher risk, out-of-school youth who may be incarcerated, homeless, or working. Another important national data source is the National Health Interview Survey carried out at regular intervals by the National Center for Health Statistics. This survey obtains baseline health data and information on varying topics. The federal governmental sponsors several more surveys, which include the National Survey of Family Growth, the National Survey of Drug Use and Health, and the University of Michigan's Monitoring the Future project, which evaluates substance use trends yearly. Information about data sources for adolescent health is readily available on the Internet (Ozer, Park, Paul, Brindis, & Irwin, 2003).

These surveys have limitations. Many continue to use differing age categories. Some do not include nonstudents; few surveys include information on the socioeconomic status of respondents. Although some have questioned whether responses on a survey vary by school or home setting, a comprehensive analysis found that such differences do not affect the validity of results (Brener, Billy, & Grady, 2003). In another analysis, adolescents showed consistency in reporting sexual and substance abuse behaviors, but were not consistent in reporting weight control activities (Rosenbaum, 2009b). Some have noted that cultural controversy has emerged over whether surveys of youth are a violation of parental confidentiality and should require active parental consent. As a result, some surveys, particularly those regarding sexual behavior, have been withdrawn from the field.

Data on Well-Being of Adolescents

Traditionally, healthcare data have focused on mortality, morbidity, and related risk behaviors. Recently, researchers have noted that positive factors about adolescents prevent and moderate harm from risky behavior. These positive aspects of youth development may in fact be more critical to the successful transition to healthy and productive adulthood than most specific risk behaviors. Many indicators such as rates of high school graduation, volunteering, or attending religious services have been used, but two constructs have been particularly identified as linked to better health and less risky behavior—parental connectedness and school engagement (Bond et al., 2007; Resnick et al., 1997).

Parental Connectedness

Adolescents who report feeling closer to their parents emotionally tend to do better in school, engage in fewer risk behaviors, and show more signs of psychological health. Thus, the degree of parental closeness reported by adolescents is one potential positive marker of adolescent well-being. Most adolescents describe feeling very close to their parents. In a study using a national database, of those adolescents living with their biological parents, 70% said they felt very close to their mothers, and 58% felt very close to their fathers (Resnick et al., 1997). Ethnic minority youth, less educated, and younger adolescents all reported more parental connectedness.

School Connectedness

The degree of being engaged in school also shows an effect on school performance, risk behaviors, and psychological health, which is similar to that of parental connectedness. In 2002, 30.9% of parents reported indicators suggesting that their adolescent had a high degree of engagement in school. Parents who were better educated and who had younger adolescents reported more school engagement (Vandivere et al., 2004). The parents perceived their youth as less highly engaged in school in 2002 than parents did in a previous study in 1997. Adolescents from families with higher incomes had a bigger decrease in the percentage who indicated that they were highly engaged in school.

Mortality

Adolescent and young adult death rates have declined slowly over the last 20 years (Figure 9–1). There are important subgroups with much worse mortality.

Mortality rates for males ages 10 to 14 years are 1.5 times female mortality rates, and males ages 15 to 19 years have a mortality rate that is 2.4 times that of females. There is also large variation by ethnicity, with Native American/Alaskan Natives and African Americans having much higher death rates. The differences among males and ethnic groups

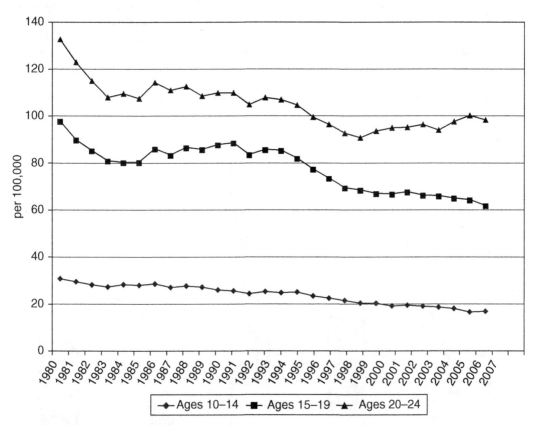

Figure 9–1 *Mortality trends, ages 10–24, 1980–2007*

Source: Centers for Disease Control and Prevention, National Center for Health Statistics. Compressed Mortality File 1979–1998. CDC WONDER On-line Database, compiled from Compressed Mortality File CMF 1968–1988, Series 20, No. 2A, 2000 and CMF 1989–1998, Series 20, No. 2E, 2003. Accessed at http://wonder.cdc.gov/cmf-icd9.html, May 17, 2011. Centers for Disease Control and Prevention, National Center for Health Statistics. Compressed Mortality File 1999–2007. CDC WONDER On-line Database, compiled from Compressed Mortality File 1999–2007 Series 20 No. 2M, 2010. Accessed at http://wonder.cdc.gov/cmf-icd10.html, May 17, 2011.

are largely accounted for by differences in injury mortality.

Injuries

Injuries, both intentional and unintentional, are the major cause of death to adolescents. Among youth ages 15 to 19 years, injuries accounted for 76% of the 13,739 deaths in 2006, and among youth ages 10 to 14 years, injuries caused 49% of the 3,414 deaths in the same year (Heron, 2010). Motor vehicle injuries are the leading cause of death for both age groups (Figure 9–2).

Males are more likely than females to die from injury, particularly among 15- to 19-year-olds. American Indians/Alaskan Natives and whites are more likely to die from motor vehicle injuries and suicide

than others. African Americans have much higher rates of homicide, although these have declined dramatically since 1993 from a high of 140 per 100,000 to 34.6 per 100,000 in 2005 among 15- to 19-year-olds (Mulye et al., 2009).

Unintentional injuries The most common causes of death from unintentional injuries are motor vehicle crashes (73% of all unintentional injuries), unintentional poisoning (7%), unintentional drowning (5%), unintentional firearm injuries (2%), and other land transportation injuries (3%) (CDC, 2010). American Indian/Alaskan Natives have nearly twice the unintentional injury rate of Caucasians and three times the unintentional injury rate of Asian American/Pacific Islanders.

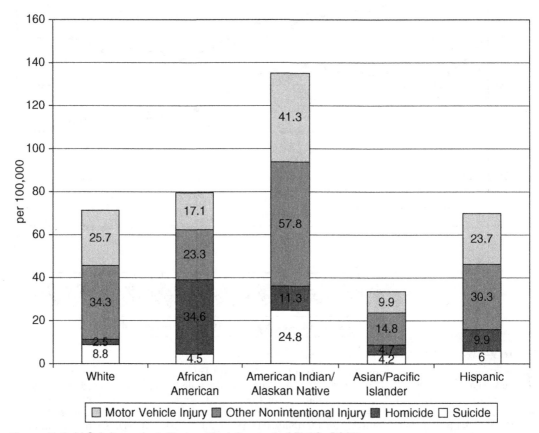

Figure 9–2 *U.S. injury mortality by ethnicity, ages 15–19, 2005.*

Source: Data from Paul-Mulye T, Park MJ, Nelson CD, Adams SH, Irwin CE, Brindis CD (2009). Trends in Adolescent and Young Adult Health in the United States. Journal of Adolescent Health, 45(1), 8–24.

Intentional injuries and violence Intentional injuries are defined as injuries resulting from interpersonal violence, including homicide, and the self-directed violence of suicide. In 2006 there were 4,302 intentional deaths of 10- to 19-year-olds, most of which were among the 15- to 19-year-olds (Heron, 2010). Although homicide deaths to youth have decreased more than 50% since 1983, the U.S. rate is still 10 to 15 times the rate of most European countries (Krug, Dahlberg, Mercy, Zwi, & Lozano, 2002). Males are much more likely to be victims, particularly black 15- to 19-year-old males, who were 17 times more likely to be killed as same-age white youth in 2000 (Ozer et al., 2003). Guns are involved in approximately three of four adolescent homicides, and three of four firearm deaths are with small handguns. Most victims knew their assailant; 60% of the shooting deaths were after an argument. Interestingly, the rate of assaults in Denmark is similar to that of the United States, but the homicide rate is approximately one-fifth that of Ohio, a comparably sized population, suggesting that the availability of guns rather than violent behavior per se is the predominant factor for increased homicide (Cohall & Cohall, 1995).

Suicide has been identified as the third leading cause of death among adolescents. Suicide rates are higher for males than for females, more frequent in rural areas and Western states, much higher among Native Americans, and somewhat higher among Hispanics and whites than among African American adolescents. Attempted suicide is even more common, with 6.3% of all adolescent students surveyed as part of the 2009 YRBSS reporting a suicide attempt and seeing a healthcare person as a result (Eaton et al., 2010) (Table 9–1). Twice as many females as males made an attempt, Hispanic females more than white or African American females. Prior history of suicide attempt, substance abuse, presence of firearms in the home, family history of suicide, antisocial behavior, and psychiatric disorders have all been associated with increased risk for completed suicide (U.S. Public Health Service, 1999).

Morbidity

Injuries cause much morbidity. It has been estimated that for every fatal injury there are 41 adolescents hospitalized for a nonfatal injury (Runyan & Gerken, 1991). In 2009 almost 4.8 million young people ages 10 to 19 were seen in hospital emergency departments for nonintentional nonfatal injuries in 2009, and 430,000 were seen for intentional injuries (National Center for Injury Prevention and Control, 2011).

Chronic Illness and Disabilities

Chronic conditions include a wide spectrum of physical and mental health problems, including hay fever, asthma, cancer, cardiovascular disease, learning disabilities, epilepsy, type II diabetes, hearing and visual impairments, leukemia, chronic kidney disease, and cystic fibrosis. Many of these disabilities result in a substantially reduced quality of life for the adolescent. Additionally, chronically ill adolescents may need significantly more health and social services.

According to the National Child Health Interview Survey, 21.4% of all 12- to 17-year-olds had an activity limitation in 2008 (Child Trends, 2011). This is somewhat higher than the 19.6% with activity limitations reported in 1998. The condition most frequently identified as a cause of functional limitation among all children aged 17 years was asthma, affecting 15% of all adolescents ages 12 to 17 years (Dey, Schiller, & Tai, 2004). Learning disability was the next highest at 10.5%. The percentage with activity limitation, emotional and behavioral problems, or being in only fair to poor health varied by income—the poorer the family background, the higher the rate of chronic symptoms (Newacheck, Hung, Park, Brindis, & Irwin, 2003a).

Mental Health

Although most adolescents and their parents don't report that "storm and stress" dominate the experience of adolescence,

Table 9–1 Health Risk Behaviors, U.S. 9th and 12th Grades, Youth Risk Behavior Surveillance Survey, 2009 (percent)

Behavior	Total	Male	Female	9th Grade	12th Grade	White	Black	Hispanic
Injury-related behaviors								
rarely or never uses a seat belt	9.7	11.5	7.7	10.6	10.1	9.5	11.7	8.8
rode within the last 30 days with a driver who had been drinking alcohol	28.3	27.8	28.8	27.5	28.2	26.2	30	34.2
carried a weapon last month	17.5	27.1	7.1	18	16.6	18.6	14.4	17.2
made a suicide attempt within last year	6.3	4.6	8.1	7.3	4.2	5	7.9	8.1
Substance use related behaviors in last 30 days								
smoked cigarettes	19.5	19.8	19.1	13.5	25.2	22.5	9.5	18
drank alcohol	41.8	40.8	42.9	31.5	51.7	44.7	33.4	42.9
had 5 or more drinks at a time	24.2	25	23.4	15.3	33.5	27.8	13.7	24.1
smoked marijuana	20.8	23.4	17.9	15.5	24.6	20.7	22.2	21.6
used cocaine	2.8	3.5	2	2.3	3	2.4	1.9	4.3
Sexual behaviors								
had intercourse in the last 3 months	34.2	32.6	35.6	21.4	49.1	32	47.7	34.6
used a condom at last intercourse	61.1	68.6	53.9	64	55	63.3	62.4	54.9
Nutrition and exercise-related behaviors								
trying to lose weight	44.4	30.5	59.3	43.5	46.4	43.7	36.8	52.1
engages in sufficient vigorous physical activity	31.9	34.6	33.3	46.7	22.4	30.6	37	40.5

Source: Eaton D., Kahn, L., Kitchen, S., Shackling, S., Ross, J., Hawkins, Lowry R., Harris, W., McManus, T., Chine, D, Lim, C., Whittle, L., Brenner, N., Wechsler, H. (2010). Youth risk behavior surveillance: United States, 2009. Morbidity Mortality Weekly Report, 59 (SS-5), 1–142.

a wide range of mental health disorders are common. From 2002 to 2004 more than 10,000 representative youth aged 13–18 were interviewed face to face with a structured format designed to identify psychiatric disorders as defined by the American Psychiatric Association's Diagnostic and Statistical Manual (DSM-IV). This study found a lifetime prevalence of some type of disorder to be 49% (Merikangas et al., 2010). The most common diagnoses were anxiety disorders (31.9%), behavioral conduct disorders (19.6%), mood disorders such as depression (14.3%), substance abuse/dependence disorders (11.4%), and eating disorders (2.7%). Of these, about one-half were found to have more than one disorder, and one in five experienced severe impairment. In this study relatively few racial or ethnic differences were noted except for higher rates of anxiety and lower rates of substance abuse among African American youth and higher rates of mood disorders among Hispanic youth. Those with behavioral conduct disorders and multiple disorders were more likely to receive treatment, but overall only one-third of those identified with a psychiatric disorder received treatment and only one-half of those with severe impairment received any treatment (Merikangas et al., 2011). Several other studies using surveys, parent data, and clinical interviews have found that about one in five youth at any given time could be considered to have a psychiatric disorder, and 1 in 10 are severely disordered (Knopf et al., 2008).

Sexual Behavior and Its Health Consequences

There has been a small decrease in sexual intercourse among adolescents over the last several years, but sexual activity is still quite common. In 2009, one in five ninth graders reported that they had had sexual intercourse, and almost half of seniors reported they had had intercourse (Eaton et al., 2010). These rates are substantially similar to youth in other comparable countries, although European youth tend to use more effective contraceptives (Santelli, Sandfort, & Orr, 2008). In addition to the decline in sexual activity among teens, there was an increase in condom use until 2003 at which point the rates of use plateaued. Among sexually active teens, 61.1% said that they used a condom at last intercourse in 2009 compared with 46% in 1991, and African American youth reported the highest rate of condom use (72.5%) (Eaton et al., 2010). Despite these improvements in safer sexual behavior, youth in the United States continue to have much more negative consequences of sexual activity than their peers in other countries.

Approximately 750,000 15- to 20-year-olds become pregnant every year (Guttmacher Institute, 2011). There has been a steady decrease in the teen pregnancy rate from the peak in 1990 to 2005 with a slight increase in 2006 (Eaton, 2010). The rates of pregnancy, birth, abortion, and miscarriage among 15- to 19-year-olds are approximately twice that of Canada or Sweden. The total number of pregnancies to non-Hispanic whites exceeds African American and Latina pregnancies, but the pregnancy rates of these two groups are three times the white rate (Guttmacher Institute, 2011). Being poor increases the birthrate among teens, with 83% of births to teens in families with incomes less than $25,000, and half of all births to teens occur in families with income less than $12,000. Approximately 59% of pregnancies result in a live birth. Approximately 27% result in an abortion, and the rest miscarry. Substantial risks have been associated with adolescent childbearing, including lower birthweight, higher mortality rates, poorer school performance, and less adequate parenting (National Campaign to Prevent Teen and Unplanned Pregnancy, 2010), although many of these effects may be more related to poverty and family background than age of the mother (Turley, 2004).

Another important health consequence of adolescent sexual activity is sexually transmitted infection, including HIV. Adolescents account for approximately one-fourth of the 15 million reported cases of sexually transmitted infections every year. Chlamydia, the most common of these diseases, has increased dramatically over the last decade, but this may be related to increased screening and less invasive testing (Ozer et al., 2003). Gonorrhea rates have generally declined but still are much more prevalent among African Americans (11 times the rate among Hispanic youth and 23 times that of white, non-Hispanic youth). Although AIDS is relatively uncommon among adolescents, the long incubation period of development from HIV infection to AIDS implies that many of those diagnosed with AIDS in their 20s contracted the disease as teens.

Tobacco, Alcohol, and Other Drug Use

The prevalence of tobacco, alcohol, and other substance use by adolescents has long been identified as a serious threat to the health of youth (Blum, 1987). Alcohol and other drug use frequently contribute to the causes of unintentional and intentional injuries, including motor vehicle-related injuries, homicide, and suicide, and may be a factor in unintended pregnancy and lead to a variety of medical, psychological, and social morbidities.

Existing data on the incidence and prevalence of tobacco, alcohol, and other drugs used by adolescents are based on self-reports. Self-reported data may not be entirely accurate because of adolescents' attempts to provide socially desirable responses. Adolescents may also report engaging in behaviors that challenge what is socially desirable.

The most frequently used drugs by adolescents are those that eventually will be legal for them to use, despite public health campaigns against them. Tobacco, alcohol, and marijuana use increased until the late 90s when rates for adolescents peaked and then steadily declined to the present. In 1991, 70% of all high school students

had tried tobacco and 12.7% were regular smokers, but in 2009 less than one-half had ever tried tobacco and 7.3% said they were regular smokers (CDC, 2010). Alcohol use has gone down slightly, but still remains at very high levels. Heavy drinking, defined as drinking within the last 30 days five or more drinks within a couple of hours has gone from 31% to 24%. Out-of-school adolescents were significantly more likely than in-school adolescents to have reported ever having smoked cigarettes (CDC, 1994). White and Hispanic students, older students, and out-of-school adolescents were significantly more likely than African American students to be current users of cigarettes. (See Table 9–1.)

Illicit substance use is not as prevalent as use of alcohol and tobacco, but a significant number of adolescents reported use of marijuana and/or cocaine. In 2009, 36.8% of students surveyed had used marijuana during their lifetime, and one in five had used marijuana in the last month. Older, male, and out-of-school youth are more likely than others to report ever having used marijuana. Overall, 6.4% of students surveyed had used cocaine during their lifetime, and 2.8% were current cocaine users. Hispanic male and female students were significantly more likely than white or African American students to have tried cocaine. Despite the stereotype of cocaine as an urban black problem, white youth were significantly more likely than African American young people to report ever having used cocaine (Eaton et al., 2010). Use of illegal substances including methamphetamine, hallucinogenics, and steroids increased in the 90s, but has generally decreased since then. Older studies have indicated that out-of-school adolescents were three times more likely than in-school adolescents to have reported ever having used cocaine (CDC, 1994). Rural substance abuse is as high or higher than other areas, particularly tobacco use and binge drinking (Atav & Spencer, 2002; Fahs et al., 1999).

Obesity, Nutrition, and Physical Activity

The nutritional and activity statuses of adolescents are important for several reasons. First, adolescent growth and development require an increase in energy and an increase in nutrients, particularly iron, calcium, and certain other minerals. Second, as adolescents make more independent food choices, patterns are developing that could play important roles in several chronic diseases in adulthood. Third, eating habits may have even more direct effects on health during adolescence, such as obesity or deficits during pregnancy. Fourth, nutrition and physical activity patterns are changing for the worse.

Obesity is a public health concern for several reasons. Rates of overweight and obesity have been increasing in the United States over the last 30 years, and adolescents are not immune to that. Between 1976 to 1980 and 2007 to 2008 among adolescents aged 12 to 19, obesity increased from 5.0% to 18.1% (Ogden & Carroll, 2010). There is much variation by ethnicity and by gender, with 14.5% of white girls, 29.2% of black girls, and 17.4% of Mexican girls being obese, and 16.7% of white boys, 19.8% of black boys and 26.8% of Mexican boys being obese.

For children and adolescences much of the concern about the increasing prevalence of obesity is that chronic diseases that previously were seen only in adults are now increasingly seen in younger populations. Autopsies of young men in their early 20s, taken during the wars in Korea and Vietnam, showed fatty streaks indicative of atherosclerosis, thus confirming that this chronic disease starts early. High blood pressure, diabetes, and fatty infiltration of the liver are all being seen in younger and younger populations due to nutritional issues and weight status.

Other nutritional concerns and irregular eating patterns can significantly affect the health status of adolescents. Skipping meals, snacking, and eating high-fat food, particularly "fast food" are all common and unhealthy eating patterns in adolescence. Additionally disordered eating include unhealthy effort for weight loss including purging and may be associated with negative body image. Diets low in calcium during adolescence may affect adult bone density. During pregnancy, nutritional needs for women increase, particularly for folic acid, but the general adolescent diet is low in this and other important nutrients. This is particularly important during the first several months when many do not know (or do not wish to know) that they are pregnant.

Although approximately two-thirds of adolescents are vigorously physically active, the percentage declines with each age group (Grunbaum et al., 2004). The percentage of vigorously active adolescents has not changed since monitoring through the YRBSS began in 1993.

Themes for Improving Adolescent Health

Analysis of adolescent health status and adolescent developmental issues has guided public health researchers, policy makers, and advocates to develop a few basic cross-cutting themes for improving the health of adolescents (Brindis et al., 1998). In addition to the U.S. Congress's Office of Technology Assistance report in 1991, numerous foundations (e.g., Carnegie Council on Adolescent Development, 1989, 1995; William T. Grant Foundation, 1988) and government-sponsored collaborations (Health Futures of Youth, 1988; Irwin & Duncan, 2002; O'Connell, Boat, & Warner, 2009) have concluded primarily the following:

1. Adolescent risk behaviors need to be addressed because of their tremendous impact on adolescent health now and throughout the life cycle.
2. Risk behavior may best be reduced by focusing on positive youth development and enhancing resilience.

3. Youth need better access to appropriate health care.
4. Research can guide our understanding of adolescent development, health status, and program effectiveness.

Undergirding all of these has been an increasing recognition that social and economic disparities are major factors in poorer health and that stigma about adolescents in general and about many adolescent subpopulations in particular inhibits adolescent growth and development.

Ubiquitousness of Adolescent Risk

Although most adolescents are on track, doing their homework, arguing about their chores, and being generally responsible, most also engage in varying degrees of risky behavior. Most concerning are those who initiate multiple risk behaviors in early adolescence (Irwin, 1990; Jessor & Jessor, 1977). Although young people are often unfairly labeled by their problems (drug users, dropouts, gangsters), research confirms what youth service providers, parents, and teenagers have long known—youth who engage in one troubling behavior often engage in other risky behaviors. The adolescent who is initially identified with one problem likely has problems in other domains. The youth with drug problems, for example, has probably had school problems, tumultuous relationships with parents, and legal troubles and is more likely to have health problems from high-risk sexual behavior. Antecedents of high-risk behavior include early school failure and behavioral problems in elementary school, smoking tobacco in late childhood and early adolescence, and early puberty in girls. All of these suggest potential for earlier interventions and for evaluations of programs for younger children that monitor behavioral outcomes well into adolescence.

Risk taking may be particularly important for adolescent development in that it may assist with developing autonomy, mastery, and intimacy. Along these lines, Donovan

and Jessor (1985) have argued that "problem behavior" should be seen as a functional aspect of development in that these behaviors may be means of achieving otherwise blocked goal attainment, may be ways of expressing opposition to adult authority, may be ways of gaining access to peers and youth culture, and may be means of confirming self-identity. From this perspective, interventions aimed at reducing risk behaviors will need to address more dramatically the developmental needs of adolescents for mastery, peer relationships, and identity (Millstein & Igra, 1996) as well as the perceptions, opportunities, and propensities for risky behavior (Boyer & Byrnes, 2009).

Resilience and Youth Development

Important concepts related to risk behavior emerging from longitudinal research are resilience and positive youth development. It has been noted that even among high-risk youth in high-risk environments, some young people succeed. One of the first such studies of high-risk children in Hawaii identified one-third of the youth as high risk because they have four or more situations thought to be unfavorable to development—family situations such as poverty, conflict, alcoholism, or mental illness. These children showed signs of emotional distress in childhood, but at 18 years old, one-third were doing well, and at 32 years old, nearly one half "loved well, worked well, played well, and expected well" (Werner, 1992, p. 263). The successful children were connected to caring and supportive adults, had positive temperament and skills, and got second chances in late adolescence through military or adult education programs. Resilience through supportive networks at a variety of levels and ages has also been noted with a variety of populations including of African American youth (Barrow, Armstrong, Vargo, & Boothroyd, 2007) and in the development of programs for psychiatric population (Luthar & Cicchetti, 2000). Others have noted that communities and youth who have many assets such as those that encourage connectedness tend to have less risky behavior and less damage from risky behaviors (Blyth, 1993; Murphey, Lamonda, Carney, & Duncan, 2004).

Healthy development of youth involves more than being risk free. Programs and policies that aim to improve adolescent health need to focus more on youth development, which has been defined as

> the ongoing growth process in which all youth are engaged in attempting (1) to meet their basic personal and social needs to be safe, feel cared for, be valued, be useful, and be spiritually grounded, and (2) to build skills and competencies that allow them to function and contribute in their daily lives.

(Pittman, O'Brien, & Kimball, 1993, p. 8)

This also leads to more focus on building assets in the community context of adolescence. A wide variety of programs such as 4-H, mentoring, recreation, and civic action groups have been built on these principles. Increasingly, the research suggests that such programs, by and large, are effective in producing positive outcomes and less negative outcomes (Eccles & Gootman, 2002; Gavin, Catalano, David-Ferdon, Gloppen, & Markham, 2010).

Access to High-Quality Health Care

Because young people and their families trust physicians and want guidance on development, sexuality, and health, healthcare visits could be an opportunity for screening, preventive health care and health promotion (Park et al., 2001). However, care is generally episodic rather than preventive. Although most parents believe their teen is getting preventive care, analysis of national provider data indicates 38% had a visit primarily for preventive care, and only 10% received anticipatory guidance on the six nationally recommended topics (Irwin, Adams, Park, & Newacheck, 2009). This may represent some slight improvement. In 1993

it was reported that only 2% of all medical office visits included discussions about smoking cessation, weight control, nutrition, or HIV transmission (Igra & Millstein, 1993).

There are both financial and nonfinancial barriers to high-quality care for adolescents. Among financial barriers is a lack of insurance coverage and/or inadequate coverage. Even those with insurance often find health insurance is inadequate to the needs of adolescents. Inadequate reimbursement rates in fee-for-service systems or time pressures in managed-care environments discourage many physicians from screening and treating adolescents who require services that are more time intensive and controversial. Approximately 30% of all adolescent health costs are paid by families out of pocket in the form of premiums, copayments, uncovered prescriptions, and uncovered services, particularly in mental health care (Newacheck, Wong, Galbraith, & Hung, 2003b). Coverage for preventive care should improve through the healthcare reforms of 2010, but it can be anticipated that funding for confidential healthcare, mental health, and substance abuse treatment services will continue to be problematic.

Many nonfinancial factors often make high-quality healthcare services difficult for adolescents. Youth who do not feel that their health concerns will remain confidential may be hesitant to seek medical care. In one survey of patients from 33 Wisconsin family planning clinics, one-half of the adolescents reported that they would stop using healthcare services if their parent's permission were required for prescriptions for oral contraceptives (Reddy, Fleming, & Swain, 2002). Only one-third of the students in a Massachusetts study knew that they could get confidential care for sexually transmitted infections. Interestingly, an even higher percentage of youth said they did not want their friends to know their health concerns, a finding that needs to be considered in the development of school-based health services and peer education programs (Cheng, Savageau,

Sattler, & DeWitt, 1993). Despite the importance of confidential care, only about 40% of parents report their 12- to 17-year-olds had time alone with the physician at the last preventive care visit (Erdman, Adams, Park, & Irwin, 2010).

Other nonfinancial impediments to high-quality health care are related to the biopsychosocial nature of adolescents' health problems. Youth and healthcare providers are often frustrated with the fragmentation of services across several different institutions—education, child welfare, juvenile justice, community mental health—each with its own priorities, cultures, and financing. Healthcare providers who work with adolescents often report that their training did not prepare them to manage these complexities. The focus on acute care within the healthcare system often makes difficult the screening, anticipatory guidance, relationship building, problem solving, and social resource locating that comprehensive high-quality care for adolescent needs.

Growing Research on Program Effectiveness

Research on adolescents and health has mushroomed. One particular area of research has been on program evaluation, with several summaries and synthesis available outlining best practices (Hawkins, Catalano, & Arthur, 2002; Moore & Zaff, 2002; Wandersman & Florin, 2003).

Most of these reviews identified degrees of evidence (i.e., "effective," "noneffective," "unproven," and "promising") for evaluating programs and established criteria for program inclusion based on the quality of evaluation and program design. One review found that effective programs were comprehensive, had multiple intervention strategies, often were implemented in multiple settings, had explicit theoretical grounding, developed positive relationships, varied in teaching methods, paid attention to timing, were socioculturally relevant, had sufficient dosage, and hired well-trained staff (Wandersman &

Florin, 2003). The Substance Abuse and Mental Health Services administration has created a registry of programs judged to be effective (available at http://www.nrepp.samhsa.gov). The nonprofit organization Child Trends (http://www.childtrends.org) has a similar search tool.

Most evaluated programs depend on community-based efforts. Reviewers have found that although community-based programs have often had positive impacts, the results have been inconsistent (Fagan, Hanson, Hawkins, & Arthur, 2008). This has been particularly so when programs expand or replicate. One difficulty has been having valid, reliable, and ethical evaluations. Some classic research requirements such as random assignment or using comparison sites can create suspicion in many communities. Another difficulty is that getting an adequate dose or amount of intervention may make it challenging to achieve significant results. Creating, maintaining, and sustaining a coalition is time consuming and often problematic because of the different agenda and cultural backgrounds of the various coalition members and researchers. As the Annie E. Casey Foundation (2001) learned through its Making Connections effort, communities change during the process; such initiatives take a long time, and issues of race, power, and equity are too often ignored but always present.

PUBLIC HEALTH PROGRAMS FOR ADOLESCENTS

Reflecting the dilemmas of the American political structure (Brindis & Ott, 2001), public health efforts to improve adolescent health have been an interaction of federal, state, and local community efforts and a mix of public and private organizational involvement. This sometimes creates a multiplicity of efforts, some duplication, much organizational complexity, diversity of opinion, difficulty reaching consensus, some contradictory efforts, and perhaps some creativity.

Federal Programs

A sometimes bewildering number of federal agencies, ranging from the Department of Agriculture to the Department of Transportation, have programs related to adolescent health. Within the Department of Health and Human Services are programs that fund direct healthcare services for poor youth through Medicaid and for low-income youth through the Child Health Insurance Program. Also within the Department of Health and Human Services are programs that address specific issues related to youth health and development, including the Substance Abuse and Mental Health Services Administration, the CDC's Division of Adolescent and School Health, and the Health Resources and Services Administration (HRSA). Particularly important for youth are programs linked to the Maternal and Child Health Bureau (MCHB) of HRSA.

MCHB

The MCHB administers Title V of the Social Security Act, which underwrites most public health work for adolescents in the United States. Using both block grants to the states and Special Projects of Regional and National Significance (SPRANS) grants for infrastructure development and demonstrations, MCHB has been the key federal agency for developing adolescent health as an area of concern. One of the sections within MCHB, the Division of Child, Adolescent and Family Health, has established Adolescent Health Coordinators in each state to develop plans for meeting adolescent healthcare needs. This office has also established national centers on adolescent health policy (NAHIC in San Francisco, the State Adolescent Health Resource Center in Minneapolis, and the School Mental Health Policy Centers in Los Angeles and Baltimore). The SPRANS program has modeled a wide variety of MCH programs such as reducing teen pregnancy and school bullying. SPRANS grants also attempt to reduce health disparity problems for high-risk populations such as homeless youth, African American males, and youth with physical disabilities.

One important part of the federal role has been to support health professional training. The epidemiology of adolescent health presented in this chapter underscores the importance of addressing the complex psychosocial mortalities and morbidities. This requires more broadly based training than traditional medically based models. Because of this need, MCHB sponsors several programs to increase interdisciplinary training. One of the prime examples is the Leadership Education in Adolescent Health at university-based sites in Baltimore, Boston, Houston, Indianapolis, Minneapolis, Rochester (New York), and San Francisco. Begun in 1978, the Leadership Education in Adolescent Health programs train graduate and postgraduate nurses, nutritionists, physicians, psychologists, and social workers to provide leadership for interdisciplinary work in adolescent health care. The MCHB also funds programs at 13 schools of public health. The Partners in Program Planning in Adolescent Health is a collaboration of several professional organizations sponsored by MCHB that aims to improve professional practice related to adolescent health.

MCHB also administers several other programs related to adolescent health, such as transition support for special healthcare needs youth, and collaborates with other federal agencies on projects such as the National Initiative to Improve Adolescent Health (discussed later).

Office of Adolescent Health

One of the continuing controversies in adolescent health is the role of the federal government in pregnancy prevention. Although all political administrations have supported efforts to reduce adolescent pregnancy, the means of doing so have been controversial. From 1996 until the beginning of the Obama administration, the federal government supported block grants to states to establish abstinence-only pregnancy prevention programs. The abstinence-only program was generally opposed by adolescent health professionals and not supported by a significant research base (Santelli et al., 2006). Instead, the Obama administration in 2008 created a separate Office of Adolescent Health within the Health Resource Services Administration with the primary purpose of supporting evidence-based pregnancy prevention. In 2010, $75 million was allocated to replicate evidence-based programs, and $25 million was allocated for demonstration programs to research the effectiveness of promising program methods. The National Campaign to Prevent Teen and Unwanted Pregnancy maintains a database of effective programs at http://www.thenationalcampaign.org.

Division of Adolescent and School Health

Within the CDC's National Center for Chronic Disease Prevention and Health Promotion, the Division of Adolescent and School Health (DASH) supports a variety of initiatives to (1) monitor adolescent health; (2) synthesize and apply research; (3) enable health interventions by states, territories, local agencies, and tribal governments as well as by nongovernmental agencies; and (4) evaluate program effectiveness. One of the main tools of DASH has been the Youth Risk Behavior Surveillance System, which is part of a large effort to assist schools to develop programs and curricula aimed at reducing a wide range of risk behaviors. In 2009, DASH had a budget of $57 million. DASH also helps coordinate school-based initiatives with a variety of other CDC chronic disease prevention efforts such as asthma control, diabetes management, and AIDS prevention.

Other Federal Efforts to Improve Adolescent Health

Other federal efforts to improve access to appropriate adolescent health care have included the Early Prevention, Screening, Diagnosis, and Treatment program (EPSDT).

This program was intended to increase access to screening and follow-up services for children and youth, including some services of particular relevance to adolescents including reproductive health and mental health. Unfortunately, even with improved funding, the program has reached only a small percentage of eligible adolescents enrolled, and few states have established mental health screening protocols.

Another area of federal initiative has been to support school-based/school-linked centers. After initial reports suggesting that such healthcare services may reduce sexual activity and pregnancy and provide acceptable and accessible mental health and substance abuse services, various agencies of the federal government joined private foundations, state governments, and local school districts in funding sites. By 2002 there were nearly 1,500 schools with school-based health centers (Center for Health and Health Care in Schools, 2003). These clinics vary in the amount of services provided and have often proven quite controversial because of some concern that they would provide reproductive healthcare services and thus increase adolescent sexual activity. Subsequent evaluations have found for some time that school health clinics do achieve accessible, acceptable, comprehensive health care for adolescents, do not increase sexual activity among the students, and may decrease pregnancy rates (U.S. Congress, 1991c).

Family Planning and Adolescent Family Life programs are other federal efforts to reduce teen pregnancy. Title X of the Public Health Service Act began in 1970 to fund family planning clinics, and Title XX of the Public Health Services Act of 1981 created the Adolescent Family Life Program, which funds both prevention programs and services for adolescents who are pregnant or parenting. Block grants to the states for MCH services and for social services are often used for adolescent pregnancy prevention efforts, as are SPRANS grants. The federal government also has created special initiatives that include teen pregnancy reduction efforts, often as part of other projects such as "Healthy Start," "Healthy Schools," "Healthy Communities," and the Community Coalition Partnership Program.

Using the Tools of Public Health

Public health workers have used a wide range of public health approaches, or conceptual tools, to improve adolescents' lives. Some examples of application of these tools include using data to develop national goals and objectives, involving research expertise to enhance healthcare services, applying the Haddon Matrix to cut down on injuries, using multiple levels of community efforts to reduce teen suicide, developing the continuum of care to reduce adolescent pregnancy, and promoting healthy lifestyles through policy changes.

Using Data to Drive National Goals and Objectives

Using data to drive goal setting, program objective planning, and funding has been one of the important public health tools of the Healthy People 2020 Health Objectives for the Nation (HP2020) initiative. The intention has been to define achievable goals with measurable objectives and to create resources to help communities, states, and federal agencies attain these goals.

For HP2020, the focus of the national objectives changed from a focus primarily on emphasizing risky behavior prevention to more broad-based efforts of comprehensive youth development. The goals include:

- Increase adolescent wellness checkups
- Increase participation in afterschool activities
- Increase adolescent-adult connections
- Improve the transition to self-sufficiency from foster care
- Improve educational achievement
- Increase the number of schools participating in the school breakfast program

- Reduce illegal drugs on school property
- Increase school safety as perceived by the parents
- Reduce student harassment related to sexual orientation and gender identity
- Reduce violent incidents in public schools
- Reduce youth participation in crimes and victimization by crimes

Healthy People 2020 has available more detailed specification of the objectives, their measurement, and evidence-based interventions on the website. The objectives will be more specifically defined by a consensus process over the next couple of years (U.S. Department of Health and Human Services, 2010b). To achieve these objectives, a collaborative planning guide has been developed (Teipel & Brinids, 2010) and several states have implemented previous aspects of this process (Healthy Teen Network, 2010). It has also been noted that there is little data on various populations of concern for many of the objectives, so the ability to focus efforts may be quite limited (Knopf, Park, Brindis, Mulye, & Irwin, 2007).

Involving Expertise to Improve Adolescent Health Services

Applying research expertise to improve adolescent health services has been an approach of the National Research Council and the Institute of Medicine. A convened group of expert researchers made recommendations to improve adolescent health services based on a review of the evidence related to adolescent health care services (O'Connell, Boat, & Warner, 2009). These recommendations to providers, agencies, insurers, and foundations are summarized as follows:

1. Coordinate primary care healthcare systems
2. Focus on disease prevention, health promotion, and behavioral health, particularly among vulnerable youth, with adequate support and funding

3. Engage community healthcare providers and institutions to develop coordinated, linked, and interdisciplinary adolescent health services

4. Provide confidentiality by supporting laws, policies, and practices that enable adolescents to access services to protect their health

5. Prepare the providers through policies and accreditation practices that encourage specific training in working with adolescents and that support adequate funding and expansion of interdisciplinary training programs

This type of panel can produce grandiose sounding recommendations, but by providing extensive and authoritative documentation of its analysis of the existing situation it can advance the discussion of key issues. As a consequence, recommendations by groups affiliated with the National Academy of Science are taken more seriously by a wide variety of policy makers in the government, legislature, and private foundations, and thus often become a basis for prioritization. Such recommendations are not sufficient to change policy in the face of competing demands placed on policy makers, but such work can help frame the discussion, provide legitimacy to certain issues such as the importance of confidentiality, identify areas for research and development, and clarify the terms of discussion.

It should be noted in this context that proving the health effectiveness or the cost benefit of the type of comprehensive health care recommended can be difficult, although not impossible (Park et al., 2001). The cost benefits of interest to those who finance health care are usually shorter term benefits. Many adolescent health behaviors, however, do not have health consequences for many years (smoking, unhealthy eating, unsafe sexual behavior). Given the high long-term costs of many of these behaviors, which may result in cancer, obesity, or HIV, even a small effect of an intervention of 5% to 7% would

be very effective for society as a whole in the long term but might not reach statistical levels of significance in shorter term studies with smaller populations (Downs & Klein, 1995).

Applying the Haddon Matrix to Reduce Injuries

Another useful tool of public health is systemic analysis as exemplified by the Haddon Matrix to reduce injuries. Even though injuries account for more than 75% of all adolescent deaths, the rate of fatal injuries has declined dramatically in past decades. Injuries include both unintentional events such as motor vehicle and bicycle crashes, drowning, and occupational safety failures, as well as intentional injuries such as homicide, suicide, and abuse. Because the frequency and severity of injury in the population are predictable, public health workers focused on primary prevention avoid use of the word "accident," preferring the term "unintentional injury." By intersecting the three time phases of the injury event (preevent, event, and postevent) with the agent, host, and environment factors from the epidemiologic model, the Haddon matrix has been a successful public health tool for identifying strategies for injury prevention. It has been used in a wide variety of situations such as playground falls, handgun injury, and cancer deaths from smoking (Runyan, 2003). Here we focus on the leading cause of adolescent death, motor vehicle crashes (Table 9–2).

Partially as a result of interventions suggested by a public health approach such as the Haddon matrix and collaborations among police, parents, engineers, media, youth, regulators, legislators, and victims, unintentional motor vehicle fatalities in the 15- to 19-year-old age group have declined by nearly one-third since 1980. Population-based strategies of benefit to all ages such as (1) improvements in highway design (e.g., interstate highways have one-third the fatality rate of rural highways), (2) automobile crash-safety design, (3) seat belt use and passive restraint

Table 9–2 Modified Haddon Matrix of Factors Related to Motor Vehicle Injury and Outcome

	Human Factors	Agent or Vehicle Factors	Physical Environment Factors	Sociocultural Environment Factors
Preevent	driver vision alcohol experience amount of travel night/weekend traffic violations	brakes, tires center of gravity jack-knife tendency speed capability ease of control	visibility of hazards road curve & grade surface divided highway signals intersection access	attitudes about alcohol enforcement of speeding laws laws re teen driving
Event	safety belt use age sex	speed on impact vehicle size automatic restraints airbags type of contact rollover	recovery areas guard rails median barriers roadside embankments speed limits	attitudes about safety belt use laws about safety belt use enforcement of safety belt use
Postevent	age physical condition severity of injury body region injured	fuel system integrity	emergency transport system quality of EMS distance to trauma center rehabilitation programs	support for trauma care systems skill of EMS personnel laws and attitudes re disability school integration

Source: Adapted from Lescohier, D., & Gallagher, S.S. (1996). Unintentional injury. In R.J. DiClemente, W.B. Hansen, & L.E. Ponton (Eds.), Handbook of adolescent risk behavior. New York: Plenum Press, and National Committee for Injury Prevention and Control, 1989.

systems (40% to 50% less fatality), and (4) enhanced emergency medical services can be derived from this type of analysis. Efforts to reduce drunk driving by raising the drinking age, lowering the permissible blood alcohol levels, making the identification of a "designated driver" the social norm, sponsoring alcohol-free events, and even restricting automobile travel time are ways to improve the human preevent factors related to injury. Efforts to increase the human factor of seat belt use during the event are only minimally successful unless they are also accompanied by a preevent social environmental intervention with legal sanctions. Interestingly, driver education classes have not been shown to improve safety and in fact may decrease

safety by enabling adolescents to drive at an earlier age (Mayhew & Simpson, 2002). All states now require graduated driver's licensing restricting hours and numbers of passengers, and these laws have been estimated to reduce the risk of fatalities of 16-year-old drivers by 19% (Vanlaar et al., 2009). The federal requirement of passive restraints and airbags is based on considering the rapid exchange of energy as the "agent" of injury at the time of the crash and may be one of the most significant factors for harm reduction (Table 9–2).

There have also been effective efforts to increase parent limit-setting and communication regarding driving behavior (Simons-Morton, Ouitmet, & Catalano, 2008). The importance of transportation in conflict with parents has a long history, as illustrated by the story told of Socrates, who asked a youth named Lysis whether his parents gratify all of his wishes. In response, Lysis complained that even though his parents seemed to want him to be happy his father would not let him ride the family's horses (quoted in Hall, 1904, p. 514).

Using Levels of Community Efforts to Reduce Teen Suicide

One conceptual tool for understanding suicide prevention used by the Institute of Medicine (IOM) was to consider universal, indicated, and targeted strategies (Goldsmith, Pellmar, Kleinman, & Bunney, 2002). Universal approaches have included public education campaigns to reduce the stigma of mental health treatment, limiting access to lethal methods such as guns, or increasing the beliefs that depression is treatable and suicide preventable. Another universal approach encouraged by the IOM is to promote connectedness among individuals, within the family, and among the community. Such an effort encourages collaboration across agencies and systems and aims to have a broad impact on a variety of health concerns, even though the primary target may be suicide prevention. Another form of universal prevention is earlier identification of youth in major distress by encouraging wide use of screening measures such as the computerized Teen Screen Program in schools (O'Connell, Boat, & Warner, 2009). Such programs are more effective than school personnel at identifying those populations and individuals at greatest risk for mental health problems including suicide (Scott et al., 2008). Those identified are then offered interviews and those indicated to have more significant problems are linked to treatment services. Teen Screen is more than a one-shot screening program. It is designed to involve considerable commitment by schools and their communities to follow up with in-person clinical interviews and to provide

accessible and acceptable services to youth and families. Initial research suggests this effort may significantly increase access to treatment and reduce suicidal behavior. The U.S. Preventive Services Task Force encourages similar efforts of screening for depression and suicide by primary care providers (Borowsky, 2010; Williams, O'Connor, Eder, & Whitlock, 2009). Other forms of universal interventions that use the school curriculum to reach adolescents have had more mixed results. Some school intervention programs have improved knowledge, attitudes, and help seeking, but documenting reduction in suicidal behavior or rates has been more difficult (Cusimano & Sameen, 2011).

One of the populations indicated to need more comprehensive interventions has been the Native American population. One evaluated program has demonstrated significant reductions in suicidal behavior through a cooperative and coordinated community planning effort that included youth, elders, and community agencies (May, Serna, Hurt, & DeBruyn, 2005). This process led to a focus not on suicide as an isolated phenomenon, but as a problem related to alcohol abuse, domestic violence, child abuse, and unemployment. Tribal leaders worked to expand social work and related mental health services. Over the 14-year evaluation period, suicide attempts were reduced from 14 per year to 3 per year in the community studied. Similar multiple-level efforts are needed for other indicated groups such as incarcerated youth, homeless youth, and nonheterosexual youth.

Targeted interventions focus on those individuals identified as having significant risk due to an algorithm of factors that typically includes previous suicidal attempts, recent or current suicidal ideation, conduct and/or depressive disorders, substance abuse, and family history of suicide. A few psychotherapy treatment modalities have some success at reducing suicidal behavior and have been replicated. These include Multi-Systemic Therapy, which provides intensive family and community services in the youth's environment (Huey et al., 2004). Also promising is Dialectical Behavioral Therapy, a variation of behavioral therapy with skills-based training for the client in mindfulness, emotional regulation, and problem solving (Comtois & Linehan, 2006).

Many other therapies, including inpatient treatment, have shown only mixed effectiveness, and evaluations have suffered from small sample sizes, lack of randomized control groups, imprecise measurements of outcome, lack of standardized treatment manuals, and unit of analysis problems.

Developing the Continuum of Care and Adolescent Pregnancy

Adolescent pregnancy is another public health problem that has become politicized, with much misinformation and distortion related to political expressions of concern. Because American sexual activity rates are similar to European rates yet U.S. pregnancy rates are substantially higher, American adolescent pregnancy rates can hardly be attributed to the nature of adolescence, to the supposed generosity of the U.S. welfare system compared with European welfare systems, or to greater promiscuity and related immoralities. Instead, the higher rates should be attributed to factors more unique to the U.S. experience. In addition to widespread poverty, inequality, and a lack of universally available and accessible healthcare services, the high U.S. teen pregnancy rate should be seen as related to American attitudes about sexuality, the sexual behavior of adolescents, and family planning. Despite the controversies regarding sex education, the National Research Council notes that most adolescent pregnancy prevention programs enjoy wide support from the majority of Americans and that even those who did not initially support these programs can often find common ground with the idea that every child should be born to a welcoming family that is ready and able to care for it (Brown & Eisenberg, 1995).

Numerous major reviews have reached general agreement on the best ways to prevent adolescent pregnancies (Hayes, 2007; Kirby, 2007; Manlove et al., 2002). Each has affirmed that there is not one strategy, but that multiple, community-wide approaches are needed based on the classic public health service continuum of health promotion and primary, secondary, and tertiary prevention.

First, echoing Marion Wright Edelman's often repeated comment that the best contraception is hope, adolescent pregnancy prevention strategies need to promote life options for at-risk adolescents by increasing employment and educational opportunities, training in specific skills, and providing support for youth in transition. One such program in 30 states and over 400 sites, the Teen Outreach Program, emphasized small discussion groups and community service. Participants in this program reduced pregnancy rates by 53% and had one-fifth the repeat pregnancy risk compared to parenting teens in the comparison groups (Allen & Philliber, 2001). School failure and school dropout also significantly decreased compared with participants in comparison groups.

Second, primary prevention programs based on comprehensive education are needed. Most current sex education programs are too short, too late, and too cognitively based. Effective programs include clear messages about sexual activity; training in social skills, assertiveness, and peer pressure resistance; and accurate, specific information on condom or contraceptive use and access. Typically, programs such as "Reducing the Risk" aimed at grades 9–12 in Arkansas and California include didactic information, role playing, and small group discussions. Replications of this program have delayed onset of sexual activity and increased condom use in other states as well (Kirby, 2002). One preventive education approach that has received significant funding over the last several years has been the encouragement of abstinence. Traditionally, public health efforts have advised young people to avoid sexual activity but have focused more on encouraging contraception and improving service delivery. Advocates for abstinence programs believe preventing sexual activity outside of marriage would be more effective and that prevention efforts that also provide information on contraception give mixed messages that undermine the abstinence message. Although the research has not generally been supportive of abstinence-only programs, some research suggests the abstinence programs may be effective with younger adolescents (Jemmott, Jemmott, & Fong, 2010).

The third approach, secondary prevention, is to increase access to contraceptives for those sizable numbers of adolescents who are already sexually active. Education about their use, confidentiality in obtaining healthcare services, readily available services such as those through school-based/linked clinics, and payment mechanisms are critical to achieve this. In a model program that integrated school educational programs and contraceptive services at a nearby clinic, 3-year pregnancy rates declined by 30% among enrolled students compared with a 58% increase among nonenrolled students (Zabin & Hayward, 1993). Studies have demonstrated that condom availability in schools does no harm and increases condom use for pregnancy prevention compared to students at schools without condoms (Blake et al., 2003).

The fourth approach, tertiary prevention, aims to improve outcomes for teen parents, usually by providing comprehensive medical, educational, and social services to teen parents. Such programs have had a variety of goals. Some have aimed to reduce low birth weight, some to improve child outcomes, and some to speed entry to the job market to avoid welfare dependency. Additionally, with nearly 25% of teen moms having a second birth before turning 20, some have focused on preventing repeat pregnancies. Results have been quite positive for some programs but not all (Klerman, 2004). Effective programs, according to one review, shared several key characteristics (Seitz & Apfel, 1999). They have goals endorsed by the participants, such as maternal and child health and well-being rather than just job entry. They provide personalized care and attention, with research suggesting the most important factor in preventing subsequent pregnancies is the relationship with the teen mom and the person working with her. These programs use schools, and they pay close attention to the timing of involvement when the mothers are most open to assistance, which is earlier in pregnancy and parenting. Others have suggested programs also need to pay close attention to the multiple relationships involved including fathers and grandparents (Beers & Hollo, 2009).

Promoting Healthy Lifestyles through Policy Change

Obesity affects health throughout the life course. Efforts to restrict food intake or encourage dieting as an individual behavior seldom work and may in fact increase obesity (Dietz & Gortmaker, 2001). Initial results from collaborative public health interventions on multiple dimensions, including family, school, neighborhood, primary care, and policy, have shown promising results. Programs that help families reduce the use of food as reward, establish family meal time, improve parental modeling, and structure more physical activity can reduce obesity (Ritchie et al., 2001). The most important physical activity is turning off the television (Dietz & Gortmaker, 2001), which is implemented at the family level but reinforced by school and primary care. School-based curricula such as the multiple-subject Planet Health program have been effective at improving diet, decreasing screen time, and increasing physical activity.

These interventions have demonstrated the importance of supportive policy in leading to sustainable change. The decline in participation in daily physical education classes from 42% in 1991 to 28.4% in 2003, and then a rise to 33.3% in 2009 (Eaton et al., 2010; Grunbaum et al., 2004) reflects a lack of supportive policy. Creating physical education programs that emphasize fitness and lifelong lifestyle activities rather than just competitive sports is also an important education policy with public health consequences.

One example of a supportive policy change is the Healthy Hunger-Free Kids Act of 2010. This act was signed into law, increasing access to healthy food for low-income children and youth at school. This law aims to set nutrition standards for what food can be served at school, increases the amount spent per meal (for higher quality food), and increases the number of students who can receive meals at school, thereby aiming to reduce obesity by offering healthier, more nutritious food to children. Other efforts to enact public health laws to control obesity have been inspired by success in tobacco control. These attempts have also have inspired similar resistance from the industries involved (Mello, Studdert, & Brennen, 2006). Many states have considered policy changes such as requiring nutrition curriculum, screening for Body Mass Index abnormalities, increasing physical education, using special taxes on junk foods, and regulating junk-food advertising aimed at children (National Conference of State Legislatures, 2010).

Special Populations and the Core Responsibilities of Public Health

Although public health uses population-based approaches, the population is heterogeneous, and certain groups of the population have worse health status, often based on being excluded from social resources, stigmatized, and blamed for their conditions. These special populations include groups such as ethnic and racial minorities, immigrants and migrants, the poor, the learning disabled, the incarcerated, pregnant and parenting youth,

the mentally ill, foster youth, maltreated youth, and youth with different sexual orientations. For youth, the multiplicity of special population identities is probably the most significant factor in risk. For example, the Native American learning-disabled youth in the foster care system who is pregnant would be considered at "multiple jeopardy." Because of the alienated and/or outcast nature of many of these groups, public health work is particularly concerned with assessing the needs of these populations, ensuring that appropriate, high-quality services are provided, and creating policies that attempt to create a link with the larger society. Sometimes the assurance function leads public health agencies to provide direct services to some of these groups to demonstrate that provision of services is feasible, to establish a beginning point for wider collaboration, or to serve groups that are considered "too difficult" for traditional healthcare providers.

Furthermore, because of the degree of social alienation experienced by many of these groups, special efforts need to be made to establish collaborative relationships for health. The population of homeless youth, for instance, is difficult to assess because many avoid contact with adults for fear of being turned over to the police and returned to their homes. Efforts to understand their health problems will need significant street outreach and work with peers. Likewise, ensuring quality may be more difficult with certain ethnic groups with traditions of alternative views of health and with traditions of not appearing to disagree with authority. Policy development regarding some particularly stigmatized groups such as the incarcerated creates many controversies beyond their immediate healthcare needs. Working with key people trusted by those within the group, recognizing existing community networks and supports, and engaging in collaborative processes around jointly identified problems have been ways that public health workers have tried to develop epidemiologic analysis, a continuum of care, and health promotion disease prevention activities for special populations.

FUTURE DIRECTIONS

Despite the widespread call for increased access to health care and improved environments for adolescents, we will continue to experience cultural conflict about the role of government, about the degree of individual versus social causation of problems, and about adolescent sexual behavior. This will make access to health care difficult for adolescents and will make broader efforts to improve adolescent health politically vulnerable. Public health initiatives have had the most success when they deliberately and systematically build a wide base at the local, state, or national level. This may be time consuming and unpredictable, but it may also lead to stronger continuing support.

Another future direction of public health work with adolescents will be efforts to include adolescent needs in any future system of healthcare reform—managed care, national health insurance, or whatever combination emerges. Particularly important is establishing and maintaining systems of confidentiality for adolescents, enabling and training providers to have a working knowledge of adolescents' needs, abilities, and limitations, and establishing primary care with risk screening, health guidance, and coordination with appropriate ameliorative programs. Identifying adolescent health indicators and adolescent-specific evaluations will be important avenues to pursue in efforts to keep healthcare systems accountable to serving adolescents. Because these problems and solutions often cross institutional boundaries, creating partnerships and a broader view of social costs will be important for implementing best practice programs in communities on a broader scale.

These dilemmas may be particularly apparent when the issues of the health needs of adolescents transitioning to adulthood are considered. What are their developmental needs? Do they need consideration in programming, training of providers, data development? Should they be considered part of the MCH area of concern (even if they are not childbearing)? How can the adult system manage the needs of young adults with special healthcare needs? How can adolescents with special healthcare needs be better prepared for the physical, cultural, vocational, and psychological transitions to the adult world? What special skills and programs will be needed to better serve this still developing group (Freed & Hudson, 2006; Park & Irwin, 2008)? Already young adults have been on the radar of policy makers with the inclusion of their healthcare insurance needs in the 2010 Patient Protection and Affordable Care Act, but in most areas of governmental policy they are considered fully responsible and independent adults, not seen as a separate group needing focused consideration.

Ultimately, adolescent health status may be affected more by broader social issues than by direct contact with the healthcare system. Factors that seem to increase health among adolescents have been described as not just the absence of maltreatment, infection, stress, or social oppression but also the presence of adults who maintain caring and connectedness with them within the community. Those wanting to improve the health of adolescents will need to find ways to institutionalize these traits and to enhance resilience, reduce harm, secure the environment, and establish a sense of engagement in the lives of adolescents. This truly is the "best and wisest adult endeavor," which makes the "age between ten and three-and-twenty" a time to celebrate rather than bemoan.

ACKNOWLEDGMENTS

This work was supported in part by grants from the Maternal and Child Health Bureau, Health Resources and Services Administration, U.S. Department of Health and Human Services (U45MC 00002 and U45MC 00023).

Special thanks to Thea Zajac, M.S.W. for research assistance.

References

Allen, J., & Philliber, S. (2001). Who benefits most from a broadly targeted prevention program? Differential efficacy across populations in the Teen Outreach Program. *Journal of Community Psychology, 29*, 637–655.

Annie E. Casey Foundation. (2001). *Change that abides: A retrospective look at community and family strengthening projects and their enduring results.* Baltimore, MD: Annie E. Casey Foundation. Retrieved October 12, 2011 from http://www.aecf .org/upload/publicationfiles/cc3622h319.pdf.

Atav, S., & Spencer, G. A. (2002). Health risk behaviors among adolescents attending rural, suburban, and urban schools. *Family Community Health, 25*, 53–64.

Balfanz, R. (2009). Can the American high school become an avenue for the advancement of all? *Future of Children, 19*, 17–36.

Barrow, F., Armstrong, M., Vargo, A., & Boothroyd, R. A. (2007). Understanding the findings of resilience-related research for fostering the development of African-American adolescents. *Child and Adolescent Psychiatric Clinics of North America, 16*, 393–313.

Baumrind, D. (1987). Rearing competent children. In C.E. Irwin, Jr. (Ed.), *Adolescent social behavior and health: New directions for child development* (No. 37). San Francisco: Jossey-Bass.

Beers, L., & Hollo, R. (2009). Approaching the adolescent-headed family: A review of teen parenting. *Current Problems in Pediatric and Adolescent Health Care, 39*, 216–233.

Blake, S. M., Ledsky, R., Goodenow, C., Sawyer, R., Lohrmann, D., & Windsor, R. (2003). Condom availability programs in Massachusetts high schools; relationships with condom use and sexual behavior—2003. *American Journal of Public Health, 93*, 955–962.

Blum, R. (1987). Contemporary threats to adolescent health in the United States. *Journal of the American Medical Association, 257*, 3390–3395.

Blyth, D. A. (1993). *Healthy communities, healthy youth: How communities contribute to positive youth development.* Minneapolis, MN: Search Institute.

Bond, L., Butler, H., Thomas, L., Carlin, J., Glover, S., Bowes, G., & Patton, G. (2007). Social and school connectedness in early secondary school as predictors of late teenage substance use, mental health, and academic outcomes. *Journal of Adolescent Health, 40*, 357.e9–18.

Borowsky, I. (2010). Expose, heed, coordinate: Priorities for mental health promotion and suicide prevention. *Pediatrics, 125*, 1064–1065.

Boyer, T. W., & Byrnes, J. P. (2009). Adolescent risk taking: Integrating personal, cognitive, and social aspects of judgment. *Journal of Applied Developmental Psychology, 30*, 23–33.

Brener, N. D., Billy, J. O., & Grady, W. R. (2003). Assessment of factors affecting the validity of self-reported health-risk behavior among adolescents: Evidence from the scientific literature. *Journal of Adolescent Health, 33*, 436–457.

Brindis, C. D., & Ott, M. A. (2001). Adolescents, health policy, and the American political process. *Journal of Adolescent Health, 30*, 9–16.

Brindis, C. D., Ozer, E. M., Handley, M., Knopf, D. K., Millstein, S. G., & Irwin, C. E., Jr. (1998). *Improving adolescent lives: An analysis and synthesis of policy recommendations.* San Francisco: University of California-San Francisco, National Adolescent Health Information Center. Retrieved October 13, 2011 from http://nahic.ucsf.edu/wp-content/uploads/2011/01/IAH_Full.pdf.

Brooks-Gunn, J., & Paikoff, R. L. (1993). "Sex is a gamble, kissing is a game": Adolescent sexuality and health promotion. In S. G. Millstein, A. C. Peterson, & E. O. Nightingale (Eds.), *Promoting the health of adolescents: New directions for the twenty-first century.* New York: Oxford University Press.

Brown, S. S., & Eisenberg, L. (1995). *The best intentions: Unintended pregnancy and the well-being of children and families.* Washington, DC: National Academy Press.

Browning, C. R., Burrington, L. A., Leventhal, T., & Brooks-Gunn, J. (2008). Neighborhood structural inequality, collective efficacy, and sexual risk behavior among urban youth. *Journal of Health and Social Behavior, 49*, 269–285.

Burt, M. R. (2002). Reasons to invest in adolescents. *Journal of Adolescent Health, 31*, 136–152.

Carnegie Council on Adolescent Development. (1989). *Turning points: Preparing American youth for the twenty-first century.* The report of the Task Force on Education of Young Adolescents. Washington, DC: Author.

Carnegie Council on Adolescent Development. (1995). *Great transitions: Preparing adolescents for a new century.* Concluding report of the Carnegie Council on Adolescent Development. New York: Carnegie Corporation of New York.

Centers for Disease Control and Prevention. (1994). Health risk behaviors among adolescents who do and do not attend school: US, 1992. *Morbidity and Mortality Weekly Report, 43,* 8.

Centers for Disease Control and Prevention, National Center for Health Statistics. Compressed Mortality File 1979-1998. CDC WONDER On-line Database, compiled from Compressed Mortality File CMF 1968-1988, Series 20, No. 2A, 2000 and CMF 1989-1998, Series 20, No. 2E, 2003. Accessed at http://wonder.cdc.gov/cmf-icd9.html on May 17, 2011 5:47:34 PM.

Centers for Disease Control and Prevention, National Center for Health Statistics. Compressed Mortality File 1999-2007. CDC WONDER On-line Database, compiled from Compressed Mortality File 1999-2007 Series 20 No. 2M, 2010. Accessed at http://wonder.cdc.gov/cmf-icd10.html on May 17, 2011 5:51:03 PM.

Centers for Disease Control and Prevention. (2010). Trends in prevalence of tobacco use, National YRBS 1991-2009. Retrieved January 11, 2011 from http://www.cdc.gov/HealthyYouth/yrbs/pdf/us_tobacco_trend_yrbs.pdf.

Center for Health and Health Care in Schools. (2003). 2002 state survey of school-based health center initiatives. Washington, DC: George Washington University. Retrieved October 13, 2011 from http://www.healthinschools.org/en/News-Room/Fact-Sheets/SBHC-Initiatives/Survey%20Narrative.aspx.

Cheng, T. L., Savageau, J. A., Sattler, A. L., & DeWitt, T. G. (1993). Confidentiality in health care: A survey of knowledge, perceptions, and attitudes among high school students. *Journal of the American Medical Association, 269,* 1404-1407.

Child Trends. (2011). Children with limitations. Washington, DC: Child Trends Data Bank. Retrieved January 11, 2011 from http://www.childtrendsdatabank.org/sites/default/files/44_tab01.pdf.

Cohall, A. T., & Cohall, R. M. (1995). Number one with a bullet. In K. K. Christoffel & C. W. Runyan (Eds.), Adolescent injury: epidemiology and prevention. *Adolescent Medicine State of the Art Reviews, 6,* 183-198.

Coles, M., Makino, K., Stanwood, N., Dozier, A., & Klein, J. (2010). How are restrictive abortion statutes associated with unintended teen birth? *Journal of Adolescent Health, 47,* 160-167.

Comtois, K., & Linehan, M. (2006). Psychosocial treatments for suicidal behavior: A practice-friendly review. *Journal of Consulting Psychology, 62,* 161-170.

Cusimano, M., & Sameen, M. (2011). The effectiveness of middle and high school-based suicide prevention programs for adolescents: A systematic review. *Injury Prevention, 17,* 43-49. doi/10.1136/ip.2009.025502.

Dey, A. N., Schiller, J. S., & Tai, D. A. (2004). Summary health statistics for U.S. children: National health interview survey, 2002. National Center for Health Statistics. *Vital and Health Statistics, 10,* 221.

Dietz, W. H., & Gortmaker, S. L. (2001). Preventing obesity in children and adolescents. *Annual Review of Public Health, 22,* 337-355.

Donovan, J. E., & Jessop, R. (1985). Structure of problem behavior in adolescent and young adulthood. *Journal of Consulting and Clinical Psychology, 53,* 890-904.

Douglas-Hall, A., & Chua, M. (2009). *Basic facts about low income adolescents.* New York: National Center for Children in Poverty.

Downs, S. M., & Klein, J. D. (1995). Clinical preventive services efficacy and adolescent risk behaviors. *Archives of Pediatric and Adolescent Medicine, 149,* 374-379.

Eaton, D., Kann, L., Kinchen, S., Shanklin, S., Ross, J., Hawkins, J., Harris, W., Lowry, R., McManus, T., Chyen, D., Lim, C., Whittle, L., Brener, N., & Wechsler, H. (2010). Youth risk behavior surveillance: United States, 2009. *Morbidity Mortality Weekly Report, 59(SS-5),* 1-142.

Eccles, J., & Gootman, J. A. (Eds.). (2002). *Community programs to promote youth development.* Washington, DC: National Academy Press.

Edelman, P., & Ladner, J. (Eds.). (1991). *Adolescence and poverty.* Washington, DC: Center for National Policy Press.

Elder, G. H., Conger, R. D., Foster, E. M., & Ardelt, M. (1992). Families under economic pressure. *Journal of Family Issues, 13,* 5-37.

English, A. (2002). Financing adolescent health care: Legal and policy issues for the coming decade. *Journal of Adolescent Health, 31,* 334-346.

English, A., & Kenney, K. E. (2003). *State minor consent laws: A summary* (2nd ed.). Chapel Hill, NC: Center for Adolescent Health & the Law.

Erdman, J., Adams, S., Park, M. J., & Irwin, C. E., Jr. (2010). Who gets confidential care in adolescence: Disparities in a national sample. *Journal of Adolescent Health, 46,* 393-395.

Fagan, A., Hanson, K., Hawkins, J., & Arthur, M. (2008). Bridging science to practice: achieving prevention program implementation fidelity in the community youth development study.

American Journal of Community Psychology, 41, 235–249.

Fahs, P. S., Smith, B. E., Atav, A. S., Britten, M. X., Collins, M. S., Morgan, L. C., & Spencer, G. A. (1999). Integrative research review of risk behaviors among adolescents in rural, suburban, and urban areas. *Journal of Adolescent Health, 24,* 230–243.

Ferguson, R. F. (2001). Test-score trends along racial lines, 1971–1996: Popular culture and community academic standards. In N. J. Smelser, W. J. Wilson, & F. Mitchell (Eds.), *America becoming: Racial trends and their consequences* (Vol. 1). Commission on Behavioral and Social Sciences and Education. Washington, DC: National Academy Press.

Freed, G., & Hudson E. (2006). Transitioning children with chronic diseases to adult care: current knowledge, practices, and directions. *Journal of Pediatrics, 148,* 824–827.

Freudenberg, N., & Ruglis, J. (2007). Reframing school dropout as a public health issue. *Prevention of Chronic Disease, 4,* A10.

Gavin, L. E., Catalano, R. F., David-Ferdon, C., Gloppen, K. M., & Markham, C. M. (2010). A review of positive youth development programs that promote adolescent sexual and reproductive health. *Journal of Adolescent Health, 46*(3, Suppl.), S75–S91.

Giedd, J. N. (2008). The teen brain: Insights from neuroimaging. *Journal of Adolescent Health, 42,* 335–343.

Goldsmith, S., Pellmar, T., Kleinman, A., & Bunney, W. (Eds.). (2002). *Reducing suicide: A national imperative.* Committee on Pathophysiology and Prevention of Adolescent and Adult Suicide. Washington, DC: National Academy Press.

Grall, T. S. (2009). *Custodial mothers and fathers and their child support, 2007.* Current Population Reports. PG0-237. Washington, DC: U.S. Department of Commerce, Economics and Statistics Administration, U.S. Census Bureau. Retrieved October 13, 2011 from http://www.census.gov/prod/2009pubs/p60-237.pdf.

Greenberg, M., Weissber, R., O'Brien, M., Zins, J., Fredericks, L., Resnik, H., & Elias, M. (2003). Enhancing school-based prevention and youth development through coordinated social, emotional, and academic learning. *American Psychologist, 58,* 466–474.

Grissmer, D. W., Kirby, S. N., Berends, M., & Williamson, S. (1995). *Student achievement and the changing American family* (RAND MR-488). Santa Monica, CA: Rand Corporation.

Grunbaum, J. A., Kann, L., Kinchen, S., Ross, J., Hawkins, J., Lowry, R., Harris, W. A., McManus, T., Chyen, D., & Collins, J. (2004). Youth risk behavior surveillance: United States, 2003. *Morbidity Mortality Weekly Report, 53*(SS-02), 1–96.

Guttmacher Institute. (2011). Facts on American teens' sexual and reproductive health.. Retrieved February 8, 2011 from http://www.guttmacher.org/pubs/FB-ATSRH.html.

Hall, G. S. (1904). *Adolescence: Its psychology, and its relations to anthropology, sex, crime, religion, and education.* New York: Appleton and Company.

Halpern, C. T. (2010). Reframing research on adolescent sexuality: Healthy sexual development as part of the life course. *Perspectives on Sexual and Reproductive Health, 42,* 6–7.

Hawkins, J. D., Catalano, R. F., & Arthur, M. W. (2002). Promoting science-based prevention in communities. *Addiction Behavior, 27,* 951–976.

Hayes, C. D. (Ed.). (1987). *Risking the future: Adolescent sexuality, pregnancy, and childbearing.* National Research Council, Panel on Adolescent Pregnancy and Childbearing, Committee on Child Development and Research, Commission on Behavioral and Social Sciences. Washington, DC: National Academy Press.

Health Futures of Youth: Proceedings of a Conference. (1988, April). *Journal of Adolescent Health Care, 9,* 1–69.

Healthy Teen Network. (2010). *Healthy People 2020 and adolescent health.* Baltimore, MD: Author. Retrieved October 13, 2011 from http://www.healthyteennetwork.org/index.asp?Type = B_PR&SEC = %7B2AE1D600-4FC6-4B4D-8822-F1D5F072ED7B%7D&DE = %7B8B323A36-B77C-450D-A79C-2B58D8D5AD8E%7D.

Heron, M. (2010). Deaths: Leading causes for 2006. *National Vital Statistics Reports, 58,* 14.

Huebner, R. C., Diaz, R., & Sanchez, J. (2009). Family rejection as a predictor of negative health outcomes in white and Latino lesbian, gay, and bisexual young adults. *Pediatrics, 123,* 346–352.

Huey, S. J., Jr., Henggeler, S. W., Rowland, M. D., Halliday-Boykins, C. A., Cunningham, P. B., Pickrel, S. G., & Edwards, J. (2004). Multisystemic therapy effects on attempted suicide by youth presenting psychiatric emergencies. *Journal of the American Academy of Child & Adolescent Psychiatry, 43,* 183–190.

Igra, V., & Millstein, S. G. (1993). Current status and approaches to improving preventive services for adolescents. *Journal of the American Medical Association, 269,* 1408–1412.

Irwin, C. E., Jr. (1987). Editor's notes: Adolescent health and behavior. In C. E. Irwin, Jr. (Ed.), *New directions for child development* (No. 37). San Francisco: Jossey-Bass.

Irwin, C. E., Jr. (1990). The theoretical concept of at-risk adolescents. *Adolescent Medicine: State of the Art Reviews, 1,* 1–14.

Irwin, C. E., Jr., & Duncan, P. M. (2002). Health futures of youth II: Pathways to adolescent health, executive summary and overview. *Journal of Adolescent Health 31*(6, Suppl.), 82–89.

Irwin, C. E., Jr., Adams, S. H., Park, M. J., & Newacheck, P. W. (2009). Preventive care for adolescents: Few get visits and fewer get services. *Pediatrics, 123(4),* e565–e572.

Jargowsky, P. A. (2003). *Stunning progress, hidden problems: The dramatic decline of concentrated poverty in the 1990s.* Living Cities Census Series. Washington, DC: Brookings Institution. Retrieved October 13, 2011 from http://www.brook.edu/es/urban/publications/jargowskypoverty.htm.

Jemmott, J. B., III, Jemmott, L. S., & Fong, G. T. (2010). Efficacy of a theory-based abstinence-only intervention over 24 months: A randomized controlled trial with young adolescents. *Archives of Pediatric and Adolescent Medicine, 164,* 152–159.

Jessor, R., & Jessor, S. (1977). *Problem behavior and psycho-social development: A longitudinal study of youth.* New York: Academic Press.

Katz, L. F., King, J. R., & Liebman, J. B. (2001). Moving to opportunity: Early results of a randomized mobility experiment. *Quarterly Journal of Economics, 116,* 607–654.

Keating, D. P., & Halpern-Felsher, B. L. (2008). Adolescent drivers. A developmental perspective on risk, proficiency, and safety. *American Journal of Preventive Medicine, 30,* S272–S277.

Kett, J. F. (1993). Discovery and invention in the history of adolescence. *Journal of Adolescent Health, 14,* 605–612.

Kirby, D. (2002). Effective approaches to reducing adolescent unprotected sex, pregnancy, and childbearing. *Journal of Sex Research, 39,* 51–57.

Kirby, D. (2007). *Emerging answers 2007: Research findings on programs to reduce teen pregnancy and sexually transmitted diseases.* Washington, DC: National Campaign to Prevent Teen and Unplanned Pregnancy.

Klerman, L. (2004). *Another chance: Preventing additional births to teen mothers.* Washington, DC: National Campaign to Prevent Teen Pregnancy.

Knopf, D., Park, M., Brindis, C., Mulye, T., & Irwin, C. (2007). What gets measured gets done: Assessing data availability for adolescent populations. *Maternal and Child Health Journal, 11,* 335–345.

Knopf, D. K., Park, M. J., & Mulye, T. (2008). *Adolescent mental health.* San Francisco: University of California, San Francisco, National Adolescent Health Information Center.

Krug, E. G., Dahlberg, L. L., Mercy, J. A., Zwi, A. B., & Lozano, R. (Eds.). (2002). *World report on violence and health.* Geneva: World Health Organization.

Lehrer, J. A., Pantell, R., Tebb, K., & Shafer, M. A. (2007). Forgone health care among U.S. adolescents: Association between risk characteristics and confidentiality concern. *Journal of Adolescent Health, 40,* 218–226.

Lenhart, A., Ling, R., Campbell, S., & Purcell, K. (2010). *Teens and mobile phones.* Washington, DC: Pew Research Center. Retrieved October 13, 2011 from http://pewinternet.org/Reports/2010/Teens-and-Mobile-Phones.aspx.

Lenhart, A., Purcell, K., Smith, A., & Zickuhr, K. (2010). *Social media and mobile Internet use by teens and young adults.* Washington, DC: Pew Research Center. Retrieved October 13, 2011 from http://pewinternet.org/Reports/2010/Social-Media-and-Young-Adults.aspx.

Lescohier, D., & Gallagher, S. S. (1996). Unintentional injury. In R. J. DiClemente, W. B. Hansen, & L. E. Ponton (Eds.), *Handbook of adolescent risk behavior.* New York: Plenum Press.

Luthar, C. C., & Cicchetti, D. (2000). The construct of resilience: implications for interventions and policy. *Developmental Psychopathology, 12,* 857–883.

Manlove, J., Terry-Humen, E., Papillor, A. R., Franzetta, K., Williams, S., & Ryan, S. (2002). *Preventing teenage pregnancy, childbearing, and sexually transmitted diseases: What the research shows.* Child Trends Research Brief. Washington, DC: Child Trends. Retrieved October 13, 2011 from http://www.childtrends.org/Files/K1Brief.pdf.

May, P., Serna, P., Hurt, L., & DeBruyn, L. (2005). Outcome evolution of a public health approach to suicide prevention in an American Indian tribal nation. *American Journal of Public Health, 95,* 1235–1244.

Mayhew, D. R., & Simpson, H. M. (2002). The safety value of driver education and training. *Injury Prevention, 8*(Suppl. 2), ii3–ii8.

Mello, M., Studdert, D., & Brennen, T. (2006). Obesity—the new frontier of public health. *New England Journal of Medicine, 354,* 2601–2610.

Merikangas, K., He, J., Burstein, M., Swanson, S., Avenevoli, S., Cui, L., Benjet, C., Georgiades, K., & Swendsen, J. (2010). Lifetime prevalence of mental disorders in U.S. adolescents: Results from the National Comorbidity Survey Replication—Adolescent Supplement (NCS-A). *Journal of the American Academy of Child and Adolescent Psychiatry, 49,* 980–989.

Merikangas, K. R., He, J., Burstein, M., Swendsen, J., Avenevoli, S., Case, B., Georgiades, K., Heaton, L., Swanson, S., & Olfson, M. (2011). Service utilization for lifetime mental disorders in U.S. adolescents: Results of the National Comorbidity Survey-Adolescent Supplement (NCS-A). *Journal of the American Academy of Child and Adolescent Psychiatry, 50,* 32–45.

Millstein, S. G., & Halpern-Felsher, B. L. (2002). Perceptions of risk and vulnerability. *Journal of Adolescent Health, 31S,* 10–37.

Millstein, S. G., & Igra, V. (1996). Theoretical models of adolescent risk-behavior. In J. L. Wallander & L. J. Siegal (Eds.), *Adolescent health problems: Behavioral perspectives.* New York: Guilford Press.

Modell, J., & Goodman, M. (1990). Historical perspective. In S. S. Feldman & G. R. Elliot (Eds.), *At the threshold: The developing adolescent.* Cambridge, MA: Harvard University Press.

Moore, K., & Zaff, J. (2002). Building a better teenager: A summary of "what works" in adolescent development. Child trends research briefs publication (#2002-57). Washington, DC: Child Trends Retrieved October 13, 2011 from http://www.childtrends.org/Files//Child_Trends-2002_11_02_RB_BuildBetterTeens.pdf.

Mulye, T. P., Park, M. J., Nelson, C. D., Adams, S. H., Irwin, C. E., Jr., & Brindis, C. D. (2009). Trends in adolescent and young adult health in the United States. *Journal of Adolescent Health, 45(1),* 8–24.

Murphey, D. A., Lamonda, K. H., Carney, J. K., & Duncan, P. (2004). Relationships of a brief measure of youth assets to health-promoting and risk behaviors. *Journal of Adolescent Health, 34,* 184–191.

National Adolescent Health Information Center. (2003). Fact sheet on demographics: Adolescents. San Francisco: University of California, San Francisco. Retrieved October 13, 2011 from http://nahic.ucsf.edu/downloads/Demographics.pdf.

National Campaign to Prevent Teen and Unplanned Pregnancy. (2010). *Linking teen pregnancy to other critical social issues.* Washington, DC: Author. Retrieved April 25, 2011 from http://www.thenationalcampaign.org/why-it-matters/pdf/introduction.pdf.

National Center for Education Statistics. (2010). *The Nation's report card: Grade 12 reading and mathematics 2009 national and pilot state results* (NES 2011-455). Washington, DC: U.S. Department of Education, Institute of Education Sciences.

National Center for Injury Prevention and Control. (2011). WISQARS. Violence-related all injury causes nonfatal injuries and rates per 100,000 and unintentional all injury causes nonfatal injuries and rates per 100,000 [online database]. Retrieved January 30, 2011 from http://webappa.cdc.gov/sasweb/ncipc/nfirates2001.html.

National Committee for Injury Prevention and Control. (1989). Injury prevention: meeting the challenge. *American Journal of Preventive Medicine 5* (3 Suppl), 123–127.

National Conference of State Legislatures. (2010). Issues and options. Health, childhood obesity, 2009 update on policy options. Retrieved February 2, 2011 from http://www.ncsl.org/default.aspx?tabid = 19776.

National Research Council. (1993). *Losing generations.* Commission on Behavioral and Social Sciences and Education. Washington, DC: National Academy Press.

Newacheck, P. W., Hung, Y. Y., Park, M. J., Brindis, C. D., & Irwin, C. E. (2003). Disparities in adolescent health and health care: Does socio-economic status matter? *Health Services Research, 38,* 1235–1252.

Newacheck, P. W., Wong, S. T., Galbraith, A. A., & Hung, Y. Y. (2003). Adolescent health care expenditures: A descriptive profile. *Journal of Adolescent Health, 32S,* 3–11.

O'Connell, M. E., Boat, T., & Warner, K. E. (Eds.). (2009). *Preventing mental, emotional and behavioral disorders among young people: Progress and possibilities.* Committee on Adolescent Health Care Services and Models of Care for Treatment, Prevention, and Healthy Development, National Research Council and Institute of Medicine. Washington, DC: National Academies Press.

Offer, D., & Schonert-Reichl, K. A. (1992). Debunking the myths of adolescence: Findings from recent research. *Journal of the American Academy of Child and Adolescent Psychiatry, 31,* 1003–1014.

Ogden, C., & Carroll, M. (2010). *Prevalence of obesity among children and adolescents: United States, trends 1963–1965 through 2007–2008.* Hyattsville,

MD: U.S. Department of Health and Human Services, Centers for Disease Control and Prevention, National Center for Health Statistics. Retrieved October 12, 2011 from http://www.cdc.gov/nchs/data/hestat/obesity_child_07_08/obesity_child_07_08.htm.

Ozer, E. M., Park, M. J., Paul, T., Brindis, C. D., & Irwin, C. E. (2003). *America's adolescents: Are they healthy?* San Francisco: University of California, San Francisco, National Adolescent Health Information Center.

Park, M. J., MacDonald, T. M., Ozer, E. M., Burg, S. J., Millstein, S. G., Brindis, C. D., & Irwin, C. E. (2001). *Investing in clinical preventive services for adolescents.* San Francisco: University of California, San Francisco, Policy Information and Analysis Center for Middle Childhood and Adolescence & the National Adolescent Health Information Center.

Park, M., & Irwin, C. (2008). Youth with special health care needs: Facilitating a healthy transition to young adulthood. *Journal of Adolescent Health, 43,* 6–7.

Pittman, K. J., O'Brien, R., & Kimball, M. (1993). *Youth development and resiliency research: Making connections to substance abuse prevention.* Washington, DC: Academy for Educational Development.

Reddy, D. M., Fleming, R., & Swain, C. (2002). Effect of mandatory parental notification on adolescent girl's use of sexual health care services. *Journal of the American Medical Association, 288,* 710–714.

Remafedi, G. (1989). The healthy sexual development of gay and lesbian adolescents. *SIECUS Report, 17,* 7–8.

Remafedi, G., Resnick, M., Blum, R., & Harris, K. M. (1992). Demography of sexual orientation in adolescences. *Pediatrics, 89*(4, Pt. 2), 714–721.

Resnick, M. D., Bearman, P. S., Blum, R. W., Bauman, K. E., Harris, K. M., Jones, J., Tabor, J., Beuhring, T., Sieving, R. E., Shew, M., Ireland, M., Bearinger, L. H., & Udry, J. R. (1997). Protecting adolescents from harm: Findings from the National Longitudinal Study of Adolescent Health. *Journal of the American Medical Association, 278,* 823–832.

Richardson, J. L., Radziszewska, B., Dent, C. W., & Flay, B. R. (1993). Relationship between after-school care of adolescents and substance use, risk taking, depressed mood and academic achievement. *Pediatrics, 92,* 32–38.

Rideout, V. J., Foehr, U. G., & Roberts, D. F. (2010). *Generation M². Media in the lives of 8- to 18-year-olds.* Menlo Park, CA: Kaiser Family Foundation. Retrieved October 13, 2011 from http://www.kff.org/entmedia/upload/8010.pdf.

Ritchie, L., Crawford, P., Woodward-Lopez, G., Ivey, S., Masch, M., & Ikeda, J. (2001). Prevention of childhood overweight: What should be done? Berkeley, CA: Center for Weight and Health. University of California, Berkeley. Retrieved October 13, 2011 from http://cwh.berkeley.edu/sites/greeneventsguide.org.cwh/files/primary_pdfs/Prev_Child_Oweight_10-28-02.pdf.

Rosenbaum, J. E. (2009a). Patient teenagers? A comparison of the sexual behavior of virginity pledges and matched non-pledgers. *Pediatrics, 123*(1), e110–e120. Retrieved from http://www.pediatrics.org/cgi/doi/10.1542/peds.2008-0407.

Rosenbaum, J. E. (2009b). Truth or consequences: The intertemporal consistency of adolescent self-report on the Youth Risk Behavior Survey. *American Journal of Epidemiology, 169,* 1388–1397. Epub 2009 Apr 10.

Runyan, C. W. (2003). Introduction: Back to the future: Revisiting Haddon's conceptualization of injury epidemiology and prevention. *Epidemiologic Reviews, 25,* 60–64.

Runyan, C. W., & Gerken, E. A. (1991). Injuries. In W. R. Hendee (Ed.), *The health of adolescents.* San Francisco: Jossey-Bass.

Santelli, J., Ott, M., Lyon, M., Rogers, J., Summers, D., & Schleifer, R. (2006). Abstinence and abstinence only education policies and programs: A position paper of the Society of Adolescent Health. *Journal of Adolescent Health, 38,* 83–87.

Santelli, J., Sandfort, T., & Orr, M. (2008). Transnational comparisons of adolescent contraceptive use: What can we learn from these comparisons? *Archives of Pediatrics & Adolescent Medicine, 162,* 92–94.

Savin-Williams, R. C., & Ream, G. L. (2007). Prevalence and stability of sexual orientation components during adolescence and young adulthood. *Archives of Sexual Behavior, 36,* 385–394.

Sayer, A. G., Hauser, S. T., Jacobson, A. M., Willett, A. B., & Cole, C. F. (1995). Developmental influences on adolescent health. In J. L. Wallander & L. J. Siegel (Eds.), *Adolescent health problems: Behavioral perspectives.* New York: Guilford Press.

Scaramella, L. V., Neppi, T. K., Ortai, L. L., & Conger, R. D. (2008). Consequences of socioeconomic disadvantage across three generations: Parenting behavior and externalizing problems. *Journal of Family Psychology, 22,* 725–733.

Scott, M. A., Wilcox, H. C., Schonfeld, S., Davies, M., Hicks, R. C., Turner, J. B., & Shaffer, D. (2008). School-based screening to identify at-risk students not already known to school professionals: The Columbia Suicide Screen. *American Journal of Public Health, 99*(2), 1–6.

Seitz, V., & Apfel, N. H. (1999). Effective interventions for adolescent mothers. *Clinical Psychology: Science and Practice, 6,* 50–66.

Shakespeare, W. (1925). A winter's tale (Act III, Scene iii). In *Complete Works.* New York: P.F. Collier and Son Company.

Sickmund, M. (2010). *Juveniles in residential placement, 1997–2008.* OJJDP Fact Sheet Washington, DC: U.S. Department of Justice, Office of Juvenile Justice and Delinquency Preventions. Retrieved October 13, 2011 from http://www.ncjrs.gov/pdffiles1/ojjdp/229379.pdf.

Simons-Morton, B., Ouimet, M., & Catalano, R. (2008). Parenting and the young driver problem. *American Journal of Preventive Medicine, 35*(3, Suppl.), S294–S303.

Smetana, J. G. (1989). Adolescents' and parents' reasoning about actual family conflict. *Child Development, 60,* 1052–1067.

Smetana, J. G. (1995). Parenting styles and conceptions of parental authority during adolescence. *Child Development, 66,* 299–316.

Steinberg, L. (2000). The family at adolescence: Transition and transformation. *Journal of Adolescent Health, 27,* 170–179.

Steinberg, L., Blatt-Eisengart, I., & Cauffman, E. (2006). Patterns of competence and adjustment among adolescents from authoritative, authoritarian, indulgent, and neglectful homes: A replication a sample of serious juvenile offenders. *Journal of Research on Adolescence, 16,* 47–58.

Steinberg, L., Mounts, N. S., Lamborn, S. D., & Dornbusch, S. M. (1991). Authoritative parenting and adolescent adjustment across varied ecological niches. *Journal of Research on Adolescence, 1,* 19–36.

Strasburger, V. C. (2004). Children, adolescents, and the media. *Current Problems Pediatric Adolescent Health Care, 34,* 54–113.

Sum, A. M., & Fogg, W. N. (1991). The adolescent poor and the transition to early adulthood. In P. Edelman & J. Ladner (Eds.), *Adolescence and poverty: Challenge for the 1990s.* Washington, DC: Center for National Policy Press.

Teipel, K. D., & Brindis, C. D. (2010). *Improving the Health of Youth—A Guide for State-Level Strategic Planning and Action.* San Francisco: State Adolescent Health Resource Center, University of Minnesota and National Adolescent Health Information and Innovation Center, University of California.

Toro, P. A., Dworsky, A., & Fowler, P. J. (2007). Homeless youth in the United States: Recent research findings and intervention approaches. In D. Dennis, G. Locke, & J. Khadduri (Eds.), *Toward Understanding Homelessness: The 2007 National Symposium on Homelessness Research.* Retrieved October 13, 2011 from http://aspe.hhs.gov/hsp/homelessness/symposium07/toro/index.htm.

Turley, R. (2004). Are children of young mothers disadvantaged because of their mother's age or family background? *Child Development, 75,* 464–475.

U.S. Congress, Office of Technology Assessment. (1991a). *Adolescent health: Vol. I: Summary and policy options* (OTA-H-468). Washington, DC: U.S. Government Printing Office.

U.S. Congress, Office of Technology Assessment. (1991b). *Adolescent health: Vol. II: Background and the effectiveness of selected prevention and treatment services* (OTA-H-468). Washington, DC: U.S. Government Printing Office.

U.S. Congress, Office of Technology Assessment. (1991c). *Adolescent health: Vol. III: Crosscutting issues in the delivery of health and related services* (OTA-H-468). Washington, DC: U.S. Government Printing Office.

U.S. Department of Health and Human Services, Administration for Children and Families. (2010a). AFCARS report. Retrieved May 8, 2011 from http://www.acf.hhs.gov/programs/cb/stats_research/afcars/tar/report17.htm.

U.S. Department of Health and Human Services. (2010b). Healthy People 2020. Topics and objectives, Adolescent health. Retrieved January 31, 2011 from http://www.healthypeople.gov/2020/topicsobjectives2020/objectiveslist.aspx?topicid = 2. http://healthypeople.gov/2020/topicsobjectives2020/overview.aspx?topicId = 2.

U.S. Public Health Service. (1999). *The Surgeon General's call to action to prevent suicide.* Washington, DC: Author.

Vandivere, S., Gallagher, M., & Moore, K. A. (2004). *Changes in children's well-being and family environments. Snapshots of America's families III.* Washington, DC: The Urban Institute. Retrieved October 13,

2011 from http://www.urban.org/publications/310912.html.

Vanlaar, W., Mayhew, D., Marcoux, K., Wets, G., Brijs, T., & Shope, J. (2009). An evaluation of graduated driver licensing programs in North America using a meta-analytic approach. *Accident Analysis Prevention, 41*, 1104–1111. Epub 2009 Jul 15.

Villani, S. (2001). Impact of media on children and adolescents: A 10-year review of the research. *Journal of the American Academy of Child Adolescent Psychiatry, 40*, 392–401.

Wandersman, A., & Florin, P. (2003). Community interventions and effective prevention. *American Psychologist, 58*, 441–448.

Werner, E. E. (1992). The children of Kauai: Resiliency and recovery in adolescence and adulthood. *Journal of Adolescent Health, 22*, 262–268.

Whitaker, A. H. (1992). An epidemiological study of anorectic and bulimia symptoms in adolescent girls: Implications for pediatricians. *Pediatric Annals, 21*, 752–759.

Williams, S. B., O'Connor, E., Eder, M., & Whitlock, E. (2009). Screening for child and adolescent depression in primary care settings: A systematic evidence review for the U.S. Preventive Services Task Force. *Pediatrics, 123*, 4, e716–e735.

William T. Grant Foundation, Commission on Work, Family, and Citizenship. (1988). *The forgotten half: Pathways to success for America's youth and young families*. Washington, DC: Author.

Zabin, L. S., & Hayward, S. C. (1993). *Adolescent sexual behavior and childbearing*. Newbury Park, CA: Sage Publications.

CROSS-CUTTING ISSUES

10

DISPARITIES IN MATERNAL AND CHILD HEALTH IN THE UNITED STATES

Diane L. Rowley, Theresa Chapple-McGruder, Dara D. Mendez, and Dorothy Browne

The demographic changes that are anticipated over the next decade magnify the importance of addressing disparities in health status. Groups currently experiencing poorer health status are expected to grow as a proportion of the total U.S. population; therefore, the future health of America as a whole will be influenced substantially by our success in improving the health status of our racial and ethnic minorities.

(Former Surgeon General David Satcher)

INTRODUCTION

Among the *Healthy People 2020* goals for the United States is the goal of achieving health equity, eliminating health disparities, and improving the health of all groups (U.S. Department of Health and Human Services, n.d.-a). *Healthy People 2020* defines *health equity* as the "attainment of the highest level of health for all people. Achieving health equity requires valuing everyone equally with focused and ongoing societal efforts to address avoidable inequalities, historical and contemporary injustices, and the elimination of health and health care disparities"; and a *health disparity* as "a particular type of health difference that is closely linked with social, economic, and/or environmental disadvantage. Health disparities adversely affect groups of people who have systematically experienced greater obstacles to health based on their racial or ethnic group; religion; socioeconomic status; gender; age; mental health; cognitive, sensory, or physical disability; sexual orientation or gender identity; geographic location; or other characteristics historically linked to discrimination or exclusion" (U.S. Department of Health and Human Services, n.d.-a). For 3 decades, *Healthy People* has provided science-based, 10-year national objectives for improving the health of all Americans. During the past 2 decades, one of *Healthy People's* overarching goals has focused on disparities. In *Healthy People 2000*, it was to reduce health disparities among racial/ethnic Americans (Stoto, Behrens, & Rosemont, 1990). In *Healthy People 2010*, it was to eliminate, not just reduce, health disparities (U.S. Department of Health and Human Services, n.d.-b). In *Healthy People 2020*, that goal was expanded even further (U.S. Department of Health and Human Services, n.d.-c).

National concern about health disparities took hold in the early 1980s as a result of a 1980 British national report on inequalities in health that documented disparities in the United Kingdom by residential area, social class, and ethnic group (Department of Health and Social Security, 1980) and a U.S. surveillance report, *Health 1983, United States* (National Center for Health Statistics [NCHS], 1983) that first documented disparities across several health outcomes. In response, the U.S. Department of Health and Human Services (USDHHS) Secretary Margaret Heckler commissioned the Minority Health Task Force in 1984, which resulted in the 1985 groundbreaking report of *Report of The Secretary's Task Force on Black and Minority Health* (USDHHS, 1985). This task force introduced the concept of *excess deaths* to denote the difference between the actual number of deaths in a subgroup and the number of deaths that would have occurred if the mortality rate of that group were the same as that for the white population. For ethnic subpopulations compared with the white majority, the task force calculated excess deaths for those younger than 70 years to be 42.3% among blacks, 14% for the Spanish surnamed, 2% among Cuban-born persons, 7.2% for those Mexican born, and 25% for Native Americans. The rate of excess deaths was particularly high, 43%, for Native Americans who were younger than 45 years. There were no excess deaths for the Asian/Pacific Islander population, suggesting that this group possesses a healthier mortality profile than all other racial or ethnic subgroups. However, the aggregation of data to obtain these larger ethnic population groups masks the heterogeneity within this grouping. That is, when the data for the Asian ethnic population are disaggregated into its component ethnic/nationality groupings, the within-group excess morbidity and mortality, masked by aggregation, becomes apparent.

The Secretary's Task Force report stimulated the establishment of the Office of Minority Health, whose stated purpose was to influence policy, promote data collection, develop strategic communications, and conduct service demonstrations and policy assessments for the improvement of minority health. National legislation now supports health disparity elimination. The Minority Health and Health Disparities Research and Education Act of 2000 authorized research, training, measurement of disparities, and dissemination of information on minority health conditions and other populations with health disparities (Minority, 2000). The Patient Protection and Affordable Care Act of 2010 improves data collection on race, ethnicity, gender, geographic location, socioeconomic status, language, and disability status to detect and monitor trends in health disparities (Patient, 2010).

In this chapter, we present changing demographics, discuss their implications for the health of the nation, and identify disparities in key maternal and child health (MCH) indicators across ethnic and racial subpopulations. When possible, we include information on other groups of people who have experienced social, economic, or environmental disadvantage that has affected their health. Although it is important to document existing disparities, it is also critical to understand the *causes* of disparities in order to move toward addressing and ultimately achieving health equity. As such, we provide an overview of emerging conceptual frameworks for understanding and eliminating health disparities. The chapter concludes with recommendations for policy, programs, research, and training and for educating MCH professionals in an effort to increase knowledge of and improve the ability to effectively reduce and ultimately eliminate disparities.

DEMOGRAPHIC CHANGES

The classification of the race and ethnic composition of the United States is based on federal reporting requirements. The number of specific racial groups required for reporting census data and other federal reports changes over time. Since the 2000 census a minimum of five racial groups are reported: American Indian/Alaska Native, Asian, Hawaiian or other Pacific Islander, Black/African American, and White. Ethnicity is a separate concept from race; currently, Hispanic origin is the only ethnic category. The census collects additional information on diversity of backgrounds among Asian and Hispanic groups and allows individuals to write in a more specific group. Individuals can select more than one racial group to indicate what the person considers herself/himself to be (Shrestha & Heisler, 2011).

The United States is becoming more ethnically and racially diverse. According to population projections, children of color will comprise 62% of all children. Between 2000 and 2050 the Asian population is expected to more than double and the Hispanic population is projected to increase from 12.6% in 2000 to 30.2% of the total population. (Shrestha & Heisler, 2011) The importance of health disparities will grow as the racial and ethnic groups that experience higher rates of poor health outcomes become a greater proportion of the population.

Race and ethnicity are both complex social constructs created to distinguish groups socially but not biologically (Ver Ploeg & Perrin, 2004). Race is based on observable phenotypic characteristics such as skin color and facial characteristics, but also is defined by common political and social history and a sense of "peoplehood" (Hatch, et al., 1993). Ethnicity is also a social construct that describes unique social characteristics of a group (culture, diet, art) or a group's social location in a diverse society (Ford & Harawa, 2010). Racial and ethnic categorizations sometimes represent overlapping concepts. For example, someone may identify as a member of different racial or ethnic groups, or as multiracial in different settings. Despite this fluidity, racial/ethnic classification is valuable because it predicts differences in quality of health care, in environmental exposures, and in health outcomes, as well as exposure to discrimination, racism, and economic deprivation (Jones, 2001; Mays, et al., 2003; Ver Ploeg & Perrin, 2004).

HEALTH STATUS OF RACIAL/ETHNIC GROUPS

Infant Health

In 2005, the United States had an infant mortality rate (IMR) of 6.86 per 1,000 live births. When compared to other developed nations, the United States ranked 29th and was tied with Poland and Slovakia (MacDorman & Mathews, 2008). Although the United States has experienced marked declines in infant mortality over the past century due to advances in sanitation, public health, and medical knowledge and technologies, the change in infant mortality from 2000 to 2007 has been marginal. The infant mortality rate was 9% lower in 2000 (6.89) than in 1995 (7.57), but the rate has declined only 2% since 2000 (MacDorman & Mathews, 2011). In 1900, the IMR was approximately 100 deaths per 1,000 live births; in 2000 it was 6.89 per 1,000 live births, and in 2008 the rate was 6.3 deaths per 1,000 live births (MacDorman & Mathews, 2011). The stagnant nature of the IMR has led the United States to be surpassed by countries such as Cuba and Hungary, with Singapore having the world's lowest IMR at 2.31 per 1,000 (United Nations, 2011).

Although the majority of infants born in this country experience healthy birth outcomes, there are segments of the country that bear a disproportional burden of adverse birth outcomes. In the United States, health disparities are based on geography, socioeconomic status, and race/ethnicity and nativity. **Figure 10-1** displays the distribution of infant mortality by state. As can be seen, the highest infant mortality rates cluster in the southern and midwestern parts of the United States, with the lowest rates in west coast states and in the northeastern part of the country (Kaiser Family Foundation, 2011).

Maternal/familial socioeconomic status has an impact on birth outcomes. Based on national data, an inverse relationship is seen such that as educational attainment increases, there is generally a decrease in the infant mortality rate. This is thought to be due

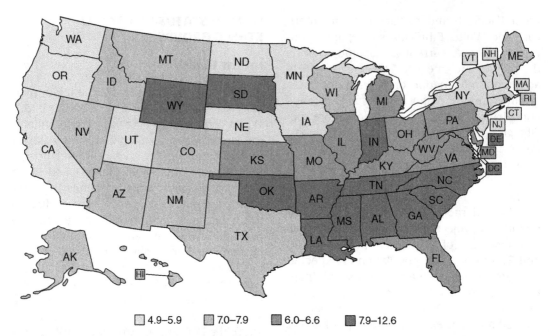

Figure 10–1 Infant mortality rate per 1,000 live births, linked files, 2004–2006.
Source: Courtesy of The Kaiser Family Foundation, statehealthfacts.org. Data Source: Matthews, TJ, M.S., et. al. Infant Mortality Statistics from the 2007 Period Linked Birth/Infant Death Data Set. Division of Vital Statistics. National Vital Statistics Report, Vol 59, No. 6, June 29, 2011. Available at http://www .statehealthfacts.org/comparemapdetail.jsp?ind = 47&cat = 2&sub = 13&yr = 89&typ = 3&sort = a. Accessed September 27th, 2012.

to the interrelationships between educational attainment, income, and financial resources (Mathews & MacDorman, 2010). However, this trend may not be observed when stratified by race/ethnicity. Educational attainment does not provide the same level of protection against adverse birth outcomes for non-Hispanic black women as it does for non-Hispanic white women (Schoendorf, 1992).

Infant mortality also varies by race/ethnicity in the United States, as indicated by the rates reported by the National Center for Health Statistics (2007) linked infant death and birth files (presented in **Table 10–1**). The linked file consists of all infant deaths occurring in 2007 that have been linked to their corresponding birth certificates, whether the birth occurred in 2006 or 2007 and is useful for computing accurate infant mortality rates by race/ethnicity. According to the most recent statistics, Hispanic infants of Central and South American descent have the lowest IMR of 4.57, whereas non-Hispanic black

infants have an IMR of 13.31 (Mathews & MacDorman, 2010). In addition, infants born to American Indian/Alaska Natives (9.22) and Puerto Rican (7.71) mothers have IMRs above the national average. For some groups infant mortality varies by maternal nativity. For non-Hispanic white, non-Hispanic black, Asian or Pacific Islander, and Mexican mothers born in the United States, infant mortality rates are higher than rates for mothers born outside the United States.

The Hispanic Paradox

The Hispanic paradox is the term used to describe lower mortality than the national average for Hispanics, despite economic disadvantages, reduced access to care, and exposure to discrimination (James, 1993). The paradox is evident among women of Mexican, Cuban, and Central American origin, but not Puerto Rican women. Explanations for the paradox include migration to the United States of women who are healthier; cultural

Table 10–1 Infant, Neonatal, and Postneonatal Mortality Rates per 1,000 Live Births and Percent Change 2000–2007 by Race and Hispanic Origin of Mother: United States, 2007 Linked File

Hispanic Origin and Race of Mother	Live Births	Infant Mortality Rate	Neonatal Mortality Rate	Postneonatal Mortality Rate	Percent Change 2000–2007
All races	4,316,233	6.75	4.42	2.33	−2.0*
American Indian or Alaska Native	49,443	9.22	4.55	4.67	11.1
Asian or Pacific Islander	254,488	4.78	3.38	1.40	−1.8
Hispanic	1,062,779	5.51	3.72	1.79	−1.4
Mexican	722,055	5.42	3.68	1.75	−0.2
Puerto Rican	68,488	7.71	5.14	2.57	−6.1
Cuban	16,981	5.18	3.65	1.53	14.1
Central and South American	169,851	4.57	3.14	1.43	−1.5
Non-Hispanic White	2,310,333	5.63	3.61	2.02	−1.2
Non-Hispanic Black	627,191	13.31	8.74	4.57	−2.1

*Significant at p < 0.05

Source: National Vital Statistics Reports, 59(6), June 29, 2011.

protective factors such as cultural support for maternity; healthy behaviors; and strong social support networks for informal prenatal care by family, friends and neighbors (Acevedo-Garcia, Soobader, & Berkman, 2007; McGlade, Saha, & Dahlstrom, 2004). The apparent advantage in birth outcome appears to diminish among infants of Mexican American women born in the United States (Acevedo-Garcia, Soobader, & Berkman, 2007).

Leading Causes of Infant Death

More than two-thirds of infant deaths in the United States occur during the neonatal period (the first 28 days of life) (Mathews & MacDorman, 2010). The U.S. neonatal mortality rate was 4.42 per 1,000 live births in 2007. However, non-Hispanic black infants were more than twice (8.74) as likely to die during the neonatal period than non-Hispanic white infants (3.61). The majority of these deaths are due to complications from preterm birth or short gestation (Mathews & MacDorman, 2010). The deaths that occur during the postneonatal period (29 to 365 days of life)

are typically due to sudden infant death syndrome or unintentional injuries. Once again, non-Hispanic black infants are more than twice as likely to die during the postneonatal period when compared to non-Hispanic whites (4.57 vs 2.02 per 1,000). Hispanics have the lowest rate of postneonatal death (1.67 per 1,000).

In 2006, the five leading causes of infant mortality accounted for 56% of all infant deaths (Mathews & MacDorman, 2010). The most common cause of infant death in 2006 was congenital malformations, deformations, and chromosomal abnormalities, which explained 21% of all infant deaths. The first four leading causes of death from 2005 to 2006 remained stable; however, death related to complications of the placenta, cord, and membranes moved from the fifth to the sixth cause of death. Although congenital malformations are the leading cause of infant death for most racial and ethnic subgroups, disorders related to short gestation and low birthweight is the leading cause for non-Hispanic blacks and Puerto Ricans (Mathews & MacDorman, 2010). See **Table 10–2.**

Table 10–2 Infant Deaths and Mortality Rates for the Five Leading Causes of Infant Death by Race and Hispanic Origin of Mother: United States, 2006 Linked File

Hispanic origin and race of mother	Causes of death (based on the International Classification of Diseases, Tenth Revision, 1992)					
	Congenital malformations, deformations, and chromosomal abnormalities (Q00–Q99)		Disorders related to short gestation and low birth weight, not elsewhere classified (P07)		Sudden infant death syndrome (R95)	
	Rank	Rate	Rank	Rate	Rank	Rate
All races	1	137.1	2	113.5	3	54.6
American Indian or Alaska Native	1	153.0	3	98.5	2	119.4
Asian or Pacific Islander	1	109.1	2	76.3	4	22.8
Hispanic	1	142.0	2	85.4	4	27.1
Mexican	1	151.4	2	81.6	4	25.5
Puerto Rican	2	122.5	1	165.8	3	55.3
Central and South American	1	117.3	2	69.6	5	15.1
Non-Hispanic White	1	126.6	2	76.8	3	55.6
Non-Hispanic Black	2	174.6	1	301.8	3	103.8

Hispanic origin and Race of mother	Newborn affected by maternal complications of pregnancy (P01)		Accidents unintentional injuries (V01-X59)		All causes	
	Rank	Rate	Rank	Rate	Rank	Rate
All races	4	39.3	5	26.8	—	668.3
American Indian or Alaska Native	6	*	4	77.5	—	827.7
Asian or Pacific Islander	3	23.6	6	12.9	—	455.1
Hispanic	3	27.9	8	14.8	—	541.1
Mexican	3	28.3	7	13.8	—	534.3
Puerto Rican	3	55.3	6	*	—	800.8
Central and South American	5	15.1	9	*	—	452.5
Non-Hispanic White	4	31.7	5	25.9	—	558.1
Non-Hispanic Black	4	89.4	6	52.8	—	1335.1

*Data excluded because it did not meet standards of reliability or precision; based on fewer than 20 deaths in the numerator

Source: Mathews, T.J., & MacDorman, M.F. (2010). Infant mortality statistics from the period linked birth/infant death data set. National vital statistics reports; vol 58 no 17. Hyattsville, MD: National Center for Health Statistics.

The ICD classification of leading causes of infant death does not capture the overwhelming contribution of prematurity (born < 37 completed weeks of gestation) to the disparity in infant mortality. If all deaths attributable to the consequences of prematurity, i.e., maternal complications; complications of placenta, cord, and membranes; respiratory distress of newborn and other respiratory diseases from the perinatal period; sepsis; intraventricular hemorrhage; and necrotizing enterocolitis—are considered, preterm related deaths account for 32% of all infant deaths, rather than 17%. Using this more analytic approach to classify cause of death, preterm related mortality among non-Hispanic black infants is higher than the total combined infant mortality rate for non-Hispanic white, Mexican, Central and South American, and Asian/Pacific Island infants; for infants born to Puerto Rican mothers it is 75% higher than non-Hispanic white infants (Callahan, et al., 2006; Mathews & MacDorman, 2010).

Childhood and Adolescence

Nationally there has been a decrease in certain health conditions unique to children and a rise in others. For instance, the percentage of children with elevated blood lead levels over 10 micrograms per deciliter is too small to provide statistically reliable estimates (Federal Interagency Forum, 2010). Adolescent smoking rates (CDC, 2010), pregnancy rates (Ventura, et al., 2011), and percentage of children with dental caries (tooth decay) continue to decrease (NCHS, 2009). However, there are increases in obesity in children (Freedman, 2011) and in children suffering from diseases that were previously associated with adults such as type 2 diabetes (CDC, 2011a). Not surprisingly, the rate of decrease or increase among these disease conditions and health behaviors differs based on race/ethnicity.

When examining health behaviors such as alcohol use, smoking, obesity, adolescent

pregnancy, and youth violence, the national picture may mask the experiences of certain segments of the population. Among all age groups in the United States, excessive use of alcohol is ranked as the third preventable cause of death (Kanny, Liu, & Brewer, 2011). Although consuming alcohol is illegal for people under the age of 21, the 2009 Youth Risk Behavior Survey found that nearly 42% of high school students had an alcoholic drink on at least one occasion in the 30 days before the survey (CDC, 2010). Non-Hispanic white teens reported the highest incidence of alcohol use (44.7%), followed by multiple-race (44.3%), Hispanic (42.9), Native American (42.8%), non-Hispanic black (33.4%), and Asian youth (18.3%).

It is estimated that 3,900 people between the ages of 12 and 17 will try their first cigarette today, with 1,000 of them becoming addicted and turning into daily smokers (Garrett, 2011). Cigarette smoking is the leading cause of preventable death in the United States. An overwhelming majority of adults currently addicted to smoking began smoking as adolescents (CDC website). Adolescent smoking rates have been on the decline (Johnston, et al., 2011); however, American Indian and Alaskan Native teens report the highest prevalence of smoking at 16.7%, followed by non-Hispanic white teens (11.3%), Hispanic teens (8.2%), non-Hispanic black teens (8.2%). Asian teens (5.2%) reported smoking three times less than American Indian teens (Garrett, 2011).

In 2005, there were approximately 740,000 pregnancies to adolescent girls in the United States. Roughly 57% of the pregnancies ended in live births, 27% ended by induced abortions, and 16% ended in fetal death (Ventura, et al., 2011). From 1990 to 2005 pregnancy rates of 15- to 19-year-old women declined for all race/ethnic groups, but disparities remained. The pregnancy rate declined 50% (from 86.6 per 1,000 women 15 to 19 to 43.3) among non-Hispanic white teenagers, 26% (from 169.7 per 1,000 to 124.9) among Hispanic teenagers (of any race), and 45% (from 223.8 per 1,000 to 122.7) among black women (Guttmacher Institute, 2010). Pregnancies among non-Hispanic whites and Hispanic adolescents were less likely to end in an induced abortion and more likely to end in a live birth when compared to pregnancies to non-Hispanic black adolescents (Ventura, et al., 2011).

The adolescent birth rate for teens 15 to 19 continuously declined every year from 1991 to 2005, with a cumulative decrease of 33%. This long-term decline was ended in 2006 and 2007 (Ventura, et al., 2011), but resumed in 2008 (Pazol, et al., 2011). During the period of decline, decreasing rates of adolescent pregnancy were seen for all racial groups and people of Hispanic origin in the United States. Rates decreased between 30% and 59%, with the highest declines among non-Hispanic blacks and American Indian and Alaskan Native population. However, birth rates for black teens and Hispanic teens were 2.3 and 2.7 times higher than non-Hispanic white teens, respectively. In 2008 birth rates for Black, Hispanic, and American Indian/Alaska Native teens aged 15 to 17 were 34.9., 46.1, and 32.5 births per 1,000 women aged 15 to 17, respectively, compared with 11.6 for white teens (Ventura, et al., 2011). Birth rates differ within Hispanic groups, with adolescent mothers of Mexican origin having a rate of 88.7 per 1,000, and adolescent mothers of Puerto Rican origin having a rate of 67.1 births per 1,000 during 2007.

Dental caries have declined significantly among school-age children since 1970, but remain the most common chronic disease in children (Dye, et al., 2007). Disparities exist in the prevalence of untreated tooth decay and use of dental sealants to prevent caries. The percentage of teens 12 to 19 years old with untreated tooth decay is 26% for black teens, 28% for Mexican American teens and 16% for white teens (Dye, et al., 2007). The percentage of teens with dental sealants is substantially lower for black and Mexican American teens, compared to white teens, 8% vs. 22% (Dye, 2007). Use of dental services

varies by race/ethnicity with one-third of black and Hispanic teens obtaining dental care in a year compared to half of white teens (Edelstein & Chinn, 2009).

Childhood obesity is defined as having a body mass index (BMI) ≥ 95th percentile of the Centers for Disease Control and Prevention (CDC) growth chart (Freedman, 2011). Childhood obesity is age specific from ages 2 to 19. The prevalence has increased over the last 30 years. Between 1976 and 1980 the prevalence of childhood obesity was 5%; in 2007 to 2008 17% of children were obese (Freedman, 2011). Obesity rates vary by sex and race/ethnicity. Overall, about one in five non-Hispanic black youth are obese (21%). National data from 2005 to 2008 indicate that non-Hispanic black females ages 2 to 19 have the highest prevalence of obesity (24%) when compared with other adolescent females, followed by 21% of Mexican American females. Non-Hispanic black females aged 12 to 19 have the highest prevalence of obesity among all races, sexes, and age groups (31%) (Freedman, 2011). Among males, a different pattern is observed such that Mexican American males were the most likely to be obese (25%), when compared with non-Hispanic black and non-Hispanic white males (18% and 15%, respectively). For every age subgroup, Mexican American males had the highest BMI when compared to non-Hispanic black and non-Hispanic white males (Freedman, 2011).

Then increased prevalence of type 2 diabetes mellitus (DM), formerly known as adult-onset diabetes, among U.S. children and adolescents is associated with the increase in of obesity. CDC estimates that about 3,700 youth are diagnosed with type 2 diabetes each year. The incidence of type 2 DM is the highest among American Indians (25.3 and 49.4 for ages 10 to 14 and 15 to 19 years, respectively), followed by African Americans (22.3 and 19.4), Asian/Pacific Islanders (11.8 and 22.7) and Hispanics (8.9 and 17.0), and is lowest (3.0 and 5.6) among non-Hispanic whites (CDC, 2011a).

Leading Causes of Child and Adolescent Mortality

In 2008, 70,651 people under the age of 25 died, with the majority of these deaths being children under the age of 1 (40%) or youth from 15 to 24 years of age (46%). Unintentional injuries were the leading cause of death, with motor vehicle injury accounting for more than half of all unintentional injury deaths for all children and youth under the age of 25. Non-Hispanic black youth (under 25 years) made up 12% of the population, but accounted for 25% of the deaths in this age group. Hispanic, American Indian/Alaskan Native, and Asian/Pacific Islander children also bore a greater burden of childhood death when compared to non-Hispanic white children (Heron, 2010).

In 2006, a total of 4,631 children between the ages of 1 and 4 died in the United States, at a rate of 28.4 per 100,000 live births. Nearly one-third (35%) of these children died from unintentional injury. Among children ages 1 to 4, the second to fifth leading causes of death included congenital malformations, (11%), malignant neoplasm (8.1%), homicide (7.9%), and heart disease (3.5%) (Heron, 2010). These leading causes of death vary by race and ethnicity. For instance, whereas unintentional injuries and congenital malformations are the first and second leading cause of death among non-Hispanic white, Hispanic, and Asian or Pacific Islander children age 1 to 4, unintentional injuries and homicide were the first and second leading causes of death among African-American children and American Indian or Alaska Native in this age group. In fact, non-Hispanic black children ages 1 to 4 were 4.8 times more likely to die from homicide than children in other racial/ethnic groups. Rates for American Indian or Alaska Native children did not meet the standard for reliability (Heron, 2010).

In 2006, there were 6,149 deaths of children aged 5 to 14, a mortality rate of 14.1 per 100,000 live births, with the top five causes of death accounting for 97% of deaths. As with the younger age group, the top cause of death was unintentional injury (33%). The remaining top causes of death were the same as that of the younger age group, although in the following order: malignant neoplasm, congenital malformations, homicides, and disease of the heart (Heron, 2010). When examining causes of death by race/ethnicity, this overall pattern was observed only for Hispanic children. For non-Hispanic whites, deaths by homicide fell to number six and suicide replaced it as number three. For non-Hispanic blacks, lower respiratory illness replaced heart disease as the fifth leading cause of death (Heron, 2010).

Of the five leading causes of death for people 15 to 24, the first three causes account for 87% of the total deaths, and all are preventable: unintentional injuries, mainly car crashes, homicide, and suicide. The fourth and fifth leading causes of death for youth aged 15 to 24 are malignant neoplasms and diseases of the heart respectively (Heron, 2010).

The five leading causes of death hold for all racial groups and youth of Hispanic origin aged 15 to 24; however, the order differs for non-Hispanic whites and blacks. The second leading cause of death for non-Hispanic whites in this age group is suicide, followed by malignant neoplasms and then homicides. For non-Hispanic blacks, the leading cause of death among youth 15 to 24 is homicide, followed by unintentional injuries (Heron, 2010).

Youth Violence

Youth are known to be both victims and perpetrators of violence. In 1993, the rate at which youth were victims of violence was at an all-time high of 44 per 1,000 persons ages 12 to 17. The all-time low was experienced in 2005 with a youth victimization rate of 11 per 1000. Victimization rates are similar for black and white youth ages 12 to 17 and are lower for Hispanic youth. From 1993 to 2003 black teens were 5 times more likely than whites to be a victim of a homicide (5 per

100,000 versus 1 per 100,000) and 7 times more likely to be the offender as white teens (14 versus 2 per 100,000) (Baum, 2005). The rate in 2008 increased to 12 per 1,000, with a 4% increase in youth murder victims (Puzzanchera, 2009). Of all the murder victims in 2008, 11% were children under the age of 18, translating to 1,740 children murdered. Of the children murdered in 2008, about 40% were black(U.S. Census, 2012).

Black youth are overrepresented in crime arrest, accounting for about 16% of the population aged 10 to 17, but arrested for 52% of violent crimes committed by youth, and 33% of property crimes commited by youth. Although white youth made up 78% of people aged 10 to 17, they accounted for only 47% of arrests in that age group. Hispanic youth are included in the white youth category. The arrest rate for robbery in 2008 was 10 times higher for black youth compared to white youth. Although the racial disparity in youth violent crimes has decreased from its high in the 1980s from black youth being arrested seven times more than whites, to a low from 1999 to 2004 of four times more, the disparity is beginning to widen again with black youth five times more likely to be arrested for a violent crime as compared to white youth (Puzzanchera, 2009).

HEALTH OF WOMEN IN THEIR REPRODUCTIVE YEARS

Pregnancy Mortality and Morbidity

Disparities are present for both pregnancy-related deaths and pregnancy complications. African American women are up to four times more likely to die of pregnancy-related causes than white women (Berg, et al., 2010). This fourfold increased risk for maternal death among African American women as compared to white women is one of the largest racial disparities among major public health indicators. Limited information is available for pregnancy-related morality among

other ethnic minority groups. Between 1991 and 1997, mortality risk among Hispanics, Asians/Pacific Islanders, and American Indians/Alaska Natives was lower than for blacks but higher than for whites; relative ratios ranged from 1.4 to 1.7. Pregnancy-related mortality was approximately 50% higher for Latina women born outside the United States compared to U.S.-born Latina women. Among Asian/Pacific Islander women born outside the United States, pregnancy-related mortality was 100% higher compared to U.S.-born Asian/Pacific Islander women (Division of Reproductive Health, 2001).

Risk factors for pregnancy-related deaths are older maternal age, lower educational attainment, high parity, and no prenatal care. All women 35 years and older have a higher risk of death than those younger than 35; however, mortality for African American women increases sharply with age, beginning with women aged 25 to 29 years. For women who are pregnant at age 35 or greater, African American women are at least five times more likely to die than white women (Callaghan & Berg, 2003). At all levels of education, the pregnancy-related mortality among African American women is three to four times that of their white counterparts. The same is true regarding the trimester in which women initiate prenatal care, and the pattern is similar regardless of the number of births a woman has had.

African American women are 40–60% more likely to be hospitalized for a pregnancy complication and once hospitalized have a longer length of stay compared to white women (Franks, 1992). Yet, African American women are 400% more likely to die of a pregnancy complication. Differences in quality of care and comorbidities may explain disparities in pregnancy-related morbidity. African American women are less likely than white women to receive surgical intervention for hemorrhage of similar severity. Pregnant African American and Latina women have higher rates of diabetes and obesity, which puts them at higher risk for preeclampsia (Tanaka, et al., 2007).

Reproductive Cancers

Breast cancer and cervical cancer are the two most common reproductive-related cancers among women in the United States. Approximately 25% of breast cancers and 40% of cervical cancer occur in reproductive age women (Camp-Sorrell, 2009). Racial differences exist in the incidence, mortality, and survival rates for these cancers. Only 5–7 % of all breast cancer occurs in women younger than 40 years of age, and although white women have a higher incidence rate of breast cancer than black women after age 40, the reverse is true among younger women, with the highest increased risk among black women younger than 30. Hispanic, Asian, and Pacific Islander women tend to have lower incidence rates of breast cancer than white women (Brinton, et al., 2008). Health disparities result from the combination of the more frequent occurrence of estrogen receptor-negative breast cancers in premenopausal black women and the lack of directed interventions against these subtypes (Agurs-Collins, et al., 2010).

Cervical cancer is usually slow growing and can be detected with a Pap smear. Pap smear use is lower among Latina women ages 18 to 44 (78% compared to 84% for non-Hispanic white and black women) (CDC). Cervical cancer is almost always caused by human papillomaviruses. Between 1992 and 2002, prior to the availability of prophylactic human papillomavirus vaccines, the average annual incidence rate of cervical cancer was highest among Hispanics (14.8, 95% CI 14.5–15.1), followed by African-American women (13.5, 95% CI 13.2–13.7). Rates among Asian or Pacific Islander (8.9, 95% CI 8.5–9.3) and white women (8.9, 95% CI 8.8–9.0) were similar (Saraiya, et al., 2007). Latina women 25 to 49 years of age continue to have higher rates of invasive cervical cancer than Write women. Moreover, 5-year relative survival rates for local and regional stages are lower for blacks than for whites (Lawson, Henson, Bobo, & Kaeser, 2000).

HIV Disease

The Human Immunodeficiency Virus (HIV) infection epidemic has become concentrated among racial/ethnic minority populations. Although black and Hispanic women constitute 24% of all U.S. women, among women aged 13 to 44, black women account for 67% of HIV infections and Latina women account for 17%. From 2003 to 2008, surveillance data from 37 states showed that, among adult and adolescent females, the rate (diagnoses of HIV infection per 100,000 population) for blacks/African Americans (56.0) was more than 19 times as high as the rate for whites (2.9), and the rate for Latina women (13.3) was more than 4 times as high as the rate for white women. Relatively few cases were diagnosed among Asian, American Indian/Alaska Native, and Native Hawaiian/other Pacific Islander women and women reporting multiple races, although the rates of diagnoses of HIV infection among females of all these races/ethnicities were higher than for white females. The rate of death (per 100,000 population) for black/African American females (25.7) was the highest among all races/ethnicities and was more than 21 times as high as the rate of death for whites (1.2). The death rate for Hispanic women (6.1) was six times higher than for white women. The rates of death for American Indians/Alaska Natives (2.9), Native Hawaiians/other Pacific Islanders (4.7), and women reporting multiple races (14.2) were higher than that for white women (CDC, 2011b).

HIV disease and AIDS rank among the top 10 leading causes of death for black and Hispanic women ages but not for non-Hispanic white women (Heron, 2010).

Effective interventions to prevent HIV infection in women at risk of HIV are lacking. Several prevention research gaps have been recognized. To strengthen future HIV prevention efforts, research needs to focus on social factors that increase vulnerability to HIV such as gender-power relationships, domestic violence or victimization, poverty, homelessness, noninjection and injection substance use, and unrecognized risk activity. This research will require community partnerships, innovative scientific initiatives, sustained support for HIV endpoint trials, and multiyear follow-up (www.hptn.org).

LGBTQ HEALTH

People who are lesbian, gay, bisexual, transgender, or queer/questioning (LGBTQ) are a diverse group from many racial/ethnic groups, socioeconomic backgrounds, and ages. Increasingly referred to as sexual and gender minorities, there are health disparities that affect LGBTQ populations as a result of structural and social inequities, discrimination, and stigma (Mayer, et al., 2008). LGBTQ persons have a disproportionate burden of disease such as substance abuse, overweight and obesity, and tobacco use (Mayer, et al., 2008). For example, bisexual women are more than two times as likely to smoke compared to their heterosexual counterparts, which has been partially attributed to social marginalization, stress, and marketing tactics of tobacco companies (Ryan, et al., 2001). Lesbians may seek routine breast and cervical cancer screening less often than heterosexual women because of discrimination within the medical community, possibly leading to an increased risk of some cancers (Mayer, et al., 2008). Transgender individuals also face specific health needs that have not been adequately addressed in the health and medical community due to structural inequities, the lack of specialized resources, and limited research or data investigating the unique health needs of the population.

LGBTQ adolescents and young adults also experience more health risk behaviors and adverse health outcomes compared to their heterosexual counterparts (Coker, Austin, & Schuster, 2010). A 1999 study found that lesbian/bisexual girls were happier with their body image than heterosexual adolescent girls, but another study found that bisexual females were more likely to purge than their heterosexual peers (Coker, Austin, & Schuster, 2010). Several state and national studies have found that there is an increased risk of suicide attempts among LGB youth compared to heterosexual youth (Coker, Austin, & Schuster, 2010). Studies have also found higher rates of experiences of violence and harassment among LGB youth compared to their peers (Coker, Austin, & Schuster, 2010). Information on suicide, violence, and harassment among transsexual and queer youth is not available. Current research has shown disparities in health outcomes among the LGBTQ adult and youth populations, yet fewer studies have examined contributors to these disparities and possible interventions to ameliorate these disparities.

CONTRIBUTORS TO HEALTH DISPARITIES

Historically, contributors to health disparities focused on documenting differences in the prevalence and incidence of disease and solutions focused on addressing health behaviors and access to health care. These solutions have demonstrated improvements in chronic disease morbidity and increased prenatal care usage, but have not translated into improvements in low birth weight. Health disparities research is shifting to exploring the root causes of health disparities and social and structural inequalities throughout the life course.

Health Behaviors

Two behavioral risk factors associated with infant mortality are maternal smoking and not putting infants to sleep on their backs. American Indian/Native Alaskan mothers have the highest rate of smoking during pregnancy, followed by non-Hispanic whites, whereas black mothers and Asian/Pacific Islander mothers have rates below the national average (CDC, 2007). Smoking during pregnancy contributes to higher rates of infant mortality among American Indian infants. Placing infants on their backs to sleep reduces mortality from Sudden Infant Death Syndrome (SIDS). A decrease in overall SIDS mortality in the United States has been attributed to the Back to Sleep Campaign that began in 1994. The campaign emphasizes putting infants on their backs to sleep and provides other recommendations for creating a safe sleep environment. Yet, since 1994 American Indian/Alaska Native infants continue to have a SIDS rate that is more than twice as high as non-Hispanic white infants, and the rate for African American infants is only slightly less than the rate for American Indians/Alaska Natives (Mathews & Mac-Dorman, 2010). African American infants have the lowest rate of being put to sleep on their backs (Colson, et al., 2009). The campaign has been criticized for being culturally neutral and therefore not addressing concerns of African American and American Indian/Alaska Native families (Hogan, Shanahan, & Rowley, 2011). In addition, low birth weight and preterm infants are at greater risk for SIDS, and the combination of non-supine sleep and prematurity may have a multiplicative effect on the risk of SIDS, causing a higher proportion of African American infants to be vulnerable to SIDS (Rowley & Hogan, *in press*).

Healthcare Access

A major public policy initiative to improve mothers' and children's healthcare access and utilization that began with Medicaid expansions in the late 1980s and continued with implementation of the Children's Health Insurance Program (CHIP) in 1997 was accompanied by expectations of reducing disparities in infant and child health. Greater access to prenatal care provided by Medicaid has not contributed to declines in infant health disparities (Dubay, Joyce, Kaestner, & Kenney, 2001; Epstein & Newhouse, 1998). One study suggests that Medicaid and CHIP expansion has contributed to declines in mortality from external causes

(unintentional injuries, homicide and suicide) for children 6 to 17 years of age, but has not resulted in a reduction in the mortality disparities between black and white children (Howell, et al., 2010). Services provided by Special Supplemental Nutrition Program for Women, Infants, and Children (WIC), i.e., supplemental food, nutrition counseling, and health services referrals for low-income pregnant women, breastfeeding mothers, nonbreastfeeding postpartum mothers, and infants and children who are found to be at nutritional risk, may be associated with reductions in infant mortality and early preterm delivery among African American women compared to white women enrolled in the program (Khanani, et al., 2010).

Access to high-quality health care remains an important goal for infants, children, and reproductive-age women. To receive high-quality care, the MCH population needs health insurance that covers a comprehensive range of benefits and providers, access to a medical home, and an appropriate set of services in the community. African American and Mexican American women and infants are more likely to be poor, and therefore a higher proportion of these groups are eligible for Medicaid or CHIP. Based on the 2002 Pregnancy Risk Assessment Monitoring System (PRAMS), Medicaid covered prenatal care for about one-third of pregnant white women (ranging from 18% to 52% across states), nearly two-thirds (range of 40% to 81%) of pregnant black women, and close to half (38% to 74%) of pregnant Hispanic women (Williams, et al., 2006). Infants born to Medicaid-eligible pregnant women can have Medicaid coverage throughout the first year of life so long as the infant remains in the mother's household and the mother remains eligible. Beginning in 2002, CHIP funds could be used to cover prenatal care and other services for pregnant women. Pregnant women who are immigrants face barriers to Medicaid or CHIP coverage for prenatal care. Most immigrants are subject to a 5-year residency requirement before they are eligible. Undocumented and temporary immigrants are not covered. An estimated 30% of the foreign-born population in the United States is undocumented (Kaiser, 2006), and there are no estimates of the annual numbers of undocumented women who deliver. Only a few states use the CHIP option of funding prenatal care without applying the immigrant test (Kaiser, 2006). Emergency Medicaid is available for deliveries and many women who receive emergency coverage may be confused about infant eligibility (Sarnoff & Hughes, 2005).

Prenatal coverage does not always result in continuous health coverage during infancy. In California, one of the most populous and diverse states, 8.7% of infants were not insured in 2001. Among infants born to Latina women, 13.7% were uninsured. The proportion of uninsured infants born to African American mothers was similar to that of infants born to white/Middle Eastern mothers. Infants born to foreign-born mothers were more likely to be uninsured compared to those of U.S.-born mothers (OR 1.89; 95% CI 1.08, 3.31) (Sarnoff & Hughes, 2005).

The American Academy of Pediatrics recommends a certain number of preventive healthcare visits for children and that these visits take place in a medical home. PRAMS found similar proportion of white and Hispanic infants completed the expected number of well-baby care visits (85.9% and 83.1%, respectively), and that fewer black infants had a sufficient number of visits (78.1%; PRAMS data were missing for > 10% of black and Hispanic respondents) (Williams, et al., 2002). Completion of recommended immunization schedule is a measurable outcome of preventive well-child care. A patchwork of public funding programs has eliminated financial barriers for vaccination and has been successful in eliminating racial/ethnic disparities in coverage. Racial disparities in coverage for the initial 4:3:1:3:3:1 vaccine series (at least four doses of diphtheria-tetanus-pertussis, three poliovirus, one measles-mumps-rubella, three hepatitis B, three Haemophilus

influenzae type B, and one varicella vaccine) declined from 2000 to 2008 to nonsignificant levels (Zhao & Luman, 2010). However, children living below poverty had lower coverage than children living at or above poverty for most vaccines (Molinari, Darling, & McCauley, 2009).

The American Academy of Pediatrics describes a medical home for children as care that is accessible, continuous, comprehensive, family centered, coordinated, compassionate, and culturally effective. It is the standard of quality for comprehensive care for all children (AAP, 2002). Young children are more likely to have a medical home than adults (Raphael, Guadagnolo, Beal, & Giardino, 2009); however, among children 4 to 35 months of age, the proportion of families that reported having a specific well-child care provider was below 50% for all families. Hispanic and African American children were significantly less likely to report having a well-child care provider (Flores, Olson, & Tomany-Korman, 2005). Hispanic and black parents were more likely than white parents to report that their child's provider never or only sometimes understood their child's specific needs (30% for Hispanic families, 15% for black families compared to 10% for white families) and that the provider had limited understanding of their child rearing practices (45–46% for Hispanic and black families compared to 34% for white families) (Flores, Olson, & Tomany-Korman, 2005), suggesting lack of culturally competent care. Furthermore, among immigrant families and other parents with limited English language proficiency, availability of medical interpreters is essential for family-centered care; however, the presence of an interpreter does not ensure the quality of care because interpreters may have differences in culture, religion, or social class that affect interaction with the provider (Mendoza, 2009).

Access to preconception care that includes risk assessment, health promotion, and clinical and psychosocial interventions are particularly important for reducing the infant mortality disparities among African American women because of their higher proportion of extreme preterm births and early fetal deaths and the inability of prenatal care to intervene with contributors to these outcomes (Besculides & Laraque, 2005). Pilot studies of preconception and interconception care that increase accessibility and availability of coordinated well-women health care, provide social and behavioral case management as an avenue, and mitigate the effects of stress and social determinants show promise (Dunlap, 2008; Livingood, et al., 2010). For preconception care to become an effective tool for reducing infant mortality disparities, it has to be more comprehensive and integrated by addressing cultural and residential factors have major influences on pregnancy outcomes and infant mortality.

Social Determinants of Health

Many explanations for social disparities in health (i.e., health differences by race/ethnicity or by socioeconomic factors like income or education) have focused on individual health behaviors (e.g., eating healthy foods), personal choices, genetic predisposition, and adequacy of health care. However, individual choices or genetic characteristics do not adequately explain existing health disparities. Barriers to optimal health exceed an individual's abilities in many cases, particularly children, who cannot choose their environments (Braveman, Egerter, Woolf, & Marks, 2011). The contexts in which individual characteristics or behaviors exist are extremely important for understanding and addressing disparities in health. For example, an individual's ability to lose weight or cease smoking or drinking is influenced by the resources available as well as factors that may limit their choices such as lack of access to grocery stores, lack of space for recreational exercise, and intensive tobacco and alcohol advertisement (Braveman, et al., 2011).

Reducing health disparities will entail addressing the root causes of individual health behaviors (Braveman, et al., 2011).

"Social determinants of health" is a phrase used to describe the context in which health and disease are determined and the related social, political, economic, and historical structures (Hogan, Rowley, Bennett, & Taylor, 2011). The social determinants of health include but are not limited to social policies, neighborhoods or communities, worksites, schools, and social relationships (Ansari, et al., 2004). There are several groups and models that describe the social determinants of health with the common theme of shifting the conversation about health, disease and disparities from individual traits or behaviors to larger societal conditions. The World Health Organization's (WHO) Commission on Social Determinants of Health (CSDH) put forward three core recommendations in order to address health inequities through the social determinants of health. The recommendations were to (1) improve daily living conditions; (2) tackle the inequitable distribution of power, money, and resources; and (3) measure and understand the problem and assess the impact of action (CSDH, 2008). In addition to the recommendations, the commission also realizes that policy has a direct influence on the stated recommendations and human health (CSHD, 2008). These recommendations take into account the unequal distribution of resources, health damaging environments, and toxic combination of poor social policies, programs, and unfair economic arrangements (CSDH, 2008). In each of these core recommendations are implications for MCH programs, which need to be more engaged in improving living standards, environmental justice, education, and economic opportunities.

Social inequalities and economic disadvantage ultimately influence the health and lives of the people living in those contexts, contributing to the disparities in health and disease. For example, housing and living environments influence health, general well-being, and fall- and burn-related injuries for families (Bambra, et al., 2010). Lead remediation programs and policies have resulted in improvements in infant and child health, although disparities in lead exposure remain (Schulz & Northridge, 2004). Improving access to care through community outreach workers and lay health advisors in community settings has shown some benefits in promoting uptake of immunization in children and adults, initiating breastfeeding, and improving self-reported health (Bambra, et al., 2010). Initiatives that provide monetary incentives and coupons to purchase fresh fruits and vegetables at farmers' markets were positively associated with weight loss and consumption of fruits and vegetables (Bambra, et al., 2010). Educational attainment and income is associated with improvements in health in general, e.g., an increase in a mother's education is related to a decrease in infant mortality rate (Mathews & MacDorman, 2010).

In order to reduce disparities, efforts should target the differential exposure to adverse environments, contexts, and social policies, not only the individual-level factors. In addition to social context, living conditions, environments and socioeconomic status as social determinants of health, social and health policies play an important role in racial/ethnic health disparities. However, these social determinants cannot be reduced to factors isolated during one point in time but have to take into account the historical, political, and economic forces that occur over time and how this influences health over many generations.

LIFE COURSE

Life course theory contributes to understanding how social determinants are underlying causes of disparities. Life course theory proposed that early exposures, critical periods of risk, the effects of cumulative exposure, and social trajectories influence health. The health of the child predicts his or her health into adulthood

(Braveman, Egerter, Woolf, & Marks, 2011). The social conditions in which infants and children live can increase their risk for chronic diseases such as diabetes, heart disease, and diabetes in adulthood (Braveman, et al., 2011). Additionally, disparities in social conditions are relevant for health across generations. The health of the mother prior to conception and adverse exposures during pregnancy can affect the health of the mother and her developing child (Hertzman & Boyce, 2010). Critical periods of risk are sensitive periods that happen during childhood and adolescence when physical and social environments have lasting effects on subsequent health. Cumulative exposures to a single recurrent factor, such as chronic poverty, or a series of exposures to different factors that affect health may be linked to health in later life. Social trajectories explain how exposure at one stage of life influences the probability of other exposures later in the life course. Taken together, social exposures that occur early in life or during a critical period can influence disease and well-being over a lifetime. The life course perspective supports shifting from single focused interventions to preventive or ameliorative interventions for women and children that are delivered in a multilayered context of family, community, and broader social forces (Shonkoff & Phillips, 2000).

IMPLICATIONS FOR MCH POLICY

A healthcare system that provides equitable care to all families who reside in the United States is an important policy need. Organizational commitment to cultural competence in health, defined as the ability of the system to provide care to patients with diverse values, beliefs and behaviors, including tailored behavior to meet patients' social, cultural and linguistic needs (Betancourt, Green, & Carrillo, 2000), will become increasingly important as the U.S. population continues to become even more diverse.

Second, interventions that reduce mortality and morbidity for the total MCH population do not reduce disparity because an *accelerated* rate of decline in the most vulnerable population groups will be necessary to achieve disparity reduction (Hogan, Rowley, Bennett, & Taylor, 2011). Specifically, we need to identify *what factors make some populations more likely to experience health disadvantages compared to other populations*, and then identify and implement ways to ameliorate these disadvantages (Hogan, Rowley, Bennett, & Taylor, 2011). For example, school-based dental sealant programs could reduce or eliminate racial and economic disparities in sealant use if programs were provided to all eligible, high-risk schools, such as those in which 50% or more of the children are eligible for free or reduced-price meals (Gooch, et al., 2009). Health disparities researchers must work collaboratively with affected communities and populations in order to have an impact (Dankwa-Mullan, et al., 2010). It needs to integrate indigenous research methodologies that can recognize and support intervention research (Wallerstein & Duran, 2010).

Third, the MCH Bureau should continue the process of applying life course theory in strategic planning of new and innovative practices, programs and policies that promote health equity across populations (Fine & Kotelchuck, 2010). This calls for working with nonhealth sectors to improve the social and physical environment at the community level. The greatest challenge is eliminating the structural barriers to health equity. These are macroeconomic policies (labor, market structure), social policies (related to housing and land), and other public policies (education, health, environment) that maintain health disparities (CSDH, 2008).

CONCLUSION

Health disparities are closely linked to historical and ongoing social disadvantage that perpetuate inequities. Public health's role, when viewed from a social justice perspective, is to implement interventions that remediate patterns of systemic disadvantage that interfere with health and well-being. Addressing disadvantage among MCH populations is particularly important because the health of women and children sets the stage for health all along the life course and contributes to eliminating disparities in adult health now and in the future.

References

Acevedo-Garcia, D., Soobader, M., & Berkman, L. (2007). Low birthweight among US Hispanic/Latino subgroups: The effect of maternal foreign-born status and education. *Social Science & Medicine, 65*(12), 2503–2516.

Agurs-Collins, T., Dunn, B. K., Browne, D., Johnson, K. A., & Lubet, R. (2010). Epidemiology of health disparities in relation to the biology of estrogen receptor-negative breast cancer. *Seminars in Oncology, 37*(4), 384–401. doi:10.1053/j.seminoncol.2010.05.002

American Academy of pediatrics Medical Home Initiatives for Children with Special Needs Project Advisory Committee. (2002). Medical home. *Pediatrics, 110*(1), 184–186.

American Academy of Pediatrics. (2008). *Recommendations for Preventive Pediatric Health Care*. Elk Grove Village, IL: American Academy of Pediatrics, Bright Futures. Retrieved October 13, 2011 from http://brightfutures.aap.org/pdfs/AAP%20Bright%20Futures%20Periodicity%20Sched%2020101107.pdf.

Ansari, Z., Carson, N. J., Ackland, M. J., Vaughan, L., & Serraglio, A. (2003). A public health model of the social determinants of health. *Sozial- Und Praventivmedizin, 48*(4), 242–251.

Bambra, C., Gibson, M., Sowden, A., Wright, K., Whitehead, M., & Petticrew, M. (2010). Tackling the wider social determinants of health and health inequalities: Evidence from systematic reviews. *Journal of Epidemiology and Community Health, 64*(4), 284–291. doi:10.1136/jech.2008.082743.

Baum, K. (2005). Juvenile victimization and offending 1993–2003. Washington, DC: U.S. Department of Justice, Bureau of Justice Statistics. Retrieved October 14, 2011 from http://bjs.ojp.usdoj.gov/index.cfm?ty=pbdetail&iid=1041.

Berg, C. J., Callaghan, W. M., Syverson, C., & Henderson, Z. (2010). Pregnancy-related mortality in the United States, 1998 to 2005. *Obstetrics and Gynecology, 116*(6), 1302–1309. doi:10.1097/AOG.0b013e3181fdfb11.

Besculides, M., & Laraque, F. (2005). Racial and ethnic disparities in perinatal mortality: Applying the perinatal periods of risk model to identify areas for intervention. *Journal of the National Medical Association, 97*(8), 1128–1132.

Betancourt, J. R., Green, A. R., & Carrillo, J. E. (2000). *Cultural competence in health care: Emerging frameworks and practical approaches.* New York: The Commonwealth Fund. Retrieved October 13, 2011 from http://www.commonwealthfund.org/Content/Publications/Fund-Reports/2002/Oct/Cultural-Competence-in-Health-Care--Emerging-Frameworks-and-Practical-Approaches.aspx.

Braveman, P. A., Egerter, S. A., Woolf, S. H., & Marks, J. S. (2011). When do we know enough to recommend action on the social determinants of health? *American Journal of Preventive Medicine, 40*(1, Suppl. 1), S58–S66.

Brinton, L. A., Sherman, M. E., Carreon, J. D., & Anderson, W. F. (2008). Recent trends in breast cancer among younger women in the United States. *Journal of the National Cancer Institute, 100*(22), 1643–1648. doi:10.1093/jnci/djn344.

Callaghan, W. M., & Berg, C. J. (2003). Pregnancy-related mortality among women aged 35 years and older, United States, 1991–1997. *Obstetrics and Gynecology, 102*(5, Pt. 1), 1015–1021. doi:10.1016/s0029-7844(03)00740-3.

Callaghan, W. M., MacDorman, M. F., Rasmussen, S. A., Qin, C., & Lackritz, E. M. (2006). The contribution of preterm birth to infant mortality rates in the United States. *Pediatrics, 118*, 1566–1573.

Camp-Sorrell, D. (2009). Cancer and its treatment effect on young breast cancer survivors. *Seminars in Oncology Nursing, 25*(4), 251–258.

Carter-Pokras, O., & Baquet, C. (2002). What is a "health disparity"? *Public Health Reports, 117*(5), 426–434.

Centers for Disease Control and Prevention (CDC). (2007). *Preventing smoking and exposure to second hand smoke before, during, and after pregnancy.* Atlanta, GA: Author. Retrieved October 13, 2011 from http://www.cdc.gov/nccdphp/publications/factsheets/Prevention/pdf/smoking.pdf.

Centers for Disease Control and Prevention. (2010). Youth risk behavior surveillance—United States, 2009. *Morbidity and Mortality Weekly Report, 59*(SS-5), 1–142.

Centers for Disease Control and Prevention. (2011a). Children and diabetes: SEARCH for diabetes in youth. Retrieved October 13, 2011 from http://www.cdc.gov/diabetes/projects/diab_children.htm.

Centers for Disease Control and Prevention. (2011b). HIV/AIDS topics. Retrieved March 3, 2011 from http://www.cdc.gov/hiv/topics.

Coker, T. R., Austin, S. B., & Schuster, M. A. (2010). The health and health care of lesbian, gay, and bisexual adolescents. *Annual Review of Public Health, 31*(1), 457–477. doi:10.1146/annurev.publhealth.012809.103636.

Colson, E. R., Rybin, D., Smith, L. A., Colton, T., Lister, G., & Corwin, M. J. (2009). Trends and factors associated with infant sleeping position: the national infant sleep position study, 1993–2007. *Archives of Pediatrics & Adolescent Medicine, 163*(12), 1122–1128.

Commission on the Social Determinants of Health (CSDH). (2008). *Closing the gap in a generation: Health equity through action on the social determinants of health. Final Report of the Commission on Social Determinants of Health.* Geneva, Switzerland: World Health Organization.

Dankwa-Mullan, I., Rhee, K. B., Stoff, D. M., Pohlhaus, J. R., Sy, F. S., Stinson, N., Jr., & Ruffin, J. (2010). Moving toward paradigm-shifting research in health disparities through translational, transformational, and transdisciplinary approaches. *American Journal of Public Health, 100*(Suppl. 1), S19–S24.

Department of Health and Social Security. (1980). *Inequalities in health. Report of a research working group.* London, England: Author.

Division of Reproductive Health. (2001). Pregnancy-related deaths among Hispanic, Asian/Pacific Islander, and American Indian/Alaska Native women—United States, 1991–1997. *Morbidity and Mortality Weekly Report, 50*(18), 361–364.

Dubay, L., Joyce, T., Kaestner, R., & Kenney, G.M. (2001). Changes in prenatal care timing and low birth weight by race and socioeconomic status: Implications for the Medicaid expansions for pregnant women. *HSR: Health Services Research, 36*(2), 373–398.

Dunlop, A. A. L. (2008). Interpregnancy primary care and social support for African-American women at risk for recurrent very-low-birthweight delivery: A pilot evaluation. *Maternal and Child Health Journal, 12*(4), 461–468.

Dye, B. A., Tan, S., Smith, V., Lewis, B. G., Barker, L. K., Thornton-Evans, G., et al. (2007). Trends in oral health status: United States, 1988–1994 and

1999–2004. National Center for Health Statistics. *Vital and Health Statistics, 11*(248).

Edelstein, B. L., & Chinn, C. H. (2009). Update on disparities in oral health and access to dental care for America's children. *Academic Pediatrics, 9*(6), 415–419.

Epstein, A. M., & Newhouse, J. P. (1998). Impact of Medicaid expansion on early prenatal care and health outcomes. *Health Care Financing Review, 19*(4), 85–94.

Federal Interagency Forum on Child and Family Statistics. (2010). *America's children in brief: Key national indicators of well-being, 2010.* Washington, DC: U.S. Government Printing Office. Retrieved October 13, 2011 from http://www.childstats.gov/americaschildren10/index.asp.

Fine, A., & Kotelchuck, M. (2010). *Rethinking MCH: The life course model as an organizing framework.* Concept paper. Washington, DC: U.S. Department of Health and Human Services, Health Resources and Services Administration, Maternal and Child Health Bureau.

Flores, G., Olson, L., & Tomany-Korman, S. C. (2005). Racial and ethnic disparities in early childhood health and health care. *Pediatrics, 115*(2), e183–e193.

Ford, C. L., & Harawa, N. T. (2010). A new conceptualization of ethnicity for social epidemiologic and health equity research. *Social Science & Medicine, 71*(2), 251–258.

Franks, A. L., Kendrick, J. S., Olson, D. R., Atrash, H. K., Saftlas, A. F., & Moien, M. (1992). Hospitalization for pregnancy complications, United States, 1986 and 1987. *American Journal of Obstetrics and Gynecology, 166*(5), 1339–1344.

Freedman, D. S. (2011, January 14). Obesity—United States, 1988–2008. *Morbidity and Mortality Weekly Report Surveillance Summaries, 60*(Suppl.), 73–77.

Garrett, B. E., Dube, S. R., Trosclair, A., Caraballo, R. S., Pechacek, T. F.; Centers for Disease Control and Prevention (CDC. (2011). Cigarette smoking–United States, 1965–2008. *MMWR Surveill Summ. 14, 60* Suppl, 109–113.

Gooch, B. F., Griffin, S. O., Gray, S. K., Kohn, W. G., Rozier, R. G., Siegal, M., et al. (2009). Preventing dental caries through school-based sealant programs: Updated recommendations and reviews of evidence. *Journal of the American Dental Association, 140*(11), 1356–1365.

Guttmacher Institute. (2010). *U.S. teenage pregnancies, births and abortions: National and state trends and trends by race and ethnicity.* Retrieved October 13, 2011 from http://www.guttmacher.org/pubs/USTPtrends.pdf.

Hannan, C., Buchanan, A. D., & Monroe, J. (2009). Maintaining the vaccine safety net. *Pediatrics, 124*(Suppl. 5), S571–S572.

Hatch, J., Moss, N., Saran, A., Presley-Cantrell, L., & Mallory, C. (1993). Community research: partnership in black communities. *American Journal of Preventive Medicine, 9*(Suppl. 6), 27–31.

Heron, M. (2010). Deaths: Leading causes for 2006. *National vital statistics reports, I*(14). Hyattsville, MD: U.S. Department of Health and Human Services, National Center for Health Statistics.

Hertzman, C., & Boyce, T. (2010). How experience gets under the skin to create gradients in developmental health. *Annual Review of Public Health, 31,* 329–347.

Hogan, V. K., Rowley, D., Bennett, T., & Taylor, K. D. (2011). Life course, social determinants, and health inequities: Toward a national plan for achieving health equity for African American infants—A concept paper. *Maternal and Child Health Journal.* DOI 10.1007/s10995-011-0847-0.

Hogan, V. K., Shanahan, M. E., & Rowley, D. L. (2011). Current approaches to reducing premature births and implications for disparity elimination. In A. Handler, J. Kennelly, & N. Peacock (Eds.), *Reducing racial/ethnic disparities in reproductive and perinatal outcomes: The evidence from population-based interventions* (pp. 181–207). New York, NY: Springer.

Howell, E., Decker, S., Hogan, S., Yemane, A., & Foster, J. (2010). Declining child mortality and continuing racial disparities in the era of the Medicaid and SCHIP insurance coverage expansions. *American Journal of Public Health, 100*(12), 2500–2506.

James, S. A. (1993). Racial and ethnic differences in infant mortality and low birth weight: A psychosocial critique. *Annals of Epidemiology, 3*(2), 130–136.

Johnston, L. D., O'Malley, P. M., Bachman, J. G., & Schulenberg, J. E. (2011). *Monitoring the Future national results on adolescent drug use: Overview of key findings, 2010.* Ann Arbor: The University of Michigan, Institute for Social Research.

Jones, C. (2001). Invited commentary: "Race," racism, and the practice of epidemiology. *American Journal of Epidemiology, 154*(4), 299–304.

Kaiser Commission on Medicaid and the uninsured. (2006). Medicaid and SCHIP eligibility for immigrants. The Henry J Kaiser Family Foundation. Retrieved from http://www.kff.org/medicaid/upload/7492.pdf.

Kaiser Family Foundation. (2011). *Infant mortality rate (deaths per 1,000 live births), linked files, 2005–2007.* Retrieved October 13, 2011 from http://www.statehealthfacts.org/comparemaptable.jsp?ind=47&cat=2 .

Kanny, D., Liu, Y., & Brewer, R. D. (2011). Binge drinking—United States, 2009. *Morbidity and Mortality Weekly Report, 60*(1), 101–104. Retrieved October 13, 2011 from http://www.cdc.gov/mmwr/preview/mmwrhtml/su6001a22.htm.

Khanani, I., Elam, J., Hearn, R., Jones, C., & Maseru, N. (2010). The impact of prenatal WIC participation on infant mortality and racial disparities. *American Journal of Public Health, 100*(Suppl. 1), S204–S209.

Lawson, H. W., Henson, R., Bobo, J. K., & Kaeser, M. K. (2000). Implementing recommendations for the early detection of breast and cervical cancer among low-income women. *Morbidity and Mortality Weekly Report. Recommendations and Reports, 49*(RR-02), 37–55. Retrieved October 13, 2011 from http://www.cdc.gov/mmwr/preview/mmwrhtml/rr4902a4.htm.

Livingood, W. C., Brady, C., Pierce, K., Atrash, H., Hou, T., & Bryant, T., III. (2010). Impact of preconception health care: Evaluation of a social determinants focused intervention. *Maternal and Child Health Journal, 14*(3), 382–391.

MacDorman, M. F., & Mathews, T. J. (2008). *Recent trends in infant mortality in the United States.* NCHS data brief, no 9. Hyattsville, MD: U.S. Department of Health and Human Services, National Center for Health Statistics.

MacDorman, M. F., & Mathews, T. J. (2011). Infant deaths—United States, 2000–2007. *Morbidity and Mortality Weekly Report, 60*(1), 49–51.

Mathews, T. J., & MacDorman, M. F. (2010). Infant mortality statistics from the period linked birth/infant death data set. *National vital statistics reports, 58*(17). Hyattsville, MD: U.S. Department of Health and Human Services, National Center for Health Statistics.

Mayer, K. H., Bradford, J. B., Makadon, H. J., Stall, R., Goldhammer, H., & Landers, S. (2008). Sexual and gender minority health: What we know and what needs to be done. *American Journal of Public Health, 98*(6), 989–995. doi:10.2105/AJPH.2007.127811.

Mays, V. M., Ponce, N. A., Washington, D. L., & Cochran, S. D. (2003). Classification of race and ethnicity: Implications for public health. *Annual Review of Public Health, 24,* 83–110.

McGlade, M. S., Saha, S., & Dahlstrom, M. E. (2004). The Latina paradox: An opportunity for restructuring prenatal care delivery. *American Journal of Public Health, 94*(12), 2062–2065.

Mendoza, F. S. (2009). Health disparities and children in immigrant families: A research agenda. *Pediatrics,124*(Suppl. 3), S187–S195.

Minority Health and Health Disparities Research and Education Act of 2000 Retrieved October 13, 2011 from http://www7.nationalacademies.org/ocga/laws/PL106_525.asp.

Molinari, N. A., Darling, N., & McCauley, M. (2009). National, state, and local area vaccination coverage among children aged 19–35 months—United States, 2008. *Morbidity and Mortality Weekly Report, 58*(33), 921–926.

National Center for Health Statistics. (1983). *Health, United States, 1983.* Hyattsville, MD: U.S. Department of Health and Human Services, National Center for Health Statistics.

National Center for Health Statistics. (2007). *Health, United States, 2007.* Hyattsville, MD: U.S. Department of Health and Human Services, National Center for Health Statistics.

National Center for Health Statistics. (2010). Health, United States, 2009 with special feature on medical technology. Hyattsville, MD: U.S. Department of Health and Human Services, National Center for Health Statistics.

Patient Protection and Affordable Care Act of 2010. Retrieved October 13, 2011 from http://docs.house.gov/energycommerce/ppacacon.pdf.

Pazol, K., Warner, L., Gavin, L., Callaghan, W. M., Spitz, A. M., Anderson, J. E., Barfield, W. D., & Kann, L. (2011). Vital signs: Teen pregnancy—United States, 1991–2009. *Morbidity and Mortality Weekly Report, 60*(13), 414–420. Retrieved October 13, 2011 from http://www.cdc.gov/mmwr/PDF/wk/mm6013.pdf.

Puzzanchera, C. (2009). *Juvenile arrests 2008.* Juvenile Justice Bulletin. Washington, DC: U.S. Department of Justice, Office of Justice Programs. Retrieved October 13, 2011 from http://www.ncjrs.gov/pdffiles1/ojjdp/228479.pdf.

Raphael, J. L., Guadagnolo, B. A., Beal, A. C., & Giardino, A. P. (2009). Racial and ethnic disparities in indicators of a primary care medical home for children. *Academic Pediatrics, 9*(4), 221–227.

Rowley, D. L., & Hogan, V. (in press). Disparities in infant mortality and effective, equitable care: Are infants suffering from benign neglect? *Annual Review of Public Health*.

Ryan, H., Wortley, P. M., Easton, A., Pederson, L., & Greenwood, G. (2001). Smoking among lesbians, gays, and bisexuals: A review of the literature. *American Journal of Preventive Medicine, 21*(2), 142–149. doi:10.1016/s0749-3797(01)00331-2.

Saraiya, M., Ahmed, F., Krishnan, S., Richards, T. B., Unger, E. R., & Lawson, H. W. (2007). Cervical cancer incidence in a prevaccine era in the United States, 1998–2002. *Obstetrics and Gynecology, 109*(2, Pt. 1), 360–370. doi:10.1097/01. AOG.0000254165.92653.e8.

Sarnoff, R., & Hughes, D. (2005). Increasing health insurance coverage in the first year of life. *Maternal and Child Health Journal, 9*(4), 343–350.

Schoendorf, K., Hogue, C. J. R., Kleinman, J. C., & Rowley, D. (1992). Mortality among infants of black as compared with white college-educated graduates. *New England Journal of Medicine, 326*(23), 1522–1526.

Schulz, A., & Northridge, M. E. (2004). Social determinants of health: Implications for environmental health promotion. *Health Education & Behavior, 31*(4), 455–471. doi:10.1177/1090198104265598.

Shonkoff, J. P., & Phillips, D. A. (Eds.). (2000). *From neurons to neighborhoods: The science of early child development*. Washington, DC: National Academy Press.

Shrestha, L. B., & Heisler, E. J. (2011). *The changing demographic profile of the United States*. Washington, DC: Congressional Research Service. Retrieved October 13, 2011 from http://www.fas.org/sgp/crs/misc/RL32701.pdf.

Stoto, M. A., Behrens, R., & Rosemont, C. (Eds.). (1990). *Healthy People 2000: Citizens chart the course*. Institute of Medicine. Washington, DC: National Academy Press.

Tanaka, M., Jaamaa, G., Kaiser, M., Hills, E., Soim, A., Zhu, M., et al. (2007). Racial disparity in hypertensive disorders of pregnancy in New York State: A 10-year longitudinal population-based study. *American Journal of Public Health, 97*(1), 163–170. doi:10.2105/AJPH.2005.068577.

United Nations. (2011). *World population prospects: The 2010 revision*. New York: United Nations, Department of Economic and Social Affairs, Population Division. Retrieved October 13, 2011 from http://esa.un.org/unpd/wpp/index.htm.

U.S. Census Bureau. (2012). Statistical Abstract of the United States: 2012 (131st Edition). Washington, DC. Retrieved from http://www.census.gov/prod/2011pubs/12statab/law.pdf.

U.S. Department of Health and Human Services. (1985). *Report of The Secretary's Task Force on Black and Minority Health* (No. 0-487-637). Washington, DC: U.S. Government Printing Office.

U.S. Department of Health and Human Services. (n.d.-a). *About healthy people*. Retrieved October 13, 2011 from http://www.healthypeople.gov/2020/about/.

U.S. Department of Health and Human Services. (n.d.-b). *Healthy People 2010*. Retrieved October 13, 2011 from http://www.healthypeople.gov/2010.

U.S. Department of Health and Human Services. (n.d.-c). *Healthy People 2020*. Retrieved October 13, 2011 from http://www.healthypeople.gov/2020/.

Ventura, S. J., Mathews, T. J., Hamilton, B. E., Sutton, P. D., & Abma, J. C. (2011). Adolescent pregnancy and childbirth—United States, 1991–2008. *Morbidity and Mortality Weekly Report, 60*(Suppl.), 105–108.

Ver Ploeg, M., & Perrin, E. (Eds). (2004). Eliminating health disparities: Measurement and data needs. Washington, DC: National Academies Press.

Wallerstein, N., & Duran, B. (2010). Community-based participatory research contributions to intervention research: The intersection of science and practice to improve health equity. *American Journal of Public Health, 100*(Suppl. 1), S40–S46.

Williams, L., Morrow, B., Schulman, H., Stephens, R., D'Angelo, D., & Fowler, C. I. (2006). *PRAMS 2002 surveillance report*. Atlanta, GA: Division of Reproductive Health, National Center for Chronic Disease Prevention and Health Promotion, Centers for Disease Control and Prevention.

Zhao, Z., & Luman, E. T. (2010). Progress toward eliminating disparities in vaccination coverage among U.S. children, 2000–2008. *American Journal of Preventive Medicine, 38*(2), 127–137.

11

WOMEN'S HEALTH: A LIFE CYCLE

Anjel Vahratian, B. Cecilia Zapata, and Siobán D. Harlow

We must recognize that, in some large measure, problems with infant ill health are a legacy of women's ill health generally. Cross-disciplinary investigations that can examine the interactions between the general health of women and childbearing are needed urgently.

(Wise, 1993, p. 14)

INTRODUCTION

At first glance, it may seem unusual to include a chapter on women's health in a textbook on maternal and child health (MCH). However, MCH advocates who approach the field from the maternal perspective seek assurance that broad women's health concerns will be promoted in public health. They note that gender discrimination and inequities may cause women's health to fall through the cracks of other disciplines and research arenas, whether they are specific to populations, diseases, or methods. With rising rates of obesity, preexisting chronic conditions such as hypertension, diabetes, and depression that place women at increased risk for adverse pregnancy outcomes, are of increasing concern. Similarly, complications of pregnancy are increasingly understood to influence a woman's long-term health and quality of life. Thus, a logical inclusion to the MCH mission may be health promotion and disease prevention, as well as early diagnosis and treatment, for women throughout the life cycle.

Proponents of a more traditional definition are concerned that the special needs of pregnant women may receive too little emphasis if MCH is defined too broadly. However, recognition of the need for a comprehensive reproductive health framework has been spreading from international to domestic MCH. Maternal outcomes are clearly influenced by a complex web of socioeconomic and environmental influences that precede a woman's pregnancy, perhaps by generations. Chronic illness and underlying health status, including psychosocial health, are important elements in the creation or exacerbation of pregnancy-related risks. Exclusion of prepregnancy and nonobstetric factors restricts our understanding of maternal health unnecessarily.

In most women's lives, the period of childbearing is much shorter than the duration of childrearing. Nevertheless, maternal outcomes are usually measured only by immediate pregnancy consequences. The mental and physical stresses and benefits of the childrearing years are seldom considered as part of maternal health. Furthermore, a growing proportion of U.S. women is delaying childbearing or is choosing not to have children. Over the past 37 years, the mean age at first birth in the United States has increased 3.6 years, from 21.4 years in 1970 to 25.0 years in 2007 (Martin, et al., 2010; Mathews & Hamilton, 2002). In an analysis of national survey data, Chandra et al. (2005) reported that among the 5.4 million women in the United States who had no children and expected none in the future, 3.8 million women chose not to have children voluntarily (6.2% of women 15 to 44 years of age). Infertility is a medical problem among U.S. couples as well, as one in six couples experience infertility (Barad & Witt, 2000).

Thus, many more "woman-years" are spent today outside the reproductive domain, and many women never enter the realm of maternity care. Because the United States lacks a universal system of health care, maternity services provide entry for many women into primary care that they might otherwise lack. Women's health concerns in MCH include continuity of care and access to services before, during, after, and independent of childbearing. It seems unreasonable to expect women to invest their trust in a healthcare system that expresses concern about them only during pregnancy.

An important insight from the international health field has been the critical role of the status of women in determining MCH outcomes. The same situation prevails in the United States. If women are not socially valued, they are likely to face limitations in reproductive decision making and hazards to their general and reproductive health status. Unless women command respect and equity in their roles as daughters, students, wives and partners, and workers, they are not likely to experience the physical and mental health advantages predictive of optimal child health. Some observers view the inclusion of women's health in MCH as yet another attempt to confine women to the maternal definition and role; nevertheless, no one can deny that any improvements in the overall determinants of women's health will benefit their offspring. The opposite, however, is not necessarily the case.

THE WOMEN'S HEALTH MOVEMENT

The M in MCH

Through the 1950s and 1960s, population growth framed MCH; thus, family planning and population control were central to MCH policies and strategies. During the decade of the 1980s, the health toll on women caused by pregnancy and human reproduction received national and international attention due to two interrelated endeavors. The first endeavor was the 1985 *Lancet* article titled, "Where Is the M in MCH?," which argued "in discussions of MCH it is commonly assumed that whatever is good for the child is good for the mother. However, not only are the causes of maternal death quite different from those of child health but so are the potential remedies" (Rosenfield & Maine, 1985, p. 83).

The second endeavor was the 1987 Safe Motherhood Conference in Nairobi, Kenya. The results were international awareness and advocacy to address the risk women faced through pregnancy, childbirth, and postpartum, as well as strategies to lower the risk of maternal mortality and fragility. Moreover, the international Conference on Population and Development held in Cairo, Egypt, in 1994, was significant for women's health and human rights by shifting from a population focus to a reproductive health framework, which encompassed family planning, maternal health, sexual health, and prevention of the human immunodeficiency virus (HIV) and sexually transmitted infections (STI). Additionally, gender equity, women's rights, and empowerment were integrated into the development goals. The long-term significance of the Cairo conference can be exemplified in the priorities of the United Nations and World Health Organization (e.g., violence against women and girls, the impact of war and terrorism on women and girls, human trafficking, sex trafficking, and unaccounted women and girls throughout the world (Rosenfield, et al., 2010).

Although most countries have experienced improvements in infant mortality, maternal mortality remains high despite public health strategies and advances in medical knowledge and technology (see **Table 11–1**).

Women's lifetime risk of dying due to pregnancy/childbirth requires a comprehensive and international approach to policies, strategies, and interventions that address women's social, political, and economic inequalities. In the United States, the M in MCH is reflected in our poor understanding of the marked differentials in maternal and infant health outcomes according to mothers' socioeconomic status, race, ethnicity, and geographic location. Both women and

Table 11–1 A Woman's Lifetime Chances of Dying Due to Pregnancy/Childbirth-Related Complications.

1 in 7,300	Developed Countries
1 in 75	Developing Countries
1 in 210	Northern Africa
1 in 22	Sub-Saharan Africa
1 in 1,200	Eastern Asia
1 in 61	South-Central Asia
1 in 130	South-East Asia
1 in 170	Western Asia
1 in 290	Latin America & the Caribbean
1 in 62	Oceania

Source: Modified from Maternal mortality: The eye of the storm by A. Foster-Rosales in: *Women's global health and human rights*, by P. Morthy and C. L. Smith (Eds.), 2010, Sudbury, MA: Jones and Bartlett Publishers. Reprinted with permission, p. 283.

children would be better served by identifying and addressing all of the women's health factors that potentially contribute to pregnancy outcomes.

A more holistic approach to maternal health requires much closer investigation of nonobstetric conditions. Human reproduction starts much earlier than conception, including appropriate nutrition and a healthy lifestyle. In a study of all of the deaths to women ages 15 to 44 years in Boston between 1980 and 1989, Katz, Holmes, Power, and Wise (1995) found that only 7 of the 1,234 total deaths were attributable to causes related to childbearing. These researchers concluded that neglect of the comprehensive health needs of women of reproductive age results in many preventable deaths. Maternal preventable deaths continue into the new millennium. For example in the United States, 623 maternal deaths were reported in 2005. It is important to note that the maternal deaths were not equally distributed among women. Black women experienced the highest rates (39.2 per 100,000 live births), which were three times the rate among white women (11.7 per 100,000 live births), and four times the rate among Latinas (9.6 per 100,000 live births) (U.S. Department of Health and Human Services, 2008). The fact that maternal mortality occurs disproportionally among different racial and ethnic groups, women of different ages, and from preventable causes, challenges the current view that the health needs of women should be defined principally in relation to childbearing and instead highlights the concept that these needs transcend reproductive care (Katz, et al., 1995, p. 1138).

A final argument for including women's health in MCH is the importance of considering pregnancy and childbearing as critical periods of risk for the development of chronic diseases later in life. This reversal of the usual paradigm creates opportunities for exploring poorly understood aspects of women's health, life expectancy, and quality of life. Beral (1985) and Green, Beral, and Moser (1988) have found that parity appears to present elevated risks for certain chronic and acute diseases in women and protection against other conditions. "These data suggest that there may be residual and cumulative effects of childbearing which influence patterns of disease in the long term" (Green, et al., 1988, p. 391).

A HISTORICAL DISCOURSE OF WOMEN'S HEALTH

Historically, interest in women's health has revolved around fertility and maternity (i.e., pregnancy, childbirth, and the postpartum period). Childbirth has symbolized the social, political, and spiritual status of women from being highly valued (the designated healers, goddesses, queens, peacemakers) to a subservient status in the patriarchal age (Brodsky, 2008). According to feminist historians, the reproductive life of Western women before the 20th century was embedded in a female culture. This provided women with sympathetic support and guidance throughout their reproductive cycle (Ruzek, 1978) and women provided most of the paid and unpaid care work (Armstrong, et al., 2008). Although social class and culture influenced women's experiences, a common value was shared—women assisted other women through the maternity process (Alexander & LaRosa, 1994). Thus, maternity was part of women's domestic and social responsibilities and women were bound together in mutual support in order to endure frequent pregnancies and childbirth, breastfeeding, and menopause. Maternity as a woman's centered experience has been summarized by Maize and Low Dog (2010) as:

Women are healers, the holders of rituals, and the determiners of family life. Mothers, sisters, daughters, wives, and friends, our many relationships often define us as powerfully as our occupations. We have experienced triumphs and losses, joys and sorrows, and we bear the hidden scars and treasured trophies as our stories. (Maize & Low Dog, 2010, p. 3)

The role of women as healers declined as men developed knowledge of human anatomy and surgical skills through embalming and later to the formal study of medicine in established medical schools, which excluded women. Midwifery, a woman-centered profession, continued to be practiced by women, whereas physicians viewed it as beneath their dignity (Brodsky, 2008) and regarded it as tedious, with unpredictable work hours (Warsh, 2010).

By the mid-18th century, the Western world started to question women's unique role in maternity care. European women began to deliver babies in hospitals with the assistance of midwives under the watchful eyes of physicians who had little experience in childbirth. French physicians took advantage of delivery hospitalizations to study childbirth as a natural process, whereas the English engaged in the development of surgical procedures and technical tools such as the forceps (Alexander & LaRosa, 1994). By the end of the 18th century, physicians attended deliveries along with midwives. This was the beginning of physician control over birthing.

It was not medical knowledge, but the introduction of drugs (e.g., opium and its derivatives and anesthetics such as ether and chloroform), cervical dilatation, labor-inducing techniques, forceps, and later surgery (cesarean) that gave rise to the medicalization of birth, which gave total control of the birthing process to the physician (Brodsky, 2008). This approach to childbirth and the powerful opposition of organized medicine brought a severe decline to midwifery and an increase of infant and maternal morbidity and mortality. It is important to note that at this juncture physicians such as Dr. Christopher Widmer, President of the Medical Board of Canada, supported the training of midwives in lying-in hospitals, whereas others voiced their strong opposition to professionally trained midwives (Warsh, 2010). Additionally, not all physicians were in support of the medicalization of birth, and Dr. Grantly Dick-Read (1933) was the first physician to challenge it. The medical establishment used his book *Natural Childbirth* (originally published in 1933) against him. He was charged with advocating cruelty to women. Ironically, the majority of physicians disregarded his knowledge of childbirth, but women expressed their appreciation for his commitment to bringing birth back to being a natural life event and not a disease (Brodsky, 2008).

By the early 1900s, the American Medical Association (AMA) became concerned about the quality of medical education, the great number of students graduating medical school, and the lack of effective licensing laws and/or regulations in many states. Licensing and reform measures enable the AMA to address the "overcrowding" in the medical field as well as to diminish the practice of midwifery. They were in direct competition with physicians for clientele (Brodsky, 2008, p. 119). More deaths were caused by these procedures at the hands of physicians than by infections in the care of midwives (Ruzek, 1978). As Brodsky explained, "hospitals didn't turn out to be the safe haven that obstetricians had proclaimed" (Brodsky, 2008, p. 131). This assertion was further supported by Dr. Matthias Nicoll, Commissioner of Health of New York State. The state had 3,000 maternal deaths in 1925. A preliminary investigation revealed that out of 696 reported deaths, 74% of the women delivered at the hospital and 26% at home. Midwives attended 16 of the home births and had one maternal death. The midwife attending that birth was later exonerated (Brodsky, 2008). These reforms were intended to limit competition and impacted midwives negatively. Additionally, the number of medical schools was reduced from 155 to 63 from 1904 to 1915 respectively (Brodsky, 2008).

In the United States, medicine became almost exclusively a white male profession by 1920. The Flexner Report (an evaluation of medical schools by the Carnegie Foundation) was responsible for the closure of six of the eight black medical schools and the majority of church-affiliated medical schools, which were more willing to train women. As childbirth moved away from the home to the hospital, women's sense of helplessness and lack of control over their bodies increased. This trend continued uninterrupted until the 1960s, when women began to question and openly express their dissatisfaction with the medical profession's approach to women's reproductive health.

By the middle of the 20th century, the birth process was a medical event in the United States. Throughout the second half of the 20th century, pregnancy and childbirth underwent a remarkable transformation due to scientific, social, and political changes. It was during this time that family-centered and women-centered childbirth movements throughout the western world regained the philosophy of birth as a natural life event (Brodsky, 2008). Midwifery regained its place in the birth process and in the 1970s and 1980s, Dr. Michael Odent, French obstetrician, became one of its most forceful international advocates:

> *Unfortunately, the role of obstetrics has never been to help women give birth. There is a big difference between the medical discipline we call "obstetrics" and something completely different, the art of midwifery. If we want to find safe alternatives to obstetrics, we must rediscover midwifery. To rediscover midwifery is the same as giving back childbirth to women. And imagine the future if surgical teams were at the service of the midwives and the women instead of controlling them. (Odent, 2009)*

The 1960s and 1970s were pivotal decades in U.S. history. The women's health movement, inspired by the civil rights movement, emerged as part of the larger political and social change activism of that time and included women, people of color, gays and lesbians, college students, organized labor, and those opposed to the Vietnam War and U.S. imperialism (Morgen, 2009). The women's health movement challenged the traditional approach to providing health care for women and affirmed that women with all their diversity, not physicians, insurance companies, organized religion, or lawmakers, had the right to control the fundamental decisions regarding their bodies and reproductive lives.

The women's health movement and the second wave of the women's liberation emerged during the 1960s and 1970s. This multifaceted women's health movement has framed beyond reproductive health. The second wave of the women's liberation movement, also inspired by the civil rights movement, offered a critique of gender inequalities and oppression in all aspects of women's lives, including their health or the lack of it. Through the lens of a gendered analysis, grassroots groups all over the country began to question women's treatment by medical professionals. The women's health movement "brought a feminist perspective to health issues affecting women. They examined power relationships among individuals and between individuals and systems" (Wilcox, 2002).

One of the main contributions of the women's health movement was the exposé of unnecessary treatments and procedures to which women were subjected, including unnecessary hysterectomies, cesarean sections, forced sterilization, mastectomies, inadequate testing of birth control products, and the exclusion of women from health services and policies affecting women. Other major contributions were the decriminalization of abortion and the expansion of women's reproductive rights; knowledge about women as biological, anatomical, physiological, and psychological beings; patients as partners with their physicians in prevention and treatment of disease; women's rightful place in the practice of medicine and health administration; women's involvement in health policy; and the development and

implementation of a fair healthcare system for people (Morgen, 2009).

Springing from women's desire to define their own sexuality and to reclaim the birthing experience, many of the earliest challenges focused on reproductive health issues. Groups such as the Boston Women's Health Collective (1984) began to develop their own knowledge base and to encourage women's self-confidence and self-reliance in health-related matters. A valuable contribution to women's health has been their book, *Our Bodies, Ourselves: A Book by and for Women.* The first edition was published in 1970 and sold millions of copies. The 1984 edition established itself as the guide for women's health and has been translated into 19 languages (Morgen, 2009), and the new edition for a new century and new generation was published in 2005 (Wells, 2009). *Our Bodies, Ourselves* has been framed by North American white feminism. To address this narrow framework, the book was rewritten in 2000 in Spanish and with collaboration from over 30 Latin American and Caribbean health groups and U.S. Latinas, with expertise in the intersection of language, gender, culture, and health promotion (Shapiro, 2009).

The women's health movement combated the unnecessary medicalization of women's lives stemming from the hegemony of the medical profession through numerous self-help activities related to gynecologic health. A national network of Feminist Women's Health Clinics developed new models of self-examination and treatment. A revival of midwifery and home birth was accompanied by pressure on hospitals to allow natural childbirth and partner's presence and participation at birth, giving more control to women and their families. Central to the changes enacted by the women's health movement was a health-promoting orientation in contrast with the prevailing disease-oriented medical model. Inherent in the framework of self-education and self-help are notions of prevention including diet, natural remedies, exercise, and stress reduction techniques to ease the discomforts of conditions ranging from menstrual cramps to pregnancy and childbirth to menopause.

As in all social movements, the beliefs and methods promoted by different segments of the women's health movement vary widely. Differences exist in the emphasis on developing alternatives to traditional medicine versus demanding changes in the healthcare system and the education of healthcare providers. Some groups have worked to create new models through their own counter institutions, whereas others have concentrated their efforts at the legislative level or targeted their demands toward professional associations, hospitals, or drug companies. For example, women's health groups have been critical advocates for the development of alternatives to radical mastectomy as well as the development of the female condom and vaginal microbicides to help reduce women's risk of contracting HIV/AIDS.

The politically charged issue of abortion illustrates the effectiveness of a dual strategy involving both approaches. Before the legalization of abortion in 1973, many women's networks made referrals to providers who were willing to perform abortions and who were known to be competent and trustworthy. At least one group, the Jane Collective in Chicago, became trained as lay abortion providers and helped thousands of women terminate their pregnancies without medical complications or economic exploitation. At the same time, broad coalitions were organizing, advocating and demonstrating to change the country's laws in order to make legal and safe abortions available to all women in the United States.

After abortion was legalized in the United States, some women in the abortion rights movement expanded their agenda to encompass more comprehensive reproductive rights. Groups such as the San Francisco-based Coalition for the Medical Rights of Women organized against sterilization abuse, to improve the quality of Pap smear screening, and to provide information to daughters

and sons whose mothers have taken DES (diethylstilbestrol). Reproductive rights represented a wide array of needs required for women to decide freely whether or not to have children. True reproductive freedom was understood to imply the guarantee of adequate income, housing, child care, health services, schools, and other necessities for bringing up children. The reproductive rights movement recognized the need to ally with other groups struggling to ensure such conditions and attempted to address social disparities in access to health and other services. In recent years, groups such as the National Black Women's Health Imperative, National Latina Health Organization, Native American Women's Health Education Resource Center, and Asian-Pacific Resource and Research Center for Women have provided new leadership to invigorate the reproductive rights movement and expand the women's health agenda to be more responsive to women in different communities and more inclusive of women of color (Fried, 1990; Kumanyika, et al., 2001; Worcester & Whatley, 1994).

At the federal level, the Office of Minority Health (OMH) was established by the U.S. Department of Health and Human Services in 1985 with a mission to improve and protect the health of racial and ethnic underrepresented populations through the development of health policies and programs to eliminate health disparities. The Office of Minority Health also advises the Secretary of Health and Human Services on public health activities involving racial and ethnic minority populations.

Attention to inequities in health outcomes and access to health care has expanded the purview of the women's health movement beyond reproductive issues and into the areas of healthcare financing, healthcare delivery systems, and medical research. Federally funded clinical research had for years excluded women, as concerns about drug toxicity in pregnancy limited women's participation in clinical trials. Diseases that affected women disproportionately were less likely to be studied. The Society for Women's Health Research, through the General Accounting Office, uncovered the lack of accountability by the National Institutes of Health (NIH) in enforcing its guidelines established in 1986 to include women as subjects in federally funded research (Greenberger & Marts, 2000a). The Society for Women's Health Research, the National Women's Health Network, and other groups were critical in changing the National Institutes of Health (NIH) policy that had excluded women from participating in clinical trials as well as in developing the congressionally mandated policy (PL 103-93), instituted in 1993, which requires the inclusion of women and minorities in federally funded clinical research. These groups were also instrumental in the formation of the Office of Research on Women's Health (ORWH) at the NIH in 1990 and directing health research to address issues of specific concern to women. The Women's Health Initiative was launched by the director of ORWH, Bernadine Healy. This large clinical trial of over 16,000 women was designed to evaluate the risks and benefits of hormone replacement therapy. The Women's Health Initiative represented a national commitment to begin to address the impact on women of all major morbidities, not just reproductive risks.

Other early research initiatives included studies to test the effectiveness of the drug tamoxifen in preventing breast cancer. Recent issues of concern have included access to emergency contraception, affordable prescription drug coverage, and HIV prevention and treatment. Campaigns to improve maternity services have recently branched out into consumer movements to force insurance companies to cover longer postpartum hospitalizations and legislative efforts to require employers to offer parental leave.

The inclusion of women and the analysis of data based on the sex of the study subjects are essential to understand all aspects of the disease process (Ramasubbu, Gurm, & Litaker, 2001; Vidaver, Lafleur, Tong, Bradshaw,

& Marts, 2000). Besides, new approaches, including paradigms for modeling women's reproductive system, are necessary to further our understanding of disease etiology (Harlow, et al., 1999). Vidaver et al. (2000, p. 503) reinforced this point in stating that "until potential differences in responses to treatment and interventions between women and men are adequately addressed, we cannot be satisfied that sex-specific adverse events are unlikely to occur." The development and refinement of the NIH guidelines in 1993 were both a response and a spur to increasing surveillance of women's health needs. In 1994, a national conference was convened under the leadership of the American Psychological Association "aimed at developing a specific agenda to address the psychosocial aspects of women's health care" (Voelker, 1994, p. 7). The Centers for Disease Control and Prevention also announced the opening of an Office of Women's Health. According to Reuben Warren, the Centers for Disease Control and Prevention's Associate Director for Minority Health, "Without an effective women's health movement, the health of the nation cannot improve" (Voelker, 1994, p. 7). A major challenge is to prioritize scientific opportunities that will close the gap in knowledge and provide tangible benefits for women (Mosca, et al., 2001). Mosca et al. (2001) identified several barriers to women's health research. These included a lack of funding, recognition, acceptance, or sensitivity by researchers and a lack of the appropriate infrastructure for interdisciplinary research.

Since the Clinton administration, changes in the Medicaid system have raised alarm about the insurance status and access to care for low-income women. Medicaid currently finances prenatal care and deliveries for a large proportion of U.S. women, and it also funds family planning and other services for many others. Lack of healthcare coverage is a threat for many women. In 2007, 7 of every 10 women aged 19 to 64 years in the United States were uninsured, underinsured, had a problem with a medical bill, or had not accessed needed care (Rustgi, Doty, & Collins, 2009). Furthermore, many low-income women experience a gap in healthcare coverage during the time after childbearing and before they are eligible for Medicare. This gap has both short- and long-term implications for the health of this population. In the short term, these women may not have access to services when they are needed. In the long term, this lack of coverage may affect the health status of low-income women over time and increase overall healthcare expenditures, as limited access to preventive health services may make this population more vulnerable to illness and disease later in life (Strobino, Grason, & Minkovitz, 2002). Of particular concern are women with conditions such as diabetes and/or hypertension that are frequently exacerbated by childbirth. The passage of the Patient Protection and Affordable Care Act in 2010 may improve low-income women's access to health care, but its implementation is incremental and uncertain as of this writing.

The women's health movement has been the most salient factor in the increase of women in clinical and academic medicine, as Morgen states, "These changes have been catalyzed and shaped by the concerted and continuing activism of the women's health movement and the institutional, cultural, and political changes the movement helped provoke and shape" (Morgen, 2009, pp. 161–162). Prior to 1970, the great majority of physicians were males, who created a gendered medical culture that viewed the few women students as anomalies (Brodsky, 2008; Rogers, 2009). Since then, the number of women physicians has increased from 25,401 or 7.6% of all physicians in 1970 to 276,417 or 30% in 2008 (Boulis & Jacobs, 2008; Morgen, 2009; Smart, 2010). The increase has been mostly among white women (70%), followed by Asian American women (18%), African American women (6.2%), Latinas (5%), and Native American/Alaskan Native women (0.02%) (Morgen,

2009). It has been suggested that physician gender may influence the quality and cost effectiveness of the treatment of disease or health conditions that are sexually related, culturally sensitive, or involve parental privacy. Research shows that male primary care physicians seem to be more confident in providing male-specific preventive screening, compared to other primary care physicians. Additionally, gender differences in medical training and experience may contribute to different treatment approaches. For example, in treating older women with an early stage of breast cancer, male surgeons tend to recommend a mastectomy, whereas female surgeons are more likely to recommend lumpectomy and adjuvant therapy (Boulis & Jacobs, 2008, p. 135). Women's health is significantly affected by the delivery of health care and its practitioners. However, women have been disproportionately encouraged to enter primary care fields and discouraged from pursuing subspecialties of surgery and medicine (Cavalcanti de Aguiar, 2009).

Recent publications suggest that the present healthcare system has deficient knowledge about treating subpopulations of women, such as lesbian, bisexual, and transgender women and women with disabilities (McDonald, McIntyre, & Anderson, 2003; Roberts, 2001; Solarz, 1999; Thierry, 1998, 2000). However these recent publications aim to improve knowledge and stimulate further research in these areas. For example, over the past decade, research on lesbian health emerged as an important field of study. A recent report on lesbian health by the Institute of Medicine identified the gaps in research and provided recommendations for future directions (Roberts, 2001; Solarz, 1999). Moreover, recent reports from the Office on Disability and Health at the Centers for Disease Control and Prevention provide further insight into the health and well-being of the 26 million women with disabilities in the United States (Thierry, 1998, 2000).

Over the last quarter century, the U.S. women's health movement has expanded its scope by forging stronger links with international women's health advocacy groups. Consciousness about the interrelationship of women here and abroad has been heightened by issues such as (1) the testing of contraceptives on women in developing countries before Food and Drug Administration (FDA) approval for U.S. distribution and (2) the international targeting of women as potential consumers of exported cigarettes while outreach increases to warn U.S. women about the hazards of smoking. At the same time, grassroots empowerment efforts by women in many parts of the globe provide inspiration for organizing efforts in the United States. International gatherings such as the meetings on international population issues in Cairo in 1994 and on women's rights in Beijing in 1995, combined with electronic communication and computer technology, have increasingly united women's efforts to improve their health and social status throughout the world.

Women's health cannot be adequately understood without discussing the role of gender on the maintenance of health and the prevention and treatment of disease (Pinn, 2003; Strickland, 1988; Verbrugge, 1989; Verbrugge & Wingard, 1987). Since the 1980s, sex and gender have been among the most applied but poorly understood concepts within health research. Sex differentials in morbidity and mortality have been widely researched. Some examples are health and well-being (Grimmell & Stern, 1992; Lane & Meleis, 1991; Low Dog & Maize, 2010; Nakano, 1990; Rathgeber & Vlassoff, 1993; Williams, Weibe, & Smith, 1992), mental health and stress (Allgood, Lewinsohn, & Hops, 1990; Anson, Levenson, & Bonneh, 1990; Avison & McAlpine, 1992; Barnett & Marshal, 1992; Costello, 1991; Desai & Jann, 2000; Gillespie & Eisler, 1992; Groer, Thomas, & Shoffner, 1992; Janes, 1990; Kane, 1991; Meisler, 1999, 2000; Napholz, 1992; Nuess & Zubenko, 1992; Radke-Yarrow, Nottelmann, Belmont, & Welsh, 1993; Woods, Lentz, & Michell, 1993; Zimmerman-Tansella & Lattanzi,

1991), cardiovascular disease (Brinton, et al., 2010; Elliott, 1994; Greenberger, 1999; Helmers, et al., 1993; Knox & Follmann, 1993; Low Dog & Maize, 2010; Ramasubbu, et al., 2001; Roger, et al., 2000; Rosser, 2009; Suarez, Harlan, Peoples, & Williams, 1993; Theorell, 1991), musculoskeletal disorders, and liver diseases (Greenberger, 1999), and use of healthcare services beyond pregnancy-related services (Ramasubbu, et al., 2001). Researchers have found sex differences at the basic level of gene expression (Greenberger, 2002; Greenberger & Marts, 2000b), and biomedical research has provided evidence of sex differences in nearly all organs and systems of the human body (Greenberger & Knab, 2002). Sex and gender have been used as synonymous terms in most of these studies. However, sex and gender have very different meanings and measure very distinct components of the continuum of health and disease.

Sex is biologically determined by the laws of genetics through the arrangement of chromosomes that result in phenotypes (groups of people with similar genetically and environmentally produced physical appearances) and genotypes (groups of people with similar genetic structures) (de los Rios, 1994; de los Rios & Gomez, 1992; Gomez, 1990; Kane, 1991; Low Dog & Maize, 2010). It can usually be measured easily by using the biological categories of male and female. Thus, sex (female or male) has a biologic base and is usually clearly defined by specific anatomic and physiologic traits.

In contrast, gender is socially determined. It is rooted in the biological differences between the sexes, but it relates to the roles assigned by society to the female and male sexes. As yet, universal measurements of gender are not well defined. Gender is expressed through relationships of power and subordination, which translate into assigned roles, norms, activities, and behaviors expected to be performed by women and men in each society (Alexander & LaRosa, 1994; Amit, Bean, McDonald, Stuart, & Stuart, 1989; Arango,

1992; Canadian Council for International Co-operation, 1991; de los Rios, 1994; de los Rios & Gomez, 1992; Gomez, 1990, 1994, 2000; J. E. Austin Associates & The Collaborative for Development Action, Inc., 1989; Kane, 1991; Moser, 1989; Rathgeber & Vlassoff, 1993). The conditions of women's and men's daily lives and their positions within society are expressed in beliefs, attitudes, and behaviors (de los Rios & Gomez, 1992; Gomez, 1990; Moser, 1989). To be a man or a woman is to be associated with different behaviors and attitudes in public and private life.

The construct of gender has been shaped by historical circumstance and is susceptible to changes in policies associated with social, economic, judicial, and political events. According to de los Rios and Gomez (1992), the core of the gender construct is the sex-based division of labor, which is expressed in the segregation of social functions on the basis of belonging to either the female or male sex. The sexual division of labor is a historical product—not a natural aspect of society (Castellanos, 1987). It is the basis by which societies ensure their social reproduction. It guarantees both the biologic reproduction (childbearing and rearing responsibilities) and the social reproduction of society, which shapes its production mode, social and political institutions, and patterns of social relationships (Castellanos, 1987; de los Rios & Gomez, 1992).

As a means of ensuring the social reproduction of society, women's lives are structured to revolve around multiple social roles, needs, and expectations (J. E. Austin Associates & The Collaborative for Development Action, Inc., 1989; Meleis & Lindgren, 2002). These roles form a dynamic web bringing together sex and gender attributes, including age and physical environments (de los Rios & Gomez, 1992). Age is directly related to the cycles in women's lives that trigger not only biological but also political and social changes at the individual and societal levels (Arango, 1992). Throughout the world, the social roles assigned to most women dictate their use of physical space (Arango, 1992; de los Rios & Gomez, 1992). The spaces where women spend most of their time are directly influenced by social class, race, ethnicity, and family dynamics. Private and public spaces (e.g., school, home, church, workplace) are the cradles of socialization for girls and women. In addition, physical environments influence women's social support and networks, which can be affective, social, or occupational in nature. However, the separations between the private and public spheres are not as clearly delineated. For example, 39% of women's fatal injuries in the workplace are due to homicide, yet many of the homicides are perpetrated by spouses or partners, bringing together the private and public (Meleis & Lindgren, 2002).

The options that shape women's lives, including marital status, religion, and political ideology, are directly linked to gender constructs. Gender relationships and identities are not universal but vary from culture to culture and sometimes from community to community. They are dynamic and change over time (de los Rios & Gomez, 1992; Gomez, 1994). The analysis of gender in research needs to take into account all these aspects as well as women's heterogeneity. The construct of gender assumes specific meaning depending upon political milieu, culture, race, ethnicity, and social class (de los Rios, 1994; de los Rios & Gomez, 1992; Gomez, 1994). Despite their heterogeneity, in most societies, women are generally disadvantaged compared with men in relationship to social and sex roles and, subsequently, with regard to services and opportunities. Thus, women are exposed more than men to gender-based violence, sexual discrimination, social displacement, and poverty (de los Rios & Gomez, 1992; Meleis & Lindgren, 2002). Women's health in the new millennium, as framed by the United Nations Fourth Conference on Women, is affected by emotional, social, cultural, spiritual and physical well-being, which in turn is influenced by the social, political, and the economic circumstances of women's lives as well as their biology. Moreover, women's health is more than data analyses by sex. A gendered approach is required to understand women's health and provide appropriate health care for women. This approach weaves the attributes that women share biologically and socially, as well as their differences among women, including their social, cultural, sexual, physical, and economic realities. Through this approach, gender is to be considered in relation to the points of intersection with the multiple factors that have an impact on women's health (Armstrong, et al., 2008).

WOMEN'S HEALTH: A LIFE CYCLE

Note: To do justice in one chapter to women's health throughout the life cycle is an impossible task. Thus, the aim of this section is to highlight aspects of women's health from a life cycle perspective.

The influence of biology, cultural roles and behaviors, and social status on health differs greatly between women and men. Women live longer than men worldwide. In addition, as life expectancy increases for both women and men, the gap tends to widen. However, the biological responsibility for human reproduction has been historically a primary cause of women's morbidity and mortality. Although reproductive mortality and morbidity are still realities for women in many countries, the differences between women's and men's health exist from the time of conception to death, and human reproduction is only part of the life cycle. The conceptualization of women's health throughout life reflects the interconnection of the different life stages and their relationship to the health of women and future generations.

In Utero

The theory of the developmental origin of adult health and disease lends support to viewing women's health from a life course perspective. The leading cause of death in women, heart disease, is a chronic disease. As this condition rarely develops in reproductive age women, our efforts at primary and secondary prevention have focused on women as they enter the menopausal transition. However, there is strong evidence to suggest that the risk for heart disease may begin *in utero*. Barker and Osmond first reported their suspicions in 1986, in an article that discussed geographical patterns of infant mortality and ischemic heart disease mortality in England and Wales (Barker & Osmond, 1986). Briefly, the authors found that the highest rates of mortality from heart disease were in less affluent areas and that trends in cardiovascular disease mortality were correlated with trends in infant mortality in these areas. The authors concluded that nutrition during the prenatal and postnatal period predisposed some children to heart disease in adulthood.

Subsequent work on this topic found that small birth size, an indicator of poor prenatal diet, was associated with the development of heart disease in midlife (Barker, 1990). Barker hypothesized that "undernutrition *in utero* and during infancy permanently changes the body's structure, physiology, and metabolism and leads to coronary heart disease and stroke in adult life" (Barker, 2007 p. 414). This hypothesis was tested and confirmed in several subsequent analyses. Rich-Edwards analyzed data from the Nurses' Health Study to examine this relationship between birth weight and nonfatal adult cardiovascular disease. This work showed that birth weight was inversely related to nonfatal adult cardiovascular disease, and that this relationship remained strong, even after adjusting for adult lifestyle factors such as cigarette smoking, body mass index, elevated cholesterol levels, and socioeconomic status (Rich-Edwards, et al., 1997). In sum, chronic diseases such as cardiovascular disease are actually part of a developmental process that occurs over the course of a woman's lifespan (Rich-Edwards, et al., 2010).

Infancy

The sex ratio estimate at conception (primary sex ratio) is 107 male embryos per every 100 female embryos (CIA Factbook, 2010). Although miscarriages in the first month of pregnancy are thought to be frequent, little is known about their sex distribution. Males are more likely to be stillborn because of difficult labor, birth injuries, and diseases or injuries of the mother, whereas deaths of females *in utero* are more likely to be caused by congenital malformations (Kane, 1991). In some countries, female fetuses are targets of abortions for the purpose of sex selection (Jha, et al., 2006). More recently, the discussion of sex selection has moved toward the use of assisted reproductive technologies and the preimplantation selection of embryos. However, its use remains controversial and subject to debate (Gleicher & Karande, 2002; Robertson, 2003). Thus, fetal survival is related to biological and genetic factors and is influenced by maternal health, personal decisions, social values, obstetrical care, and other environmental factors (Bandyopadhyay, 2003).

More males than females are born. The sex ratio of live births (secondary sex ratio) is approximately 102–106 males to 100 females (World Health Organization, 2011). However, this ratio is not universal. In some Asian countries, including China and India, the ratio is higher than average; in some African countries, it is lower (Kane, 1991; United Nations, 2000; World Health Organization, 2011). The sex ratio difference could be due to selective abortion, sex differences in risk for fetal mortality, or ineffective birth registration systems. People may not register births that are followed by the death of the infant (Bandyopadhyay, 2003). Parents may be less likely to register an infant girl in countries where girl children are less valued than males, as a girl has a lower chance of

survival in such countries. Presently, there are 100 million females unaccounted for worldwide, and sex preference may be the reason. The preference for a son is associated with the perception of women's meager economic potential. Both women and men have expressed a strong preference for boys in many countries. However, the son preference is especially prevalent in Hindu, Moslem, and Chinese societies (Bandyopadhyay, 2003; Kane, 1991) (**Table 11–2**).

Infants of both sexes are at risk of dying during the early weeks after birth. The causes of death are related to complications of pregnancy, childbirth, congenital abnormalities, prematurity, low weight for gestational age, and inadequate postnatal care. Infant mortality in general is also associated with poverty, social inequities, and a lack of access to adequate sources of health care (Kane, 1991).

Childhood

Death rates begin to fall after the first year of life. The risk of dying is two times higher for children ages 1 to 4 years than children ages 5 to 14 years (Arias, MacDorman, Strobino, & Guyer, 2003; Kane, 1991). In developed

Table 11–2 Sex Ratio at Birth—Five Countries with Strong Preference for Sons.

Country	Boys Born per 100 Girls
China	118
Egypt	105
India	108
Pakistan	105
Republic of Korea	110

Source: United Nations Department of Economic and Social Affairs, Population Division, Population Estimates and Projections Section. *World population prospects,* The 2010 Revision. [Online Database], Detailed indicators. Retrieved May 16, 2011 from http://esa.un.org/unpd/wpp/unpp/panel_indicators.htm.

countries boys die at a higher rate than girls, primarily because of a higher mortality rate due to intentional and unintentional injuries (Kishor, 1993). In countries with strong son preferences, child survival has been documented to favor boys (Li, et al., 2004). According to the World Health Organization (WHO, 1992, p. 20), "Gender discrimination is found throughout the world, from birth onwards. Research on disease prevalence, health care utilization and family resource allocation indicates that girls are treated differently from boys, with negative results that last for a lifetime." In societies with son preference, baby girls may be breastfed for a shorter time and thus may be exposed at an early age to contaminated or poor quality foods. In addition, a daughter may get less food and less medical and preventive health care (Frongillo & Bégin, 1993; Kane, 1991; Shrestha, 1990; Singh, 1990; United Nations, 2000). It has been argued by some that better feeding and caring for boys is not so much discrimination against girls as it is a way to compensate for boys' biological disadvantages. However, it is difficult to accept these practices as an impartial way to deal with boys' vulnerabilities.

Health information about school-aged children (5 to 14 years old) is limited, as studies and reports rarely address sex differentials among school-age children. Selwyn (1990) found in reviewing community surveys that the incidence rates of acute and upper respiratory infections were only slightly higher for boys than girls, but boys were very often the main users of inpatient or outpatient hospital services for those conditions. In England, boys 0 to 14 years old have higher total rates of hospitalization than girls (Kane, 1991). The main causes of illness and hospitalization among school-aged children across the world are infectious and parasitic diseases; upper and lower respiratory infections; congenital anomalies; signs, symptoms, and ill-defined conditions; and injury and poisoning. Evidence suggests that many countries underreport illness episodes for school-aged

girls, suggesting that illness among boys tends to be taken more seriously than sickness among girls (Williams, Baumslag, & Jelliffe, 1994).

Children are frequent targets of violence, abuse, and neglect. In 2009, 3.6 million children in the United States were the subjects of a child protective services investigation or assessment, of which 20% were found to have experienced abuse or neglect (U.S. Department of Health and Human Services, 2010). Girls (51.1%) are slightly more likely than boys (48.2%) to be victims of maltreatment. Research indicates that as abused children become adolescents, they have elevated risks of substance use, suicide attempts, aggressive behavior, anorexia and bulimia, pregnancy, depression, and running away.

In some countries, girls and young women experience cultural practices that place them at risk of morbidity and mortality (Almroth-Berggren, Almroth, Hassanei, El Hadi, & Lithell, 2001; Toubia, 1994). The practice of female genital mutilation is one example. Worldwide, approximately 100 to 140 million women and girls have undergone genital mutilation (Almroth-Berggren, et al., 2001; World Health Organization, 2000). This practice is widespread and has been documented in 28 African countries as well as in Malaysia, Indonesia, Yemen, along the Persian Gulf, among some communities in Mexico, Brazil, Peru, and among migrants from these regions to Europe, North America, and Australia (Almroth-Berggren, et al., 2001; Crossete, 1995). England and France have responded by outlawing genital mutilation. It is now recognized internationally as a violation of the human rights women and girls (WHO Study Group, 2000). Egypt banned the practice in 2008, as did Uganda in 2010.

There is not a set age for this cultural practice, which ranges from infancy to adulthood, but it is most commonly practiced from infancy to age 15. The procedures are traditionally performed by women known to the girl, in her home, and without anesthesia. However, it is increasingly practiced by medical professionals. In 1994, the International Federation of Gynecology and Obstetrics passed a resolution opposing the medicalization of this procedure. There are three types of female circumcision: (1) clitoridectomy—the removal of the skin over the clitoris or the tip of the clitoris; (2) excision—removal of the entire clitoris and the labia minora without closing the vulva; and (3) infibulation—encompassing the two previous mutilations plus removing part of the labia majora and stitching it together, leaving just a small opening to allow the release of urine and menstrual fluid (Shell-Ducan & Hernlund, 2000; Smyke, 1993; Toubia, 1994).

Girls and women undergoing these procedures experience short- and long-term effects. Soon after the surgery, women may experience pain, shock, hemorrhage, retention of urine, infection, fever, or tetanus. Death may be an outcome if the girl or woman does not have appropriate medical care to deal with complications. Throughout the life cycle, women subsequently experience pelvic infections, sometimes so severe that the fallopian tubes get blocked, and chronic pain. Urinary tract infections are common, and women develop cysts and scar tissue. Most women experience problems with the flow of menstrual blood. The first intercourse is extremely painful for women who have undergone infibulation. If the vaginal opening is too small, the husband or midwife has to cut the scar to enlarge the opening. Female genital mutilation increases the risk of labor complications, cesarean section, postpartum hemorrhage and neonatal death (WHO, 2006). These women also tend to have labor complications. The most common is obstructed labor, which may bring additional complications (hemorrhage, tearing of the perineal tissue, urinary or rectal fistulae, and possible prolapsed uterus) (Toubia, 1994). Giving birth does not free infibulated women; they are stitched back into their prebirth status. Though most circumcised women do not feel free to talk about sexual

matters, a few understandably have reported unresponsiveness and anxiety connected with intercourse (Toubia, 1994).

Tradition is the main reason for the perpetuation of a practice that inflicts pain, suffering, adverse health sequelae, and sometimes even death of girls and women. For some women and men, it is a symbol of belonging and shared heritage (Shell-Ducan & Hernlund, 2000). For example, in the western part of Sierra Leone, 90% of women are circumcised (Smyke, 1993). In this region, female circumcision is the ritual of passage into women's secret societies, and the desire to be accepted into the society outweighs other considerations. Another reason often given is religion. However, according to Muslim and Christian scholars, nowhere in the Qur'an or the Bible is there a female circumcision requirement (Smyke, 1993). Parents often state that they have the girl's best interest in mind—a girl who does not undergo the procedure will be socially unacceptable without a chance for marriage. The cultural issue has been challenged by Dr. Nafis Sadikon, who stated at the Fourth World Women's Conference, "The function of culture and tradition is to provide a framework for human well-being. If they are used against us, we will reject them" (Crossete, 1995, p. 18). Many African and Asian women reject the claim that female genital mutilation must be understood in a cultural context. Furthermore, women health professionals from Africa have been outspoken against the practice of female circumcision. The Inter-African Committee on Traditional Practices Affecting the Health of Women and Children has been established to unite and to empower Africans working to abolish female circumcision and other dangerous cultural practices.

Teen Years

Adolescence has been recognized as the most turbulent stage in the life cycle because of the extent of physiologic changes and social role development (Cothran & White, 2002; Muuss, 1988). Young women and men go through drastic biological changes during their adolescence. The sex hormones responsible for these major changes—estrogens and androgens—are present in both sexes (Whatley, 1994). Women tend to have higher levels of estrogens than androgens and men the reverse; however, there is not a defined ratio of these hormones, and there is a great deal of individual variation. Unfortunately, much emphasis has been placed on the differences and very little on the similarities between adolescent boys and girls. Consequently, sexuality becomes defined in terms of hormones and culturally circumscribed sex roles, instead of common areas such as affection, love, and sexual rights and responsibilities.

Although they are the least likely to die of natural causes, adolescents are notorious for their risk-taking behavior (Banister & Schreiber, 2001). Injury and poisoning are *the* major causes of death in the teen years. Morbidity associated with risk-taking behavior is exemplified by the high rates of sexually transmitted infections (STIs) and the spread of HIV/AIDS among young people. (In order to be consistent with the new terminology recommended by the World Health Organization, the term sexually transmitted disease has been replaced with STIs in this chapter.)

An estimated 19 million new STI cases occur among the U.S. population each year, of which 48% occur in adolescents aged 15 to 24 years of age (Weinstock, et al., 2004). The most reported STI in the United States is chlamydia, with 3 million new cases annually (Weinstock, et al., 2004). Teen females have the highest rate of infection, as young women aged 15 to 19 years account for 46% of chlamydia cases in the United States (Cothran & White, 2002). The cost of the infection is estimated to be $2 million per year. One of the consequences of untreated chlamydia is the subsequent development of pelvic inflammatory disease. Human papillomavirus (HPV) is a common STI in the United States, as it is estimated that 6.2 million new HPV infections occur each year (Weinstock, et al., 2004). Both STIs are preventable and diagnosable. Frequent screening has been recommended to ensure early diagnosis. HPV is now known to be the principal cause of cervical cancer, and two vaccines have been approved by the U.S. Food and Drug Administration to prevent the most high-risk types of HPV.

STIs present greater risk and complications to women than men. Women experience pain, infertility, increased risk of ectopic pregnancy, pelvic inflammatory disease, and psychological distress. As most societies have a sexual double standard for women and men, STIs can be a source of shame and embarrassment for women. When a woman finds out that she has STI, she may experience denial, hurt, feelings of victimization, anger, fear, shame, or loss of control over her sexuality. Infection and the ensuing distress are compounded by the fact that women are more likely than men to live in poverty, and they have less access to comprehensive health care, including diagnostic screening, treatment, and follow-up services for STIs (Williams, et al., 1994; World Health Organization, 1992). Worldwide, 1 in 20 adolescents contract an STI each year (Bearinger, et al., 2007). Moreover, adolescents and young adults account for 40% of all new HIV infections worldwide (World Health Organization, 2010).

Teenagers face difficult gender role expectations. Appearance can be a source of unhealthy practices among teenagers. For example, in the United States and European cultures, tall and well-muscled physiques are socially desirable for males; women are exhorted to be thin (Alexander & LaRosa, 1994; Hoskins, 2002; Mahowald, 1993). Unfortunately, some adolescents pay a high price for such characteristics and consequently develop serious health problems. Young men may seek growth hormone therapy to increase their height and/or steroidal treatment to increase their muscle mass. Young women may develop anorexia nervosa or bulimia nervosa in attempting to keep their weight down. Both eating disorders are identified with extreme preoccupation with food and body figure and image (Alexander & LaRosa, 1994; Hoskins, 2002). Anorexics may purge after eating even a small portion of food, whereas bulimics tend to starve themselves before a binge. Anorexia is very difficult to cure. It is a physically and psychologically debilitating disease. According to research in the United States, the feeling of being "fat" increases with age among young women from 50% in 14-year-olds to 70% in 18-year-olds (Mahowald, 1993). In sum, teenagers today are faced with a range of choices that were not even dreamed of two generations ago. At the same time, adolescents experience high levels of alienation, depression, injuries, and death. Furthermore, teenagers are being targeted as consumers for cigarettes, illicit drugs, alcohol, cars, and daring sports and physical activities, which increase the risk of injury and illness in the short term and may lead to chronic disease in adulthood.

Middle Years

In their middle years, women and men assume a number of new social roles and responsibilities and are the main contributors to the economic well-being of their societies. This stage of the life cycle has traditionally been associated with issues of human reproduction, marriage, and career. In the last hundred years, women's time spent in childbearing has been reduced from half to one-sixth of their lives. It was not so long ago that women could not expect to live long enough to enjoy their grandchildren. Presently, in many cultures, women survive pregnancy and childbirth and have increased life spans, partly because of the implementation of public health interventions and partly because of access to advances in medicine and medical technology.

Besides pregnancy, women of reproductive age may experience health conditions that affect the uterus. Among those conditions are fibroids, endometriosis, heavy bleeding during the menstrual cycle, and pelvic pain. Currently, the medical field has deficient knowledge about these conditions and lacks holistic approaches to effectively deal with them. Fibroids and excessively heavy bleeding are among the leading causes of hysterectomy in the United States. Among women in their forties, one in 45 will be diagnosed with endometriosis, one in 24 with heavy bleeding, and one in 12 with uterine fibroids (Merrill, et al., 2008). Hysterectomy is the most common nonobstetric surgery for women, approximately 45% of U.S. women having had a hysterectomy by age 70. Damage to the pelvic floor muscles and ligaments secondary to pregnancy and childbirth may lead to urinary incontinence and uterine prolapse in many women. One in 61 women in their 40s and one in 13 women in their 60s are diagnosed with prolapse (Merrill, et al., 2008). Among women 20 years of age and older, 50% report symptoms of urinary incontinence or involuntary loss of urine, with the prevalence of significant incontinence increasing with age (Dooley, et al., 2008). In the United States, white and Mexican American women are more likely than black women to report stress incontinence, defined as urine loss occurring with physical activity, such as sneezing, coughing, or exercise. Black and Mexican-American women are more likely than White women to report urge incontinence, defined as sudden urge to urinate and frequent urination. Women with higher parity and obese women are more likely to report incontinence of urine.

STIs remain a health condition of concern in adult women, with 177 million cases reported of the four major STIs (trichomoniasis, chlamydia, gonorrhea, and syphilis) among women worldwide (World Health Organization, 2001). Untreated STIs have serious short- and long-term consequences for women's general health. For example, untreated infections and pelvic inflammatory disease are considered to be the major causes of disease-related infertility. Worldwide, there are approximately 50 to 80 million people with infertility problems (United Nations, 2000) with approximately 9% of couples experiencing infertility, or difficulty conceiving after one year of trying to get pregnant (Boivin, et al., 2007). Although male factors account for about half of the burden of infertility, women often bear the burden of infertility and are usually the targets for screening and treatment (Vayena, Rowe, & Griffin, 2002).

Women assume multiple roles in most societies today, and in 2008 they comprised 40% of the world's labor force (International Labour Office, 2009). In 2010, women comprised 46.8% of the U.S. labor force (U.S. Department of Labor, 2010). In addition, more women are remaining in the labor force during their childbearing years. Women are responsible for 50% of production in industrialized countries and 60% in the developing world (Meleis & Lindgren, 2002). They also contribute $16 trillion dollars to the global economy with their unremunerated work (Meleis & Lindgren, 2002). Furthermore, women work more hours than men, often juggling responsibilities in both paid and unpaid positions. However, women earn less than men, especially in cases in which women are the head of household (United Nations, 2000). International data show a direct relationship between female family headship and poverty (Williams, et al., 1994).

In general, both having a paid job and being married have health benefits for women and men. Men, however, tend to benefit more from being married (Haber, 1991; Klonoff & Landrine, 1991; Martikainen, 1995; Rosenfeld, 1992). According to Kane (1991), paid work and marriage generally have a synergistic and positive effect on the health status of women and men, but unemployed married men have worse health outcomes than unemployed unmarried men.

In contrast, women who are either single and employed or married and unemployed have more acute and chronic disabilities than married and employed women. These findings suggest that multiple roles may be related to women's status in the household. In African and Latin American countries where women are responsible for childbearing, at least 70% of food production, and approximately 50% of animal husbandry, the interactions among overwork, pregnancy, and malnutrition has serious health consequences. Women's work encompasses three roles: social production, social capital, and financial capital (Meleis & Lindgren, 2002).

Women everywhere work long hours. The workday of women in most countries is 16 hours. Despite modern appliances, Western housewives spend 56 hours per week working, whereas their counterparts in Pakistan works just 6 hours more (62 hours) per week (Williams, et al., 1994). Furthermore, it is important to note that the distribution of health and illness is influenced by social class, race and ethnicity, geographic location, and social indicators such as education, access to health services, occupational hazards, environmental factors, and a range of personal circumstances.

Women are responsible for the biological reproduction of humankind, and the experience of reproduction can have long-term consequences for women's health. In addition to the pelvic floor damage that can lead to incontinence and uterine prolapse discussed above, chronic illnesses developed during pregnancy, such as gestational diabetes and hypertension, place a woman at higher risk of developing these conditions later in life (Rich-Edwards, et al., 2010; Sattar & Greer, 2002). When these conditions are preexisting, they are frequently exacerbated by pregnancy. For example, women who developed gestational diabetes during pregnancy have up to a 45% chance that it will recur in a subsequent pregnancy and up to a 63% chance of developing Type II diabetes later in their lifetime (Centers for Disease Control and

Prevention, 2001). Furthermore, Peters and colleagues showed that a pregnancy complicated by gestational diabetes may accelerate the development of Type II diabetes in some women (Peters, et al., 1996). A similar association exists for hypertensive diseases during pregnancy and the development of cardiovascular disease. Women who developed preeclampsia during pregnancy have a 3.7 times increased risk of developing hypertension after a mean follow-up of 14 years and a 2.2 times increased risk of developing ischemic heart disease after a mean follow-up of 12 years. Thus, pregnancy may be viewed as a "stress test" for future chronic disease risk (Sattar & Greer, 2002).

This stress test is challenged further by the rising rates of obesity among women of reproductive age. Nearly one in four women 20–44 years of age in the United States is overweight (body mass index [BMI] 25.0–29.9 kg/m^2) and 23.0% were obese (BMI $\geq$ 30 kg/m^2) (Vahratian, 2009). Among those who were obese, 10.3% met the criteria for class II or III obesity (BMI $\geq$ 35 kg/m^2). Women who are obese prior to pregnancy have an increased risk for developing pregnancy complications such as gestational diabetes, gestational hypertension, and preeclampsia. They are also more likely to experience high postpartum weight retention, which places them at increased risk for Type II diabetes and cardiovascular disease later in life. Given the current epidemics of obesity and diabetes and the high prevalence of hypertension in African-Americans, increased attention to preventive health measures are critical during pregnancy.

Transitional Years

Significant changes in women's life patterns have occurred in the last 100 years. As mentioned earlier, women's life expectancy surpasses that of men in most countries, and women currently have approximately 30 years more to live compared with women a century ago. Thus, a considerable proportion of women's lives are spent in the postreproductive years. In 2009, there were an estimated 63 million women 45 years old and older in the United States (U.S. Census, 2010). Approximately 26% of women are between the ages of 54 and 64 years in the United States (U.S. Census, 2010). An interesting phenomenon affecting women's health is that the increase of women's life expectancy has not changed the average age for the onset of menopause (Baron-Hall & Vidaver, 2000), with the median age at menopause in the United States at 51.4 years (Gold, et al., 2001). The menopausal transition is characterized by two phases. During the early transition, which begins an average 5 to 7 years before the final menstrual period, women's menstrual cycles become more variable. The late menstrual transition is characterized by the occurrence of long menstrual cycles of 60 days of more that occur on average 2 years before menopause (Harlow, et al., 2006, 2007, 2008). The final menstrual period, or menopause, is defined as 12 consecutive months of no menses. Women who are currently experiencing the menopausal transition are challenging how society deals with the natural process of aging. Aging is a major phobia in the United States, whereas in some societies women's status increases with age.

Menopause (natural or surgically induced) has been until recently a social taboo—women talked about it only in whispers (Mingo, Herman, & Jasperse, 2000). Not long ago, physicians viewed menopause as the "death of the woman in the woman" (Braus, 1993). Avis and McKinlay (1995) conducted the first large prospective cohort study on menopause in the United States. They found that the majority of women undergoing natural menopause did not seek medical help, and their attitudes were overwhelmingly positive or neutral.

The menopausal transition does, however, represent a critical period for women as it is associated with time-limited risk of symptoms such as hot flashes, sleep disturbances, and depression, as well as accelerated change in bone mineral density, lipids, and physical functioning that can influence a woman's quality of life and likelihood of healthy aging (Matthews, et al., 2009; Neer, 2010; Sowers, et al., 2007). Some women experienced transitional depression, with the rate of depression increasing during the late transition and declining once again as women reach menopause and transition to postmenopause (Avis, et al., 2001; Bromberger, et al., 2010; Cohen, et al., 2006; Mingo, et al., 2000). Women with a history of depression are at particular risk during this period.

Endocrine changes of menopause are the main causes of physical and psychological symptoms (e.g., hot flashes, vaginal atrophy, weight gain, insomnia, mood changes, and depression), but not all women experience these symptoms. However, all women do experience an increase in follicle stimulating hormone beginning in the early transition and accelerating in the late transition as well as a dramatic decline in estrogen levels during the late transition (Burger, et al., 2007; Sowers, et al., 2006, 2008a, 2008b). Low estrogen levels and rapid decline in estrogen have been associated with an accelerated loss of bone mineral density (Neer, 2010), and adverse changes in lipid profiles have been documented to occur in the year immediately preceding and after the final menstrual period (Matthews, et al., 2009).

By the 1990s, hormone replacement therapy (HRT) had become the "magic bullet" to combat these risks, as it had been argued that HRT maintained the high-density lipoprotein and low-density lipoprotein levels at the premenopausal stage. In 1991, the Women's Health Initiative clinical trials were designed to test the effect of estrogen plus progestin on the risk of coronary heart disease and invasive breast cancer. Between 1993 and 1998, the Women's Health Initiative randomized 16,608 healthy postmenopausal women with an intact uterus to receive either estrogen plus progestin or a placebo (Women's Health Initiative Study

Group, 1998). However, this trial stopped on May 31, 2002, when the data and safety monitoring board concluded that evidence for breast cancer harm, along with evidence for some increase in coronary heart disease, stroke, and pulmonary embolism, outweighed the evidence of benefit for fractures and possible benefit for colon cancer over the average 5.2-year follow-up period (Writing Group for the Women's Health Initiative Investigators, 2002, p. 325).

It is important to note that the trial tested only one drug regimen, conjugated equine estrogen, 0.625 mg/day, plus medroxyprogesterone acetate, 2.5 mg/day, in postmenopausal women with an intact uterus (Writing Group for the Women's Health Initiative Investigators, 2002). The results of this trial generated an ongoing debate in the scientific literature, the medical community, and in the popular media about whether postmenopausal women should continue to take HRT. Presently, there is insufficient evidence that the results from this trial can be generalized to all forms of hormonal replacement therapy and a lack of consensus in the scientific community about the use of HRT remains (Dixon, 2002; Fletcher & Colditz, 2002; Stevenson & Whitehead, 2002; Warren, 2004). There are also questions on when to initiate hormone therapy, as some findings show that that hormone therapy should be initiated in the early transition before adverse changes in lipid profiles and arterial elasticity occur.

Over the past 2 decades, a considerable body of research from several large prospective studies of the menopausal transition has improved scientific understanding of menopause-related issues. Continuing attention to these emerging results are critical for decision-making regarding issues on the quality of life and health for a growing number of women worldwide.

Older Women

Older women live longer and are poorer than older men. Worldwide, millions of older women experience poverty, social isolation, and ill health. For example, nearly 60% of women aged 60 years or more are widowed in Northern Africa and Central Asia. In Northern Africa, this trend is due in part to women marrying older men, whereas in Central Asia, it is due in part to higher levels of male mortality (United Nations, 2000). In 2009, 13% of the U.S. population was 65 years of age and older (U.S. Census, 2010). Women constitute 58% of the older population and are more likely than men to live alone (U.S. Census, 2010). Thirteen percent of U.S. women aged 65 years and older live in poverty. However, a higher percentage of Latina and African American women age 65 years and over live in poverty (Kramarow, et al., 1999). According to Arendell and Estes (1991, p. 62), "Being old, female, and a member of a minority group represents a triple jeopardy." A consequence of longevity is the onset of diseases such as osteoporosis. Women reach their peak bone mass in their mid to late 20s (Meisler, 2000). This is also the time when women are engaged in dieting and other weight-control activities. Osteoporosis is the major public health risk for 28 million people, and 80% of them are women. Unfortunately, one of every two women over 50 years of age will have an osteoporosis-related fracture in her lifetime. Most of the time it is a hip fracture, which has long-lasting consequences in both quality of life and medical cost (Meisler, 2000).

Societal views on older women are not necessarily shared by the women themselves. Most older women do not consider themselves old if they are in good health (Moen, Dempster-McClain, & Williams, 1992). For this population, health is the key to remaining active and to participating meaningfully in society. Older women are organizing themselves and joining forces with women of all ages to improve their lives and to create a world where women can hold their rightful place in society.

FINAL THOUGHTS

Because women's health is heavily influenced by socioeconomic, environmental, and political trends as well as gender dynamics and other social relationships, new issues are constantly rising to the fore. In the last 2 decades, technological and political changes have had a tremendous impact, making available new means of reproduction such as in vitro fertilization and surrogacy and restricting access to abortion and family planning services as legislative mandates and funding have fluctuated. New legal and ethical dilemmas have arisen with the development and approval of long-acting hormonal contraceptives such as intrauterine devices, shots, and implants, which offer new forms of coitus-independent protection but also new potential for coercion in reproductive decision making.

Women continue to comprise an increasing proportion of the population affected by HIV infection. The tragedies of women's vulnerability to HIV/AIDS and their role in perinatal transmission have accentuated stark disparities in health—disproportionate numbers of poor women of color and their children are affected by HIV. The plague of substance abuse in these women's communities and soaring rates of other sexually transmitted diseases enhance their risk of HIV infection. Models of appropriate drug treatment services for women now exist, but moral judgments compound class and racial discrimination in restricting resource allocation for such badly needed services.

Little is known about the health effects of the combination of work and family responsibilities that most women now assume, and the concentration of women in low-wage, low-status occupations creates additional physical and psychological stresses. Advocacy by and for women continues to seek redress for health inequities and to pursue the long-term goal of universal health care for all women and their families.

References

Alexander, L. L., & LaRosa, J. H. (1994). *New dimensions in women's health*. Boston and London: Jones & Bartlett Publishers.

Allgood, M. B., Lewinsohn, P. M., & Hops, H. (1990). Sex differences and adolescent depression. *Journal of Abnormal Psychology, 99*, 56–63.

Almroth-Berggren, V., Almroth, L., Hassanei, O. M., El Hadi, N., & Lithell, U.-B. (2001). Reinfibulation among women in a rural area of central Sudan. *Health Care for Women International, 22*, 711–721.

Amit, H. R., Bean, W., MacDonald, A. A., Stuart, C., & Stuart, R. (1989). *A handbook for social/gender analysis*. Ottawa, Canada: Canadian International Development Agency, Social and Human Resources Development Division.

Anson, O., Levenson, A., & Bonneh, D. Y. (1990). Gender and health on the Kibbutz. *Sex-Roles, 22*, 213–235.

Arango, Y. (1992). Autocuidado: Una toma de decisión de la mujer frente a su salud. In Y. Arango (Ed.), *Mujer, salud y autocuidado: Memorias* (pp. 81–101). Washington, DC: Pan American Health Organization.

Arendell, T., & Estes, C. L. (1991). Older women in the post-Reagan era. *International Journal of Health Services, 21*, 59–73.

Arias, E., MacDorman, M. F., Strobino, D. M., & Guyer, B. (2003). Annual summary of vital statistics: 2002. *Pediatrics, 112*, 1215–1230.

Armstrong, P., Armstrong, H., & Scott-Dixon, K. (2008). *Critical health care: The invisible women in health care services*. Toronto: University of Toronto Press.

Avis, N. E., & McKinlay, S. M. (1995). The Massachusetts women's health study: An epidemiologic investigation of the menopause. *Journal of the American Medical Women's Association, 50*, 45–49.

Avis, N. E., Crawford, S., Stellato, R., & Longcope, C. (2001). Longitudinal study of hormone levels and depression among women transitioning through menopause. *Climacteric, 4*, 243–249.

Avison, W. R., & McAlpine, D. D. (1992). Gender differences in symptoms of depression among adolescents. *Journal of Health and Social Behavior, 33*, 77–96.

Bandyopadhyay, M. (2003). Missing girls and son preference in rural India: Looking beyond popular myth. *Health Care for Women International, 24*, 910–926.

Banister, E., & Schreiber, R. (2001). Young women's health concerns: Revealing paradox. *Health Care for Women International, 22*, 633–647.

Barad, D. H., & Witt, B. R. (2000). Multiple pregnancies and assisted reproductive technologies. *Journal of Women's Health & Gender-Based Medicine, 9*, 101–107.

Barker, D. J. P. (1990). The fetal and infant origins of adult disease: The womb may be more important than the home. *British Medical Journal, 301*, 111.

Barker, D. J. P. (2007). The origins of the developmental origins theory. *Journal of Internal Medicine, 261*, 412–417.

Barker, D. J. P., & Osmond, C. (1986). Infant mortality, childhood nutrition, and ischemic heart disease in England and Wales. *Lancet, 1*, 1077–1081.

Barnett, R. C., & Marshal, N. L. (1992). Worker and mother roles, spill over effects, and psychological distress. *Women and Health, 18*, 9–40.

Baron-Hall, D., & Vidaver, R. M. (2000). The first annual conference on sex and gene expression. *Journal of Women's Health & Gender-Based Medicine, 9*, 955–958.

Bearinger, L. H., Sieving, R. E., Ferguson, J., & Sharma, V. (2007). Global perspectives on the sexual and reproductive health of adolescents: patterns, prevention and potential. *Lancet, 369*, 1220–1231.

Beral, V. (1985). Long term effects of childbearing on health. *Journal of Epidemiology and Community Health, 39*, 343–346.

Boivin, J., Buntin, L., Collins, J. A., & Nygren, K. G. (2007). International estimates of infertility prevalence and treatment-seeking: Potential need and demand for infertility medical care. *Human Reproduction, 22*, 1506–1512.

Boston Women's Health Collective. (1984). *Our bodies ourselves: A book by and for women*. New York: Simon and Shuster.

Boulis, A. K., & Jacobs, J. A. (2008). *The changing face of medicine: women doctors and the evolution of health care in America*. Ithaca and London: Cornell University Press.

Braus, P. (1993). Facing M. *American Demographics, 15*, 44–48.

Brinton, E. A., Hopkins, P. N., & Sankaran, G. (2010). Cardiovascular disease in women: Risk factors and risk reduction. In P. Murthy and C. L. Smith (Eds.), *Women's global health and human rights* (pp. 161–175). Sudbury, MA: Jones & Bartlett Learning.

Brodsky, P. L. (2008). *The control of childbirth.* Jefferson, NC: McFarland & Company, Inc., Publishers.

Bromberger, J. T., Schott, L. L., Kravitz, H. M., Sowers, M., Avis, N. E., Gold, E. B., Randolph, J. F., & Matthews, K. A. (2010). Longitudinal change in reproductive hormones and depressive symptoms across the menopausal transition: Results from the Study of Women Health across the Nation (SWAN). *Archives of General Psychiatry, 67,* 598–607.

Burger, H. G., Hale, G. E., Robertson, D. M., & Dennerstein, L. (2007). A review of hormonal changes during the menopausal transition: focus on findings from the Melbourne Women's Midlife Health Project. *Human Reproduction, 13,* 559–565.

Canadian Council for International Co-operation. (1991). *Two halves make a whole: Balancing gender relations in development.* Ottawa, Canada: MATCH International, and Association Québécoise des Organismes de Coopération Internationale.

Castellanos, P. (1987). Sobre el concepto de salud-enfermedad: Un punto de vista epidemiologico. Fifth World Congress of Social Medicine. Medellin, Colombia, Mimeo.

Cavalcanti de Aguiar, A. (2009). Medicine and women's studies: Possibilities for enhancing women's health care. In S. V. Rosser (Ed.), *Diversity and women's health* (pp. 247–267). Baltimore: Johns Hopkins University Press.

Centers for Disease Control and Prevention. (2001). Diabetes and women's health across the life stages. Retrieved May 16, 2011 from http://www.cdc.gov/diabetes/pubs/women/index.htm#2.

Central Intelligence Agency. (2010). The world factbook. Retrieved October 18, 2011 from https://www.cia.gov/library/publications/the-world-factbook/.

Chandra, A., Martinez, G. M., Mosher, W. D., Abma, J. C., & Jones, J. (2005). Fertility, family planning, and reproductive health of U.S. women: Data from the 2002 National Survey of Family Growth. National Center for Health Statistics. *Vital Health Statistics 23*(25).

Cohen, L. S., Soares, C. N., Vitonis, A. F., Otto, M. W., & Harlow, B. L. (2006). Risk for new onset of depression during the menopausal transition: The Harvard study of moods and cycles. *Archives of General Psychiatry, 63,* 385–390.

Costello, E. J. (1991). Married with children: Predictors of mental and physical health in middle-aged women. *Psychiatry, 54,* 292–305.

Cothran, M. M., & White, J. P. (2002). Adolescent behavior and sexually transmitted disease: The dilemma of human papillomavirus. *Health Care for Women International, 23,* 306–319.

Crossete, B. (1995, December 10). Female genital mutilation by immigrants is becoming cause for concern in the US. *The New York Times,* p. 18.

de los Rios, R. (1994). Gender, health, and development: An approach in the making. In E. Gomez (Ed.), *Gender, women, and health in the Americas* (pp. 3–17). Washington, DC: Pan American Health Organization.

de los Rios, R., & Gomez, E. (1992). Mujer en la salud y el desarrolo. In Y. Arango (Ed.), *Mujer, salud y autocuidado: Memorias* (pp. 107–123). Washington, DC: Pan American Health Organization.

Desai, H. D., & Jann, M. W. (2000). Major depression in women: A review of the literature. *Journal of the American Pharmaceutical Association, 40,* 525–537.

Dick-Read, G. (1933). *Natural childbirth.* London: Heinemann Medical Books.

Dixon, J. M. (2002). Message about hormone replacement therapy is unclear. *British Medical Journal, 325,* 1036.

Dooley, Y., Kenton, K., Cao, G., Luke, A., Durazo-Arvizu, R., Kramer, H., & Brubaker, L. (2008). Urinary incontinence prevalence: Results from the National Health and Nutrition Examination Survey. *Journal of Urology, 179,* 656–661.

Elliott, S. J. (1994). Psychosocial stress, women and heart health: A critical review. *Social Science & Medicine, 40,* 105–115.

Fletcher, S. W., & Colditz, G. A. (2002). Failure of estrogen plus progestin therapy for prevention. *Journal of the American Medical Association, 288,* 366–368.

Foster-Rosales, A. (2010). Maternal mortality: The eye of the storm. In P. Murthy and C. L. Smith (Eds.), *Women's global health and human rights* (pp. 279–286). Sudbury, MA: Jones & Bartlett Learning.

Fried, M. G. (Ed.). (1990). *From abortion to reproductive freedom: Transforming a movement.* Boston: South End Press.

Frongillo, E. A., Jr., & Bégin, F. (1993). Gender bias in food intake favors male preschool Guatemalan children. *Journal of Nutrition, 123,* 189–196.

Gillespie, B. L., & Eisler, R. M. (1992). Development of the feminine gender role stress scale: A cognitive-behavioral measure of stress, appraisal, and coping for women. *Behavioral Analysis and Modification, 16,* 426–438.

Gleicher, N., & Karande, V. (2002). Gender selection for nonmedical indications. *Fertility & Sterility, 78,* 460–462.

Gold, E. B., Bromberger, J., Crawford, S., Samuels, S., Greendale, G. A., Harlow, S. D., & Skurnick, J. (2001). Factors associated with age at natural menopause in a multiethnic sample of midlife women. *American Journal of Epidemiology, 153,* 865–874.

Gomez, E. (1990). *Perfil epidemiologico de la salud de la mujer en la region de las Americas* (pp. 1–3, 221–237). Washington, DC: Pan American Health Organization.

Gomez, E. (1994). Introduction. In E. Gomez (Ed.), *Gender, women, and health in the Americas* (pp. ix–xviii). Washington, DC: Pan American Health Organization.

Gomez, E. G. (2000). *Equity, gender and health policy reform in Latin America and the Caribbean.* Washington, DC: Pan American Health Organization: Women, Health and Development Program.

Green, A., Beral, V., & Moser, K. (1988). Mortality in women in relation to their childbearing history. *British Medical Journal, 297,* 391–395.

Greenberger, P. (1999). News from the society for women's health research: SAM IX: More information on sex-based differences. *Journal of Women's Health & Gender-Based Medicine, 8,* 1223–1224.

Greenberger, P. E. (2002). Advances in sex-based analysis. *Journal of Women's Health & Gender-Based Medicine, 11,* 199–200.

Greenberger, P. E., & Knab, S. (2002). News from the society for women's health research: Subgroup analysis in clinical trials: Detecting sex differences. *Journal of Women's Health & Gender-Based Medicine, 11,* 7–9.

Greenberger, P., & Marts, S. A. (2000a). Women in NIH-funded research studies: There's good news, and there's bad news. *Journal of Women's Health & Gender-Based Medicine, 9,* 463–464.

Greenberger, P. E., & Marts, S. (2000b). Hormones, chromosomes, and the future of sex-based biology. *Journal of Women's Health & Gender-Based Medicine, 9,* 937–938.

Grimmell, D., & Stern, G. S. (1992). The relationship between gender role ideals and psychological well-being. *Sex Roles, 27,* 487–497.

Groer, M. W., Thomas, S. P., & Shoffner, D. (1992). Adolescent stress and coping: A longitudinal study. *Research in Nursing and Health, 15,* 209–217.

Haber, L. C. (1991). The effect of employment on the relationship between gender-role preference and self-esteem in married women. *Journal of Advanced Nursing, 16,* 606–613.

Harlow, S. D., Bainbridge, K., Howard, D., Myntti, C., Potter, L., Sussman, N., Van Olphen, J., Williamson, N., & Young, E. (1999). Methods and measures: Emerging strategies in women's health research. *Journal of Women's Health, 8,* 139–147.

Harlow, S. D., Cain, K., Crawford, S., Dennerstein, L., Little, R., Mitchell, E. S., Nan, B., Randolph, J. F., Jr., Taffe, J., & Yosef, M. (2006). Evaluation of four proposed bleeding criteria for the onset of late menopausal transition. *Journal of Clinical Endocrinology and Metabolism, 91,* 3432–3438.

Harlow, S. D., Crawford, S., Dennerstein, L., Burger, H. G., Mitchell, E. S., & Sowers, M. F. (2007). Recommendations from a multi-study evaluation of proposed criteria for staging reproductive aging. *Climacteric, 10,* 112–119.

Harlow, S. D., Mitchell, E. S., Crawford, S., Nan, B., Little, R., & Taffe, J. (2008). The ReSTAGE Collaboration: Defining optimal bleeding criteria for the onset of early menopausal transition. *Fertility and Sterility, 89,* 129–140.

Helmers, K. F., Krantz, D. S., Howell, R. H., Klein, J., Bairey, C. N., & Rozanski, A. (1993). Hostility and myocardial ischemia in coronary artery disease patients: Evaluation by gender and ischemic index. *Psychosomatic Medicine, 55,* 29–36.

Hoskins, M. L. (2002). Girls' identity dilemmas: Spaces defined by definitions of worth. *Health Care for Women International, 23,* 231–247.

International Labour Office. (2009). *Global employment trends for women.* Geneva: International Labour Office.

Janes, C. R. (1990). Migration, changing gender roles and stress: The Samoan case. *Medical Anthropology, 12,* 217–248.

J. E. Austin Associates & The Collaborative for Development Action, Inc. (1989). Gender analysis for project design: UNFPA training manual. Cambridge, MA: Author.

Jha, P., Kumar, R., Vasa, P., Dhingra, N., Thiruchelvam, D., & Moineddin, R. (2006). Low male-to-female sex ratio of children born in India: National survey of 1.1 million households. *Lancet, 367,* 211–218.

Kane, P. (1991). *Women's health: From womb to tomb.* New York: St. Martin's Press.

Katz, M. E., Holmes, M. D., Power, K. L., & Wise, P. H. (1995). Mortality rates among 15- to 44-year-old women in Boston: Looking beyond reproductive status. *American Journal of Public Health, 85,* 1135–1138.

Kishor, S. (1993). "May God give sons to all": Gender and child mortality in India. *American Sociological Review, 58,* 247–265.

Klonoff, E. A., & Landrine, H. (1991). Sex roles, occupational roles, and symptom-reporting: A test of competing hypothesis on sex difference. *Journal of Behavioral Medicine, 15,* 355–364.

Knox, S. S., & Follmann, D. (1993). Gender difference in the psychosocial variance of Framingham and Bortner Type A measures. *Journal of Psychosomatic Research, 37,* 709–716.

Kramarow, E., Lentzner, H., Rooks, R., Weeks, J., & Saydah, S. (1999). *Health and aging chartbook. Health, United States, 1999.* Hyattsville, MD: National Center for Health Statistics.

Kumanyika, S. K., Morssimk, C. B., & Nestle, M. (2001). Minority women and advocacy for women's health. *American Public Health Journal, 91,* 1383–1388.

Lane, S. D., & Meleis, A. (1991). Roles, work, health perceptions and health resources of women: A study in an Egyptian delta hamlet. *Social Science & Medicine, 33,* 1197–1208.

Li, S., Zhu, C., & Feldman, M. W. (2004). Gender differences in child survival in contemporary rural China: A county study. *Journal of Biological Sciences, 36,* 83–104.

Low Dog, T., & Maize, V. (2010). Women's health: An epilogue. In V. Maize, & T. Low Dog (Eds.), *Integrative women's health* (pp. 660–670). New York: Oxford University Press.

Mahowald, M. B. (1993). *Women and children in health care: An unequal majority* (pp. 242–254). New York: Oxford University Press.

Maize, V., & Low Dog, T. (2010). Philosophy of integrative women's health. In V. Maize, & T. Low Dog (Eds.), *Integrative women's health* (pp. 3–6). New York: Oxford University Press.

Martikainen, P. (1995). Women's employment, marriage, motherhood and mortality: A test of multiple role and role accumulation hypotheses. *Social Science & Medicine, 40,* 199–212.

Martin, J. A., Hamilton, B. E., Sutton, P. D., Ventura, S. J., Mathews, T. J., Kirmeyer, S., & Osterman, M. J. K. (2010). Births: Final data for 2007. *National vital statistics reports, 58*(24). Hyattsville, MD: National Center for Health Statistics.

Mathews, T. J., & Hamilton, B. E. (2002). Mean age of mother, 1970–2000. *National Vital Statistics Reports, 51,* 1–13. Retrieved October 18, 2011 from http://www.cdc.gov/nchs/data/nvsr/nvsr51/nvsr51_01.pdf.

Matthews, K. A., Crawford, S. L., Chae, C. U., Everson-Rose, S. A., Sowers, M. F., Sternfeld, B., & Sutton-Tyrrell, K. (2009). Are changes in cardiovascular disease risk factors in midlife women due to chronological aging or to the menopausal transition? *Journal of the American College of Cardiology, 54,* 2366–2373.

McDonald, C., McIntyre, M., & Anderson, B. (2003). The view from somewhere: Locating lesbian experience in women's health. *Health Care for Women International, 24,* 697–711.

Meisler, J. G. (1999). Toward optimal health: The experts respond to depression. *Journal of Women's Health & Gender-Based Medicine, 8,* 1141–1146.

Meisler, J. G. (2000). Toward optimal health: The experts discuss chronic fatigue syndrome. *Journal of Women's Health & Gender-Based Medicine, 9,* 477–482.

Meleis, A. I., & Lindgren, T. G. (2002). Man works from sun to sun, but woman's work is never done: Insights on research and policy. *Health Care for Women International, 23,* 742–753.

Merrill, R. M., Layman, A. B., Oderda, G., & Asche, C. (2008). Risk estimates of hysterectomy and selected conditions commonly treated with hysterectomy. *Annals of Epidemiology, 18,* 253–260.

Mingo, C., Herman, C. J., & Jasperse, M. (2000). Women's stories: Ethnic variations in women's attitudes and experiences of menopause, hysterectomy, and hormonal replacement therapy. *Journal of Women's Health & Gender-Based Medicine, 9,* S-27–S-38.

Moen, P., Dempster-McClain, D., & Williams, R. M. (1992). Successful aging: A life-course perspective on women's multiple roles and health. *American Journal of Sociology, 97,* 1612–1638.

Morgen, S. (2009). Women physicians and the twentieth-century women's health movement. In E. S. More, E. Fee, & M. Parry (Eds.), *Women physicians and the cultures of medicine* (pp. 161–183). Baltimore: Johns Hopkins University Press.

Mosca, L., Allen, C., Fernandez-Repollet, E., Kim, C., Lee, M., McAuley, J. W., & McLaughlin, M. (2001). Setting a local research agenda for women's health: The National Centers of Excellence in Women's Health. *Journal of Women's Health & Gender-Based Medicine, 10,* 927–935.

Moser, C. O. (1989). Gender planning in the third world: Meeting practical and strategic gender needs. *World Development, 17,* 1799–1825.

Muuss, R. E. (1988). Carol Gilligan's theory of sex differences in the development of moral reasoning during adolescence. *Adolescence, XXIII*, 229–243.

Nakano, K. (1990). Type A behavior, hardiness, and psychological well-being in Japanese women. *Psychological Reports, 67*, 367–370.

Napholz, L. (1992). Locus of control and depression as a function of sex role orientation [abstract]. *Acta-Psiquiatrica y Psicologica de America Latina, 38*, 205–212.

Neer, R. M. (2010). Bone loss across the menopausal transition. *Annals of the New York Academy of Sciences, 1192*, 66–71.

Nuess, W. S., & Zubenko, G. S. (1992). Correlates of persistent depression symptoms in widows. *American Journal of Psychiatry, 149*, 346–351.

Odent, M. (2009). Rediscovering midwifery. Retrieved May 16, 2011 from http://Fullmoonsdaughter.com/blog/tag/michael-odent/.

Peters, R. K., Kjos, S. L., Xiang, A., & Buchanan, T. A. (1996). Long-term diabetogenic effect of single pregnancy in women with previous gestational diabetes mellitus. *Lancet, 347*, 227–230.

Pinn, V. W. (2003). Sex and gender factors in medical studies: Implications for health and clinical practice. *New England Journal of Medicine, 289*, 397–400.

Radke-Yarrow, M., Nottelmann, E., Belmont, B., & Welsh, J. D. (1993). Affective interactions of depressed and nondepressed mothers and their children. *Journal of Abnormal Child Psychology, 21*, 683–695.

Ramasubbu, K., Gurm, H., & Litaker, D. (2001). Gender bias in clinical trials: Do double standards still apply? *Journal of Women's Health & Gender-Based Medicine, 10*, 757–764.

Rathgeber, E. M., & Vlassoff, C. (1993). Gender and tropical diseases: A new research focus. *Social Science & Medicine, 37*, 513–520.

Rich-Edwards, J. W., McElrath, T. F., Karumanchi, S. A., & Seely, E. W. (2010). Breathing life into the lifecourse approach: Pregnancy history and cardiovascular disease in women. *Hypertension, 56*, 331–334.

Rich-Edwards, J. W., Stampfer, M. J., Manson, J. E., Rosner, B., Hankinson, S. E., Colditz, G. A., Willett, W. C., & Hennekens, C. H. (1997). Birth weight and risk of cardiovascular disease in a cohort of women followed up since 1976. *British Medical Journal, 315*, 396–400.

Roberts, S. J. (2001). Lesbian health research: A review and recommendations for future research. *Health Care for Women International, 22*, 537–352.

Robertson, J. A. (2003). Extending preimplantation genetic diagnosis: Medical and non-medical uses. *Journal of Medical Ethics, 29*, 213–216.

Roger, V. L., Farkouh, M. E., Weston, S. A., Reeder, G. S., Jacobsen, S. J., Zinsmeister, A. R., Yawn, B. P., Kopecky, S. L., & Gabriel, S. E. (2000). Sex differences in evaluation and outcome of unstable angina. *Journal of the American Medical Association, 283*, 646–652.

Rogers, N. (2009). Feminists fight the culture of exclusion in medical education, 1970–1990. In E. S. More, E. Fee, & M. Parry (Eds.), *Women physicians and the cultures of medicine* (pp. 205–241). Baltimore: Johns Hopkins University Press.

Rosenfeld, J. A. (1992). Maternal work outside the home and its effect on women and their families. *Journal of the American Medical Women's Association, 47*, 47–53.

Rosenfield, A., Min, C., & Bardfield, J. (2010). Global women's health and human rights. In P. Murthy & C. L. Smith (Eds.), Women's global health and human rights (pp. 3–7). Sudbury, MA: Jones & Bartlett Learning.

Rosenfield, A., & Maine, D. (1985). Maternal mortality: A neglected tragedy: Where is the M in MCH? *The Lancet, 2*, 83–85.

Rosser, S. V. (2009). Ignored, overlooked, or subsumed: Research on lesbian health care. In S. V. Rosser (Ed.), *Diversity and women's health* (pp. 113–133). Baltimore: The Johns Hopkins University Press.

Rustgi, S. D., Doty, M. M., & Collins, S. R. (2009). *Women at risk: Why many women are forgoing needed health care.* New York: The Commonwealth Fund. Retrieved October 18, 2011 from http://www.commonwealthfund.org/~/media/Files/Publications/Issue%20Brief/2009/May/Women%20at%20Risk/PDF_1262_Rustgi_women_at_risk_issue_brief_Final.pdf.

Ruzek, S. B. (1978). *The women's health movement.* New York: Praeger Publishers.

Sattar, N., & Greer, I. A. (2002). Pregnancy complications and maternal cardiovascular risk: Opportunities for intervention and screening? *British Medical Journal, 325*, 157–160.

Selwyn, B. J. (1990). The epidemiology of acute respiratory tract infection in young children: Comparison of findings from several developing countries. *Review of Infectious Diseases, 12*(Suppl. 8), S877.

Shapiro, E. R. (2009). Because words are not enough: Latina re-visionings of transnational collaborations using health promotion for gender justice and social change. In S. V. Rosser (Ed.), *Diversity and women's health* (pp. 64–94). Baltimore: Johns Hopkins University Press.

Shell-Ducan, B., & Hernlund, Y. (2000). *Female "circumcision" in Africa: Culture, controversy, and change.* Boulder, CO: Lynne Rienner Publishers.

Shrestha, N. M. (1990). The girl child. *Asian-Pacific Journal of Public Health, 4,* 205–208.

Singh, I. (1990). Sociocultural factors affecting girl children in Nepal. *Asian-Pacific Journal of Public Health, 4,* 251–254.

Smart, D. R. (2010). *Physician characteristics and distributions in the US: 2010 edition.* Table 1.1, Total Physicians by Age, Activity and Sex, 2008. Chicago, IL: American Medical Association, p. 8.

Smyke, P. (1993). *Women and health* (2nd ed.). Atlantic Highlands, NJ: Zed Books Ltd.

Solarz, A. L., & Committee on Lesbian Health Research Priorities, Neurosciences and Behavioral Health Program, Health Sciences Policy Program, Health Sciences Section, Institute of Medicine (Ed.). (1999). *Lesbian health: Current assessment and directions for the future.* New York: National Academy Press.

Sowers, M. F., Jannausch, M., McConnell, D., Little, R., Greendale, G. A., Finkelstein, J. S., Neer, R. M., Johnston, J., & Ettinger, B. (2006). Hormone predictors of bone mineral density changes during the menopausal transition. *Journal of Clinical Endocrinology and Metabolism, 91,* 1261–1267.

Sowers, M. F., Tomey, K., Jannausch, M., Eyvazza-deh, A., Nan, B., & Randolph Jr., J. F. (2007). Physical functioning and menopause states. *Obstetrics and Gynecology, 110,* 1290–1296.

Sowers, M. F., Zheng, H., McConnell, D., Nan, B., Harlow, S. D., & Randolph Jr., J. F. (2008a). Follicle stimulating hormone and its rate of change in defining menopause transition stages. *Journal of Clinical Endocrinology and Metabolism, 93,* 3958–3964.

Sowers, M. F., Zheng, H., McConnell, D., Nan, B., Harlow, S. D., & Randolph, Jr., J. F. (2008b). Estradiol rates of change in relation to the final menstrual period in a population-based cohort of women. *Journal of Clinical Endocrinology and Metabolism, 93,* 3847–4852.

Stevenson, J. C., & Whitehead, M. I. (2002). Hormone replacement therapy: Findings of women's health initiative trial need not alarm users. *British Medical Journal, 325,* 113–114.

Strickland, B. R. (1988). Sex-related differences in health and illness. *Psychology of Women Quarterly, 12,* 381–399.

Strobino, D. M., Grason, H., & Minkovitz, C. (2002). Charting a course for the future of women's health in the United States: Concepts, findings, and recommendations. *Social Science & Medicine, 54,* 839–848.

Suarez, E. C., Harlan, E., Peoples, M. C., & Williams, R. B., Jr. (1993). Cardiovascular and emotional responses in women: The role of hostility and harassment. *Health Psychology, 12,* 459–468.

Theorell, T. (1991). Cardiovascular health in women: Results from epidemiological and psychosocial studies in Sweden [abstract]. In M. Frankenhaeuser, U. Lundberg, & M. A. Chesney (Eds.), *Women, work and health: Stress and opportunities.* New York: Plenum Press.

Thierry, J. M. (1998). Promoting the health and wellness of women with disabilities. *Journal of Women's Health, 7,* 505–507.

Thierry, J. M. (2000). Increasing breast and cervical cancer screening among women with disabilities. *Journal of Women's Health & Gender-Based Medicine, 9,* 9–12.

Toubia, N. (1994). Female circumcision as a public health issue. *New England Journal of Medicine, 331,* 712–716.

United Nations. (2000). *The world's women 2000: Trends and statistics.* New York: United Nations Department of Economic and Social Affairs.

United Nations. (2010). Power and decision-making (chapter 5). In *The world's women 2010: Trends and statistics* (pp. 111–124). Retrieved May 16, 2011 from http://unstats.un.org/unsd/demographic/products/Worldswomen/wwPower&dec2010.htm.

U.S. Census. (2010). Population estimates: National-characteristics; National sex and age. Retrieved May 16, 2011 from http://www.census.gov/popest/national/asrh/NC-EST2009-sa.html.

U.S. Department of Health and Human Services, Health Resources and Services Administration. (2008). Women's health USA 2008. Retrieved October 18, 2011 from http://mchb.hrsa.gov/whusa08/hstat/mh/pages/237mm.html.

U.S. Department of Health and Human Services, Administration on Children, Youth and Families, Children's Bureau. (2010). *Child maltreatment 2009.* Washington, DC: U.S. Government Printing Office.

U.S. Department of Labor. (2010). Quick stats on women workers, 2010. Retrieved October 18,

2011 from http://www.dol.gov/wb/factsheets/QS-womenwork2010.htm.

Vahratian, A. (2009). Prevalence of overweight and obesity among women of childbearing age: Results from the 2002 National Survey of Family Growth. *Maternal and Child Health Journal, 13*, 268–273.

Vayena, E., Rowe, P. J., & Griffin, P. D. (Eds.). (2002). *Current practices and controversies in assisted reproduction: Report of a WHO meeting on "medical, ethical, and social aspects of assisted reproduction."* Geneva: World Health Organization. Retrieved May 16, 2011 from http://www.who.int/reproductivehealth/publications/infertility/9241590300/en.

Verbrugge, L. M. (1989). The twain meet: Empirical explanations of sex differences in health and mortality. *Journal of Health and Social Behavior, 30*, 282–304.

Verbrugge, L. M., & Wingard, D. L. (1987). Sex differentials in health and mortality. *Women & Health, 12*, 103–144.

Vidaver, R. M., Lafleur, B., Tong, C., Bradshaw, R., & Marts, S. A. (2000). Women subjects in NIH-funded clinical research literature: Lack of progress in both representation and analysis by sex. *Journal of Women's Health & Gender-Based Medicine, 9*, 495–504.

Voelker, R. (1994). A new agenda for women's health. *Journal of the American Medical Association, 272*, 7.

Warren, M. P. (2004). A comparative review of the risks and benefits of hormone replacement therapy regimens. *American Journal of Obstetrics and Gynecology, 190*, 1141–1167.

Warsh, C. K. (2010). *Prescribed norms: Women's health in Canada and the United States since 1800* (p. 86). Toronto: University of Toronto Press.

Weinstock, H., Berman, S., & Cates, W., Jr. (2004). Sexually transmitted diseases among American youth: Incidence and prevalence estimates, 2000. *Perspectives on Sexual and Reproductive Health, 36*, 6–10.

Wells, S. (2009). Narrative forms in "Our Bodies, Ourselves." In E. S. More, E. Fee, and M. Parry (Eds.), *Women physicians and the cultures of medicine* (pp. 184–204). Baltimore: Johns Hopkins University Press.

Whatley, M. H. (1994). Male and female hormones: Misinterpretation of biology in school health and sex education. In N. Worcester & M. Whatley (Eds.), *Women's health: Readings on social, economic, and political issues* (2nd ed., pp. 97–103). Dubuque, IA: Kendall/Hunt Publishing Company.

Wilcox, J. (2002). The face of women's health: Helen Rodrigrez-Trias. *American Journal of Public Health, 92*, 566–669.

Williams, C. D., Baumslag, N., & Jelliffe, D. B. (1994). *Mother and child health: Delivering the services* (3rd ed.). New York: Oxford University Press.

Williams, P. G., Weibe, D. J., & Smith, T. W. (1992). Coping processes as mediators of the relationship between hardiness and health. *Journal of Behavioral Medicine, 15*, 237–255.

Wise, P. (1993). Confronting racial disparities in infant mortality: Reconciling science and politics. *American Journal of Preventive Medicine, 9*, 7–16.

Women's Health Initiative Study Group. (1998). Design of the Women's Health Initiative clinical trial and observational study. *Controlled Clinical Trials, 19*, 61–109.

Woods, N. F., Lentz, M., & Michell, E. (1993). The new woman: Health-promotion and health-damaging. *Health Care for Women International, 14*, 389–405.

Worcester, N., & Whatley, M. H. (Eds.). (1994). *Women's health: Readings on social, economic, and political issues* (2nd ed.). Dubuque, IO: Kendall/Hunt Publishing Company.

World Health Organization. (1992). *Women's health: Across age and frontier.* Geneva: Author.

World Health Organization. (2000). *Female genital mutilation.* Fact Sheet No. 241. Geneva: World Health Organization. Retrieved May 16, 2011 from http://www.who.int/mediacentre/factsheets/fs241/en./

World Health Organization. (2001). *Global prevalence and incidence of selected curable sexually transmitted infections: Overview & estimates.* Geneva: Author.

World Health Organization. (2010). Young people: Health risks and solutions. Retrieved May 16, 2011 from http://www.who.int/mediacentre/factsheets/fs345/en/index.html.

World Health Organization. (2011). *Preventing gender-based sex selection.* Geneva: Author. Retrieved May 16, 2011 from http://whqlibdoc.who.int/publications/2011/9789241501460_eng.pdf.

World Health Organization Study Group on Female Genital Mutilation and Obstetric Outcome. (2006). Female genital mutilation and obstetric outcome:

WHO collaborative perspective study in six African Countries. *Lancet, 367,* 1835–1841.

Writing Group for the Women's Health Initiative Investigators. (2002). Risks and benefits of estrogen plus progestin in healthy menopausal women: Principal results from the Women's Health Initiative randomized controlled trial. *Journal of the American Medical Association, 288,* 321–333.

Zimmerman-Tansella, C., & Lattanzi, M. (1991). The Ryle Marital Patterns Test as a predictor of symptoms of anxiety and depression in couples in the community. *Social Psychiatry and Psychiatric Epidemiology, 26,* 221–229.

12

CHILDREN WITH SPECIAL HEALTH CARE NEEDS

Anita M. Farel

We have new goals for the decade ahead: to expand the cadre of families and youth from diverse cultures, obtain funding for F2FHIC (Family-to-Family Health Information Centers) for tribal entities and territories, and strengthen partnerships among family run organizations in every state. Families and professionals, working in partnership, can and will meet the challenges before us.

(Nora Wells. National Center for Family/Professional
Partnerships Celebrate 2010, Title V 75th anniversary)

Increased understanding of the impact of a broad array of childhood chronic conditions, and of ways to address the needs of these children and their families, has shaped public policies and programs. Approximately one of every seven children in the United States younger than 18 years of age lives with a special health care need. This chapter provides an overview of the evolution of public policy guiding the development of programs and service delivery systems to meet the needs of this population and their families, the epidemiology of chronic childhood conditions, persistent issues, and promising strategies.

EVOLUTION OF PUBLIC POLICY: LEGISLATIVE HISTORY

Initially, programs for Children with Special Health Care Needs (CSHCN) were referred to as Crippled Children's Services (CCS) when Maternal and Child Health (MCH) and Crippled Children's Services programs were simultaneously initiated in 1935 as part of Title V of the Social Security Act. Since that time, the federal government has played an active role in financing, organizing, and delivering services for children with special needs.

In contrast to Maternal and Child Health programs, which had a clear mandate to develop public health programs for all mothers and children and a firm seat in each state's capitol, decisions about which chronic health conditions could best be treated were left to state discretion.

Although Crippled Children's Services incorporated a broad vision of how the needs of children with, or at risk for, chronic conditions could be addressed, funds for the program were dispersed primarily for children who would benefit most from treatment. The program for crippled children was oriented toward *direct* services and depended primarily on the private sector to provide specialty care. Because the effects of polio were of paramount concern, most Crippled Children's

Services programs emphasized treatment for orthopedic conditions, such as those that affected child survivors of polio.

Medical advances in the 1940s and 1950s continued to broaden the focus of CCS programs to include newly treatable pediatric conditions, such as rheumatic heart conditions and congenital cardiac anomalies. Through the 1940s, 80% of all children served were treated for orthopedic conditions, but by 1959, the development of the polio vaccine reduced this segment to less than 50%. Other medical and surgical advances continued to modify the context within which the state programs operated, broadening perceptions about the population that could be served and the range of services that could be offered.

During the first 3 decades of its existence, Title V was the sole source of federal funding for children with chronic conditions. However, in 1965 the enactment of Medicaid (Title XIX of the Social Security Act) provided states with a source of funding for medical care for needy children that alleviated many of the reimbursement and direct service provision functions of CCS programs. State programs were thus relieved of some of the financing concerns that had dominated program planning and consequently were able to focus their efforts on the original Title V mandate—to extend and improve services through planning programs for children with chronic health conditions. An amendment to Medicaid in 1967, the Early and Periodic Screening, Diagnosis, and Treatment program, strengthened Medicaid's preventive care component for children. Starting in the 1960s with Medicaid legislation and associated program development, the following decades would see many strides in legislation and thus program and policy development for this population.

Since the early 1970s, the Supplemental Security Income (SSI) childhood disability program (Title XVI of the Social Security Act), which is administered by the Social Security Administration at the federal level, has provided monthly cash payments to low-income children with disabilities. In almost all states, SSI eligibility automatically qualifies a child for Medicaid benefits. A child (birth to 21 years of age) is considered disabled if the physical, mental, or chronic medical condition has lasted or is expected to last at least 12 months or to result in death. Whereas the Medicaid program directly reimburses providers, the SSI monthly cash benefit is sent directly to the family to help defray costs incurred in caring for a child with special needs, such as transportation for specialty care, special equipment, or respite care.

In the 1970s, Developmental Disabilities (DD) legislation (Developmental Disabilities Amendments of 1970, PL 91-517; Developmentally Disabled Assistance and Bill of Rights Act of 1975, PL 94-103) generated a multifaceted mandate to identify services for individuals with developmental disabilities and to establish state DD councils. By 1978, developmental disabilities were defined functionally and included all conditions attributable to mental or physical impairment manifested before the age of 22 years that resulted in substantial functional limitations in three or more areas of major life activity (self-care, receptive and expressive language, learning, mobility, self-direction, capacity for independent living, economic self-sufficiency) (Rehabilitation, Comprehensive Services, and Developmental Disabilities Amendments of 1978, PL 95-602). Under DD legislation, each state DD council, composed of individuals with disabilities, parents of children with disabilities, and representatives from diverse state agencies, including Title V, education, and social services, developed a comprehensive state plan that identified services needed by the population with disabilities. Through several arms of this legislation (primarily the state DD councils and Protection and Advocacy agencies), service delivery systems for children with developmental disabilities and their families became increasingly organized and monitored.

Across the country, deliberate and persistent attempts to enroll children with special needs in schools culminated in a landmark lawsuit in 1972 (*Pennsylvania Association for Retarded Children v. Pennsylvania*, 343 F Supp. 279 E.D. Pa. 1972). In 1975, the U.S. Congress determined that children with disabilities did not receive appropriate educational services and enacted the Education for All Handicapped Children Act (1975). Renamed the Individuals with Disabilities Education Act (IDEA) (20 U.S.C. § 1400[a]) in 1990, the law guarantees a free, appropriate public education (referred to as FAPE) for all school-age children with disabilities. Multidisciplinary assessments were mandated for all children who may need special services. An Individualized Education Plan (IEP), which identifies needed services, must be developed by a multidisciplinary group that includes teachers, counselors, and allied health professionals. Parents or guardians are encouraged to be a part of this process. As a result of this legislation, new collaborative relationships among teachers, families, and health care professionals were forged. At the same time, schools began to assume certain responsibilities previously relegated to the health services sector, such as administering medications and treatment recommendations.

Since the passage of special education legislation in 1975, states had been encouraged to plan for extending services from school age to birth based on evidence that potential developmental problems could be prevented or corrected the earlier intervention started. Early intervention (EI) focuses on reducing the impact of or eliminating developmental delay and helping identified children and their families make the transition to preschool and kindergarten programs. Early intervention services address the developmental needs of children with disabilities in one or more developmental areas: physical, cognitive, communication, social/emotional, and adaptive development. Multiple funding sources have been tapped to help implement these services. In most states, the state health agency takes the lead in overseeing the implementation of the EI program.

Finally, in recognition of the increasingly broad childhood population with special needs, the program title, Crippled Children's Services, was changed to the program for Children with Special Health Care Needs (CSHCN) in 1985. Many state programs had continued to broaden their focus to include children with other physical disabilities, sensory impairments, developmental disabilities, and chronic physical illnesses. The focus of care also broadened from the child's condition to the family and stimulated the development of service delivery systems that were based on a family—professional partnership. There was growing recognition that care was best delivered through a comprehensive, coordinated, multidisciplinary, and multiagency approach centered on the child, family, and community.

Definitions of the CSHCN population that were based solely on conditions or diagnostic lists were rejected as being too unwieldy. Definitions based on functional status alone were eliminated because they would not include children whose disabilities have been alleviated by treatment or the continued use of special services. The following definition achieved consensus and was incorporated into federal legislation: "Children with special health care needs are those who have or are at increased risk for chronic physical, developmental, behavioral, or emotional conditions and who also require health and related services of a type or amount beyond that required by children generally" (McPherson, et al., 1998). Although very broad, this definition is consistent with the population described in diverse federal laws and provides state programs with useful guidance for strategic planning.

Continued medical advances, escalating professional specialization, program expansion, and increasingly fragmented services threatened to undermine the ability of state Title V programs to offer comprehensive and continuous services. In 1989, the Omnibus Budget Reconciliation Act (OBRA '89) redirected the mission of the CSHCN program. This legislation reinforced the leadership role of state Title V programs in developing community-based systems of services for all children with special health care needs, regardless of socioeconomic status, and in implementing the program's mission to promote and provide family-centered, community-based, coordinated, comprehensive, and culturally competent services. Explicitly acknowledging the diverse conditions comprising the population of children with special health care needs, 30% of the MCH Services Block Grant was to be directed toward "children with disabilities; chronic illnesses and conditions; and health-related educational and behavioral problems" (OBRA '89).

OBRA '89 also included the requirement that any medically necessary service required to treat a condition identified through an Early and Periodic Screening, Diagnosis, and Treatment screen must be provided, even if the service were an optional one that the state had not otherwise chosen to cover in its Medicaid program (42 U.S.C. § 1396d [r] [5]).

Although the SSI program experienced periods of heightened attention and languished at other times, it was greatly expanded in the wake of OBRA '89 and the 1990 Supreme Court decision, *Sullivan v. Zebley*. As a result of the Zebley decision, the *functional status* of children from low-income families, who had previously not been eligible for SSI because they were evaluated against stricter disability criteria than low-income adults, was included in the disability assessment. Although a child's impairment must be comparable in severity to one that would prevent an adult from working, comparability under the new law was interpreted to mean an impairment that substantially reduces the child's ability to function independently and effectively in an age-appropriate manner (Perrin & Stein, 1991). As a result of the outreach to potentially eligible children and their families mandated by OBRA '89, the increased number

of childhood impairment listings (from 4 to 11 general categories), and the rising rate of childhood poverty in the early 1990s, there was a threefold increase in SSI recipients, from approximately 300,000 in 1989 to almost 900,000 over the following 5 years (National Commission on Childhood Disability, 1995). In 1989, approximately 51% of the children enrolled in SSI had physical impairments; by 1994, children with physical impairments comprised approximately 39% of children enrolled, whereas children with mental impairments, including mental retardation, accounted for over 61% of enrollment. A child's disability determination is based on information solicited from physicians, psychologists, schools, teachers, therapists, social workers, parents, friends, relatives, the child, and others who may be able to provide useful information about the child's impairment(s) and functioning.

Alarmed by the rapidly increasing SSI enrollment, Congress passed the Personal Responsibility and Work Opportunity Reconciliation (Welfare Reform) Act of 1997 (PL 104–193) that dramatically redesigned the SSI program by cutting the cash assistance program for children with disabilities and restricting eligibility. This legislation established a definition of childhood disability based on more restrictive medical listings. In order to qualify for benefits, a child must have a "medically determinable physical or mental impairment which results in marked and severe functional limitations" of substantial duration (Schulzinger, 1998). The Individualized Functional Assessment was eliminated.

EPIDEMIOLOGY OF SPECIAL HEALTH CARE NEEDS

Not all chronic conditions impose the same burden on the child and family. Some conditions require frequent hospitalizations or are more disruptive for a family, whereas others may be managed more easily. The effect of different conditions on developmental progress would also thus be expected to vary. These considerations have stimulated efforts to classify children with chronic health conditions according to such variables as impact on the family, use of medical services, or the child's functional status. In other words, although they may live with distinct illnesses and disabilities, the daily experiences of children with special health care needs and their families may be very similar. For example, diabetes and sickle cell anemia have very different etiologies and treatment protocols, but children affected by these conditions have in common school absences and the need for careful monitoring. Conditions also have different ramifications depending on the child's age and stage of development. Children with compromised lung development as a result of preterm birth usually require less specialized medical attention as they mature, but the developmental delay often associated with this birth outcome may require special education services when the child enters school.

The means for preventing some conditions are known. For example, the large decline in spina bifida has been attributed to daily consumption of folic acid (Centers for Disease Control and Prevention, 2002a). Estimated to affect 1 in 1,000 births, fetal alcohol syndrome, which has been associated with mental retardation, birth defects, central nervous system impairment, and other cognitive and behavioral abnormalities, is preventable if alcohol is not consumed during pregnancy (Centers for Disease Control and Prevention, 2002b). However, the means for primary prevention of most chronic conditions are unknown or fraught with ethical or technical challenges.

Ruth Stein and her colleagues (1993) developed a conceptual framework that builds on the organizing principle of noncategorical care for understanding the needs of children with chronic conditions. This framework cuts across diagnostic categories and provides a means to estimate the impact of chronic health conditions on children and their families. In lieu of specific diagnoses, the framework uses consequences of chronic ongoing conditions to identify children along such parameters as disability or functional limitation, dependency on medications, special diets, medical technology, assistive devices, and personal assistance, and needs for services. The concepts of noncategorical care and understanding the impact of a chronic health condition are critical components for strategic planning and developing service delivery systems for CSHCN.

National Survey of Children with Special Health Care Needs

Planning health care services and developing responsive health care policies for children and youth with chronic conditions require valid and reliable prevalence estimates. National population-based surveys are the most useful data source about chronic conditions in childhood. The National Survey of CSHCN provides national and state-level estimates of the prevalence and impact of special needs from the unique perspective of families (http://www.cshcndata.org/Content/Default.aspx). Results from this survey, first conducted in 2001 and repeated in 2005–2006 and 2009–2010, are useful for trend analysis, program planning, and evaluation. This survey provides uniform state and national data essential for generating baseline estimates for federal and state Title V Maternal and Child Health programs. Thus, for the first time, each state has data for planning and evaluating programs for children and youth with special needs and their families.

A CSHCN screener (Bethell, et al., 2002) based on the MCH Bureau's definition was used to identify and select 750 children from each state and the District of Columbia. The screener operationalizes the broad definition of the population. Parents, or guardians, completed a battery of questions designed to collect information about the prevalence of CSHCN, the health insurance coverage they have, the health services they use, and the impact of their child's health conditions on the family. The interview was conducted in 12 languages.

Estimates based on the National Survey of CSHCN indicate that approximately 13% (or 9 million children) have childhood chronic conditions leading to special health care needs (van Dyck, et al., 2002). Improvements in the ability to diagnose some conditions (e.g., asthma and hearing impairments) and improved survival generated by medical advances (e.g., cystic fibrosis) and therapeutic regimens (e.g., HIV) are credited with increasing the prevalence of certain conditions. Changes in prevalence rates for some chronic conditions and disabilities also speak to the success of programs with legislatively mandated outreach and child-find components.

Minority Children and Youth with Special Needs

Hispanic and other ethnic minority populations are expected to continue to increase. If current trends continue, the Bureau of the Census projects that minority racial and ethnic groups will together account for almost half of the U.S. total population by 2050 (U.S. Census Bureau, 2008). The commitment to culturally competent service systems requires understanding cultural variations in the use of health care and the impact and prevalence of chronic health and disabling conditions among minority populations. Health care practices and attitudes about illness and disability vary among different cultures.

Certain health conditions clearly have a disproportionate impact on children in minority populations. For example, asthma is the most common chronic childhood disease and leading cause of disability among children in the United States (Centers for Disease Control and Prevention, 2000). African American children with asthma are less likely to receive adequate asthma therapy compared with white children—a finding that persists for children enrolled in Medicaid (Cooper &

Hickson, 2001). In 1997, 67.5% of black children diagnosed with asthma reported having an asthma attack in the past year compared to 52.2% of white, non-Hispanic children and 51.3% of Hispanic children. Disparities in activity limitation caused by asthma are even more significant for black children living in poverty (Centers for Disease Control and Prevention, 2000).

Data from the National Health Interview Survey revealed that differences in disability prevalence among black and white non-Hispanic children could be entirely explained by socioeconomic status (Newacheck, Stein, Bauman, & Hung, 2003). The prevalence of disability increased for both black and white children over the 40-year period studied—possibly the result of an increase in disease prevalence and severity, changes in awareness of health problems, better detection and ascertainment of health conditions by health professionals and educators, shifts in attitudes and beliefs about health limitations, and other factors. However, largely because of their exposure to poverty, black children had higher rates of disability.

Latinos constitute the fastest growing minority group in the United States. Latinos currently comprise approximately 11% of the population and will reach 14% by 2020. It is estimated that by the year 2020, one in five children in the United States will be Latino/Latina (Zambrana & Logie, 2000).

In addition to differences in language, minority groups may vary in their attitudes and beliefs about disability, standard medical practice, and use of professional services. In an effort to conduct a cultural validation of a measure of disability among children living in Puerto Rico, Gannotti and Handwerker (2002) assessed Puerto Rican parents' understanding of their child's disability. Although Puerto Rico must provide educational and rehabilitation services to infants, toddlers, and children with disabilities under the IDEA, shortages of qualified professionals, accessible buildings, equipment, and transportation impede the implementation of services

(Mulero & Font, 1997). The authors found that parental expectations and child care customs delayed mastery of diverse skills compared to children with disabilities in the United States. Puerto Rican children may have appeared to their parents as more disabled than might be expected given their actual level of impairment. For example, parents assumed that children with a disability would be more dependent on family members for many activities of daily living and therefore put relatively little emphasis on facilitating their child's independence through early intervention programs. Although a goal of EI is to make children with disabilities more capable and independent, constraints on achieving this goal may be imposed by the assumptions and orientation of parents. Because these assumptions are associated with the parents' cultural background, interventions, to be effective, must take account of this context.

Ngui and Flores (2006) examined racial/ethnic disparities in parent-reported satisfaction with care and ease of using health care services among children with chronic health conditions and identified factors that contribute to these disparities. Interview language had a strong influence on disparities in satisfaction and ease of service use among Hispanic parents of CSHCN. The authors note that interview language is a crude proxy for language barriers that undermine access to services for Latino children with chronic health conditions. More than one-third of minority parents reported that health care services for their child were not easy to use.

Disentangling the relative contribution of income and racial or ethnic background to disparities in health outcomes for CSHCN has significant implications for program and policy development. For minority families, obstacles such as lack of transportation and language barriers may result in missed appointments, reliance on episodic health care, emergency room visits, and poor adherence to treatment regimens.

MENTAL HEALTH

Mental health conditions generate substantial disability in childhood and constitute a rising proportion of children who are affected by a chronic disabling condition. Most reports about unmet mental health needs use data from surveys of parents that are not supplemented by professional assessments of child functioning.

In 1999, the U.S. Surgeon General reported that as many as 11% of all children in the United States have a mental disorder that significantly undermines their day-to-day functioning (USDHHS, 1999). This report galvanized the dissemination of several research initiatives to counter the lack of national data on children's mental health.

Results from the National Survey of Children's Health (NSCH) were used to assess the prevalence of mental health conditions among children aged 2 to 17 years (USDHHS, 2010). Parents were asked whether their child had been diagnosed with, and still had, any of 16 specific conditions, 7 of which were related to emotions, behavior, or development (depression, anxiety, Attention Deficit Disorder/Attention Deficit Hyperactivity Disorder, conduct disorders, autism spectrum disorders, developmental delay, Tourette Syndrome). Over 11% of children aged 2 to 17 years were reported to have at least one of these seven conditions at the time of the survey. Boys (65.7%) were more likely to be diagnosed with these conditions, more than half (51%) of those diagnosed were 12 to 17 years old. Among children with at least one emotional, behavioral, or developmental condition, 24.8% had family incomes below the federal poverty level.

In addition to emotional, behavioral, and developmental conditions, many children may also have chronic physical health conditions. The survey asked parents whether their children had been diagnosed with any of the following conditions: asthma; diabetes; bone, joint, or muscle problems; hearing problems; vision problems; epilepsy or seizure disorder; and brain injury or concussion. One-third (33.3%) of children who have an emotional, behavioral, or developmental condition have, in addition, at least one of those physical health conditions

An array of services, including screening, counseling, behavior and talk therapies, and medications, can help children with emotional, behavioral, or developmental conditions. According to the NSCH, of children with one or more emotional, behavioral, or developmental conditions, 45.6% were treated by a mental health professional. More than one-quarter (28.5%) of children with three or more conditions did not receive any mental health services.

The adequacy of insurance coverage for services and costs related to children's mental health conditions is uneven. Parents whose children were currently insured were asked whether they have reasonable out-of-pocket costs, benefits, and access to services that meet their needs, and ability to see the health care providers they need regarding the services and costs associated with their child's health insurance. Overall, 29.4% of children with emotional or behavioral problems lacked adequate insurance. Among children with three or more emotional, developmental, or behavioral conditions who had insurance, 36.9% did not have adequate coverage.

Of the three criteria for adequacy of insurance, reasonable costs seem to present the most significant barrier to families of children with emotional, behavioral, or developmental conditions. Of children with at least one condition, 21.1% of parents reported that out-of-pocket costs for their children's care were never or sometimes reasonable; 12.0% reported that their child's plan never or sometimes offered benefits and covered services that met their child's needs; and 9.0% reported that their child's insurance never or sometimes offered access to the providers they needed. These figures are not mutually exclusive, and the parents of some children may have reported more than one of these problems with their child's coverage.

Merikangas and colleagues (2010) used the National Comorbidity Survey—Adolescent Supplement (NCS-A) to assess the prevalence of DSM-IV mental disorders, their comorbidity across broad classes of disorder, and their sociodemographic correlates among U.S. adolescents 13 to 18 years of age. According to the report, approximately one in every four to five youth in the United States meets criteria for a mental disorder with severe impairment across their lifetime. One in 10 has a serious emotional disturbance. Among affected adolescents, 50% of disorders had their onset by age 6 for anxiety disorders, by age 11 for behavior disorders, by age 13 for mood disorders, and by age 15 for substance use disorders. Prevalence of all mood disorders increased uniformly with age, with a nearly twofold increase from the 13- to 14-year age group to the 17- to 18-year age group. The probability that mental disorders in adults first emerge in childhood reinforces the importance of incorporating prevention and early intervention with treatment.

The financial burden for families with a child with mental health care needs differs in several important ways from families with children with solely special medical care needs. There are inequities in coverage under private insurance: mental health services are usually offered on a more limited basis than more typical medical services. Mental health services are associated with higher cost-sharing and special coverage limits. Although a federal parity law to eliminate these differences was enacted in 2010 (http://www.hhs.gov/news/press/2010pres/01/20100129a.html), it does not address the soaring prescription drug costs for the treatment of mental health conditions and only marginally affects the labor market and time costs of caring for a child with a mental health condition. Apart from insurance, the national shortage of child psychiatrists and the characteristics of mental illness (e.g., stigma, less stability than many other childhood disorders) challenge service delivery systems (Busch & Barry, 2009).

Using three national household surveys (National Survey of American Families, National Health Interview Survey, and Community Tracking Survey), Kataoka, Zhang, and Wells (2002) analyzed rates of mental health service use by children and adolescents 3 to 17 years of age and differences by ethnicity and insurance status. From 1996 to 1998, 2%–3% of children 3 to 5 years old and 6%–9% of youth 6 to 17 years old used mental health services. The rate of unmet need was reported to be greater among Latino than white children and among uninsured than publicly insured children.

A study of unmet mental health needs and access to services found that even though perceived need for mental health treatment was greatest among CSHCN with a chronic emotional, behavioral, developmental condition, mental healthcare needs were also reported for children with solely a chronic medical condition. The fact that Spanish-interviewing Hispanic parents but not English-interviewing Hispanic parents reported greater unmet need relative to white non-Hispanic children suggests that language is important for understanding potential access disparities for family members of children with chronic health, mental health, and developmental problems and emphasizes the importance of studying Hispanic subgroups (Inkelas, et al., 2007).

The risk factors associated with mental illness, as well as mental illness itself, increase the risk for development of a chronic condition. Yet to date, effective public health interventions are not widely practiced.

FINANCING CARE

The burden of illness falls disproportionately on those who lack resources to pay for health care. Insurance coverage is essential for ensuring appropriate and timely access to care for children and youth with special health care needs. Young children with disabilities are significantly more likely to live in poverty than their peers without disabilities.

Exposure to poverty creates additional risk for adverse outcomes for these children. Risks for poor physical health, diminished cognitive abilities, emotional and behavioral problems, and lower educational attainment are all increased by poverty.

An array of public programs, including SSI, Medicaid, and the Children's Health Insurance Program, provide an important source of insurance for children with special health care needs. Although almost one-third of children with special health care needs are covered by these programs, many eligible children are not enrolled (Kaiser Commission on Medicaid and the Uninsured, 2002).

Families in the United States largely bear the high costs associated with their children's disabilities, and there is evidence that having a child with special needs dramatically reduces a family's economic status. Although health insurance offers more secure access to needed care and improvements in the quality of life for affected children, the deterioration of employer-based health insurance, state deficits that erode public programs, economic contractions at the state level that include the risk that employers will switch to less expensive health insurance plans all place CSHCN at risk for underinsurance (Newacheck, et al., 2009). Families are more likely to pay a higher percentage of their income for their child's care (Parish, et al., 2008), and parents are more likely to have cut back or stopped working all together (Okumura, et al., 2009). Additional costs are generated by more than the cost of health services. For example, lower levels of maternal employment, higher rates of divorce/separation associated with raising a child with special needs, higher co-pays, and greater employee contributions to premiums for family coverage all contribute to the impoverishment of families and reduce a family's chances for regaining financial stability.

Emerson (2004) raised the question whether poverty may lead to disability among children. In other words, not only does having a CSHCN increase the likelihood of economic hardship. Economic hardship itself may lead to disability among children by increasing the likelihood of exposure to environmental hazards and inadequate health care during pregnancy. Both these factors must be understood in order to design effective social policy and to develop health services for CSHCN.

In a time of dramatic economic downturn, reports about material hardship among families with children with chronic illnesses and or disabilities have particular resonance in discussions about health care reform. However, insurance is but one element in a comprehensive strategy to provide financial security for families with CSHCN (Chen & Newacheck, 2006). Depending on the definition used, the prevalence of underinsurance has been estimated to range from 7%–53% of the population. Recent data from the National Survey of CSHCN documented that approximately one-third of CSHCN were underinsured (Kogan, et al., 2005). A significant proportion of the participating families reported that health insurance benefits did not meet the child's needs and that the coverage did not allow them to see needed providers. There are several reports of children with chronic conditions having periods of no insurance during a given year. The authors argue that for this population, underinsurance is a larger problem than absence of insurance. They cite evidence for higher rates of supplemental insurance purchased by families to provide "wraparound" services for this population as well as the inadequacy of appropriate depth and breadth of covered services for privately insured children.

Another area in which health insurance may not be sufficient is if a child does not have access to needed care for elevated needs. Although specialty care is not only for children with special needs, most children with special needs use specialty care. Skinner and Mayer (2007) reviewed research conducted between 1992 and 2006 to examine the impact of insurance status on children's access to specialty care. They report that children with public insurance have better access to specialty care than uninsured children but poorer access than children with private insurance. They conclude that insurance should be structured to optimize access to specialty care for children but that more information is needed about specific health plans and health outcomes in order to recommend a particular structure of health insurance coverage. Current research does not show which arrangements best improve the health of children who need specialty care.

Children's Health Insurance Program (CHIP)

In 1997, the State Children's Health Insurance Program extended health insurance to children in families with incomes below 200% of the federal poverty level who are not eligible for Medicaid, 17% of whom were estimated to have special health care needs. This program, Title XXI of the Social Security Act, was the largest single expansion in health insurance coverage for children since Medicaid. Funded as a capped block grant to states, the Children's Health Insurance Program, referred to as CHIP, has great potential for removing one of the barriers to care for children with special health care needs by expanding access to insurance. In passing this legislation, Congress gave states substantial flexibility in designing their programs. For example, states can choose to use Medicaid or a separate state health plan, or a combination of both, to expand insurance coverage. Within certain guidelines, states can choose eligibility levels, benefit coverage, and other program characteristics allowing wide variation in the approaches taken across states.

As a result of CHIP, declines in uninsurance rates have been highest for minority children (Kenney & Yee, 2007). Using information from telephone interviews with families, Szilagyi and colleagues (2004) reported that enrollment in New York's CHIP program was associated with improved access and quality of care and that more care for CSHCN was taking place in the child's usual source of primary care. Similar positive outcomes from New York's program were reported by Davidoff et al. (2005), who used data from the National Health Interview Survey. According to this research, SCHIP generated a 9.8% increase in the proportion of children with chronic conditions reporting public insurance and a 6.4 percentage point decline in the proportion that was uninsured. Although early published reports that examined SCHIP enrollment among CSHCN described mixed results, Yu and Dick (2009) found a slight increase in SCHIP eligibility among CSHCN between 2001 and 2005. Noting that the SCHIP had become a relatively mature program by 2005, the authors assert that state policies that included presumptive eligibility stimulated SCHIP enrollment whereas states that required assets tests reduced enrollment.

Two promising strategies for organizing effective service delivery systems for CSHCN are the Medical Home and Transition Planning for youth with special health care needs.

Medical Home

The need for an ongoing source of health care for all children has been identified as a priority for child healthcare reform at the national and local level. Families with children with chronic conditions in particular need help navigating the complex and often fragmented health care delivery system in order to obtain needed services. A number of leaders in health care have advanced the medical home model of primary care to optimize the accessibility, continuity, and coordination of services for this population. This strategy for continuous access to quality, comprehensive, and coordinated care has as its foundation a partnership between families and providers and a single point of entry to a system of care that facilitates access to medical and nonmedical services. The six attributes comprising a medical home include having (1) a usual place for sick/well care;

(2) a personal doctor or nurse; (3) no difficulty in obtaining needed referrals; (4) needed care coordination; (5) family-centered care; and (6) services for making transitions to all aspects of adult life that are associated with treatment adherence, use of preventive health services, and reduction of healthcare disparities. These attributes of care also frame a set of six core objectives for CSHCN that are used for measuring the performance of state Title V programs and achieving the Healthy People 2020 goals.

Using a medical home approach for delivering services has revealed numerous benefits. Kogan et al. (2010) analyzed 30 studies for evidence supporting the national goal that CSHCN receive care from a medical home. Although none of the studies examined all six attributes of the medical home, most described a positive relationship between the medical home and outcomes such as better health status, timeliness of care, and family-centered care.

However, in a unique study examining geographic disparities in access to the medical home, Singh et al. (2009) reported that, although prevalence varies across the states, 53% of CSHCN do not have access to a medical home. Using the National Survey of CSHCN to analyze the quality of a medical home (children receiving needed services), Benedict (2008) reported that, among children who needed therapeutic and supportive services, less than one-quarter had a high-quality medical home. Nageswaran (2009) reported similar findings for families who needed respite care, a specific supportive service recommended by the American Academy of Pediatrics. Supportive services (e.g., transportation, respite care) are essential for families to be able to raise their children in their homes and communities. Many professional organizations, including the American Academy of Pediatrics, the Academic Pediatric Association, the Society for Teachers in Family Medicine, and the Society of General Internal Medicine, promote the development of a more robust evidence base and evidence-based implementation of the medical home model (Stille, et al., 2010).

Transition Planning for Youth with Special Needs

Chronic health and disabling conditions that continue through adolescence compound the complex tasks of achieving independence. Adolescents with chronic conditions experience ongoing health problems that require continuing interaction with the health care system through adulthood. Adequate insurance coverage (defined as whether the family feels its insurance covers the services needed, including covering a reasonable share of costs and being able to see the providers they feel are best for their child) is associated with fewer problems obtaining referrals and a greater likelihood of having a personal doctor or nurse. However, achievements in medical technology that have improved survival, and public attitudes that have enlightened community responsiveness for many children with chronic conditions, have not been translated into comprehensive services for adolescents with special needs.

Youth with chronic conditions need developmentally appropriate support to understand and manage their conditions and to negotiate the changes in policies, providers, and programs inherent in the move from pediatric to adult health care systems. The majority of young adult (17–25 years of age) respondents (those with limitations in activities of daily living or work, use of assistive devices, learning disabilities, developmental problems) to the 2001 Survey of Income and Program Participation reported gaps in insurance coverage, and many were uninsured for a substantial portion of the study period (Callahan & Cooper, 2007)

Results from the 2005–2006 National Survey of CSHCN revealed that less than half (41%) of youth with SHCN met the core outcome measure for transition to adult health care, work, and independence (Lotstein, et al., 2009). The American Academy of Pediatrics, the American Academy of Family Physicians, and the American College of Physicians-American Society of Internal Medicine (2002) developed a joint statement that specified steps necessary for ensuring an effective transition. Steps for medical providers included securing a primary care provider with responsibility for transition planning, creating a written health care transition plan by age 14, and ensuring continuous health insurance coverage.

Despite evidence-based recommendations, few pediatric practices initiate planning for transition early in adolescence. Most practices do not organize their office systems or care processes to disseminate educational materials. There are likely numerous reasons including limited staff training or technical support in transition planning and financial barriers. It may also be due to the lack of an identified staff member responsible for transition planning and the emotional uneasiness pediatricians, adolescents and their parents experience when anticipating a change in providers (McManus, et al., 2008).

A paramount concern for adolescents who live with chronic conditions is making a successful transition from school to work, achieving a maximum level of independence, securing financial support, completing job training, and having adult health care services. As a result, it is essential to ensure continued access to health care and benefits and to strengthen coordination among the public programs with mandates to serve this population.

CIVIL RIGHTS FOR CHILDREN AND YOUTH WITH SPECIAL HEALTH CARE NEEDS

Several legislative initiatives address specifically the civil rights of individuals with disabilities and have implications for protecting the interests of children and youth with special needs. Section 504 of the Rehabilitation Act of 1973 (PL 93-112) is neither an education law nor a federal grant program. Paralleling the language in the Civil Rights

Act of 1964, Section 504 established rights and entitlements for persons with disabilities. For example, under this law, acts of discrimination and failure to provide an appropriate public education for eligible students are perceived as violations of basic civil rights and can be addressed through this legislation. Section 504 has the potential to cover a broader spectrum of students and scope of activities than IDEA. The definition of who qualifies as an "individual with a disability" is more inclusive than IDEA, and many children who are not considered eligible for special education or related services under IDEA are covered under Section 504. Students who fit the Section 504 definition are those with a disability (physical or mental) that substantially limits one or more major life activities. Students who "have a history of" or are "regarded as" having a disability are included. For example, students with ADHD, or students with physical disabilities or sensory impairments who may need only accommodations for physical access or alternative methods of communication, qualify for services through Section 504 even if they do not meet the criteria specified under special education legislation.

In amendments to DD legislation in 1975, Congress established Protection and Advocacy systems in every state to pursue legal, administrative, and other appropriate remedies to protect the rights of persons with disabilities. Over the course of the implementation of special education legislation, some families have used state Protection and Advocacy programs to assist with developing an Individualized Education Plan for their children.

The Americans with Disabilities Act of 1990 was designed to protect people with mental or physical disabilities from discrimination based on disability. The Americans with Disabilities Act requires public facilities, including child care centers, to make reasonable modifications in policies, practices, and procedures to accommodate individuals with special needs. Necessary changes for child care centers may include curriculum adaptations, removal of physical barriers, additional staff training, alteration of staffing patterns, and adaptive equipment.

CONCLUSION

A sizable number of children and youth live with chronic conditions. Improved understanding of this diverse population of children and their families, propelled by the dissemination and analysis of new population-based national surveys, has generated clearer understanding of the characteristics of appropriate services and has inspired legislative, policy, and programmatic commitments to the health and welfare of this population. This understanding has bolstered the urgency of improving linkages among health, mental health, education and social services, developing stronger partnerships between private and public service sectors, and sustaining community-based services. Assuring comprehensive and continuous care at each developmental stage across the life course requires that current deliberations and decisions about the financing of care for CSHCN are monitored and that leadership roles at state and community levels are reinforced.

References

American Academy of Pediatrics, American Academy of Family Physicians, American College of Physicians-American Society of Internal Medicine. (2002). A consensus statement on health care transitions for young adults with special health care needs. *Pediatrics, 110*(6), 1304–1306.

Benedict, R. E. (2008). Quality medical homes: Meeting children's needs for therapeutic and supportive services. *Pediatrics, 121*(1), e127–e134.

Bethell, C. D., Read, D., Neff, J., Blumberg, S. J., Stein, R. E. K., Sharp, V., & Newacheck, P. W. (2002). Comparison of the children with special health care needs screener to the questionnaire for identifying children with chronic conditions. *Ambulatory Pediatrics, 2,* 49–57.

Busch, S. H., & Barry, C. L. (2009). Does private insurance adequately protect families of children with mental health disorders? *Pediatrics, 124*(4), S399–S406.

Callahan, S. T., & Cooper, W. O. (2007). Continuity of health coverage among young adults with disabilities. *Pediatrics, 119*(6), 1175–1180.

Centers for Disease Control and Prevention. (2000). Measuring childhood asthma prevalence before and after the 1997 redesign of the national health interview survey: United States. *Morbidity Mortality Weekly Report, 49,* 908–911. Retrieved March 23, 2004 from http://www.cdc.gov/mmwr/preview/mmwrhtml/mm4940a2.htm.

Centers for Disease Control and Prevention. (2002a). Folic acid and prevention of spina bifida and anencephaly, 10 years after the U.S. public health service recommendation. *Morbidity and Mortality Weekly Report, 51*(RR-13), 1–3.

Centers for Disease Control and Prevention. (2002b). Alcohol use among women of childbearing age: United States, 1991–1999. *Morbidity Mortality Weekly Report, 51*(13), 273–276.

Chen, A. Y., & Newacheck, P. W. (2006). Insurance coverage and financial burden for families of children with special health care needs. *Ambulatory Pediatrics, 6*(4), 204–209.

Cooper, W., & Hickson, G. B. (2001). Corticosteroid prescription filling for children covered by Medicaid following an emergency department visit or a hospitalization for asthma. *Archives of Pediatrics and Adolescent Medicine, 155,* 1111–1115.

Davidoff, A., Kenney, G., & Dubay, L. (2005). Effects of the State Children's Health Insurance Program expansions on children with chronic health conditions. *Pediatrics, 116*(1), e34–e42.

Developmental Disabilities Services and Facilities Construction Amendments of 1970, Pub. L. No. 91-517, 84 Stat. 1316 (1970).

Developmentally Disabled Assistance and Bill of Rights Act, Pub. L. No. 94-103, 89 Stat. 486 (1975).

Education for all Handicapped Children Act, Pub. L. No. 94-142 (1975).

Education of the Handicapped Act Amendments of 1986, Pub. L. No. 99-457, 100 Stat. 1145 (1986).

Emerson, E. (2004). Poverty and children with intellectual disabilities in the world's richer countries. *Journal of Intellectual and Developmental Disability, 29*(4), 319–338.

Gannotti, M. E., & Handwerker, W. P. (2002). Puerto Rican understandings of child disability: Methods for the cultural validation of standardized measures of child health. *Social Science & Medicine, 55,* 2093–2105.

Inkelas, M., Raghavan, R., Larson, K., Kuo, A. A., & Ortega, A. N. (2007). Unmet mental health need and access to services for children with special health care needs and their families. *Ambulatory Pediatrics, 7*(6), 431–438.

Kaiser Commission on Medicaid and the Uninsured. (2002, February). Health insurance coverage in America: 2000 data update. Menlo Park, CA: The Henry J. Kaiser Family Foundation. Retrieved March 26, 2011 from http://www.kff.org/uninsured/4007-index.cfm.

Kataoka, S. H., Zhang, L., & Wells, K. B. (2002). Unmet need for mental health care among US children: Variation by ethnicity and insurance status. *American Journal of Psychiatry, 159,* 1548–1555.

Kenney, G., & Yee, J. (2007). SCHIP at a crossroads: Experiences to date and challenges ahead. *Health Affairs, 26*(2), 256–369.

Kogan, M. D., Newacheck, P. W., Honberg, L., & Strickland, B. (2005). Association between underinsurance and access to care among children with special health care needs in the United States. *Pediatrics, 116*(5), 1162–1169.

Kogan, M. D., Strickland, B. B., & Newacheck, P. W. (2010). Building systems of care: Findings from the national survey of children with special health care needs. *Pediatrics, 124*(4), S333–S336.

Lotstein D. S., Ghandour, R., Cash, A., McGuire, E., Strickland, B., & Newacheck P. W. (2009). Planning for health care transitions: Results from the 2005 2006 National Survey of Children with Special Health Care Needs. *Pediatrics, 123,* e145–e152.

McManus, M., Fox, H., O'Connor, K., Chapman, T., & MacKinnon, J. (2008). *Pediatric perspectives and practices on transitioning adolescents with special needs to adult health care.* Fact Sheet No. 6. Washington, DC: National Alliance to Advance Adolescent Health.

McPherson, M., Arango, P., Fox, H., Lauver, C., McManus, M., Perrin, J. M., Shonkoff, J. P., & Strickland, B. (1998). A new definition of children with special health care needs. *Pediatrics, 102,* 137–141.

Merikangas, K. R., He, J., Burstein, M., Swanson, S., Avenevoli, S., Cui, L., Benjet, C., Georgiades, K., & Swendsen, J. (2010). Lifetime prevalence of mental disorders in U.S. adolescents: Results from the national comorbidity survey replication-adolescent supplement (NCS-A). *Journal of* the American Academy of Child & Adolescent Psychiatry, 49(10), 980–989.

Mulero, A., & Font, A. (1997). Pediatric physical therapy services in Puerto Rico. *Pediatric Physical Therapy, 7*, 172–174.

Nageswaran, S. (2009). Respite care for children with special health care needs. *Archives of Pediatrics & Adolescent Medicine, 163*(1), 49–54.

National Commission on Childhood Disability. (1995, October). Supplemental Security Income for children with disabilities report to Congress. Washington, DC: U.S. Government Printing Office.

Newacheck, P. W., Houtrow, A. J., Romm, D. L., Kuhlthau, K. A., Bloom, S. R., Van Cleave, J. M., & Perrin, J. M. (2009). The future of health insurance for children with special health care needs. *Pediatrics, 123*(5), e940–e947.

Newacheck, P. W., Stein, R. E. K., Bauman, L., & Hung, Y. Y. (2003). Disparities in the prevalence of disability between black and white children. *Archives of Pediatrics and Adolescent Medicine, 157*, 244–248.

Ngui, E. M., & Flores, G. (2006). Satisfaction with care and ease of using health care services among parents of children with special health care needs: The roles of race/ethnicity, insurance, language, and adequacy of family-centered care. *Pediatrics, 117*(4), 1184–1196.

Okumura, M. J., Van Cleave, J., Gnanasekaran, S., & Houtrow, A. (2009). Understanding factors associated with work loss for families caring for CSHCN. *Pediatrics, 124*(4). S392–S398.

Parish, S. L., Rose, R. A., Grinstein-Weiss, M., Richman, E. L., & Andrews, M. E. (2008). Material hardship in U.S. families raising children with disabilities. *Exception Children, 75*(1), 71–92.

Pennsylvania Association for Retarded Children v. Pennsylvania, 343 R Supp. 279 E.D. Pa. (1972).

Perrin, J., & Stein, R. E. K. (1991). Reinterpreting disability: Changes in Supplemental Security Income for children. *Pediatrics, 87*, 1047–1051.

Personal Responsibility and Work Opportunity Reconciliation Act of 1996, Pub. L. No. 104-193, 110 Stat. 2105 (1996).

Rehabilitation, Comprehensive Services, and Developmental Disabilities Amendments of 1978, Pub. L. 95-602, 92 Stat. 2955 (1978).

Schulzinger, R. (1998). *Advocate's guide to SSI for children* (3rd ed.). Washington, DC: Judge David L. Bazelon Center for Mental Health Law.

Skinner, A. C., & Mayer, M. L. (2007). Effects of insurance status on children's access to specify

care: a systematic review of the literature. *BioMed Central, 7*(194), 1–12.

Singh, G. K., Strickland, B. B., Ghandour, R. M., & van Dyck, P. C. (2009). Geographic disparities in access to the medical home among US CSHCN. *Pediatrics, 124*(4), S352–S360.

Stein, R. E. K., Bauman, L. J., Westbrook, L. E., Coupey, S. M., & Ireys, H. T. (1993). Framework for identifying children who have chronic conditions: The case for a new definition. *Journal of Pediatrics, 122*, 342–347.

Stille, C., Turchi, R., Antonelli, R., Cabana, M. D., Cheng, T. L., Laraque, D., Perrin, J., & Academic Pediatric Association Task Force on Family-Centered Medical Home. (2010). The family-centered medical home: Specific considerations for child health research and policy. *Academic Pediatrics, 10*(4), 211–217.

Sullivan v. Zebley, 88-1377 (U.S. Supreme Court, 20 February) (1990).

Szilagyi, P. G., Dick, A. W., Klein, J. D., & Shone, L. P. (2004). Improved access and quality of care after enrollment in the New York State Children's Health Insurance Program (SCHIP). *Pediatrics, 113*(5), e395–e404.

U.S. Census Bureau. (2008). National population projections released 2008. Retrieved March 26, 2011 from http://www.census.gov/population/www/projections/summarytables.html.

U.S. Department of Health and Human Services (USDHHS). (1999). *Mental health: A report of the Surgeon General*. Rockville, MD: Substance Abuse and Mental Health Services Administration, Center for Mental Health Services, National Institutes of Health, National Institute of Mental Health.

U.S. Department of Health and Human Services, Health Resources and Services Administration, Maternal and Child Health Bureau (USDHHS). (2010). *The National Survey of Children's Health 2007*. Rockville, MD: Author.

van Dyck, P. C., McPherson, M., Strickland, B. B., Nesseler, K., Blumberg, S. J., Cynamon, M. L., & Newacheck, P. W. (2002). The national survey of children with special health care needs. *Ambulatory Pediatrics, 2*, 29–37.

Yu, H., & Dick, A. W. (2009). Recent trends in state children's health insurance program eligibility and coverage for CSHCN. *Pediatrics, 124*(4), S337–S342.

Zambrana, R. E., & Logie, L. A. (2000). Latino child health: Need for inclusion in the US national discourse. *American Journal of Public Health, 90*, 1827–1833.

13

WOMEN, CHILDREN, AND ENVIRONMENTAL HEALTH

Jack K. Leiss

We are conducting a vast toxicologic experiment in our society, in which our children and our children's children are the experimental subjects.

(Herbert L. Needleman, cited in Weiss & Landrigan, 2000)

I learned a valuable lesson that night: the entire debate about scientific studies, about the health risks for children, was merely a shadow play. The real decision had been made by DuPont's economists.

(Needleman, 2000)

INTRODUCTION

Environmental chemical exposures can have a profound impact on the health of women, children, and their families. These exposures act by disrupting the biochemical processes that are the basis of human physiology. Evidence suggests that they are affecting the full range of health outcomes that are of concern to the MCH community (Leiss & Kotch, 2010).

Children are especially vulnerable to harm from environmental exposures because their organs and body systems are developing. By disrupting the development of an organ or system, the exposure can result in permanent structural damage or functional disability that affects the child throughout her lifetime. The harm can be subtle (e.g., small deficits in intelligence) or obvious (e.g., violent behavior). It can become manifest at or near the time of exposure (e.g., as birth defects) or later in life (e.g., as hypertension during pregnancy). In general, the prenatal period is thought to be the time of greatest vulnerability because

the basic structure and function of many organs and systems, including the brain, are determined during that time. Development continues through adolescence, however, and at various times during infancy, childhood, and adolescence, particular organs and body systems may be at heightened vulnerability (Dietert, 2009; Faustman, Silbernagel, Fenske, Burbacher, & Ponce, 2000).

Discussions of MCH problems and environmental health often include lack of safe drinking water, malnutrition, vector-borne diseases, and comparable conditions that are major causes of childhood morbidity and mortality in developing countries. The causes, consequences, and prevention of these conditions are qualitatively different from those of the issues addressed in this chapter, and therefore they are not discussed here. Rather, this chapter focuses on involuntary exposures to chemicals and physical agents (e.g., radiation, noise) that are present in the environment as a result of human activity.

NINE THEMES IN MCH ENVIRONMENTAL HEALTH

The subject of this chapter is pertinent to most other MCH topics and virtually all of public health. It encompasses a vast range of chemical and physical agents, environmental processes, exposure pathways, physiological processes, health outcomes, scientific disciplines, and policy perspectives. In this section, this diverse material is summarized into themes that integrate the subject matter across its various dimensions. For brevity, maternal exposures are included in general references to children's exposures. Some environmental exposures, such as radiation, are potentially harmful because of their physical rather than their chemical properties. For simplicity in presentation, these agents are included in general references to chemicals.

1. Children's exposure to environmental chemicals is pervasive, extensive, and intensive.

Pervasive exposure means that children are exposed virtually everywhere they are. Table 13–1 lists some of the places in which children's exposures have been documented. The list includes places that serve the general population, places that are principally intended for occupancy by children, places where children spend most of their time, and the womb. Children are also exposed to chemicals at work; worldwide, 300 million

Table 13–1. Places in Which Children's Exposure to Environmental Chemicals Has Been Documented.

Womb	Child care
Hospital	School
Home	School bus
Yard	Playground
Car	Sports field

children work, mostly but not only in developing countries (Diallo, Hagemann, Etienne, Gurbuzer, & Mehran, 2010).

The pervasiveness of children's exposure can be attributed to three conditions. First, the general environment—the air, the food supply, and the water supply throughout the world—is suffused with chemicals produced by human activity. MCH populations living in this environment cannot avoid exposure. Even when chemicals are put into the environment in distant locations, they can become distributed around the globe, thus exposing women and children who live in regions in which those chemicals are neither produced nor used (Sandau, Ayotte, Dewailly, Duffe, & Norstrom, 2002).

Second, many products that are intentionally introduced into children's environments produce exposure to chemicals. These include pesticides; cleaners and disinfectants; laundry products; air fresheners; clothes and shoes; bedding; appliances and electronic devices; toys; arts and crafts; plastic products; cosmetics and personal care products; baby care products; tobacco smoke; vaccines, drugs, and medical treatments; indoor fuels (primarily in developing countries); building materials; and military armaments and weapons. Many of these products are intended specifically for children and are marketed to or for children.

Third, children are subject not only to their own direct exposures, but also to the exposures of their parents and other household members. Maternal exposures become fetal exposures for chemicals that cross the placenta. The mother's exposures become the nursing child's exposures for chemicals that enter breast milk. The household's working members' occupational exposures become the mother's or child's exposures for chemicals that are inadvertently brought home from the workplace, for example, on the worker's clothes. (This source of household exposure is called "take-home toxins" in the occupational health literature.) Furthermore, children are subject to their parents' preconception exposures. The mother's preconception exposures that remain in her body and subsequently cross the placenta or enter her breast milk become the child's prenatal or postnatal exposures. Certain chemicals to which the father may be exposed can damage the sperm before conception or be carried in the sperm to the zygote, thus exposing the developing embryo and fetus. Finally, the pregnant woman's preconception and post-conception exposures can affect the infant indirectly, as well as the woman herself, by their effects on the woman's health during and after pregnancy.

Extensive exposure means that children are exposed to many different chemicals simultaneously. These include a long list of metals, dioxins, solvents, pesticides, pharmaceuticals, plasticizers, endocrine disrupters, carcinogens, and other volatile organic compounds and persistent organic pollutants. (See Table 13–2.) Dozens of different chemicals have been found in cord blood, breast milk, placenta, and the blood and urine of various maternal and child populations around the world. Moreover, only the specific chemicals for which tests were conducted could have been detected, and these represent only a tiny fraction of the tens of thousands of industrial chemicals in use in the world today. Consequently, the number of different chemicals to which children everywhere are exposed is likely much greater than studies to date indicate, and the actual extent of children's exposure to environmental chemicals is unknown.

Intensive exposure means that children are exposed to high levels of environmental chemicals. The appropriate criteria for gauging the intensity of children's environmental exposure levels are (1) environmental or biological levels that have been shown to be harmful in human or animal studies, (2) environmental contaminant levels deemed harmful by regulatory agencies, and (3) environmental contaminant levels used by regulatory agencies to determine safe exposure

Table 13–2 Some Environmental Chemicals and Physical Agents to Which Children Are Exposed.

AFCA[1]	Nitrates
Air pollutants	Noise
Arsenic	Organotins
Bisphenol A	PAHs[3]
Cadmium	PBDEs[4]
DEA[2]	PCBs[5]
Dioxins	PCP[6]
Fluoride	Perchlorate
Formaldehyde	Pesticides
Ionizing radiation	PFCs[7]
Lead	Phthalates
Manganese	Solvents
Mercury	Tobacco smoke
Nanoparticles	Triclosan

[1] artificial food color and additives
[2] diethanolamine
[3] polycyclic aromatic hydrocarbons
[4] polybrominated diphenyl ethers
[5] polychlorinated biphenyls
[6] pentachlorophenol
[7] perfluorinated compounds

limits (e.g., assumptions about the amount of mercury in particular types of fish used to set recommended quantities of fish consumption for pregnant women). For most of the chemicals that are prevalent in children's environments, not even one of these criteria has been set, and children's exposure levels are unknown. Consequently, there is no basis for concluding that exposure levels are low. Regarding those chemicals for which these criteria have been set and for which children's exposure levels are known, the exposure levels exceed one or more of the criteria for many of the chemicals. Thus, children's exposure levels are known to be high for some chemicals and known to be low for few, if any, chemicals.

2. Currently, scientific research is able to provide only a limited understanding of how environmental exposures are affecting women's and children's health.

Given the pervasive, extensive, and intensive exposure described previously, it is important to understand how these exposures are affecting the health of MCH populations. Although scientific study of this question has expanded greatly in recent years, advances in understanding these effects have been inhibited by several problems. Following is a brief overview of some of the major issues.

What to Look for

Scientific studies are most productive when they are guided by *a priori* hypotheses about the causal association between a given exposure and a given outcome. However, for many of the chemicals to which MCH populations are exposed, there has been or continues to be a lack of prior understanding about what the effect of the exposure *could* be. In some cases, erroneous notions of how particular chemicals act in the body have actively inhibited progress in studying the effects of those chemicals (Rudel, 1997).

Misconstrued Exposures

Almost all research to date on the health effects of children's environmental exposures has examined the effects of exposure to a single chemical. However, the effects of exposure to different chemicals in combination may bear little relation to the effects of exposure to those same chemicals singly or in a different combination. Even the order in which sequential exposure to different chemicals occurs may be important for determining the health effects of those exposures (Ashauer, Boxall, & Brown, 2007). Given the extensive nature of children's environmental exposures (see Theme 1), the effects of exposure to an individual chemical, or even to a limited combination of chemicals, may be irrelevant for understanding the impact of actual environmental exposures on MCH populations (Kortenkamp, 2007; Richard, Moslemi, Sipahutar, Benachour, & Seralini, 2005; Suk, Olden, & Yang, 2002).

Poorly Understood Outcomes

For some health outcomes, advances in understanding possible causal associations have been slow due to a limited understanding of the outcome itself (e.g., autism; Hertz-Picciotto & Delwiche, 2009).

Subtle Effects

Some harmful effects may be difficult to measure or detect because of their subtle manifestation. However, subtle effects are not necessarily trivial; they can have strong impacts on both individual and population health (Counter, 2003; Davidson, et al., 2006).

Multiplicity and Complexity of Effects

Individual chemicals may cause diverse effects, such as cancer and neurodevelopmental disability. Moreover, some chemicals cause one effect at lower doses and a different effect at higher doses. Similarly, for some chemicals, the effect of a short-term, high-dose exposure (used in many toxicological tests) is quite different from the effect of a long-term, low-dose exposure (typical of many environmental exposures to MCH populations). Additionally, some chemicals cause one outcome if the fetus is exposed at a particular stage of its development but a different outcome if exposure occurs at a different stage. (This phenomenon is called "windows of vulnerability.") Some exposures may be harmful to children with a particular genetic profile but not to those with a different genetic profile. (This phenomenon is called "gene-environment interaction.") Furthermore, the effect of an exposure on the developing fetus may be influenced not only by the genetic profile of the fetus itself, but also by the genetic profiles of the mother or the father. For many chemicals, progress in understanding the health effects of exposure has been inhibited (or is still being inhibited) by the need to first conceptualize, identify, distinguish, and measure these complex factors (Myers, Zoeller, & Vom Saal, 2009; Scinicariello, Murray, Smith, Wilbur, & Fowler, 2005; Weiss, 2007).

Whom to Look at

Related to the previous point is the difficulty of identifying the appropriate study population for investigating a particular exposure-effect association. As mentioned earlier, a particular association may be limited to children who have (or whose father or mother has) a specific genetic profile or to those who were exposed during a narrow period of their development. Similarly, nutritional factors, psychological stress, other social exposures, and other chemical exposures can be strong determinants of the effects of a particular exposure ("effect modification"). If these issues are not incorporated into selection of the study population, which may be difficult or impossible even if the issues are recognized, the study may fail to detect the effect even if it exists (Weiss & Bellinger, 2006).

Lack of Reference Groups

Epidemiologic and toxicological studies are based on comparing the outcome in an exposed group to the outcome in an unexposed group. However, because of the pervasive nature of children's environmental exposures, it can be difficult to find an unexposed group for a particular study. Similarly, because of the pervasive contamination of the general environment, even in the controlled conditions of an experimental laboratory it may be difficult to obtain and maintain an unexposed group of animals for a toxicological study (Thigpen, et al., 2004).

Methods Not Available

For many of the problems raised by children's environmental exposures, the toxicological, epidemiologic, or other methods needed to study the problems do not exist (Colborn, 2009; Savitz, 2001).

3. Environmental chemical exposures are having a severe adverse impact on the health of women and children worldwide.

Although knowledge of how environmental exposures are affecting women and children is lacking for many exposures, outcomes, and population groups, numerous associations between particular exposures and adverse outcomes have been found. It is important for prevention to know whether these associations are causal. For this purpose, exposures can be classified as proven harmful; found to be harmful in some studies, but the evidence is insufficient to prove causality yet too strong to be dismissed as noncausal; or unknown because the research has not been done (and perhaps cannot be done). Theoretically, a body of research could establish that a particular chemical is safe, i.e., causes no harmful effects at environmental exposure levels. However, given the huge number of different combinations of chemicals (see Theme 1) and other relevant variables (e.g., stress, nutritional factors) to which MCH populations are exposed, the likelihood of different effects from different combinations of exposures and for different segments of the population, and the limited ability to identify these effects through scientific research (see Theme 2), it may be impossible with current methods and resources to study a particular chemical for all of its likely harmful effects.

Even limiting the discussion to the exposures that have been proven harmful or for which the evidence of harm is quite strong, the known impact is profound. Environmental exposures are having harmful effects on children at every stage of their development, from preconception through adolescence, and on into adulthood (and parenting). Furthermore, environmental exposures are having adverse effects with regard to all of the crosscutting MCH issues, including breastfeeding, nutrition, and obesity; oral health; health disparities, both within and between countries; children and youth with special health care needs; and women's health across the life span. Table 13–3 lists some of the MCH outcomes for which there is substantial scientific evidence that they are caused by environmental exposures (Lanphear & Bearer, 2005).

Although the effects of numerous chemicals have been studied, these represent only a fraction of the chemicals, and an even smaller fraction of the combinations of chemicals, to which MCH populations are exposed. Furthermore, these studies examined only a limited set of the potential harmful effects of these chemicals. Along with the fact that even the quantity and chemical composition of children's exposures are largely unknown (see Theme 1), the overall picture is one of pervasive, extensive, and intensive exposure to chemicals known to be harmful or, at best, not known to be safe. A growing body of evidence suggests that the unknown (as well as the known) effects of these exposures are having a profound impact on children's health at the population level throughout the world (Grandjean & Landrigan, 2006; Royal Commission on Environmental Pollution, 2003).

Table 13–3 Some MCH Outcomes that Are Known or Thought[1] to Be Caused by Environmental Exposures.

Asthma
Autism
Birth defects
Cancer
Cognitive and intellectual deficits, including learning disabilities
Complications of pregnancy, including hypertension
Disrupted sexual development
DNA damage
Fetal death and miscarriage
Impaired fetal growth, including preterm birth
Impaired immune function
Impaired lactation
Infant death
Infertility
Neurobehavioral deficits, including delinquency, violence, and ADHD[2]
Obesity
Reduced respiratory function
Thyroid disorders during and after pregnancy

[1]That is, the scientific evidence is strong but not conclusive.
[2]attention deficit hyperactivity disorder

4. Medical care, health education, and environmental remediation are generally ineffective at reducing the harmful effects of chemical exposures to MCH populations, whereas preventing the introduction of chemicals into the environment prevents both exposure and its adverse effects.

For most of the MCH outcomes that are known or thought to be caused by environmental exposures, treatment can often do little more than alleviate symptoms (e.g., for asthma), prevent adverse secondary outcomes (e.g., for women with preeclampsia related to lifetime lead exposure), or enable adaptive behaviors (e.g., for learning disabilities). For conditions that are less well understood, such as multiple chemical sensitivity or disrupted sexual development, even less can be done (Woolf, 2000). Although treatment for some conditions (e.g., childhood cancer) is often successful, the overall impact of medical care on alleviating the adverse effects of environmental exposures to MCH populations is limited.

Similarly, prevention efforts often focus on educating the public, and parents in particular, on how to protect children from exposure to chemicals that are pervasive in the environment, for example, by staying out of a room for a limited period of time after it has been sprayed with pesticides or keeping children indoors when air pollution exceeds certain limits (EPA, 2010b). Yet there is no scientific basis for believing that this approach is effective, and there is no evidence that it prevents exposure or adverse outcomes in MCH populations (with a few possible exceptions, e.g., environmental tobacco smoke). Likewise, screening programs that identify children after they have been exposed do little to improve population health, particularly if there is no effective treatment for the harmful effects of the exposure (Lanphear, 2005). Community interventions that aim to reduce exposure by removing the chemicals from the individual child's environment (e.g., lead abatement of individual homes) without removing them from the general environment (in this case, the housing stock) have been singularly unsuccessful at reducing population exposure levels (Brown, McLaine, Dixon, & Simon, 2006; Elias & Gulson, 2003). Moreover, these various approaches have seldom been evaluated for possible harmful effects of the intervention itself.

Finally, considerable resources are devoted to removing high concentrations of chemicals from particular locations (e.g., cleaning up toxic waste sites) to prevent further exposure to neighboring populations. Regardless of the benefits of these actions for local residents, this approach does little to address the problems discussed in Themes 1 and 3.

In contrast, stopping the introduction of harmful chemicals into the environment has been effective in reducing population exposure levels. For example, lowering the amount of lead in gasoline has markedly reduced population lead levels in several countries (Thomas, Socolow, Fanelli, & Spiro, 1999). Similarly, banning the use of certain persistent organic pollutants (e.g., polychlorinated biphenyls [PCBs]) has markedly reduced the levels of these chemicals in breast milk (Lignell, Aune, Darnerud, Cnattingius, & Glynn, 2009).

5. Regulation of environmental chemicals has failed to protect children's health.

The policy mechanism for protecting MCH (and other) populations from harmful environmental exposures is regulation of the manufacture, sale, and use of potentially harmful chemicals. In the United States, the three regulatory agencies that are most relevant for women's and children's environmental health are the Environmental Protection Agency (EPA), the Consumer Product Safety Commission (CPSC), and the Food and Drug Administration (FDA).

All three of these agencies describe their mission as protecting public health (CPSC, 2010a; EPA, 2010a; FDA, 2009). However, if the proverbial visitor from Mars who has no prior knowledge of our society were to observe environmental regulation in the United States, it might easily conclude that the purpose of regulation is to enable the introduction of harmful chemicals into the environment. A brief description of the major features of this system with regard to the protection of women's and children's health is provided next, followed by case studies of regulatory decisions by these three agencies.

1. *There are few restrictions on the manufacture, sale, or use of chemicals that have not been proven to be harmful.* Chemicals sold as pesticides (insecticides, herbicides, fungicides, etc.) are required by the EPA to undergo only minimal toxicity testing before they are allowed to be marketed and used; chemicals that are not sold as pesticides can be marketed and used without any toxicity testing. It is the intended use of the chemical, not its toxicity, that determines how it is regulated by the EPA.

The CPSC is responsible for ensuring that consumer products are safe. However, except for acute injury, the agency gives little attention to the adverse health effects of chemicals in consumer products.

New drugs and medical devices must meet safety standards specified by the FDA and therefore represent a partial exception to the rule. However, the integrity of controlled randomized trials for new drugs, the primary mechanism for evaluating drug safety, has become questionable (DeAngelis & Fontanarosa, 2010; Drazen & Wood, 2010). Furthermore, the chemical ingredients of cosmetics and personal care products, which are nominally under the purview of the FDA, are not regulated, are not required to meet any safety standards, and can be marketed without undergoing any toxicity testing.

2. *Once populations are exposed to a particular chemical, its manufacture, sale, or use may be restricted if it can be proven that people have been or will be harmed by it.* The regulatory criteria for establishing that a chemical has been proven to be harmful are extreme. Often, considerable illness, injury, and death must occur in order for the criteria to be met. Furthermore, because proof of harm depends on evidence of illness, injury, or death, in many cases restricting continued exposure to MCH populations can only begin after the population has experienced demonstrable harm. Given current limitations on the ability of scientific research to detect the harmful effects of environmental exposures (see Theme 2), it may be impossible to prove that a given chemical is harmful according to the regulatory criteria, even if the chemical is having a profound negative impact on women's and children's health. (See Theme 3.) Moreover, the convoluted process of establishing that a chemical is harmful according to regulatory criteria includes many stages at which the industry being regulated can delay, overturn, or halt the process. For example, one of the many ways in

which this happens is that in evaluating the evidence that a particular chemical is harmful, the regulatory agency often gives greater credence to studies funded by the industry that is being regulated than to studies funded by other sources (Ivory, 2010).

3. *Once a chemical is ruled to be harmful, the process of restricting its sale and use is long and drawn out.* It often takes years or decades to determine what restrictions will be imposed, during which time manufacture and use of the chemical and the resulting exposure can continue. Often, the final restrictions limit specific uses of the chemical but allow its continued release into the environment and exposure of the population from other uses.

4. *The process of determining the harm caused by a chemical and considering whether to restrict its sale or use is applied to one chemical at a time.* The entire process takes years and requires millions of dollars in research resources for each chemical. Although the federal government supports research in this area both internally and through academic institutions, the number of chemicals that can be studied is small compared to the extensive exposure of MCH populations (see Theme 1), and the range of harmful effects that can be studied for each chemical is limited (see Themes 2 and 3). Thus, most chemicals remain in use with little or no reduction in their harmful effects on MCH populations.

An obfuscatory rhetoric, which may be used by regulatory agencies, the industries they are regulating, or public commentators, accompanies this process.

- *"If it wasn't safe, we (they) would have regulated it."* Regulatory inaction with regard to a particular exposure is often used as evidence that the exposure poses no harm.

- *"The problem is with the consumer, not the chemical."* The harmful effects of a particular exposure are often dismissed as irrelevant because, it is argued, they were caused by improper use of the product.
- *"The exposure is trivial."* Opponents of a restriction often claim that a particular exposure is too small to have any effect on health. Similarly, it is frequently argued that population exposure to the chemical is greater from sources other than the use in question and that the public health benefits of restrictions on that use would be negligible. These arguments often directly contradict the scientific evidence, or at least are not supported by the evidence, but they are not officially rejected until the regulatory criteria for proof of harm are met.
- *"The harmful effect is greater than previously thought. (We didn't know.)"* When new studies produce evidence of harmful effects, the findings are often presented as a new discovery that could not have been acted on earlier. In fact, it is often the case that the harm was recognized earlier by some but the evidence was not given credence in the regulatory arena, or that substantial evidence of harm was acknowledged yet did not satisfy the regulatory criteria for proof of harm.
- *"Action has been (is being) taken."* New restrictions on the sale and use of harmful chemicals, and in particular bans on sale and use, are usually announced with great fanfare as a significant move to protect the public's health. However, the restrictions are often less than what they seem. A ban frequently includes a period of months or years during which the chemical is allowed to be manufactured, sold, and used before the actual ban takes effect; that is, a "ban" often allows the chemical to be sold and used for months or years after the agency has determined that such sale and use is harmful to public health. Secondly, the restrictions may limit the sale and use of the chemical for one purpose, but because sale and use for another purpose are not restricted, there may be little or no actual reduction in population exposure. Finally, a restricted chemical is often simply replaced with a different chemical, such that population exposure shifts from a chemical whose harmful effects have been proven according to regulatory criteria to one for which the scientific evidence does not meet those criteria (although the harm may be great) or for which the effects are unknown. Thus, the restriction may have little impact on overall population exposure to harmful chemicals. If the substitute chemical has greater harmful effects than the restricted chemical, restrictions based on a proof-of-harm, one-chemical-at-a-time approach to regulation could cause a worsening of MCH environmental health rather than an improvement.

Three Case Studies

FDA: Phthalate exposure in neonatal intensive care

The class of chemicals known as phthalates are endocrine disrupters that are contained in polyvinyl chloride (PVC) plastics, among other sources. One type of phthalate, di-(2-ethylhexyl) phthalate (DEHP), is approved by the FDA for use in medical devices as a consequence of its being in use before the FDA was given authority to regulate devices (i.e., 1976). In order to restrict its use, FDA would have to rule that such use was harmful (as opposed to the manufacturer having to show that it was safe, which is the criterion for new devices).

Beginning in the 1970s, evidence began to accumulate that (1) exposure to DEHP could disrupt sexual development (among other adverse outcomes), especially in males;

(2) that DEHP moves from plastic medical devices (such as intravenous bags and infusion lines) into the fluids they contain; and (3) that neonates who receive intensive therapeutic interventions could receive a higher dose of DEHP than was considered safe. Based on this information, the organization Health Care Without Harm (HCWH) petitioned the FDA in 1999 to require manufacturers of medical devices to include the DEHP content on the device label, so that providers could select non-DEHP devices for neonatal intensive care.

The FDA denied HCWH's petition in 2001 (FDA, 2001a). Instead, based on its own risk assessment (FDA, 2001b), FDA issued a Public Health Notification in 2002 in which it advised healthcare providers that "precautions should be taken to limit the exposure of the developing male to DEHP" (FDA, 2002). In the notification, FDA recommended that providers consider "alternatives when [selected] procedures are to be performed on male neonates, pregnant women who are carrying male fetuses, and peripubertal males." However, manufacturers were not required to include the DEHP content on the device label (HCWH, 2002).

The mild, suggestive language of the Public Health Notification contrasts with the findings of FDA's own safety assessment, in which it determined that the amount of DEHP to which some populations of neonates were exposed could exceed the safe dose by a factor of 20 (FDA, 2001b). Furthermore, by not requiring that device labels include the DEHP content, FDA effectively ensured that few providers would be able to comply with the agency's own patient safety recommendations. Theoretically, each provider could contact the suppliers and manufacturers of the different brands of the various devices and inquire about the devices' DEHP content. However, this process requires an inordinate amount of resources. It is beyond the capacity of many providers, whose patients instead are likely to be exposed to high levels of DEHP. Consequently, HCWH petitioned

the FDA again, in July 2007, to require labeling of the DEHP content of medical devices (FDA, 2007a). Included with the petition was documentation showing that without the labeling, many providers would not be able to identify DEHP-free devices for purchase (FDA, 2007b). As of September 2010, 11 years after the original petition and 9 years after FDA's own risk assessment, FDA had not responded to the 2007 petition.

CPSC: Arsenic exposure from CCA-wood play structures

Chromated copper arsenic (CCA) is a pesticide that is used as a wood preservative. It is 22% arsenic, which is an endocrine disrupter and human carcinogen and is associated with diverse adverse health outcomes. In the 1970s, CCA-treated ("pressure-treated") wood began to be used for wooden play structures in schools, parks, and residences, and CCA wood quickly became ubiquitous on playgrounds. EPA began a review of the safety of CCA wood in 1978, which lasted 10 years, and ultimately decided not to restrict its use. However, in the 1980s, scientific evidence began to accumulate showing that exposure to arsenic causes a variety of serious adverse health outcomes.

In 1990, CPSC conducted an analysis and concluded that, under conservative (i.e., higher exposure) assumptions, children would have a 21 per million risk of getting skin cancer (a very high risk by public health standards) from playing on CCA-wood play structures (CPSC, 1990). No regulatory action was taken at that time. Throughout the 1990s, scientific evidence continued to accumulate regarding associations between arsenic exposure and adverse health effects, and particular risks to children were identified. Furthermore, it was shown that children's exposure to CCA from play equipment and their consequent risk of cancer were orders of magnitude greater than the exposure levels and risk assumptions used in the 1990 CPSC analysis. Based on this information, two organizations, the Environmental

Working Group (EWG) and the Healthy Building Network (HBN), petitioned CPSC in 2001 to immediately ban the use of CCA wood in play equipment (CPSC, 2001). They subsequently extended the request to include a recall of all existing CCA-wood play structures (CPSC, 2003e).

In February 2003, CPSC reported the results of another analysis, which found that the lifetime risk of lung and bladder cancer from playing on CCA-wood play structures in early childhood was between 2 and 100 per million (CPSC, 2003c). CPSC noted that risks 100 times lower than that estimate (i.e., 1 per million) were its criterion for "regulatory consideration." In addition, in November 2003, EPA reported the results of an analysis that showed that, among young children who lived in a warm climate in the United States, half the population had a greater than 10 per million lifetime risk of cancer as a result of exposure to arsenic from CCA-wood play structures (EPA, 2003).

Nevertheless, in November 2003, CPSC denied the 2001 EWG/HBN petition (CPSC, 2003b). The basis for the denial was that action taken by EPA in the interim had made restrictions on CCA-wood play equipment by CPSC unnecessary and inconsequential. The EPA action, announced in February 2002, did result in cessation of the manufacture of CCA wood for use in residential settings (including play structures) by December 31, 2003 (EPA, 2002). However, the sale of CCA wood for this purpose was allowed to continue from existing stocks for another year, i.e., 3 years after the EWG/HBN petition and 14 years after the CPSC first determined that children had very high risk of cancer from this exposure. Furthermore, although the EPA action did eventually stop the introduction of new CCA-wood play structures into children's environments, CPSC did not recall existing structures and has done nothing to prevent children's continued exposure to chemicals that it has concluded are pervasive in children's environments and are very harmful. Moreover, CPSC's public information about CCA wood (as well as EPA's) implies that the agency has fulfilled its public health obligation and places further responsibility for preventing children's exposure on parents and caregivers (CPSC, 2003a, 2010b). After downplaying the risk posed by children's exposure to CCA ("Although the lifetime health risk from exposure to CCA-treated wood may be comparatively small…"), the agency recommends the "prudent" action of "thoroughly wash[ing] children's hands with soap and water immediately after playing on CCA pressure-treated wood playground equipment" (CPSC, 2003d). The absence of any scientific evidence that this "action" is effective in preventing exposure or protecting children's health contrasts sharply with the strong evidence of intensive exposure and severe harm found in CPSC's own risk assessments.

EPA: The Food Quality Protection Act

In the mid-1990s, several developments converged to produce legislation specifically aimed at protecting children from the harmful effects of pesticides in food. These developments included recognition of substantial increases in childhood morbidity and mortality thought to be caused by environmental exposures; recognition that many of these health outcomes (e.g., behavioral disorders) were not taken into account in regulatory decisions; and recognition that children had both higher exposure levels to environmental chemicals and greater vulnerability to the harmful effects of those exposures than were taken into account in regulatory decisions (Colborn, Dumanoski, & Myers, 1996; National Research Council, 1993).

The resulting legislation was the Food Quality Protection Act of 1996 (FQPA; Food Quality Protection Act of 1996, 1996). Among its provisions, the FQPA required EPA, when setting permissible levels of pesticide use on food, to (1) use a criterion of "safety," defined as "a reasonable certainty that no harm will result to infants and children from aggregate exposure to the pesticide" from all sources (i.e., from all types of food, not just individual items, and from nonfood sources such as home pesticide use); (2) "assess the... cumulative effects on infants and children of [pesticides] and other substances that have a common mechanism of toxicity" (i.e., take exposure to these other chemicals into account when assessing the risk from use on food of a particular pesticide); and (3) apply "an additional tenfold margin of safety...with respect to exposure and toxicity to infants and children" (i.e., reduce permissible levels to 10% of what is otherwise deemed safe) unless reliable evidence shows that a different factor is appropriate for protecting infants and children. In addition, EPA was required to include endocrine disruption as a toxic endpoint when determining permissible levels of use for pesticides and to reevaluate within ten years the permissible levels for all pesticides for which EPA had set permissible levels before enactment of FQPA.

The FQPA represented a groundbreaking redirection of regulatory policy in the United States in the interests of protecting children's health. Its passage was a cause for celebration among children's environmental health advocates. However, its implementation has fallen short of its promise, and interested organizations have had to sue EPA several times to force compliance with the law, with limited success. Among the many ways in which implementation of FQPA falls short of its intent, the testing program that EPA instituted for assessing the endocrine-disrupting effects of pesticides cannot detect harmful effects on major organs and cannot detect important serious adverse health outcomes (Colborn, 2009). Furthermore, for numerous pesticides, the permissible level of use has been set without a tenfold margin of safety for infant and child exposures even when toxicity tests indicated that even that margin would be insufficient (National Research Council, 2006; Thayer & Houlihan, 2004). Moreover, despite the criterion of safety stipulated in the FQPA, the proof-of-harm approach continues to dominate pesticide

regulation. Fifteen years after its passage, implementation of FQPA may have reduced children's exposure to particular pesticides, but it has done little to reduce children's overall exposure to harmful pesticides or even to ensure that their food is free of these exposures (Watnick, 1999).

Other Approaches to Regulation

In developing countries, pesticides that are used on export crops are generally regulated in accordance with recent international agreements that limit the types and amounts of permissible pesticide residues on food (Galt, 2008). However, even for these crops, regulatory practices may not protect MCH populations from exposure through handling and application of the pesticides. For nonexport crops, pesticide use is generally subject to few regulations. For other chemicals, documentation of regulatory practices is sparse, but sporadic and anecdotal evidence suggests that regulation is lax (Blacksmith Institute, 2007; Nweke & Sanders, 2009).

The European Union is in the process of implementing a new chemical regulation policy adopted in 2006. The new policy, called Registration, Evaluation and Authorisation of Chemicals (REACH), is an attempt to replace the regulatory approach described previously with one that is more protective of public health (Williams, Panko, & Paustenbach, 2009). In particular, REACH is intended to place the primary responsibility for establishing the safety of a chemical on the manufacturer. As such, it represents a radical departure from the regulatory approach used in the United States. However, the extent to which these goals will be achieved through REACH remains to be seen (Koch & Ashford, 2006; Rudén & Hansson, 2010).

Weiss (2001) has argued that regulatory decisions about environmental exposures should incorporate formal ethical assessments along with risk assessments. This approach is compatible with the Precautionary Principle, which has been proposed as an alternative to the proof-of-harm approach that currently characterizes environmental regulation in the United States. Under the Precautionary Principle, regulatory approval for use of a chemical would be determined, among other criteria, by scientific evidence that the use was safe, i.e., would not be harmful to public health. The practicability of the Precautionary Principle, as well as procedures for its general application, are currently being debated (Petrenko & McArthur, 2010). However, there are numerous instances of its application in practice. One is the response of the Australian Pesticides and Veterinary Medicines Authority (APVMA) to the exposure of children to harmful chemicals from CCA-wood playground equipment. In contrast to the regulatory inaction of the CPSC described earlier, APVMA announced in July 2003 that, by the end of 2003, CCA could no longer be used to treat wood used in playground equipment "unless there is conclusive proof that continued use is safe" (APVMA, 2003). The APVMA stated that "while scientific opinion on whether CCA poses a significant hazard was divided, the Board considered that they should take a highly protective approach in this instance ... Suppliers of CCA products had called for its retention unless there was conclusive scientific evidence that CCA poses an unacceptable risk to the community ... the APVMA did not support this approach. ... it was up to the [suppliers] to prove their products were safe." (APVMA, 2003; APVMA did not have the authority to recall existing CCA playground equipment.)

6. Disparities in exposure and health outcomes characterize MCH environmental health both within and between countries.

There are two dimensions of disparity in MCH environmental health, disparity in exposure and disparity in health outcomes caused by exposure. Some harmful exposures are greater among more advantaged social groups, especially exposures that result from a more affluent lifestyle. In addition, some exposures are evenly distributed across social groups. However, such situations are atypical. Although disparities in environmental exposure are more complex than a simple dichotomy between minority vs. majority race/ethnicity or low vs. high socioeconomic status (SES), more advantaged groups generally have lower exposure.

Most of the findings on disparities in exposure come from the United States, but comparable disparities have been found in Europe and in some developing countries. In general, the places where racial/ethnic minorities and lower SES populations live have higher levels of harmful environmental chemicals than the places where racial/ethnic majorities and higher SES populations live. This is true for geographic areas such as neighborhoods as well as for smaller environments such as houses. It is also true for places that are intended especially for children, such as schools. Higher levels of harmful chemicals in the environment would be expected to result in greater exposure for the women and children who live in these environments. Not surprisingly, MCH populations who live in these more contaminated environments do have higher levels of environmental chemicals in their organs and tissues (i.e., higher body burdens) compared to MCH populations who live in less contaminated environments. Moreover, because women and children form a larger percentage of the population among racial/ethnic minorities and lower SES groups compared to racial/ethnic majorities and higher SES groups, the overall racial and SES disparities in exposure result in even larger disparities for MCH populations. A relative lack of political and economic power, racism, and racial discrimination seem to be the social factors underlying these disparities (Mohai, Pellow, & Roberts, 2009).

Internationally, MCH populations in developing countries generally have greater exposure to harmful chemicals than MCH populations in developed countries. At least four interrelated conditions create the situation in which this greater exposure occurs. First, the political and economic policies of developing countries, including policies that affect the environmental exposures of MCH populations, are to a large degree subject to the interests of developed countries and transnational corporations. Second, developing countries do not have sufficient financial resources for addressing the numerous social and economic problems of their populations, one of which is harmful environmental exposures. Third, governmental and social institutions in developing countries have limited technical, legal, organizational, political, and social capacity for controlling environmental exposures. And fourth, most wars and armed conflicts are conducted in developing countries (d'Harcourt & Purdin, 2009; Gross, 1974; Harari, Morales, & Harari, 2005; Jansen, 2008; New York Times, 1992; Reed, 2002).

As a result of these conditions, several factors commonly found in developing countries lead to the greater exposure of MCH populations there. Some of these factors are outlined next (Ecobichon, 2001; Harari, Morales, & Harari, 2005; Mahdavi, 2010; McCann, 1996; Ni & Zeng, 2009; Nweke & Sanders, 2009).

1. Much of the enormous amount of hazardous waste produced in developed countries is disposed of in developing countries.

2. Some harmful chemicals that have been banned in developed countries are still in use in developing countries. Examples include leaded paint, certain pesticides that are used primarily on crops not intended for export, DDT for preventing malaria (in some countries), and leaded gasoline (in some countries).

3. Some harmful chemicals that are no longer in use in developing countries, but which continued to be used for some time in those countries after they had been banned in developed countries, persist in the environment and constitute a continuing source of exposure.

For example, although many developing countries have banned leaded gasoline, those bans were generally enacted several years after leaded gasoline was banned in developed countries. Similarly, some pesticides that were banned for use in developed countries continued to be manufactured there and exported to developing countries, where they were applied to both export and domestic crops. (This arrangement has largely been replaced by production of these pesticides within developing countries for use on domestic crops [Galt, 2008]; see Theme 5.) In addition, there are large stockpiles of old pesticides in developing countries that are difficult to destroy safely but constitute a potential severely harmful exposure from unsafe disposal or unintentional release into the environment.

4. Regulations governing harmful chemicals in developing countries are weaker and enforcement is more lax than in developed countries. Many steps taken in developed countries to reduce harmful environmental exposures have not yet been taken in developing countries.

5. The general population has a low level of knowledge about harmful chemicals and how exposures occur.

6. Considerable economic activity consists of cottage industries in which production takes place at home (e.g., making pottery or recycling lead-acid batteries). These production processes often use or generate harmful chemicals to which women and children who participate in the work or live in the household are exposed.

7. The proportion of women and children, including very young children, who participate in the agricultural and industrial workforce is larger and occupational health regulations and enforcement are weaker in developing countries compared to developed countries. In addition to greater exposures

in the workplace, this situation leads to greater exposures from take-home toxins (see Theme 1) brought home from the workplace by male as well as female working household members.

8. Military weapons release harmful chemicals into the environments of populations who live in conflict areas, and sometimes the chemicals themselves are released directly into the environment as weapons. In addition to the many other ways in which armed conflict hurts women and children, it can cause intensive exposure to harmful chemicals that continues for generations after the fighting has ended (Nhu, et al., 2009; Press TV, 2010; Rohter, 2000).

Given that women and children of minority race/ethnicity and lower SES have greater exposure to harmful environmental chemicals, as discussed previously, it would be expected that they also have higher rates of adverse health outcomes caused by these exposures. In fact, this is the case for many outcomes known or thought to be caused by environmental chemicals (see Theme 3). In addition, as mentioned under Theme 2, poor nutrition, psychosocial stress, and exposures to other chemicals can interact with a particular chemical exposure to exacerbate the adverse effects of that exposure, causing populations subject to these factors to have even higher rates of the harmful outcomes of the chemical exposure. Because women and children of minority race/ethnicity and lower SES do have greater exposure to these vulnerability factors (in addition to greater exposure to harmful chemicals), it is not surprising that stronger adverse effects for some environmental exposures have been found in these populations compared to the same level of exposure in women and children of majority race/ethnicity and higher SES. Moreover, biological mechanisms that could explain these types of interactions have been identified, which supports the conclusion that the combined chemical and

social exposures that racial/ethnic minority and lower SES populations experience make them more vulnerable to the harmful effects of particular chemicals. Although there are still gaps in knowledge about this issue, the evidence suggests that disparities in many MCH outcomes are caused, in part, by greater exposure to harmful chemicals combined with increased vulnerability to that exposure among racial/ethnic minorities and lower SES groups (Dilworth-Bart & Moore, 2006; Evans & Kantrowitz, 2002; Gee & Payne-Sturges, 2004; Hubbs-Tait, Nation, Krebs, & Bellinger, 2005; Wright, 2009).

7. There is general ignorance and misinformation about children's environmental health in all sectors of society, including parents, school officials, political leaders, the medical community, and public health professionals.

Protecting children from harmful environmental exposures requires that private citizens, local officials, and public health and medical professionals be knowledgeable about the presence of harmful chemicals in the environment, how children become exposed, the effects of exposure, and how to prevent exposure and its adverse outcomes. This is especially true because, given the weak regulatory protection described under Theme 5, the burden of protecting children from harmful exposures falls to a great degree on parents, local officials, and women's and children's advocates. However, the predominant message to the public from both government and private sources is that environmental exposures are harmless, that use of the chemicals is beneficial and necessary, and that minor, "common-sense" precautions are sufficient to protect children's health. This misleading information inhibits action by the above groups that could be effective in reducing exposures and adverse outcomes.

Some of the misleading messages commonly given by public and private sources are described next. Much of this rhetoric is similar to the rhetoric that accompanies the regulatory process (see Theme 5), although the motivation behind the messages may be quite different (Khokha, 2010; McCown, 2007; McKenna, 2003; NYCDOH, 2010; OAG, 2003; Rust, 2008).

Harmlessness

1. *"It has been approved."* The fact that a chemical is allowed by a regulatory agency to be sold and used is presented as verification that the use is safe ("If it wasn't safe, they wouldn't let us use it."). However, as discussed in Theme 5, regulatory decisions are poor indicators of a chemical's safety.
2. *"Laws and regulations provide adequate protection."* Rules that are in place to govern the use of harmful chemicals are cited as protecting MCH populations from harmful exposures. However, even if all existing rules were followed, women and children would still experience pervasive, extensive, and intensive exposure to these chemicals. Furthermore, violations or evasions of the rules that do exist are frequent and preclude the possibility that the rules provide adequate protection.
3. *"There is no evidence of harm."* The absence of definitive evidence that a particular chemical causes a particular effect is used to imply that lack of proof of harm equates with proof of no harm. In addition to the fallacy of this logic, lack of evidence of harm actually often equates with lack of scientific study of the exposure-outcome association.
4. *"Exposures are too low to matter."* Exposure levels are often vaguely described as low without specifying what level is harmful or to whom it is harmful. This argument may emphasize the seemingly small concentrations of the chemical to which people are exposed (e.g., a few

parts per billion) and that such tiny concentrations could not possibly have any biological effect. These statements are usually without scientific basis and often directly contradict the scientific evidence.

5. *"Risks are small."* The statement that risks are small is often bolstered by the statement that the chemical has been in use for a long time or has been studied extensively, implying that, if risks were not small, this would have become apparent by now. However, the set of risks that have been studied and that are known to be small is often a limited subset of the risks that are of concern for women's and children's health. The purported extensive study of the chemical usually does not include chronic low dose exposure, endocrine disrupting effects, long-term developmental deficits, or the effects of mixtures of the chemical with other common environmental and social exposures. Furthermore, without identifying the mechanism that would have detected the adverse effects of a chemical that has been in use for a long time if it were harmful (e.g., a specific surveillance program), this argument is purely speculative.

Beneficence

Some potentially harmful chemicals do have important public health or medical benefits. For example, DEHP provides the plasticity that is needed for some devices used in neonatal intensive care. (See case study under Theme 5.) Flame retardants may prevent deaths and injuries from fire. However, presenting this information along with the message that the chemicals are harmless as used is misleading. It undermines efforts to understand risks as well as benefits and to find similarly beneficial but less harmful alternatives.

Necessity

Many MCH environmental health issues involve competing necessities. Preventing death and injury from fire and preventing cognitive impairment and disrupted sexual development from exposure to flame retardants are both necessary to protect the health of MCH populations (Talsness, 2008). Consequently, presenting continued use of a chemical as an unqualified necessity inhibits constructive action—a choice between two necessary alternatives cannot be decided on the basis of necessity. More important, presenting the options as a choice between mutually exclusive alternatives undermines efforts to find safe solutions for the full range of MCH health needs.

On the other hand, some claims of necessity for continuing use of a harmful chemical are not justified by the scientific evidence. An example of this may be the claim that continued use of pesticides and chemical fertilizers is necessary to ensure an adequate global food supply (Badgley, et al., 2007; Lotter, Seidel, & Liebhardt, 2003).

Sufficiency of Minor Precautions

Both government and private sources emphasize minor safety measures that parents and other adults can take to protect children from harmful chemicals, with the implication that a few common-sense precautions are all that is necessary to protect children's health (e.g., EPA, 2010b). Although this advice may seem reasonable, it is seldom based on scientific evidence of the effectiveness of the advice at reducing population exposure or adverse health effects (with some possible exceptions, e.g., acute poisoning). Furthermore, it seldom takes into account the potential harm that the advice could cause.

For example, numerous government and private sources advise parents to restrict their children's outdoor activity on "air quality action days," when the concentration of harmful chemicals in the air exceeds specified levels. In addition, schools are advised to restrict the outdoor activity of some or all children on these days. Actions by school officials may include flying colored flags to announce air pollution levels, restricting an individual child's activity based on his or her symptoms, and restricting the entire student body's activity based on pollution levels. This program of advice constitutes a public health intervention (as distinguished from components of an individual child's medically supervised asthma management plan) promulgated by the federal government and numerous other public and private organizations (AIRNow, 2010). However, it is not based on scientific studies of the effectiveness of this approach in reducing either children's harmful exposures or the adverse health outcomes of these exposures (including asthma attacks), and it ignores evidence that this approach is not effective. Furthermore, the potential harm caused by this intervention to children with asthma and their families—including exacerbation of asthma symptoms—as well as to the general MCH population has not been studied. Thus, this "common-sense" approach to protecting children from harmful environmental exposures is actually a public health intervention that has not been evaluated according to prevailing standards of public health practice (CDC, 2006; Goldstein, 2001).

Similarly, government and private sources advise parents to keep children, toys, and pets out of areas that have been treated with pesticides for a short period of time after treatment to prevent children's exposure to the chemicals. School policies may include applying pesticides when children are not on the premises, notifying parents before pesticides are applied if the parents request such notification, and routinely notifying all parents before pesticides are applied. These "common-sense" precautions ignore the fact that children's greatest exposure may occur well after the pesticides have been applied, after the chemicals volatize and become concentrated in the air and settle on toys, desks, and other surfaces. The effectiveness of the recommended actions at preventing exposure and harm has not been established, and the potential harm caused by the recommendations has not been studied (Gurunathan, et al., 1998).

8. Grassroots activism and community-based advocacy are important forces for improving women's and children's environmental health.

Numerous local, national, and international nonprofit groups (nongovernmental organizations [NGOs]) are working to advance MCH environmental health. The membership, scope, methods, and objectives of these groups are quite diverse. They may focus on a particular health issue (e.g., asthma), a particular population group (e.g., mothers), or a particular environmental problem (e.g., contamination of the food supply). They may or may not work closely with scientists and public health professionals. They may concentrate on empowering local communities or on influencing national policies. A common thread among these diverse groups is the shared goal of protecting children from harmful environmental exposures.

These groups have been responsible for a number of important advances in MCH environmental health, including mobilizing physicians and other professional groups around this issue (McKenna, 2003). They often respond to new scientific findings sooner than regulatory agencies and legislatures, and frequently their work is one of the reasons these bodies do eventually move to protect women's and children's health. Furthermore, these groups are often able to act through media campaigns, litigation, and consumer mobilization to influence the practices of manufacturers and suppliers without waiting for regulatory or legislative action (Brown, et al., 2003; Weiss & Yan, 2008). However, these groups may also give misinformation or erroneous advice that reflects the problems described in Theme 7, and their actions may sometimes actually impede improvements in MCH environmental health (Needleman, 1998).

9. The current approach to MCH environmental health by government, industry, and the many organizations and individuals that manufacture, use, or control harmful environmental chemicals does not conform with widely accepted ethical standards.

Children do not volunteer to receive pervasive, extensive, and intensive exposure to chemicals of known toxicity or unknown safety (see Theme 1). They are forced to accept these exposures beginning with conception. Children do not give informed consent to be human subjects in an experiment in which they are exposed to harmful chemicals to test the effects of those exposures on themselves and other humans (see Theme 3). Children do not give consent to be used as biological instruments for measuring whether environmental concentrations of various chemicals have yet to reach harmful levels (see Theme 5); neither do they give consent to be used as biological instruments for detecting the presence of harmful chemicals in the environment, as in screening programs that locate environmental hazards by measuring the levels of chemicals in children's bodies (e.g., lead; Mielke, 2002). Children of racial/ethnic minorities and lower SES do not volunteer to accept higher exposures to harmful chemicals so that other children and their families can have lower exposures; children of other racial/ethnic and SES groups do not give consent to be protected by imposing higher exposures on children and families of racial/ethnic minorities and lower SES. Although the foregoing conditions characterize MCH environmental health, children, and for the most part their parents also, have no voice in the regulatory and policy decisions that force these conditions on them. This arrangement violates the ethical principles of justice, beneficence, respect for persons, and nonmaleficence, as well as the notion that adult society has an obligation to protect and nurture children (Gilbert, 2005; Jarvie & Malone, 2008; Weiss, 2001).

CONCLUSION

Like poverty, exposure to environmental chemicals is having a profound negative impact on all aspects of women's and children's health (Leiss & Kotch, 2010). In fact, the impacts of the physical environment and the social environment on women's and children's health cannot be separated. Harmful chemical exposures and harmful social exposures occur together, cause each other, and characterize the same population groups. They act through the same physiological pathways and cause the same adverse health outcomes (Weiss & Bellinger, 2006; Wright, 2009).

The fundamental unity of the physical and social environments for MCH is illustrated by taking a life course approach to the case of pregnancy and lead. Over the course or her lifetime, beginning in childhood, a woman may accumulate lead in her bones from environmental exposures. During pregnancy, a portion of this bone lead is transferred to the bloodstream and may cause hypertension and related health problems. In addition to affecting the mother's health directly, maternal lead causes adverse birth outcomes as well as neurobehavioral deficits in the child. Furthermore, part of the maternal lead burden is transferred to the fetus. Thus, the child may begin to accumulate lead in utero, which, in the case of a daughter, may affect her health during her own pregnancies as well as the health of her children.

Like lead, maternal stress is associated with hypertension in pregnancy, adverse birth outcomes, impaired fetal growth, and impaired neurobehavioral development of the child. Moreover, early life exposure to each of these toxicants (lead and stress) can cause permanent structural changes to the developing brain that increase the harm caused by subsequent exposures of both types (i.e., increased vulnerability; Weiss & Bellinger, 2006). This suggests that lead and stress interact over the life course to cause hypertension in pregnancy, adverse birth outcomes, and impaired development

of the offspring. Moreover, the same populations—racial/ethnic minorities and lower SES groups—have greater exposure to both environmental chemicals and psychosocial stressors; greater vulnerability to both types of exposures because of other chemical and adverse social exposures; and higher rates of adverse MCH outcomes thought to be caused by these exposures.

The foregoing suggests that harmful chemical exposures and adverse social exposures, rather than being qualitatively different from each other, are closely related aspects of a single toxic physical-social environment. This is the environment in which many disadvantaged MCH populations live. Thus, disparities among MCH populations can be seen as the product of disparities in cumulative lifetime exposure to this toxic physical-social environment combined with biological as well as social transmission of its exposures, vulnerabilities, and adverse health outcomes to successive generations.

Although the effects of chemical and social exposures are not separable, they are currently seen as separate areas for intervention. With regard to harmful chemical and physical agents, the fundamental feature of women's and children's environmental health is the pervasive, extensive, and intensive exposure described in Theme 1. All of the other issues stem from exposure. Consequently, the most pressing need is for policies that prevent harmful chemical exposures to MCH populations and for research on how to achieve such policies (see Theme 5). Secondly, there is a need to educate the public, medical and public health professionals, and officials at all levels of government on how MCH environmental exposures occur, how they affect health, and the limitations of current scientific knowledge and public policy (see Theme 7). Finally, there is a need to develop research methods that address the limitations described in Theme 2 and are capable of increasing understanding of the physical-social environment described above and its effect on women's and children's health.

References

AIRNow. (2010). Partners. Retrieved November 10, 2010 from http://www.airnow.gov/index.cfm?action = partnerslist.index.

Ashauer, R., Boxall, A. B. A., & Brown, C. D. (2007). Modeling combined effects of pulsed exposure to carbaryl and chlorpyrifos on gammarus pulex. *Environmental Science & Technology, 41*, 5535–5541.

Australian Pesticides and Veterinary Medicines Authority (APVMA). (2003). Copper chrome arsenate (CCA)/APVMA puts industry on notice. Retrieved October 13, 2010 from http://www.apvma.gov.au/news_media/media_releases/archive/2003/mr0306.php.

Badgley, C., Moghtader, J., Quintero, E., Zakem, E., Chappell, M. J., Aviles-Vazquez, K., Samulon, A., & Perfecto, I. (2007). Organic agriculture and the global food supply. *Renewable Agriculture and Food Systems, 22*, 86–108.

Blacksmith Institute. (2007). *The world's worst polluted places.* New York, NY: Blacksmith Institute. Retrieved October 11, 2010 from http://www.worstpolluted.org/.

Brown, M. J., McLaine, P., Dixon, S., & Simon, P. (2006). A randomized, community-based trial of home visiting to reduce blood lead levels in children. *Pediatrics, 117*, 147–153.

Brown, P., Mayer, B., Zavestoski, S., Luebke, T., Mandelbaum, J., & McCormick, S. (2003). The health politics of asthma: Environmental justice and collective illness experience in the United States. *Social Science & Medicine, 57*, 453–464.

Centers for Disease Control and Prevention (CDC). (2006). *Strategies for addressing asthma within a coordinated school health program, with updated resources.* Atlanta, GA: Centers for Disease Control and Prevention, National Center for Chronic Disease Prevention and Health Promotion. Retrieved November 1, 2010 from http://www.cdc.gov/HealthyYouth/asthma/pdf/strategies.pdf.

Colborn, T. (2009, April 27). EPA's new pesticide testing is outdated, crude. *Environmental Health News.* Retrieved September 7, 2010 from http://www.environmentalhealthnews.org/ehs/editorial/epa2019s-new-pesticide-testing-is-outdated-crude.

Colborn, T., Dumanoski, D., & Myers, J. P. (1996). *Our stolen future: Are we threatening our fertility, intelligence, and survival? A scientific detective story.* New York, NY: Dutton.

Consumer Product Safety Commission (CPSC). (1990). *Dislodgeable arsenic on playground equipment wood and the estimated risk of skin cancer.* Retrieved September 2, 2010 from http://www.cpsc.gov/LIBRARY/FOIA/Foia00/brief/woodpla2.pdf.

Consumer Product Safety Commission (CPSC). (2001). *Petition to the United States Consumer Product Safety Commission to ban arsenic treated wood in playground equipment and review the safety of arsenic treated wood for general use.* Retrieved September 2, 2010 from http://www.cpsc.gov/LIBRARY/FOIA/Foia01/petition/Arsenic.pdf.

Consumer Product Safety Commission (CPSC). (2003a). CPSC denies petition to ban CCA pressure-treated wood playground equipment. Retrieved September 2, 2010 from http://www.cpsc.gov/CPSCPUB/PREREL/prhtml04/04026.html.

Consumer Product Safety Commission (CPSC). (2003b). Letter to Richard Wiles and Bill Walsh (December 3, 2003). Retrieved September 2, 2010 from http://www.cpsc.gov/LIBRARY/FOIA/FOIA04/petition/Playgrd.pdf.

Consumer Product Safety Commission (CPSC). (2003c). *Petition to ban chromated copper arsenate (CCA)-treated wood in playground equipment (Petition HP 01-3).* Retrieved September 29, 2010 from http://www.cpsc.gov/LIBRARY/FOIA/FOIA03/brief/cca1.pdf.

Consumer Product Safety Commission (CPSC). (2003d). Statement of Chairman Hal Stratton regarding No. HP-01-03, a petition for a ban on use of CCA *treated wood in playground equipment.* Retrieved September 2, 2010 from http://www.cpsc.gov/CPSCPUB/PREREL/prhtml04/04026stratton.html.

Consumer Product Safety Commission (CPSC). (2003e). *Testimony before the Consumer Product Safety Commission. Ban Petition HP01-3. Jane Houlihan, March 17, 2003.* Retrieved September 2, 2010 from http://www.cpsc.gov/LIBRARY/FOIA/FOIA03/pubcom/CCAwoodpt1.pdf.

Consumer Product Safety Commission (CPSC). (2010a). CPSC overview. Retrieved November 11, 2010 from http://www.cpsc.gov/about/about.html.

Consumer Product Safety Commission (CPSC). (2010b). Fact sheet. Chromated *copper arsenate (CCA)-treated wood used in playground equipment.*

Retrieved September 2, 2010 from http://www.cpsc.gov/phth/ccafact.html.

Counter, S. A. (2003). Neurophysiological anomalies in brainstem responses of mercury-exposed children of Andean gold miners. *Journal of Occupational and Environmental Medicine, 45*, 87–95.

d'Harcourt, E., & Purdin, S. (2009). Impact of wars and conflict on maternal and child health. In J. Ehiri (Ed.), *Maternal and Child health: Global challenges, programs, and policies* (pp. 121–133). New York, NY: Springer.

Davidson, P. W., Weiss, B., Beck, C., Cory-Slechta, D. A., Orlando, M., Loiselle, D., Young, E. C., Sloane-Reeves, J., & Myers, G. J. (2006). Development and validation of a test battery to assess subtle neurodevelopmental differences in children. *Neurotoxicology, 27*, 951–969.

DeAngelis, C. D., & Fontanarosa, P. B. (2010). Ensuring integrity in industry-sponsored research: Primum non nocere, revisited. *Journal of the American Medical Association, 303*, 1196–1198.

Diallo, Y., Hagemann, F., Etienne, A., Gurbuzer, Y., & Mehran, F. (2010). *Global child labour developments: Measuring trends from 2004 to 2008.* Geneva: International Labour Office, International Programme on the Elimination of Child Labour (IPEC).

Dietert, R. R. (2009). Developmental immunotoxicology: Focus on health risks. *Chemical Research in Toxicology, 22*, 17–23.

Dilworth-Bart, J. E., & Moore, C. F. (2006). Mercy mercy me: Social injustice and the prevention of environmental pollutant exposures among ethnic minority and poor children. *Child Development, 77*, 247–265.

Drazen, J. M., & Wood, A. J. J. (2010). Don't mess with the DSMB. *New England Journal of Medicine, 363*, 477–478.

Ecobichon, D. J. (2001). Pesticide use in developing countries. *Toxicology, 160*, 27–33.

Elias, R. W., & Gulson, B. (2003). Overview of lead remediation effectiveness. *The Science of the Total Environment, 303*, 1–13.

Environmental Protection Agency (EPA). (2002). Chromated copper arsenate (CCA): Cancellation of residential uses of CCA-treated wood. Retrieved October 12, 2010 from http://www.epa.gov/pesticides/antimicrobials/reregistration/cca/residential_use_cancellation.htm.

Environmental Protection Agency (EPA). (2003). *A probabilistic risk assessment for children who contact CCA-treated playsets and decks.* Retrieved September 2, 2010 from http://www.epa.gov/scipoly/sap/meetings/2003/december3/shedsprobabalisticriskassessmentnov03.pdf.

Environmental Protection Agency (EPA). (2010a). Human health. Retrieved November 11, 2010 from http://www.epa.gov/ebtpages/humanhealth.html.

Environmental Protection Agency (EPA). (2010b). Ten tips to protect children from pesticide and lead poisoning. Retrieved March 31, 2011 from http://www.epa.gov/pesticides/factsheets/child-ten-tips.htm.

Evans, G. W., & Kantrowitz, E. (2002). Socioeconomic status and health: The potential role of environmental risk exposure. *Annual Review of Public Health, 23*, 303–331.

Faustman, E. M., Silbernagel, S. M., Fenske, R. A., Burbacher, T. M., & Ponce, R. A. (2000). Mechanisms underlying children's susceptibility to environmental toxicants. *Environmental Health Perspectives, 108*(Suppl. 1), 13–21.

Food and Drug Administration (FDA). (2001a). *Letter to Sanford J. Lewis re: Docket Number 99P-2077/CP1 (September 5, 2001).* Retrieved September 2, 2010 from http://www.fda.gov/ohrms/dockets/dailys/01/Sep01/091101/pdn0001.pdf.

Food and Drug Administration (FDA). (2001b). *Safety assessment of Di(2-ethylhexyl)phthalate (DEHP) released from PVC medical devices.* Retrieved September 2, 2010 from http://www.fda.gov/downloads/MedicalDevices/DeviceRegulationandGuidance/GuidanceDocuments/UCM080457.pdf.

Food and Drug Administration (FDA). (2002). *FDA public health notification: PVC devices containing the plasticizer DEHP.* Retrieved September 2, 2010 from http://www.fda.gov/MedicalDevices/Safety/AlertsandNotices/PublicHealthNotifications/UCM062182.

Food and Drug Administration (FDA). (2007a). *Citizen petition for a Food and Drug Administration regulation or guideline to label medical devices that leach DEHP plasticizers.* Retrieved September 2, 2010 from http://www.fda.gov/ohrms/dockets/dockets/07p0320/07p-0320-cp00001-01-vol1.pdf.

Food and Drug Administration (FDA). (2007b). *Exhibit 3, Supporting letters.* Retrieved September 2, 2010 from http://www.fda.gov/ohrms/dockets/dockets/07p0320/07p-0320-cp00001-05-Exhibit-03-vol2.pdf.

Food and Drug Administration (FDA). (2009). What we do. Retrieved November 11, 2010 from http://www.fda.gov/AboutFDA/WhatWeDo/default.htm.

Food Quality Protection Act of 1996, Pub. L. 104-170, 7 U.S.C. 136 (1996).

Galt, R. E. (2008). Beyond the circle of poison: Significant shifts in the global pesticide complex, 1976–2008. *Global Environmental Change, 18*, 786–799.

Gee, G. C., & Payne-Sturges, D. C. (2004). Environmental health disparities: A framework integrating psychosocial and environmental concepts. *Environmental Health Perspectives, 112*, 1645–1653.

Gilbert, S. G. (2005). Ethical, legal, and social issues: Our children's future. *Neurotoxicology, 26*, 521–530.

Goldstein, B. D. (2001). The precautionary principle also applies to public health actions. *American Journal of Public Health, 91*, 1358–1361.

Grandjean, P., & Landrigan, P. J. (2006). Developmental neurotoxicity of industrial chemicals. *Lancet, 368*, 2167–2178.

Gross, B. M. (1974). Destructive decision-making in developing countries. *Policy Sciences, 5*, 213–236.

Gurunathan, S., Robson, M., Freeman, N., Buckley, B., Roy, A., Meyer, R., Bukowski, J., & Lioy, P. J. (1998). Accumulation of chlorpyrifos on residential surfaces and toys accessible to children. *Environmental Health Perspectives, 106*, 9–16.

Harari, A. R., Morales, R. F., & Harari, F. H. (2005). Major concerns in developing countries: Applications of the Precautionary Principle in Ecuador. *Human and Ecological Risk Assessment: An International Journal, 11*, 249–254.

Health Care Without Harm (HCWH). (2002). *Letter to Food and Drug Administration re: medical devices made with polyvinylchloride (PVC) using the plasticizer di-(2-Ethylhexy~phthalate (DEHP); Draft guidance for industry and FDA (December 4, 2002).* Retrieved September 2, 2010 from http://www.fda.gov/ohrms/dockets/dailys/02/Dec02/120502/02d-0325-c000018-01-vol1.pdf.

Hertz-Picciotto, I., & Delwiche, L. (2009). The rise in autism and the role of age at diagnosis. *Epidemiology, 20*, 84–90.

Hubbs-Tait, L., Nation, J. R., Krebs, N. F., & Bellinger, D. C. (2005). Neurotoxicants, micronutrients, and social environments: Individual and combined effects on children's development. *Psychological Science in the Public Interest, 6*, 57–121.

Ivory, D. (2010, July 8). Weighing safety of weed killer in drinking water, EPA relies heavily on industry-backed studies. *Huffington Post.* Retrieved October 18, 2011 from http://www.huffingtonpost.com/2010/07/08/weighing-safety-of-weed-k_n_639120.html.

Jansen, K. (2008). The unspeakable ban: The translation of global pesticide governance into Honduran national regulation. *World Development, 36*, 575–589.

Jarvie, J. A., & Malone, R. E. (2008). Children's secondhand smoke exposure in private homes and cars: An ethical analysis. *American Journal of Public Health, 98*, 2140–2145.

Khokha, S. (2010, February 28). "Pesticide drift" eluding efforts to combat it. *NPR.* Retrieved October 27, 2010 from http://www.npr.org/templates/story/story.php?storyId=123817702.

Koch, L., & Ashford, N. A. (2006). Rethinking the role of information in chemicals policy: Implications for TSCA and REACH. *Journal of Cleaner Production, 14*, 31–46.

Kortenkamp, A. (2007). Ten years of mixing cocktails: A review of combination effects of endocrine-disrupting chemicals. *Environmental Health Perspectives, 115*, 98–105.

Lanphear, B. P. (2005). Childhood lead poisoning prevention: Too little, too late. *Journal of the American Medical Association, 293*, 2274–2276.

Lanphear, B. P., & Bearer, C. F. (2005). Biomarkers in paediatric research and practice. *Archives of Disease in Childhood, 90*, 594–600.

Leiss, J. K., & Kotch, J. B. (2010). The importance of children's environmental health for the field of maternal and child health: A wake-up call. *Maternal and Child Health Journal, 14*, 307–317.

Lignell, S., Aune, M., Darnerud, P. O., Cnattingius, S., & Glynn, A. (2009). Persistent organochlorine and organobromine compounds in mother's milk from Sweden 1996–2006: Compound-specific temporal trends. *Environmental Research, 109*, 760–767.

Lotter, D. W., Seidel, R., & Liebhardt, W. (2003). The performance of organic and conventional cropping systems in an extreme climate year. *American Journal of Alternative Agriculture, 18*, 146–154.

Mahdavi, A. (2010). Problems of pesticide/chemical regulations in developing countries. *Toxicology Letters, 196*(Suppl. 1), S93.

McCann, M. (1996). Hazards in cottage industries in developing countries. *American Journal of Industrial Medicine, 30*, 125–129.

McCown, D. (2007, July 20). Company that sprayed kids likely will face fine. *SWVAToday.* Retrieved October 27, 2010 from http://www.swvatoday.com/news/article/company_that_sprayed_kids_likely_will_face_fine/373/.

McKenna, B. (2003, August/September). How green is your pediatrician? *From the ground up.* Retrieved October 18, 2011 from http://www.ecocenter.org/

newsletters/from-the-ground-up/august-september-2003/how-green-your-pediatrician.

Mielke, H. W. (2002). Research ethics in pediatric environmental health: Lessons from lead. *Neurotoxicology and Teratology, 24,* 467–469.

Mohai, P., Pellow, D., & Roberts, J. T. (2009). Environmental justice. *Annual Review of Environment and Resources, 34,* 405–430.

Myers, J. P., Zoeller, R. T., & Vom Saal, F. S. (2009). A clash of old and new scientific concepts in toxicity, with important implications for public health. *Environmental Health Perspectives, 117,* 1652–1655.

National Research Council. (1993). *Pesticides in the diets of infants and children.* Washington, DC: National Academy Press.

National Research Council. (2006). *Toxicity testing for assessment of environmental agents. Interim report.* Washington, DC: National Academy Press.

Needleman, H. L. (1998). Childhood lead poisoning: The promise and abandonment of primary prevention. *American Journal of Public Health, 88,* 1871–1877.

Needleman, H. L. (2000). The removal of lead from gasoline: Historical and personal reflections. *Environmental Research, 84,* 20–35.

New York City Department of Health (NYCDOH). (2010). *2010 health advisory #22: Pesticide spraying notification to reduce mosquito activity and control West Nile Virus in Queens.* New York: New York City Department of Health and Mental Hygiene.

New York Times. (1992, February 7). Furor on memo at World Bank.

Nhu, D. D., Kido, T., Naganuma, R., Sawano, N., Tawara, K., Nishijo, M., Nakagawa, H., Hung, N. N., & Thom, L. T. H. (2009). A GIS study of dioxin contamination in a Vietnamese region sprayed with herbicide. *Environmental Health and Preventive Medicine, 14,* 353–360.

Ni, H. G., & Zeng, E. Y. (2009). Law enforcement and global collaboration are the keys to containing e-waste tsunami in China. *Environmental Science & Technology, 43,* 3991–3994.

Nweke, O. C., & Sanders, W. H., III. (2009). Modern environmental health hazards: A public health issue of increasing significance in Africa. *Environmental Health Perspectives, 117,* 863–870.

Office of the Attorney General (OAG). (2003). Dow subsidiary to pay $2 million for making false safety claims in pesticide ads. (Press release). Retrieved October 18, 2011 from http://www.oag.state.ny.us/media_center/2003/dec/dec15a_03.html.

Petrenko, A., & McArthur, D. (2010). Between same-sex marriages and the large hadron collider: Making sense of the Precautionary Principle. *Science and Engineering Ethics, 16,* 591–610.

Press TV. (2010, July 23). UK admits using DU ammunition in Iraq. Retrieved September 13, 2010 from http://edition.presstv.ir/detail/135896.html.

Reed, D. (2002). Resource extraction industries in developing countries. *Journal of Business Ethics, 39,* 199–226.

Richard, S., Moslemi, S., Sipahutar, H., Benachour, N., & Seralini, G. E. (2005). Differential effects of glyphosate and Roundup on human placental cells and aromatase. *Environmental Health Perspectives, 113,* 716–720.

Rohter, L. (2000, May 1). To Colombians, drug war is toxic enemy. *New York Times.*

Royal Commission on Environmental Pollution. (2003). *Twenty-fourth report. Chemicals in products: Safeguarding the environment and human health.* Cm 5827. Retrieved October 18, 2011 from http://www.ecehh.org/downloads/process_download.php?file=rcep/24-chemicals/24-chemicals.pdf.

Rudel, R. (1997). Predicting health effects of exposures to compounds with estrogenic activity: Methodological issues. *Environmental Health Perspectives, 105*(Suppl. 3), 655–663.

Rudén, C., & Hansson, S. O. (2010). Registration, Evaluation, and Authorization of Chemicals (REACH) is but the first step–how far will it take us? Six further steps to improve the European chemicals legislation. *Environmental Health Perspectives, 118,* 6–10.

Rust, S. (2008, November 15). BPA leaches from "safe" products. *Journal Sentinel.* Retrieved October 27, 2010 from http://www.jsonline.com/watchdog/watchdogreports/34532034.html.

Sandau, C. D., Ayotte, P., Dewailly, É., Duffe, J., & Norstrom, R. J. (2002). Pentachlorophenol and hydroxylated polychlorinated biphenyl metabolites in umbilical cord plasma of neonates from coastal populations in Québec. *Environmental Health Perspectives, 110,* 411–417.

Savitz, D. A. (2001). Environmental exposures and childhood cancer: Our best may not be good enough. *American Journal of Public Health, 91,* 562–563.

Scinicariello, F., Murray, H. E., Smith, L., Wilbur, S., & Fowler, B. A. (2005). Genetic factors that might lead to different responses in individuals exposed to perchlorate. *Environmental Health Perspectives, 113,* 1479–1484.

Suk, W. A., Olden, K., & Yang, R. S. H. (2002). Chemical mixtures research: Significance and future perspectives. *Environmental Health Perspectives, 110*(Suppl. 6), 891–892.

Talsness, C. E. (2008). Overview of toxicological aspects of polybrominated diphenyl ethers: A flame-retardant additive in several consumer products. *Environmental Research, 108,* 158–167.

Thayer, K., & Houlihan, J. (2004). Pesticides, human health, and the food quality protection act. *William and Mary Environmental Law and Policy Review, 28,* 257–312.

Thigpen, J. E., Setchell, K. D. R., Saunders, H. E., Haseman, J. K., Grant, M. G., & Forsythe, D. B. (2004). Selecting the appropriate rodent diet for endocrine disruptor research and testing studies. *ILAR Journal, 45,* 401–416.

Thomas, V. M., Socolow, R. H., Fanelli, J. J., & Spiro, T. G. (1999). Effects of reducing lead in gasoline: an analysis of the international experience. *Environmental Science & Technology, 33,* 3942–3948.

Watnick, V. (1999). Risk assessment: Obfuscation of policy decisions in pesticide regulation and the EPA's dismantling of the Food Quality Protection Act's safeguards for children. *Arizona State Law Journal, 31,* 1315–1372.

Weiss, B. (2001). Ethics assessment as an adjunct to risk assessment in the evaluation of developmental neurotoxicants. *Environmental Health Perspectives, 109*(Suppl. 6), 905–908.

Weiss, B. (2007). Why methylmercury remains a conundrum 50 years after Minamata. *Toxicological Sciences, 97,* 223–225.

Weiss, B., & Bellinger, D.C. (2006). Social ecology of children's vulnerability to environmental pollutants. *Environmental Health Perspectives, 114,* 1479–1485.

Weiss, B., & Landrigan, P. J. (2000). The developing brain and the environment: An introduction. *Environmental Health Perspectives, 108*(Suppl. 3), 373–374.

Weiss, J., & Yan, H. (2008, May 21). Debate on plastic's safety moves to consumer. *The Deseret News (Salt Lake City, UT).*

Williams, E. S., Panko, J., & Paustenbach, D. J. (2009). The European Union's REACH regulation: A review of its history and requirements. *Critical Reviews in Toxicology, 39,* 553–575.

Woolf, A. (2000). A 4-year-old girl with manifestations of multiple chemical sensitivities. *Environmental Health Perspectives, 108,* 1219.

Wright, R. J. (2009). Moving towards making social toxins mainstream in children's environmental health. *Current Opinion in Pediatrics, 21,* 222–229.

14

ISSUES IN MATERNAL AND CHILD NUTRITION

Barbara Laraia, Bethany Hendrickson, and Sara Benjamin Neelon

Our lives are not in the lap of the gods, but in the lap of our cooks.

(Yutang, 1937)

INTRODUCTION

Nutrition is a critical component in any discussion of the health status of the maternal and child health (MCH) population. Physical growth is anticipated and desired in all subgroups of children and among pregnant women. Women who are between pregnancies or who do not become pregnant during their childbearing years focus on achieving or maintaining their optimal nutrition status. Good nutrition is biologically central to growth in that it provides the elements for building and repairing tissue and is required for the metabolic processes that mediate tissue development. If there is not adequate repair or growth, the body becomes dysfunctional. An inadequately nourished child becomes a sick child, one who is absent from or listens poorly in school. If prolonged, inadequate nutrition during pregnancy and early childhood can affect the brain's development and functioning. In older children and adults, malnutrition can give rise to cardiovascular disease, and an excess of certain nutrients can accelerate the disease process in cancer-prone sites.

Underlying the following discussion, but beyond the scope of this textbook, is the aspect of nutritional sciences that provides a variety of tools that are used to assess nutritional status of an individual. These include the measurement and assessment of dietary intake, mineral and nutrient stores, energy expenditure and metabolism, and growth. Briefly, measures of dietary intake include 24-hour recall, 3-day food records, food frequency questionnaires, and dietary history techniques, which may or may not adequately measure the nutrient status of a given individual. Expanding beyond dietary assessment to create a more comprehensive picture of one's overall nutrient status, biochemical measures of serum levels such as hemoglobin, hematocrit, cholesterol, triglycerides, vitamin A, protein, and glucose are used to assess under and over nutrition. Additional measures are used less frequently due to their considerable cost to provide a better understanding of disease processes. These include measurement of energy expenditure using doubly labeled water; measures of metabolism, such as bioelectrical impedance, dual-energy X-ray absorptiometry (dexa scan) to measure fat and muscle; and measures of bone health such as bone densitometry. Finally, we more commonly rely on measures of growth, such as height and weight or body mass index (BMI = weight in kilograms/height in meters squared), tracking these using a growth chart (http://www.cdc.gov/growthcharts/), as important proxies for adequate nutritional intake and development, especially for children and pregnant women (de Onis, Garza, Onyango, & Borghi, 2007).

The knowledge base of nutrition is expanding at an accelerated rate with the application of technology to all phases of research into dietary intake, metabolism, eating behavior, and food composition. Each of these areas is relevant to MCH issues. The reader is referred to the maternal and child nutrition texts noted in the bibliography, which are regularly updated for a discussion of the full range of nutrition topics in these populations.

This chapter is organized around five broad themes. First, the two federal nutrition policies—Dietary Guidelines for Americans and Food Guides—are reviewed. Second, the history of hunger or food insecurity in the United States, which has fueled much of federal policy and food and nutrition programs that exist in the United States is reviewed. Third, four major federal food and nutrition programs are reviewed that have a direct impact on maternal and child dietary intake. Fourth, we review the literature pertaining to breastfeeding prevalence and programs that promote the initiation and duration of breastfeeding. Lastly, obesity in the United States is reviewed.

GUIDING PRINCIPLES OF PUBLIC HEALTH NUTRITION

Nutrition Policies and Guidance

Nutrition policies and guidance are implemented in the United States with the goal of disseminating science to the population as well as providing nutritional direction for healthy individuals, groups, and institutions such as schools, government entitlement programs, and hospitals. Although based on scientific data, the end message can often be muddled due to the influence of agriculture policy, food policy, and politics. This section reviews the history and application of two nutrition policies—Dietary Guidelines for Americans and the Food Guides.

Dietary Guidance

The Dietary Guidelines for Americans are an official statement of the U.S. government's nutrition policy. The Dietary Guidelines present the Dietary Reference Intakes (DRIs). The Recommended Dietary Allowances (RDAs), the precursor to DRIs, were adopted in 1941 after the National Nutrition Conference and were published by the Food and Nutrition Board of the National Academy of Sciences. The DRIs are reviewed every 10 years. They are the standard against which dietary adequacy is measured and include the vitamins, minerals, and calories for which there are enough data to establish a recommended daily dietary intake for various age and gender groups. One or two nutrients are added with each revision as the scientific literature provides adequate evidence of the critical role of those nutrients and the amount the human body requires.

Although the recommendations may appear simple and uncontroversial, the language of these guidelines is highly debated and finely tuned. For example, in 1977, a Senate committee chaired by Senator George McGovern issued dietary goals for the United States, one of which was to reduce saturated fat. To achieve this goal the committee suggested that the recommendation be to "reduce consumption of meat." This caused a backlash from the meat industry, which protested and persuaded Congress to hold hearings. As a result, Senator McGovern's committee reworded the advice to "choose meats, poultry and fish which will reduce saturated fat intake." This set a precedent. When the first dietary guidelines appeared in 1980, they used saturated fat as a euphemism for meat, and subsequent editions have continued to use nutrients as euphemisms for "eat less" foods. As New York University Professor Marion Nestle points out:

Then came obesity. To prevent weight gain, people must eat less (sometimes much less), move more, or do both. This puts federal agencies in a quandary. If they name specific foods in "eat less" categories, they risk industry wrath, and this is something no centrist-leaning government can afford. (Nestle, 2011)

The most recent edition of the guidelines, *The* Dietary Guidelines for Americans, 2010 (U.S. Department of Agriculture & U.S. Department of Health and Human Services, 2010), includes 23 key recommendations for the general population and 6 additional key recommendations for specific population groups, such as pregnant women. (See Table 14–1.)

Implications for MCH

Although the Dietary Guidelines are available to the public, they are not widely distributed nor largely sought out. They do, however, provide useful direction for providers and agencies dealing with a maternal and child population. The DRIs are used as the criteria for nutrient adequacy in the meals served in the School Meals Program and for menu systems used in the Supplemental Nutrition Assistance Program (SNAP, formerly the Food Stamp Program). There are several caveats for the use of these standards. They are for healthy individuals. They are for groups of people, and they should be compared with dietary data that include several days of intake, not a single day, or a large sample.

Food Guides

A food guide is the consumer information that advises people about their food selection over the course of a day. Food guides were first developed in the United States in 1923. They were developed to help lay people ascertain whether they were eating enough of the right

foods to prevent nutrition deficiencies. During the war years, food was scarce, and careful planning was necessary in order to maintain nutrition adequacy in the population. In fact, it was the discovery after the war that more men than expected failed their physical examinations because of undernutrition that led to the establishment of the National School Lunch and Milk Programs to prevent this problem in the future (U.S. Congress, 1945).

In the 1950s, when the food guide grouping was reorganized and simplified from seven groups—milk, vegetables, fruits, eggs, meat (fish, poultry, cheese), cereal, and butter—to four—dairy, grains, fruits and vegetables, and meat, the food guide became known as the Basic Four and was central for nutrition education in schools. Nearly every adult was taught the Basic Four, and it was used by food companies in advertising and packaging. It was not until the early 1970s that nutritionists recognized that excess food intake rather than deficiencies was the primary dietary problem in the United States. Because the Basic Four did not include fat or sugar, people assumed that they could eat as much of these as they wanted. The shift to address excess dietary intake began with the publication of Dietary Goals by the Senate Select Committee on Hunger in 1977 (U.S. Senate Select Committee on Nutrition and Human Needs, 1977). It was not until the 1980s, when the administrative arms of the government, the U.S. Department of Agriculture (USDA) and the U.S. Department of Health and Human Services (U.S. DHHS), officially released the Dietary Guidelines, establishing them as policy, which programs began to teach moderation energetically. However, the Dietary Guidelines are not helpful in planning a meal, a day's intake of food, or a weekly food list. For that reason, the USDA released the Food Pyramid in 1992, which provides dietary guidance to those who wish to eat for their own health and to assist others in doing so (Figure 14–1). The Basic Four Food Groups were the prevailing instructions for a number of years but were replaced in 1993 by the Food Guide Pyramid; in 2005 by MyPyramid,

Table 14–1 Dietary Guidelines for Americans, 2010[1]

DIETARY GUIDELINES FOR AMERICANS 2010

Balancing calories to manage weight

- Prevent and/or reduce overweight and obesity through improved eating and physical activity behaviors.
- Control total calorie intake to manage body weight. For people who are overweight or obese, this will mean consuming fewer calories from foods and beverages.
- Increase physical activity and reduce time spent in sedentary behaviors.
- Maintain appropriate calorie balance during each stage of life—childhood, adolescence, adulthood, pregnancy and breastfeeding, and older age.

Foods and food components to reduce

- Reduce daily sodium intake to less than 2,300 milligrams (mg) and further reduce intake to 1,500 mg among persons who are 51 and older and those of any age who are African American or have hypertension, diabetes, or chronic kidney disease. The 1,500 mg recommendation applies to about half of the U.S. population, including children, and the majority of adults.
- Consume less than 10% of calories from saturated fatty acids by replacing them with monounsaturated and polyunsaturated fatty acids.
- Consume less than 300 mg per day of dietary cholesterol.
- Keep *trans* fatty acid consumption as low as possible by limiting foods that contain synthetic sources of *trans* fats, such as partially hydrogenated oils, and by limiting other solid fats.
- Reduce the intake of calories from solid fats and added sugars.
- Limit the consumption of foods that contain refined grains, especially refined grain foods that contain solid fats, added sugars, and sodium.
- If alcohol is consumed, it should be consumed in moderation—up to one drink per day for women and two drinks per day for men—and only by adults of legal drinking age

Foods and nutrients to increase

Individuals should meet the following recommendations as part of a healthy eating pattern while staying within their calorie needs.

- Increase vegetable and fruit intake.
- Eat a variety of vegetables, especially dark-green and red and orange vegetables and beans and peas.
- Consume at least half of all grains as whole grains. Increase whole-grain intake by replacing refined grains with whole grains.
- Increase intake of fat-free or low-fat milk and milk products, such as milk, yogurt, cheese, or fortified soy beverages.
- Choose a variety of protein foods, which include seafood, lean meat and poultry, eggs, beans and peas, soy products, and unsalted nuts and seeds.
- Increase the amount and variety of seafood consumed by choosing seafood in place of some meat and poultry.
- Replace protein foods that are higher in solid fats with choices that are lower in solid fats and calories and/or are sources of oils.

(Continued)

Table 14–1 (Continued)

- Use oils to replace solid fats where possible.

- Choose foods that provide more potassium, dietary fiber, calcium, and vitamin D, which are nutrients of concern in American diets. These foods include vegetables, fruits, whole grains, and milk and milk products.

Recommendations for specific population groups

Women capable of becoming pregnant

- Choose foods that supply heme iron, which is more readily absorbed by the body, additional iron sources, and enhancers of iron

- Consume 400 micrograms (mcg) per day of synthetic folic acid (from fortified foods and/or supplements) in addition to food forms of folate from a varied diet.

Women who are pregnant or breastfeeding

- Consume 8 to 12 ounces of seafood per week from a variety of seafood types.

- Due to their high methyl mercury content, limit white (albacore) tuna to 6 ounces per week and do not eat the following four types of fish: tilefish, shark, swordfish, and king mackerel.

- If pregnant, take an iron supplement, as recommended by an obstetrician or other healthcare provider.

---

[1]U.S. Department of Agriculture and U.S. Department of Health and Human Services. Dietary guidelines for Americans; 2010. Retrieved March 28, 2011 from http://www.cnpp.usda.gov/DGAs2010-PolicyDocument.htm.

(USDA, 2011b), which emphasizes physical activity and includes a personalized web-based diet component; and most recently, in 2011, by MyPlate (USDA, 2011a).

As with the *Dietary Guidelines for Americans*, the changes in the Food Guide Pyramid were scrutinized and debated at every turn. Agricultural interests had a substantial influence on the changes (Nestle, 1993). Two commodity groups—dairy and meat—resisted the efforts to limit consumption of their foods even though scientific evidence showed a strong association between animal fat, notably saturated fat, and cardiovascular disease. Initially, dietary cholesterol alone was the focus for dietary change, and people were advised to eat no more than three or four eggs per week. As studies demonstrating the relationship between saturated fat and cardiovascular disease proliferated, nutritionists began advising individuals to reduce cholesterol and saturated fat by selecting reduced fat milk, preferably skim milk, and low-fat yogurt and limiting meat

intake to two to three servings of two to three ounces per day, and red meat to only three times per week. By 2005, the total amount of meat, eggs, and nuts available for consumption (unadjusted for waste and spoilage) grew from 225 pounds in 1970 to about 242 pounds per person (Wells & Buzby, 2008). This 8% increase, however, was not distributed equally across the meat group. For example, between 1970 and 2005, per capita poultry availability more than doubled, from 34 pounds per person to 74 pounds per person, significantly contributing to the increase in meat intake. In contrast, red meat availability (beef, veal, pork, and lamb) faced a major decline. Since its peak of 133 pounds per person in 1976, red meat availability fell to 110 pounds per person in 2005. Part of the rise in poultry, particularly chicken, results from the emphasis on leaner meat products as well as chicken industry's catering to consumers' and foodservice operators' demand for value-added, brand-name, and convenience products (Buzby & Farah,

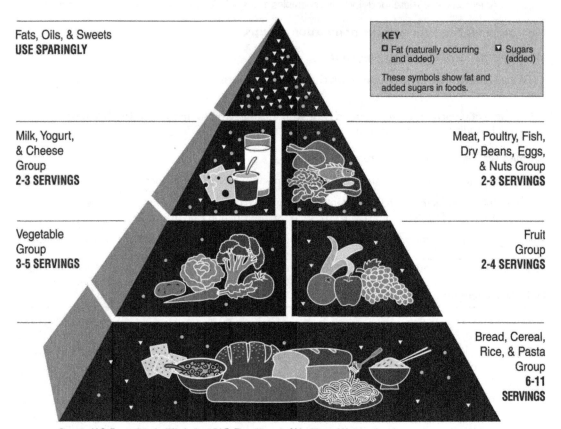

Food Guide Pyramid
A Guide to Daily Food Choices

Fats, Oils, & Sweets
USE SPARINGLY

KEY
□ Fat (naturally occurring   ◩ Sugars
and added)   (added)

These symbols show fat and
added sugars in foods.

Milk, Yogurt,
& Cheese
Group
2-3 SERVINGS

Meat, Poultry, Fish,
Dry Beans, Eggs,
& Nuts Group
2-3 SERVINGS

Vegetable
Group
3-5 SERVINGS

Fruit
Group
2-4 SERVINGS

Bread, Cereal,
Rice, & Pasta
Group
**6-11
SERVINGS**

Source: U.S. Department of Agriculture/U.S. Department of Health and Human Services

Figure 14–1 The Food Pyramid.

2006). Additionally, the trend in milk intake as a beverage was toward lower fat milk. Beverage milk availability decreased 33% between 1970 and 2005. Within the beverage milk category, whole-milk availability dropped 73% whereas lower fat milk rose 143%.

The original pyramid was criticized for not keeping up with the science and for making a number of blanket claims supporting its categorizations, such as, all fats are to be avoided as much as possible; all complex carbohydrates are good; all protein is the same; dairy products are essential; additionally, there was no recommendation for exercise. Heeding this criticism, in 2005 the USDA unveiled MyPyramid, which included physical activity and emphasized personalization and an individualized approach to improving diet and lifestyle. MyPyramid also introduced an online program where users could tailor their diets according to age, weight, height, and activity level (USDA, 2011b). Alas, criticism continued and in 2011, MyPyramid was replaced with MyPlate (Figure 14–2). The newest guide uses the image of a plate to divide four categories of food with fruits and vegetables taking up half of the plate and, protein and grains taking up the other half. A fifth category, dairy, appears on the side of the plate. MyPlate has been touted as an improvement over the complicated pyramid design as it provides a widely recognized reference to an item found in most American's households.

Implications for MCH

The latest version of the food guide, MyPlate, can be a useful addition for MCH populations working on building a healthier diet. Providers should become familiar with the associated MyPlate website (http://www.choosemyplate .gov/) and encourage their clients to use the tool as one way to assess nutrient needs. Users are able to enter their height, weight, age, and activity level as well as if they are pregnant or lactating in the interactive tools section of the website and with serving sizes of each food group to try to meet in order to maintain one's current weight. This may not be as useful with low literacy populations or for those without Internet access; additional nutrition counseling would be necessary.

Dietary guidelines and food guides provide useful tools for individuals as well as direction for public and private institutions. Although they are informed by rigorous scientific method, the end messages to the population at large often become less clear when outside interests influence the communication. Therefore, these tools can be an excellent starting point for women, children, and providers of this population. However, it may take more nutritional education or consultation with a doctor or nutritionist to better personalize and incorporate these guidelines into everyday life.

HUNGER IN AMERICA

The issue of food access and availability is emotionally, morally, and economically charged. There have been several moments in U.S. history when a significant number of citizens have not been able to acquire enough calories from the types of food that support health. One continues to see hunger among families with chil-

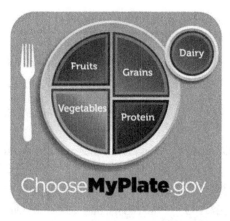

Figure 14–2 The MyPlate Food Guide, 2011. *Source:* USDA, 2011b.

dren, and they confront a variety of additional social and environmental problems, including poverty, lack of nutrition education, the disintegration of families and communities, and inadequate accessibility to service programs.

Hunger from the 1930s to 1960s

Hunger has existed throughout U.S. history. The nation has grappled with being hungry as the pioneers built this country, through war and famine, and as a result of poverty. It is in more recent history—1930s to present—that the country has struggled to make sense of why a nation with so much still cannot meet the needs of the least of its citizens. (See Table 14–2.)

It was during the Depression of the 1930s that federal domestic food assistance was first developed as a way to meet the needs of the unemployed and to answer the emotional outrage that the problem of hunger created. Communities battled the problem by starting soup kitchens, canneries, gleaning projects, and food baskets. However, this was not enough. The agricultural sector had been concerned about large food surpluses throughout the 1920s. In the 1930s, food rotted, whereas many Americans went hungry. The government tried to control the agricultural problem by depressing the prices of farm surpluses. Eventually the disposal

Table 14–2 Selected Events in the History of Federal Policies to Address Hunger in the U.S.

1930	U.S. Department of Agriculture (USDA) and Federal Emergency Relief Administration distribute surplus agricultural commodities as food relief through Federal Surplus Relief Corporation.
1933	Congress creates the Agricultural Adjustment Administration to control farm prices and production and the Federal Surplus Relief Corporation to distribute surplus farm products to needy families.
1935–1942	Congress provides for continued operation of Federal Surplus Commodities Corporation, which, under USDA, purchases commodities for distribution to state welfare agencies.
1936–1942	The Amendments to Agricultural Act permit food donations to school lunches.
1939–1943	The Federal Surplus Commodities Corporation initiates an experimental FSP.
1946	The National School Lunch Program is established.
1954	Special Milk Program is established.
1955	The USDA determines that the average low-income family spends one-third of after-tax income on food.
1961	President Kennedy expands use of surplus food for needy people at home and abroad and announces eight pilot FSPs.
1964	Congress establishes the national FSP. The Social Security Administration establishes poverty line at three times the cost of USDA's lowest cost Economy Food Plan. Since 1969, values are adjusted according to the Consumer Price Index.
1966	The Child Nutrition Act passes. President Johnson outlines Food for Freedom program.
1968–1977	The Senate establishes Select Committee on Nutrition and Human Needs to lead nation's antihunger efforts.
1968–1970	Ten-State and Preschool Nutrition Surveys and Hunger, USA report evidence of malnutrition among children in poverty.
1969	President Nixon announces the "war on hunger" and holds a White House Conference on Food, Nutrition, and Health. The USDA establishes the Food and Nutrition Service to administer federal food assistance programs.
1971	Results of the Ten-State Survey released to Congress indicate a high risk of malnutrition among low-income groups.
1972	Congress authorizes the Special Supplemental Food Program for WIC.
1975	School Breakfast Program is initiated and becomes permanent.
1977	Food and Agricultural Act and Child Nutrition and National School Lunch Amendments are passed.
1981	The USDA establishes a small demonstration project for commodity distribution, the Special Supplemental Dairy Distribution Program.
1981–1982	Congress passes the Omnibus Budget Reconciliation Acts, Omnibus Farm Bill, and Tax Equity and Fiscal Responsibility Act, which eliminate, restrict, and reduce food and income benefits.
1983	The Special Supplemental Dairy Distribution Program becomes institutionalized as the Temporary Emergency Food Assistance Program.

(Continued)

Table 14–2 (Continued)

1984	President's Task Force on Food Assistance finds little evidence of widespread or increasing undernutrition but concludes that hunger exists and is intolerable in the U.S.
1986	The General Accounting Office finds that method flaws discredit findings of the Physician Task Force on Hunger that hunger is prevalent in counties with low food stamp participation rates.
1988	The U.S. DHHS publishes Surgeon General's Report on Nutrition and Health, which states that lack of access to an appropriate diet should not be a health problem for any American. Congress passes the Hunger Prevention Act, increasing eligibility and benefits for Food Stamps, Child Care, and Temporary Emergency Food Assistance Program programs.
1989	The House Select Committee on Hunger holds hearings on food security in the U.S.
1991	Mickey Leland Childhood Hunger Relief Act (HR-1202, S-757) is introduced.

Source: Nestle, M., & Guttmacher, S. (1992). Hunger in the US: Rationale, methods, and policy implications of state hunger surveys. Journal of Nutrition Education, 24, 18S–22S.

of farm surpluses was initiated, backed by the Agriculture Department, to maintain the income of large-scale commercial farmers. The agriculture committees in Congress appropriated money, coined "farmers' money," to support this disposal. This became "the paradox of want amid plenty."

The first attempt at federal food assistance was through the Red Cross during the Hoover Administration (1929–1933). This measure was resisted by both Hoover and the Congress until they were confronted by the cost of surplus storage; the waste caused by rodents, insects, and decay; and the outrage of the American people. Finally, wheat from the Farm Board was distributed to the unemployed.

During the Roosevelt Administration (1933–1945), a continuous food assistance program was created. Congress had made many unsuccessful attempts at trying to deal with the problems of both hunger and surplus food. In the end, Roosevelt announced that the government would purchase a "wide variety" of surplus and have it distributed to the unemployed. The surplus commodity procurement and distribution project was formed and lasted for 30 years. Even today the fundamental problem exists of focusing on surplus crops and not on the nutritional needs of the citizenry (Poppendieck, 1992).

During the 1930s, 1940s, and 1950s, the government continued to address hunger and nutrition through the distribution of surplus agricultural commodities. After World War II, President Kennedy, in response to a campaign promise, outlined a program to expand food distribution by piloting a food stamp program (FSP) in eight counties. In 1964, under President Johnson, the FSP became permanent, and in 1966, the School Breakfast Program was established. The 1960s brought about much change, but the single most powerful event that caused the public to refocus its concern over hunger was the release by the Field Foundation of *Hunger, USA* in 1968 (Citizen's Board of Inquiry into Hunger and Malnutrition, 1968). This report, and its accompanying television documentary, showed widespread malnutrition and hunger in the rural South, and once again, raised national recognition of hunger.

Hunger Held in Abeyance—1970s

The Select Committee on Nutrition and Human Needs, chaired by Senator McGovern, was appointed by the Senate the same year that *Hunger, USA* was released. Its charter was to eliminate hunger. Food assistance for families, children, and the older population was expanded. The Special Supplemental Food

Program for Women, Infants, and Children (WIC) and congregate and home-delivered meal programs were initiated, and the School Lunch Program was expanded. In 1978, the Field Foundation sent its hunger investigation teams back to the same sites they had visited in 1968–1969. They found that hunger had greatly diminished and that nutrition programs were reaching the at-risk communities they had studied. As a result, hunger was considered to be virtually abolished in America during the 1970s (Brown & Allen, 1988; Nestle & Guttmacher, 1992).

Reemergence of Hunger—1980s

During the early 1980s, many studies and reports documented a resurgence of hunger in America, especially among families with children. Among the organizations reporting on hunger were the U.S. Conference of Mayors, the USDA, the U.S. General Accounting Office, the United Church of Christ, the Salvation Army, the Working Group on Hunger and Poverty of the National Council of Churches, Bread for the World, the Citizens Commission on Hunger in New England, the Save the Children Foundation, Second Harvest, the Food Research and Action Center (FRAC), and the Physicians' Task Force on Hunger in America. A faltering U.S. economy, accompanied by cuts in federal assistance programs, had increased the demand on emergency food during this time. President Ronald Reagan appointed a Task Force on Food Assistance in 1983 as a result of the attention that many of these studies and reports drew to this issue. The task force confirmed that serious hunger exists in America, but stated that it could not determine to what extent (Brown & Allen, 1988).

One of the largest obstacles in studying hunger was the lack of a clear definition and an acceptable measure of hunger. In 1984, the Connecticut Association for Human Services—with the help of a distinguished panel of child health and research experts—developed a scientifically valid design for a study of hunger among low-income families with children

under 12 years of age. A national replication of this study, known as the Community Childhood Hunger Identification Project (CCHIP), was initiated in 18 sites across the United States under the coordination of FRAC (Food Research and Action Center, 1995).

Beginning in the late 1980s, advocates, academics, and government officials worked to define, operationalize, and measure the extent of hunger in the United States. The first CCHIP study was conducted between February 1989 and August 1990. What made it unique was the use of a uniform definition of hunger applied to a nationwide study. Hunger was defined as "the mental and physical condition that comes from not eating enough food due to insufficient economic, family or community resources" (FRAC, 1995, p. 2). An eight-item indicator was used to estimate the prevalence of hunger among U.S. children. Twelve percent of families with children younger than 12 years old in the United States experienced hunger, with an additional 28% of families estimated to be at risk of hunger. The series of CCHIP studies found child hunger to be associated with poor school attendance, poor concentration, fatigue, irritability, dizziness, frequent headaches, ear infections, frequent colds, and unwanted weight loss (FRAC, 1995). In 1990, the Office of Life Science published the definitions for food security, food insecurity, and hunger. Working with these definitions, questionnaires were developed to assist in the measurement of child and household hunger.

Food security is the access by all people at all times to enough food for an active, healthy life. Food security includes at a minimum: (1) the ready availability of nutritionally adequate and safe foods and (2) an assured ability to acquire acceptable food in socially acceptable ways (e.g., without resorting to emergency food supplies, scavenging, stealing, and other coping strategies). Food insecurity exists whenever the availability of nutritionally adequate and safe foods or the ability to acquire acceptable foods in socially acceptable ways is limited or uncertain. Hunger is the uneasy or painful sensation caused by a lack of food. Hunger and malnutrition are potential, although not necessary, consequences of food insecurity (Anderson, 1990, p. 1560).

The Cornell/Radimer scale was also created during this time and was developed from qualitative studies with low-income women from upstate New York. Three dimensions of food insecurity were identified: physiologic, social, and psychologic. Indicators of food insecurity included worrying about having enough meals, skipping meals, and inability to acquire foods in socially acceptable ways. Hunger was defined as "the inability to acquire or consume an adequate quality or sufficient quantity of food in socially acceptable ways, or the uncertainty that one will be able to do so" (Radimer, Olson, Greene, Campbell, & Habicht, 1992, p. 395). The CCHIP and Cornell/Radimer questions were piloted with other questions in the 1995 Current Population Survey. An 18-item scale was created that could categorize households as food secure, food insecure, food insecure with moderate hunger, and food insecure with severe hunger (Carlson, Andrews, & Bickel, 1999; Hamilton, et al., 1997). (See Table 14–3.)

Table 14–3 USDA Core Food Security Module

---

1. "I worried whether our food would run out before I got money to buy more." Was that often true, sometimes true, or never true for your household in the last 12 months?

2. "The food that I bought just didn't last, and I didn't have money to get more."

3. "I couldn't afford to eat balanced meals."

4. "I relied on only a few kinds of low-cost food to feed our children because we were running out of money to buy food."

5. "I couldn't feed our children a balanced meal because I couldn't afford that."

6. "Our children were not eating enough because we just couldn't afford enough food."

7. In the last 12 months, did you ever cut the size of your meals or skip meals because there wasn't enough money for food?

8. How often did this happen—almost every month, some months, or only 1 or 2 months?

9. In the last 12 months, did you ever eat less than you felt you should because there wasn't enough money to buy food?

10. In the last 12 months, were you ever hungry but didn't eat because you couldn't afford enough food?

11. In the last 12 months, did you lose weight because you didn't have enough money for food?

12. In the last 12 months, did you ever not eat for a whole day because there wasn't enough money for food?

13. How often did this happen—almost every month, some months, or only 1 or 2 months?

14. In the last 12 months, did you ever cut the size of any of the children's meals because there wasn't enough money for food?

15. In the last 12 months, did any of the children ever skip meals because there wasn't enough money for food?

16. How often did this happen—almost every month, some months, or only 1 or 2 months?

17. In the last 12 months, were the children ever hungry but you just couldn't afford more food?

18. In the last 12 months, did any of the children ever not eat for a whole day because there wasn't enough money for food?

Source: Bickel, Gary, Mark Nord, Cristofer Price, William Hamilton, and John Cook: Guide to Measuring Household Food Security, Revised 2000. U.S. Department of Agriculture, Food and Nutrition Service, Alexandria VA. March, 2000.

Since the piloting of the 18-item food security scale, the USDA has monitored the prevalence of food security in the United States. In 1995, there was a 12% prevalence rate of food insecurity. Of that, 4% were food insecure with hunger. The economic downturn, beginning in 2007, produced job loss and financially burdened families contributing to decreased food security. By 2009, food insecurity rates rose to 14.7%, with very low food security (previously classified as food insecurity with hunger) seen in 5.7% of households, the highest levels recorded since the first household food security survey was conducted (Nord, Coleman-Jensen, Andrews, & Carlson, 2010). The Healthy People 2020 Goals are to reduce household food insecurity from 14.67% to 6% or less as well as reduce very low food security in children from 1.3% to 0.2% (U.S. DHHS, 2010).

Hypothesized to act through both nutritional deprivation as well as a component of family stress, food insecurity has several consequences in childhood. Food insufficiency has been associated with poor dietary intake, iron deficiency (Eicher-Miller, Mason, Weaver, McCabe, & Boushey, 2009), frequent headaches, and stomachaches among children (Alaimo, Briefel, Frongillo, & Olson, 1998). In addition, it is associated with repeating a grade, poor cognitive ability, poor development (Jyoti, Frongillo, & Jones, 2005), poor academic performance, emotional problems (Belsky, Moffitt, Arseneault, Melchior, & Caspi, 2010), and poor mental health (Slopen, Fitzmaurice, Williams, & Gilman, 2010) among children and adolescents (Jyoti, et al., 2005). Food insecurity, however, has inconsistently been associated with overweight among children. A small number of studies have found an association with food insecurity and obesity and weight gain (Bronte-Tinkew, Zaslow, Capps, Horowitz, & McNamara, 2007; Kaiser, et al., 2002; Olson & Strawderman, 2008; Whitaker & Orzol, 2006; Winicki & Jemison, 2003). However, the majority of the studies found

no association or evidence that children in food-insecure households are less likely to be obese than children in food-secure households (Beydoun & Wang, 2010; Casey, et al., 2006; Feinberg, Kavanagh, Young, & Prudent, 2008; Gundersen, Lohman, Eisenmann, Garasky, & Stewart, 2008; Martin & Ferris, 2007; Matheson, Varady, Varady, & Killen, 2002; Webb, Schiff, Currivan, & Villamar, 2008).

In adult women, food insecurity has also been associated with increased body mass (Olson, 1999) and an increase in overweight and a risk of obesity (Adams, Grummer-Strawn, & Chavez, 2003; Hanson, Sobal, & Frongillo, 2007; Kaiser, Townsend, Melgar-Quinonez, Fujii, & Crawford, 2004; Lyons, Park, & Nelson, 2008; Townsend, Peerson, Love, Achterberg, & Murphy, 2001; Wilde & Peterman, 2006). Depending on the measure used, however, this relationship does not always hold up. Using a one-item, "concern about having enough food," from the Behavior Risk Factor Surveillance System (BRFSS), concern about enough food was inconsistently associated with obesity among adults (Centers for Disease Control and Prevention [CDC], 2003; Laraia, Siega-Riz, & Evensen, 2004). An association between food insecurity and being overweight has not been found for men; however, food insecurity has been associated with being underweight in men (Vozoris & Tarasuk, 2003). Additionally, food security has been associated with increased diabetes prevalence (Gucciardi, Vogt, DeMelo, & Stewart, 2009; Seligman, Bindman, Vittinghoff, Kanaya, & Kushel, 2007) and poor diabetes management (Seligman, Davis, Schillinger, & Wolf, 2010), especially with the loss of food stamps (Nelson, Brown, & Lurie, 1998), as well as hypertension and hyperlipidemia (Seligman, Laraia, & Kushel, 2010). It has also been associated with elevated gestational weight gain and gestational diabetes during pregnancy (Seligman, et al., 2010). Finally, food insecurity has been associated with poor mental health among women (Casey, et al., 2004) and pregnant women (Laraia, Siega-Riz, Gundersen, & Dole, 2006).

The phenomenon of food insecurity in U.S. households seems to be one that influences health in a variety of ways, although the pathways are not clearly understood.

Implications for MCH

Hunger affects children physically, mentally, emotionally, and psychologically. If hunger persists, potential healthcare needs and the decrease in productivity that accompany prolonged hunger can have long-lasting, irreversible effects. Combating hunger starts at the local level. People can take several actions to help fight against hunger: find out where soup kitchens and food banks are located; investigate other food programs, such as gleaning projects and food rescue programs; and, most important, know that although people do not want to be poor and hungry, they often need professionals' support to break barriers. For those who meet the requirements, breaking the barriers to access federal assistance programs, such as SNAP or WIC, is an important step in combating hunger. A qualitative study of hunger conducted in North Carolina found that barriers to getting help and relieving hunger included pride, the stigma of poverty, transportation, staff attitudes at social services, and discrimination. During the focus groups that the North Carolina Hunger Project held, participants frequently cited the desire for all of the public assistance programs to be more supportive of men and women who are making an effort. They also stated that as soon as they "get ahead" their benefits are cut immediately, often leaving them further behind.

FEDERAL FOOD AND NUTRITION PROGRAMS TO COMBAT HUNGER

Supplemental Nutrition Assistance Program (SNAP)

The Supplemental Nutrition Assistance Program (SNAP), previously known as the Federal Food Stamp Program, is the primary government program designed to improve the nutrition of low-income individuals and families. The program aims "to alleviate hunger and malnutrition ... by increasing food purchasing power for all eligible households who apply for participation," as stated in the Food Stamp Act of 1977, as amended by P.L. 108-269. In 2010, over 40 million individuals, or nearly one in eight Americans, participated in SNAP, up from 1 in 50 in the 1970s (USDA, 2011c). To be eligible for food stamps, a household without an elderly or disabled member must have a monthly gross income at or below 130% of the federal poverty guideline. The federal poverty guideline is based on the Thrifty Food Plan, a market basket of food that serves as a national standard for a nutritionally balanced diet at low cost. In addition, the cost of the Thrifty Food Plan is used to determine maximum food stamp allotments. The amount is revised each year after July when the annual poverty income guidelines are released by the U.S. Department of Labor. At the food stamp office, the household's net income is calculated, and the program assumes that 30% of the income is spent on food. In 2008, the average monthly benefit was about $101 per person and about $227 per family, or a little over $3.30 per person per day (USDA, 2011d). "Certification" of the household can be for 1 to 24 months. Before the expiration of the certification, the household is notified, and a household member may make an appointment with the program to apply for recertification. SNAP benefits can be used to purchase most foods at participating stores. They may not be used to purchase items such as diapers, cigarettes, household cleaning supplies, pet food, prepared foods, or alcoholic beverages. Participating stores are interviewed and monitored by the USDA. If a store is found to be violating the rules, it will be discontinued from the SNAP benefits. If the store also redeems WIC vouchers, the WIC program becomes discontinued automatically.

The amount of money issued to the recipient is often not enough to cover all food expenses; however, the benefits are meant to be a supplement to the recipient's personal income. The program assumes that the difference between the Thrifty Food Plan amount and the food stamp value issued is spent on food. In fact, the money available in a household is frequently used for emergencies that arise such as transportation to employment or to a healthcare appointment, school fees for trips or special services, and household bills such as telephone, heat, and/or power. In addition, the Thrifty Food Plan requires economical food purchasing, planning, and time for preparation, as many of the menus use recipes requiring preparation "from scratch." When middle- or upper-class individuals follow the menus and recipes prescribed for food stamp participants, their comments include that they are possible to do, but that the menus are boring, there is no allowance for eating out, every household member must carry lunch made at home, and that preparing the meals required too much time.

Periodically, it is recommended that the program be "cashed out," that is, included in the welfare benefit a household receives. However, recipients, particularly mothers, insist that the program retain the food coupons or debit cards so the benefit must be spent on food; therefore, the recipient could not be forced to yield to pressures that it be spent on other expenses. As it is now, the value of the food stamp benefit issued is less than the cost of the Thrifty Food Plan, and thus, it is not surprising that households, particularly those who are eating at emergency food locations, report that the food stamps do not last the month.

Although studies have found SNAP benefits to be effective at reducing food insecurity (Mykerezi & Mills, 2010; Nord & Golla, 2009), there has been some scrutiny that food stamps may increase overweight and obesity in participants of the program. A 2009 study found that people never receiving food stamps had lower rates of obesity than those who had been on them at some point in their lives, even after accounting for differences in socioeconomic status. This effect was most striking for white women where a two-unit increase in BMI was found (Zagorsky & Smith, 2009); others have shown a similar effect in women (Townsend, Peerson, Love, Achterberg, & Murphy, 2001). However, other studies have shown a more modest effect. This association, that one who is lacking in resources to obtain food would experience the effects of overconsumption, seems paradoxical. One theory, sometimes referred to as the "food stamp cycle," explains this by a 3-week period of overeating when food stamps and money are available, followed by a 1-week period of involuntary food restriction when resources have been depleted, followed by overeating when the monthly food stamp allotment has been restored, and so on (Wilde & Ranney, 2000). Over the course of the month, in one study, food consumption was shown to go down 10%–15%, suggesting that some recipients may eat well in the beginning of the month but cut consumption as the month goes on. This kind of "binge–starvation" cycle has been linked to changes in metabolism, insulin resistance, and, ultimately, increases in BMI (Dietz, 1995). Due to these concerns, the USDA convened an Institute of Medicine (IOM) workshop that focused on food insecurity and obesity, the results of which suggest that, although there is an association between household food insecurity and obesity, the coexistence of these two issues is probably driven by underlying poverty rather than a causal relationship (Troy, Miller, & Olson, 2011).

One in three people eligible for SNAP does not participate in the program. Because of the ability of the program to alleviate food insecurity and supplement the income of a financially struggling family, it is crucial that those eligible, especially women and others taking care of children, enroll. Implementing SNAP/Food Stamps policies that improve program access, ensuring staff capacity to process applications, and mounting outreach campaigns to get the word out to the public are some of the ways to help communities maximize the federal recovery dollars available to help local families and businesses (FRAC, 2010).

School Nutrition Programs

Congress established the National School Lunch Program in 1946, recognizing that a large proportion of children were not receiving an adequate lunch and possibly less than desirable breakfasts and dinners. Congress passed laws and allocated funds to establish a program to make low-priced milk available in all schools and a hot lunch in as many schools as possible. This program has grown so that in 2009, 31.3 million children in public and private schools participate in the National School Lunch Program (National School Lunch Program, 2011). Most of the support the USDA provides to schools in the National School Lunch Program comes in the form of a cash reimbursement for each meal served. School districts are subsidized for all lunches. Some children receive a free lunch and some a reduced-price lunch based on the ability to pay. Children whose families have annual incomes at or below 130% of the federal poverty line can receive free meals; those with incomes between 130% and 185% of poverty can receive reduced price lunch; and those with income greater than 185% pay a higher price set by the school district.

Until 1995, participating school districts planned menus that followed the USDA criteria, and they were evaluated for approval by the state education agency. The guidelines required that a menu consist of five items—a protein food, bread, vegetable or fruit, dessert, and milk. In the 1970s, plate waste (food being thrown away) in the school meal program was reaching unacceptable levels. There were efforts to design menus that children liked; however, this did not totally rectify the problem. Now the school meal regulations allow children to select three of the five items on the menu rather than requiring them to take all five, knowing that they are going to throw away at least two. One strength of the current program is the requirement that meals meet national nutrition standards based on nutritional research.

The meals are required to meet one-third of the Recommended Dietary Allowances of protein, vitamin A, vitamin C, iron, calcium, and calories and no more than 30% of calories from fat, with less than 10% of calories from saturated fat (National School Lunch Program, 2011). Although nearly all lunch programs are meeting the requirements for vitamins and minerals, most are exceeding the requirements for fat, saturated fat, and sodium. In 2004, over two-thirds of public schools served school lunches that exceeded the recommendation for fat and saturated fat, with sodium intakes exceeding limits by 200% (Rees, Richards, & Gregory, 2008). The reason fat, salt, and sugar are a problem is because their high satiety value (feeling full), and choosing highly palatable foods may replace foods that are nutrient dense, such as fruits and vegetables. Although this is a dilemma for the school meal program, the problem extends well beyond the schools. The concerns are that there are a substantial number of young people now, and there will be more in the future, who have poor food habits and are less likely to try new foods. They have developed a one or two taste palate. Indeed, the population with these food habits is deficient in vitamins and minerals that are critical for their health. It also makes them more susceptible to cardiovascular disease and cancer at an early age. This is a problem that every MCH professional needs to deal with, whether through parents, teachers, physicians, or the children themselves.

Schools reach over 95% of children in the United States. Despite the excess in certain nutrients, School Lunch Program participants are more likely than nonparticipants to consume more milk, vegetables, and whole grains as well as fewer sweets and snack foods (Cole & Fox, 2008). Efforts by the schools and the USDA's National School Lunch Program need to focus on improving the school nutrition environment and improving enrollment of the hundreds of thousands of students they feed each year. MCH providers should encourage those who qualify to enroll in the School Lunch Program along with advocating for healthier meals in the schools through getting involved in parent groups and other organizations that support improvements to the program.

Child and Adult Care Food Program (CACFP)

The Child and Adult Care Food Program (CACFP) is a federal nutrition program organized under the National School Lunch Act and administered by the U.S. Department of Agriculture and designated state agencies (http://www.fns.usda.gov/cnd/care/). CACFP provides more than $2 billion in reimbursement for meals and snacks served to over 3.2 million children in child care and after school programs. Child care programs are eligible to participate if they serve children from low-income families or children with a specified disability or chronic health condition. Both child care centers and family child care homes are eligible to participate, but homes must work with a sponsoring agency. All Head Start programs not participating in the National School Lunch and Breakfast Program must participate in CACFP.

For children enrolled in participating child care centers, CACFP provides reimbursement to the program for two meals and one snack or one meal and two snacks daily. Meals and snacks served to children are reimbursed at rates based on the type of meal served (i.e., breakfast, lunch, or dinner) and the child's eligibility for free, reduced-price, or paid meals and snacks. Similarly, meals and snacks served to children in family child care homes are reimbursed based on two tiers of eligibility. Tier I reimbursement rates support family child care homes located in low-income areas and for low-income child care providers, whereas Tier II rates apply to all other participating family child care homes. CACFP also reimburses child care programs for exclusively breastfed infants. Thus, childcare programs can receive funding through this program and still support breastfeeding mothers with children in child care. In addition to reimbursement for meals and snacks, CACFP provides nutrition education for child care providers, regulates meal patterns and portion sizes, and offers sample menus to help child care programs comply with nutrition standards. Child care programs not eligible to participate in CACFP are still encouraged to follow CACFP guidelines for healthy meals and snacks.

CACFP is an important federal program that states can use to help promote healthy eating and decrease obesity in young children in child care. In addition, Healthy People 2020 included, for the first time, a nutrition objective specifically targeting child care settings to "increase the number of states with nutrition standards for foods and beverages provided to preschool-aged children in child care from 24 states to 35 states" (U.S. DHHS, 2010). Because child care is governed primarily by states and not the federal government, regulations for child care programs vary considerably by state. Improving state regulations can help ensure that minimum standards for health promotion are required in most child care programs. Several policy reviews have found that most states lack strong regulations related to nutrition and obesity prevention and that family child care homes had the fewest and most general regulations (Benjamin, Copeland, et al., 2009; Benjamin, Cradock, Walker, Slining, & Gillman, 2008; Benjamin, Taveras, et al., 2009; Kaphingst & Story, 2009). To learn more about nutrition standards governing child care within states visit http://www .childhealthpolicy.org.

Special Supplemental Nutrition Program for Women, Infants, and Children (WIC)

Assurance of food availability to low-income or disenfranchised populations is a growing concern in the United States. Nutrition problems—either deficiencies or excesses—have been identified but are difficult to combat because of the many barriers to food access. There may not be enough money to purchase the food or the population may live in a neighborhood where the food is not sold or is too high priced. These factors were described in more detail previously in this chapter. At the 1969 White House Conference on Food, Nutrition, and Health, this problem was made very clear and led to the expansion of the FSP and to the Special Supplemental Food Program for Women, Infants, and Children (WIC), renamed in 1994 under the Healthy Meals for Healthy Americans Act to the Special Supplemental Nutrition Program for Women, Infants, and Children in order to emphasize its role as a nutrition program. Studies have demonstrated the effect of inadequate nutrition during pregnancy on birth outcomes, including lower birth weight and prematurity. Inadequate nutritional intake by newborns and older infants also puts normal development at risk because of the rapid brain growth that occurs from birth until 2 years of age. Along with the possibility of nutritionally compromised brain growth, the most common nutrient deficiency of children below 5 years of age, iron deficiency, may further jeopardize cognitive development. Therefore, children less than 5 years of age are included in the WIC population because of the potential harm that undernutrition has on growth and learning.

The WIC program was designed to give a woman and/or a child's caretaker a voucher or "check" with a list of approved foods and amounts to be purchased at participating food stores. A certain amount of food is approved for the certified person for 6 months, at which time she needs to return for recertification. For pregnant women and children, up until 2009, those foods were milk, eggs, cheese, cereal, peanut butter or dry beans, and fruit juice. The determination is based on their concentration of the target nutrients—protein, iron, calcium, and vitamin C. Breastfeeding mothers may continue to get food supplements for up to 6 months postpartum. Infants may be given the infant formula that meets their needs, and foods are added progressively up to age 1 year. Each participant or caretaker in the program must have two nutrition education program contacts every 6 months, when she must return to the agency for recertification. If the food supply is not limited among these participants, after 6 or 12 months on the program, the nutritional risk is often rectified. However, if the participant leaves the program, she is likely to be back in several months because her low income puts her at nutritional risk again.

Eligibility for WIC is met in most states if the pregnant woman, infant, or child has an income below 185% of poverty and has a nutritional risk factor that includes specific medical conditions, such as anemia, or an inadequate diet. Nearly half of all babies born in the United States participate in WIC. In 2007, approximately 56% of eligible pregnant women were being served (Jacknowitz & Tiehen, 2010). The WIC program requires referral for medical services, and thus, many programs are associated with primary health care for women and children.

WIC was controversial from its inception (Brown, Gershoff, & Cook, 1992). Although the purchase of foods included in the program supported domestic agriculture, critics of the program protested the "free lunch" appearance. In order to answer questions about the benefits of the WIC program, a large, national evaluation was funded by the USDA and was designed and conducted by Dr. David Rush and the Research Triangle Institute. The study demonstrated that infants whose mothers were on the WIC program weighed an additional 28 grams at birth, a statistically significant difference. In addition, other studies showed that a $1 investment in WIC was worth $3 of Medicaid money saved in hospital costs that the lower weight infants would have incurred without WIC (Buescher, Larson, Nelson, & Lenihan, 1993).

Improvements in the offerings to WIC clients have come in various ways. In 1992, the

Farmer's Market Nutrition Program (FMNP) was established to provide fresh, nutritious, unprepared, locally grown fruits and vegetables through farmers' markets to WIC participants. WIC also saw a major revamping to its food package in 2009 due largely in response to the Institute of Medicine's (IOM) report; *WIC Food Packages: Time for a Change*. The report recommended revisions to the food packages that match current dietary guidance for infants and young children, encourage consumption of fruits and vegetables, emphasize whole grains, lower saturated fat, and appeal to diverse populations (IOM, 2005). In response to this report as well as feedback from participants and WIC staff, the food package was revamped in 2009 to reflect these recommendations. Recognizing this population's increased risk of overweight and obesity, the amount of milk, cheese, eggs, peanut butter, fruit juice, and, in some cases, infant formula was reduced and vouchers to purchase fruits and vegetables were added. More culturally appropriate foods such as corn tortillas, tofu, bulgur, and lentils were also included.

Implications for MCH

Participants in WIC like the program, and thus, it becomes a good entry point for the population that MCH programs want to serve. For this reason, immunization, injury prevention, and early intervention programs have paired up with WIC to increase its health promotion potential. Sometimes abuse of the program or lack of participation by eligible people may come to the attention of an MCH staff person. Referral of eligible people and notification of possible abuses to the WIC staff can lead to important improvements in the program. If a health facility for children or pregnant women does not have a WIC program or does not know where to refer clients to find one, advocacy by MCH personnel on behalf of the program is needed.

Programs such as SNAP, the National School Lunch Program, CACFP, and WIC are all in place to provide a safety net for families at risk of food insecurity and/or nutritional inadequacy. Although each of these programs has its limitations, they can fill a crucial gap, especially for women and children who have specific nutritional needs.

BREASTFEEDING

The issue of breastfeeding has become very complex in America's recent history. Although no longer an established practice in the United States, breastfeeding is widely agreed to be the best form of nourishment for a baby. Not only does breast milk have all of the necessary nutrients in the correct proportion, it also has antibacterial factors and immunoglobulins to protect the infant. These biologically active constituents of breast milk are absent from formula. Since the advent of formula at the turn of the century, rates of breastfeeding have fluctuated greatly. The industrial revolution, urbanization, glass bottles, rubber nipples, pasteurization, and refrigeration are only some of the forces that have influenced the increased use of "artificial" feeding (Thulier, 2009).

Currently, the American Academy of Pediatrics (AAP), the American Dietetic Association (ADA), and the Surgeon General all endorse breastfeeding as the optimal feeding method for healthy infants. The AAP supports exclusive breastfeeding for the first 6 months of life (Gartner, et al., 2005). The definition of exclusive breastfeeding is that no other form of milk or food be used for the first 6 months and that breastfeeding continue until 1 year (or until the infant is weaned). In other words, no formula, cow's milk, or other milk substitute is recommended during the first year of life. Many studies have looked at breastfeeding using loosely constructed definitions; any breastfeeding, breastfeeding and formula feeding, or breastfeeding for 3 to 6 months are all considered "breastfeeding." To see the effect of breastfeeding more clearly, however, many studies have used a more robust definition of exclusive breastfeeding.

Breastfeeding rates have increased over the past 2 decades and the Healthy People 2020 objectives for breastfeeding are to increase the categories ever breastfed from 74% to 81.9%, breastfed at 6 months from 43.5% to 60.6%, and breastfed at 12 months from 22.7% to 34.1% (U.S. DHHS, 2010). Based on the National Immunization Survey, an assessment of Healthy People 2010 breastfeeding goals found that there was a low prevalence of breastfeeding among single mothers with children, mothers who were less educated, mothers who participated in WIC, and those living in nonwestern states and in areas of high newborn risk. Conversely, women who were Hispanic, college educated, or lived in the West had higher breastfeeding rates. Women who had a college education were the only group that was on target to meet the Healthy People 2010 objectives for initiating breastfeeding (84%), breastfeeding at 6 months (52%), and breastfeeding at 12 months (25%); however, no group met the goal for exclusive breastfeeding at 6 months (Forste & Hoffman, 2008). Among women who were employed, women with professional positions were 20% more likely to initiate breastfeeding than administrative workers. However, those employed full time, regardless of job type, were 10% less likely to initiate breastfeeding and 19% less likely to breastfeed longer than 6 months compared to those not employed (Ogbuanu, Glover, Probst, Hussey, & Liu, 2011). Rassin et al. (1993) found a decrease in breastfeeding among Hispanic women with increased acculturation in the United States. Since the new objectives were released, breastfeeding has remained constant among most racial groups but may be decreasing among black mothers (Li & Grummer-Strawn, 2002; Li, Zhao, Mokdad, Barker, & Grummer-Strawn, 2003).

Barriers to Breastfeeding

Many of the initial barriers to breastfeeding occur before a woman becomes pregnant and while she is pregnant. Attitudes and beliefs before delivery are the best predictors of breastfeeding initiation. In one study that interviewed WIC participants, perceived barriers to breastfeeding included preferring to know how much the baby is being fed, which is easier to do when feeding with a bottle, not wanting to breastfeed in public, concern about insufficient milk, painful breastfeeding, relations with men and sexuality issues, and smoking (McCann, Baydar, & Williams, 2007).

Hospital policies, such as separating baby and mother after birth, lead to a more difficult time breastfeeding. The early introduction of bottles has been shown to interfere with the prolactin reflex and also to reduce the duration of breastfeeding. Prolactin is the hormone that stimulates the breast's milk-producing alveoli and is released in response to its stimulation. This let-down reflex may be interrupted because of interference with proper infant sucking. The sucking movement has been said to be different for a bottle and for a breast, leading to difficulty or "nipple confusion" for the baby. Poor suckling may also occur when a baby is more easily rewarded by the rapid flow of breastmilk or formula from a bottle (Newman, 1990).

The World Health Organization/United Nations International Children's Emergency Fund's (WHO/UNICEF, 1989) "Ten Steps to Successful Breastfeeding" can be used by hospitals and birthing centers as a standard of practice for more successful breastfeeding outcomes. Based on these guidelines and other criteria (such as no free formula samples), a hospital can work toward a "Baby Friendly" UNICEF designation. First, a self-appraisal tool is used to establish how baby friendly an institution is to start. This assessment tool can then be used to work toward a more baby-friendly state. After the majority of the questions of the assessment tool are answered "yes," the institution can proceed with an external assessment conducted by a multidisciplinary professional team with expertise in breastfeeding and lactation. After the team observes and questions the administrators, staff, and patients, the

344   CHAPTER 14: Issues in Maternal and Child Nutrition

institution can be designated a baby-friendly place by UNICEF. If the institution does not meet the baby-friendly external assessment criteria, which are an 80% adherence to the UNICEF criteria (Table 14-4) and at least a 75% exclusive breastfeeding rate, the administrators can sign a certificate of commitment to put in place the necessary changes by a specified date (Jones & Green, 1993).

In a meta-analysis by Pérez-Escamilla, Pollitt, Lonnerdal, and Dewey (1994), hospital-based breastfeeding interventions, such as the ones that follow the WHO/UNICEF recommendations, are found to have a beneficial effect on lactation success. This was found strongly among first-time mothers. Their results showed that commercial discharge packs had a negative effect on successful breastfeeding. Rooming-in and breastfeeding support had a positive effect on breastfeeding among first-time mothers. Finally, breastfeeding on demand had a positive effect on successful lactation (Pérez-Escamilla, et al., 1994). Apart from hospital policies and protocols, societal and political influences also have a bearing on breastfeeding success. The value placed on breastfeeding is reflected in workplace policies and state legislation. The presence of women in the workforce has increased since the industrial revolution, and it continues to climb at a fast pace. In 1977, 32% of women with a child who is younger than 1 year of age worked outside the home. In 1989, the percentage had increased to 52%, and by 1998, the number rose to 59%. Employment of mothers of infants and young children could be detrimental to successful breastfeeding. However, a paucity of conclusive evidence shows that this is true. What has been shown is that some types of work interfere with breastfeeding more than others. A study by Kurinij, Shiono, Ezrine, and Rhoads (1989) of women from Washington, DC, showed that both black and white women returning to a professional job had a longer duration of breast-feeding after leaving the hospital compared with women returning to sales or technical jobs. The authors suggest that professional women have more control over their situation and can achieve a balance between the demands of the job and the demands of breastfeeding, whereas the women who hold clerical, sales, or technical positions have little control over their environment and have more difficulty acclimating to the demands of the job and of breastfeeding (Kurinij, et al., 1989).

Contraindications

Physiologically, almost all women can breastfeed. Ninety-nine percent of women who try breastfeeding are successful. There are very rare instances when a woman cannot breastfeed because of pathophysiologic reasons. There are other reasons, however, that a woman may not be able to breastfeed or should be advised against breastfeeding. Four such contraindications are most notable. The first three are that breastfeeding is not appropriate when a mother is addicted to drugs such as cocaine or PCP, when a mother takes more than a minimal amount of alcohol, or when a mother is receiving certain therapeutic or diagnostic agents, such as radioactive elements and cancer chemotherapy.

In addition, women in the United States infected with human immunodeficiency virus (HIV) should not breastfeed to avoid transmission of HIV to a child who may not be infected (Gartner, et al., 2005). Mother-to-child transmission of HIV has declined in the United States, especially among those prescribed antiretroviral therapy during pregnancy or in the postpartum period (Aldrovandi & Kuhn, 2010; Birkhead, et al., 2010). However, this is not the case in situations in which there is an otherwise high infant morbidity and mortality due to infectious diseases and malnutrition, and for women living in a developing country without access to antiretroviral medications

(Gartner, et al., 2005; Kennedy, et al., 1990). Mother-to-child transmission of HIV can occur during pregnancy, labor, or delivery or through breastfeeding. Without specific interventions, HIV-infected women will pass the virus to their infants during pregnancy or delivery in about 15%–25% of cases; and an additional 5%–20% of infants may become infected postnatally during breastfeeding, for an overall risk of 30%–45%. Breastfeeding may thus be responsible for one-third to one-half of HIV infections in infants when interventions are not available (WHO, 2008). In any case, where high infant death rates are attributable to infectious diseases, namely diarrhea, the mortality rate from bottle feeding can be as high as 15/100,000, with a relative risk of 4, producing twice as many deaths (Kennedy, et al., 1990). Therefore, because the risk of not breastfeeding outweighs the risk of infection with HIV, breastfeeding should be promoted, even where the HIV epidemic is severe (WHO, 2010). Additional investigation is needed to define clearly the risks attributable to breastfeeding and the timing of transmission through breastfeeding (ADA, 2001).

For more information on breastfeeding rates among U.S. states and policies to support breastfeeding mothers, download the latest CDC Breastfeeding Report Card at http://www.cdc.gov/breastfeeding/data/reportcard.htm.

THE OTHER EXTREME—OBESITY IN AMERICA

Obesity, once a sign of wealth, is now a growing concern in most industrialized countries because it is a risk factor for many chronic diseases. In fact, many developing countries are also experiencing a rapid increase in the prevalence of obesity, especially among groups with low socioeconomic status and among women (Monteiro, Moura, Conde, & Popkin, 2004; Prentice, 2006). Obesity is associated with a variety of adverse health conditions that include Type II diabetes mellitus (Freedman, Serdula, Srinivasan, & Berenson, 1999; Pinhas-Hamiel, et al., 1996), hypertension and hyperlipidemia (Freedman, et al., 1999; Morrison, Sprecher, Barton, Waclawiw, & Daniels, 1999), asthma and sleep apnea (Barlow, 2007; Cleland, Schmidt, Dwyer, & Venn, 2008; Landhuis, Poulton, Welch, & Hancox, 2008; Parsons, Manor, & Power, 2008; Wells & Buzby, 2008), early maturation (Hoppe & Ogden, 1997; Oberrieder, Walker, Monroe, & Adeyanju, 1995; Price, Desmond, Krol, Snyder, & O'Connell, 1987), and psychosocial stress (Dietz, 1998; French, Story, & Perry, 1995; Laraia, Siega-Riz, Dole, & London, 2008; Puhl & Latner, 2007; Puhl, Moss-Racusin, & Schwartz, 2007).

Prevalence and Incidence

Rates of overweight and obesity have increased rapidly over the past 3 decades and have now reached epidemic proportions (Flegal, Carroll, Kuczmarski, & Johnson, 1998; Mokdad, et al., 1999). By 2008, 68% of the U.S. adult population was either overweight or obese, with low-income populations and ethnic minorities disproportionately affected. For adults, overweight is usually defined by a BMI of 25 to 30. Obesity is indicated by a BMI of greater than 30. Current data show that nearly 34% of adults 20 years of age and over—about 59 million people—have a BMI greater than or equal to 30, compared with 23% in 1994. Approximately 36% of U.S. adult females and 32% of U.S. adult males are obese (Flegal, Carroll, Ogden, & Curtin, 2010). In the past 10 years these numbers have remained fairly constant for most groups, and it appears as of this writing that the prevalence of overweight and obesity is reaching a plateau, although large changes in the future cannot be ruled out (Flegal, et al., 2010).

For children, the CDC defines overweight as a BMI at or above the 85th percentile and lower than the 95th percentile, and obesity as a BMI at or above the 95th percentile for children of the same age and sex on the CDC growth charts (Barlow, 2007). The prevalence of overweight among children and adolescents nearly tripled between 1980 and 2008. Among preschool children aged 2 to 5 years, obesity increased from 5% to 10% and among those aged 6 to 11 from 7% to 20% between 1976 to 1980 and 2007 to 2008. Among adolescents aged 12 to 19, obesity increased from 5% to 18% during the same period (Ogden, Carroll, Curtin, Lamb, & Flegal, 2010). The trend is especially alarming since obese children may be at increased risk of becoming obese adults. A review of 25 studies published since 2001 found that all consistently reported an increased risk of overweight and obese youth becoming overweight adults (Singh, Mulder, Twisk, Van Mechelen, & Chinapaw, 2008).

The environmental effects that are strongest are found within the family. Sixty to 70% of obese adolescents have one or both parents who are obese. Furthermore, 40% of obese adolescents have obese siblings. Many people think that obese children may have metabolic or glandular disorders, but in reality, less than 1% have these severe types of problems (Dietz & Robinson, 1993).

There is no clear understanding of why obesity occurs, and unfortunately, there is no one successful treatment for obesity. Many theories purport to account for the increase in obesity in recent history, and most are sketchy at best. The majority of these cite both a genetic and an environmental component to obesity. One theory is that obesity has increased with an increase of available calories per capita while there has been a decrease in energy expenditure. Available calories increased from 3,100 calories per capita from 1950 to 1959 to 3,900 calories in 2006 (USDA, 2010). During this time, the percentage of calories available from fat remained consistently 40% to 43% of the diet. Per capita egg consumption decreased until the mid-1990s, at which point it leveled

off, and dairy consumption has declined by 38% since the 1950s, mostly because of a decrease in milk consumption. The greatest increase in per capita consumption has been in caloric sweeteners. Americans have become conspicuous consumers of sugar and sweet-tasting foods and beverages. Per capita consumption of caloric sweeteners— mainly sucrose (table sugar made from cane and beets) and corn sweeteners (notably high-fructose corn syrup)—increased 26% between 1966 and 2005 (Wells & Buzby, 2008). The increase in the amount of food available and the increase in the amount of food consumed have a direct impact on weight management in America.

Studies have shown diet to be directly linked to obesity, to chronic diseases such as cardiovascular disease, and to some cancers. Although for most of its history the United States has been concerned that its citizens get enough food, the concern now focuses on "optimal" intake, which may be an emphasis on consuming less food. Current dietary recommendations suggest no greater than 30% of calories in the diet be from fat. Moreover, studies show that a diet containing less than 20% of calories from fat can reverse disease processes. Needless to say, this greatly differs from the 40% to 43% fat diet that many Americans currently are eating (Wells & Buzby, 2008).

The greatest environmental influences on children are their parents. In a study by Klesges, Stein, Eck, Isbell, and Klesges (1991), the impact of parental influences on food selection in young children was evaluated. A wide range of foods was offered to children for lunch under three conditions: (1) independent of their mothers, (2) then again with the understanding that their mothers would monitor their selection, and finally, (3) mothers were allowed to modify the choices of their children. This study showed that, when children chose foods freely, their diets were less nutritious than when there was a threat of their mothers watching or when their mothers modified the diet. Twenty-five percent of calories came from added sugar when children selected their own lunches. The meals were more nutritious when modified by the mothers. These were lower in total calories, lower in calories from saturated fats, and had lower sodium content. Nevertheless, even though these meals were lower in total calories and saturated fat, foods highest in nutrient content still were not selected. The overall results reveal first that children do not choose nutritious foods on their own and second that mothers focus on lowering calories but not on increasing high nutrient-dense foods (Klesges, et al., 1991). Beyond food selection, parents influence children's eating behavior in other ways. Verbal prompting at mealtime, adult eating behavior, and the use of food for rewards and punishments all directly influence behavior.

Inactivity and a sedentary lifestyle also contribute to obesity. More frequent television viewing has been associated with greater BMI gains and obesity (Cleland, et al., 2008; Landhuis, et al., 2008; Parsons, et al., 2007). This may be explained by an increase in the number of inactive hours, as well as the effect on children of televised high-calorie food commercials. National surveys of U.S. families have found that patterns of viewing start very young: 75% of babies, toddlers, and preschoolers watch TV for an average of more than an hour per day despite American Academy of Pediatrics' recommendations discouraging any screen media use before the age of 2 (American Academy of Pediatrics, 2001). Additionally, nearly one-third live in households where the television set is on all or most of the time, and an additional 30% live in homes where the television is on during meals (Rideout & Hamel, 2006). A study by Kotz and Story (1994) reviewed a total of 997 commercials selling a product during 52.5 hours of Saturday morning children's television. Of the commercials, 57% were for food, 33% were for toys, and 10% were for other items. Of the food advertisements, 44% were for foods that contained fats and sweets; 36% were for breads, cereals, rice, and pasta. Of the latter group, 23% were for high-sugar cereals. Fast-food restaurants comprised 11% of the commercials, and milk, cheese, yogurt, meats, eggs, nuts, and frozen meals totaled less than 10% of all commercials. Needless to say, the overall picture of food commercials does not comply with the USDA Food Guide Pyramid's recommendations. Food commercials encourage consumption of the foods that are least necessary in one's diet, namely, fats and sweets. Television viewing has been associated with not only an increased consumption of advertised foods, but an increase in children's requests for and parent purchase of these foods (Chamberlain, 2006).

As mentioned, obesity is associated with coronary heart disease, hypertension, non-insulin-dependent diabetes mellitus, certain cancers, and gallbladder disease. Both adults and children can experience hypercholesterolemia, hypertriglyceridemia, Blount's disease and other bone diseases, and respiratory complications directly related to obesity. Obesity is also associated with psychosocial problems. Problems with body image and discrimination have been well documented. A seminal study conducted by Stunkard and Burt (1967) showed that the development of a negative body image takes place most often during adolescence. Although other studies have shown that overweight individuals have no greater psychological disturbances than do nonobese persons, all studies have shown evidence of a strong prejudice against obese persons as young as 6 years old. Children have reported words such as "lazy," "dirty," "stupid," "ugly," and "lies" when describing silhouettes of obese children (Wadden & Stunkard, 1985). Multiple studies have documented explicit negative attitudes about obesity among physicians, nurses, dieticians, and medical students as well as in job hiring (Hoppe & Ogden, 1997; Oberrieder, et al., 1995; Price, et al., 1987; Swami, Chan, Wong, Furnham, & Tovee, 2008). These attitudes include the following: obese people lack self-control and are lazy, obesity is caused by character flaws, and failure to lose weight is due only to noncompliance. Gortmaker, Must, Perrin, Sobol, and Dietz (1993) found social and economic consequences of obesity in adolescence. Obese women were less often married, had lower incomes, and a higher rate of poverty than nonobese women when controlling for socioeconomic status and aptitude.

Obesity Interventions

Studies have shown that there is no easy treatment for obesity. One of the most effective approaches thus far is a family-based behavioral intervention, which employs nutrition, exercise, and parent/child involvement (Epstein, Paluch, Roemmich, & Beecher, 2007). The absence of a successful treatment for obesity makes preventive measures even more important. Reducing excessive caloric intake by reducing fat in school lunches, decreasing television viewing time, and implementing nutrition education for families is a good beginning. Furthermore, the amount of exercise must also increase. Daily physical education during primary and secondary school is very important. Decreasing the amount of television viewing time will aid in a decrease in sedentary activity and lower exposure to inappropriate food commercials. Interactive nutrition education during school can help to reinforce and shape a child's eating habits. Having children involved in the solution is necessary in order to create the most effective change possible. Optimal diet and exercise are still the best preventive tools!

The challenge of the food environment

Challenges in preventing overweight and obesity are expected to continue for the foreseeable future. While many of the programs, guidelines and recommendations discussed in this chapter lay the groundwork for healthier women and children, those living in the U.S. are up against an environment that does little to support a healthy lifestyle. Active discussions on the best ways to improve the food environment to make healthy choices by "default," or by passive decision making, and ways families and individuals can work to improve health are ongoing and include the First Lady Michelle Obama's "Let's Move" initiative (http://www.letsmove.gov/). A significant challenge that must be confronted is that obesity continues to be framed as an issue of personal responsibility. Solutions are often targeted at individual change, as is the case with some suggestions to prevent obesity stated earlier in this chapter. Further evidence is the multi-billion dollar weight loss industry that includes numerous diet pills, one on one counseling, meal delivery plans, and surgery (The US Weight Loss and Diet Control Market, 2011). Another current strategy is to use celebrities to revamp schools and communities through cooking lessons, which have resulted in a backlash of women concerned with food fascism (Fox 2011). Unfortunately, these individual approaches are often met with minimal impact or success.

A growing body of research focuses on the extent to which the larger social environment may play a direct role in food purchases, dietary intake and obesity. One feature of the neighborhood environment is the presence (or absence) of supermarkets and other food stores and restaurants. Differential access to food is seen in some low income and minority neighborhoods where fewer supermarkets and more liquor and convenience stores are commonly found compared with higher income neighborhoods where the reverse is often true (Moore 2006). The lack of supermarkets near one's home is associated with participants reporting less healthy diets when compared to those who have supermarkets nearby (Moore, 2008).

Presence of a supermarket has been associated with a better diet in pregnant women (Laraia, 2004) but not in adolescents (Boone-Heinonen, 2011) and a lower prevalence of obesity in adults (Morland, 2006). Research findings suggest that children and adults who eat outside of the home consume more fat, more calories, more fried foods, more soft drinks and fewer fruits and vegetables than those who eat at home (Poti & Popkin, 2011; French, Harnack & Jeffrey, 2000; Zoumas-Morse, Rock, Sobo & Neuhouser, 2001). Fast food restaurants populate black and low income neighborhoods more so than white and higher income neighborhoods further differentiating the types of food available (Block, Scribner & DeSalvo, 2004; Powell, Chaloupka & Bao, 2007). Children in California with fast food near their schools ate less fruits and vegetables, consumed more soda and were more likely to be overweight than those without fast food nearby (Davis & Carpenter, 2009).

Using a bioethics framework to improve nutrition and address the issue of obesity in the school system, Crawford et al. suggest a more stringent guideline to help make decisions about available foods in schools (Crawford 2011). Since children are not autonomous agents at school, school authorities should be responsible for offering limited choices of foods from which the child can select that provide nutritional benefit. The approach incorporates a social justice component that demands that individuals are treated fairly. Children, especially children from low-income areas who are at greatest nutritional risk, are at greatest need for healthful foods and at great susceptibility to be dependent upon foods offered at school. While government or policy approaches to create a "health as default" environment may contrast with individualistic ideals common in the U.S., Schwartz and Brownell argue that, "an environment that creates ill health in children usurps an individual's liberty and interferes with the right of children to be healthy and happy. An environment that maximizes health enhances liberty" (2007, p. 86).

Local approaches to improve the food environment such as community supported agriculture, farmer's markets in inner cities and rooftop gardens, farm to school programs, gardens in schoolyards, and local biking and walking trails have all been suggested; however, substantial funding is necessary to evaluate these programs (Schwartz & Brownell 2007). Others propose more broad legislative and regulatory action such as taxes on sodas and junk food (Brownell & Frieden, 2009), restrictions on food marketing to children (McGinnis, 2006), requirements for nutrition standards on competitive foods sold in schools (Koplan, Liverman, & Kraak, 2005) and a restructuring of farm subsidies to promote fruit and vegetable production. A food environment that substantially impacts health will likely require broad regulatory and legislative action.

CONCLUSION

Women and children face substantial diet related challenges. The nutritional needs of the MCH population have been met with updated federal guidelines and programs, new policies and rejuvenated advocacy. Programs to address food insecurity, such as WIC, SNAP, and School Meal Programs are crucial resources for women and children to maintain consistent food intake. Strong promotion of breastfeeding and the creation of a supportive environment to do so will continue to provide countless benefits to children and should be a priority for all MCH providers to encourage. Challenges in preventing overweight and obesity are expected to continue for the foreseeable future. Active discussions on the best ways to improve the food environment to make healthy choices the "default" and ways families and individuals can work to improve health are ongoing. Providers are encouraged to participate and pay attention to changes in policy and programs that best promote the health of the MCH population.

References

American Dietetic Association (ADA). (2001). Breaking the barriers to breastfeeding: Position of ADA. *Journal of the American Dietetic Association, 101*, 1213.

Adams, E. J., Grummer-Strawn, L., & Chavez, G. (2003). Food insecurity is associated with increased risk of obesity in California women. *Journal of Nutrition, 133*, 1070–1074.

Alaimo, K., Briefel, R. R., Frongillo, E. A., & Olson, C. M. (1998). Food insufficiency exists in the United States: Results from the Third National Health and Nutrition Examination Survey (NHANES II). *American Journal of Public Health, 88*, 419–425.

Aldrovandi, G. M., & Kuhn, L. (2010). What infants and breasts can teach us about natural protection from HIV infection. *Journal of Infectious Diseases, 202*(Suppl. 3), S366–S370.

American Academy of Pediatrics (AAP) . (2001). Children, adolescents, and television. *Pediatrics, 107*, 423–426.

Anderson, S. A. (1990). Core indicators of nutritional state for difficult-to-sample populations. *Journal of Nutrition, 120*, 1559S–1600S.

Anonymous. (1993). Position of the American Dietetic Association: Promotion and support of breast-feeding. *Journal of the American Dietetic Association, 93*, 467–469.

Barlow, S. E. (2007, December). Expert committee recommendations regarding the prevention, assessment, and treatment of child and adolescent overweight and obesity: Summary report. *Pediatrics, 120*(Suppl.), S164–S192.

Belsky, D. W., Moffitt, T. E., Arseneault, L., Melchior, M., & Caspi, A. (2010). Context and sequelae of food insecurity in children's development. *American Journal of Epidemiology, 172*(7), 809–818.

Benjamin, S. E., Copeland, K. A., Cradock, A., Neelon, B., Walker, E., Slining, M. M., & Gillman, M. W. (2009). Menus in child care: A comparison of state regulations with national standards. *Journal of the American Dietetic Association, 109*(1), 109–115.

Benjamin, S. E., Cradock, A., Walker, E. M., Slining, M., & Gillman, M. W. (2008). Obesity prevention in child care: A review of U.S. state regulations. *BMC Public Health, 8*, 188.

Benjamin, S. E., Taveras, E. M., Cradock, A. L., Walker, E. M., Slining, M. M., & Gillman, M. W. (2009). State and regional variation in regulations related to feeding infants in child care. *Pediatrics, 124*(1), e104–e111.

Beydoun, M., & Wang, Y. (2010). Pathways linking socioeconomic status to obesity through depression and lifestyle factors amount young US adults. *Journal of Affective Disorders, 123*(1-3), 52–63.

Birkhead, G. S., Pulver, W. P., Warren, B. L., Klein, S. J., Parker, M. M., Caggana, M., & Smith, L. C. (2010). Progress in prevention of mother-to-child transmission of HIV in New York State: 1988–2008. *Journal of Public Health Management and Practice, 16*(6), 481–491.

Block, J. P., Scribner, R. A., & DeSalvo, K. B. (2004) Fast food, race/ethnicity, and income: a geographic analysis. *American Journal of Preventive Medicine. 27(3)*, 211-7.

Boone-Heinonen, J., Gordon-Larsen, P., Kiefe, C. I., Shikany, J. M., Lewis, C. E., & Popkin, B. M. (2011). Fast Food Restaurants and Food Stores. Longitudinal Associations With Diet in Young to Middle-aged Adults: The CARDIA Study. *Archives of Internal Medicine, 171(13)*, 1162–1170.

Bronte-Tinkew, J., Zaslow, M., Capps, R., Horowitz, A., & McNamara, M. (2007). Food insecurity works through depression, parenting, and infant feeding to influence overweight and health in toddlers. *Journal of Nutrition, 137*(9), 2160–2165.

Brown, J. L., & Allen, D. (1988). Hunger in America. *Annual Review of Public Health, 9*, 503–526.

Brown, J. L., Gershoff, S. N., & Cook, J. T. (1992). The politics of hunger: When science and ideology clash. *International Journal of Health Services, 22*, 221–237.

Brownell, K., & Frieden, T. (2009) Ounces of prevention–The public policy case for taxes on sugared beverages. *New England Journal of Medicine, 360*, 1805–1808.

Buescher, P. A., Larson, L. C., Nelson, M. D., & Lenihan, A. J. (1993). Prenatal WIC participants can reduce low birth weight and newborn medicine costs: A cost-benefit analysis of WIC participants in North Carolina. *Journal of the American Dietetic Association, 93*, 163–166.

Buzby, J. C., & Farah, H. A. (2006). Chicken consumption continues long run rise. *Amber Waves, 4*, 5.

Carlson, S. J., Andrews, M. S., & Bickel, G. W. (1999). Measuring food insecurity and hunger in the United States: Development of a national benchmark measure and prevalence estimates. *Journal of Nutrition, 129*(2S Suppl.), 510S–516S.

Casey, P., Goolsby, S., Berkowitz, C., Frank, D., Cook, J., Cutts, D., et al. (2004). Children's Sentinel Nutritional Assessment Program Study Group: Maternal depression, changing public assistance, food security, and child health status. *Pediatrics, 113*, 298–304.

Casey, P. H., Simpson, P. M., Gossett, J. M., Bogle, M. L., Champagne, C. M., Connell, C., et al. (2006). The association of child and household food insecurity with childhood overweight status. *Pediatrics, 118*(5), e1406–e1413.

Centers for Disease Control and Prevention (CDC). (2003). Self-reported concern about food security associated with obesity: Washington, 1995–1999, *Morbidity and Mortality Weekly Report, 52*, 840–842.

Chamberlain, J. (2006). Does children's screen time predict requests for advertised products? Cross-sectional and prospective analyses. *Archives of Pediatrics & Adolescent Medicine, 106*, 363–368.

Citizen's Board of Inquiry into Hunger and Malnutrition. (1968). *Hunger, USA*. Boston: Beacon Press.

Cleland, V., Schmidt, M., Dwyer, T., & Venn, A. (2008). Television viewing and abdominal obesity in young adults: Is the association mediated by food and beverage consumption during viewing time or reduced leisure-time physical activity? *American Journal of Clinical Nutrition, 87*(5), 1148–1155.

Cole, N., & Fox, M. K. (2008). *Diet quality of American school-age children by school lunch participation status: Data from the National Health and Nutrition Examination Survey, 1999–2004*. Alexandria, VA: U.S. Department of Agriculture, Food and Nutrition Service, Office of Research, Nutrition and Analysis.

Crawford, P. B., Gosliner, W., & Kayman, H. (2011) The ethical basis for promoting nutritional health in public schools in the United States. *Preventing Chronic Disease, 8*, A98.

Davis, B., & Carpenter, C. (2009) Proximity of fast-food restaurants to schools and adolescent obesity. *American Journal of Public Health, 99*(3), 505–510.

de Onis, M., Garza, C., Onyango, A. W., & Borghi, E. (2007). Comparison of the WHO child growth standards and the CDC 2000 growth charts. *Journal of Nutrition, 137*(1), 144–148.

Dietz, W. H. (1995). Does hunger cause obesity? *Pediatrics, 95*, 766–767.

Dietz, W. H. (1998). Health consequences of obesity in youth: Childhood predictors of adult disease. *Pediatrics, 101*(3, Pt. 2), 518–525.

Dietz, W. H., & Robinson, T. N. (1993). Assessment and treatment of childhood obesity. *Pediatrics in Review, 14*, 337–343.

Eicher-Miller, H. A., Mason, A. C., Weaver, C. M., McCabe, G. P., & Boushey, C. J. (2009). Food insecurity is associated with iron deficiency anemia in US adolescents. *American Journal of Clinical Nutrition, 90*(5), 1358–1371.

Epstein, L. H., Paluch, R. A., Roemmich, J. N., & Beecher, M. D. (2007). Family-based obesity treatment, then and now: Twenty-five years of pediatric obesity treatment. *Health Psychology, 26*(4), 381–391.

Feinberg, E., Kavanagh, P., Young, R., & Prudent, N. (2008). Food insecurity and compensatory feeding practices among urban black families. *Pediatrics, 122*(4), e854–e860.

Flegal, K. M., Carroll, M. D., Ogden, C. L., & Curtin, L. R. (2010). Prevalence and trends in obesity among US adults, 1999–2008. *Journal of the American Medical Association, 303*(3), 235–241.

Flegal, K. M., Carroll, R. J., Kuczmarski, R. J., & Johnson, C. L. (1998). Overweight and obesity in the United States: Prevalence and trends, 1960–1994. *International Journal of Obesity Related Metabolic Disorders, 22*, 39–47.

Food Research and Action Center (FRAC). (1995). Community Childhood Hunger Identification Project: A survey of childhood hunger in the US. Washington, DC: Food Research and Action Center.

Food Research and Action Center. (2010). SNAP/Food Stamp Monthly Participation Data. Retrieved March 26, 2011 from http://frac.org/reports-and-resources/snapfood-stamp-monthly-participation-data/.

Food Stamp Act of 1977, as amended. Pub. L. No. 108-269, § 2 [U.S.C. 2011] (2004).

Forste, R., & Hoffman, J. P. (2008). Are US mothers meeting the Healthy People 2010 breastfeeding targets for initiation, duration, and exclusivity? The 2003 and 2004 National Immunization Surveys. *Journal of Human Lactation, 24*(3), 278–288.

Fox, R., & Smith, G. (2011). Sinner Ladies and the gospel of good taste: geographies of food, class and care. *Health Place, 17*(2), 403–12.

Freedman, D. S., Serdula, M. K., Srinivasan, S. R., & Berenson, G. S. (1999). Relation of circumferences and skinfold thicknesses to lipid and insulin concentrations in children and adolescents: The Bogalusa Heart Study. *American Journal of Clinical Nutrition, 69*(2), 308–317.

French, S. A., Story, M., & Perry, C. L. (1995). Self-esteem and obesity in children and adolescents: A literature review. *Obesity Research, 3*(5), 479–490.

French, S. A., Harnack, L., & Jeffrey, R. W. (2000) Fast food restaurant use among young women in the pound of prevention study: Dietary, Behavioral and Demographic correlates. *International Journal of Obesity and Related Metabolic Disorders, 24*(10), 1353–1359.

Gartner, L. M., Morton, J., Lawrence, R. A., Naylor, A. J., O'Hare, D., Schanler, R. J., et al. (2005). American Academy of Pediatrics Section on Breastfeeding: Breastfeeding and the use of human milk. *Pediatrics, 115*(2), 496–506.

Gortmaker, S. L., Must, A., Perrin, J. M., Sobol, A. M., & Dietz, W. H. (1993). Social and economic consequences of overweight in adolescence and young adulthood. *New England Journal of Medicine, 329*, 1008–1012.

Gucciardi, E., Vogt, J. A., DeMelo, M., & Stewart, D. E. (2009). Exploration of the relationship between household food insecurity and diabetes in Canada. *Diabetes Care, 32*(12), 2218–2224.

Gundersen, C., Lohman, B., Eisenmann, J., Garasky, S., & Stewart, S. (2008). Child-specific food insecurity and overweight are not associated in a sample of 10- to 15-year old low-income youth. *Journal of Nutrition, 138*(2), 371–378.

Hamilton, W. L., Cook, J. T., Thompson, W. W., Buron, L. F., Frongillo, E. A., Olson, C. M., et al. (1997). *Household food security in the United States in 1995: Summary report of the Food Security Measurement Project.* Alexandria, VA: U.S. Department of Agriculture, Food and Consumer Service.

Hanson, K. L., Sobal, J., & Frongillo, E. A. (2007). Gender and marital status clarify associations between food insecurity and body weight. *Journal of Nutrition, 137*(6), 1460–1465.

Hoppe, R., & Ogden, J. (1997). Practice nurses' beliefs about obesity and weight related interventions in primary care. *International Journal of Obesity Related Metabolic Disorders, 21*(2), 1416.

Institute of Medicine. (2005). *WIC food packages: Time for a change.* Washington, DC: National Academies Press.

Jacknowitz, A., & Tiehen, L. (2010). *WIC participation patterns: An investigation of delayed entry and early exit* (No. EER-109). Washington, DC: U.S. Department of Agriculture, Economic Research Service.

Jones, F., & Green, M. (1993). Baby friendly care. *The Canadian Nurse, 89*, 36–39.

Jyoti, D. F., Frongillo, E. A., & Jones, S. J. (2005). Food insecurity affects school children's academic performance, weight gain, and social skills. *Journal of Nutrition, 135*(12), 2831–2839.

Kaiser, L., Melgar-Quinonez, H., Lamp, C., Johns, M., Sutherlin, J., & Harwood, J. (2002). Food security and nutritional outcomes of preschool-age Mexican-American children. *Journal of the American Dietetic Association, 102*(7), 924–929.

Kaiser, L. L., Townsend, M. S., Melgar-Quinonez, H. R., Fujii, M. L., & Crawford, P. B. (2004). Choice of instrument influences relations between food insecurity and obesity in Latino women. *American Journal of Clinical Nutrition, 80*(5), 1372–1378.

Kaphingst, K. M., & Story, M. (2009). Child care as an untapped setting for obesity prevention: State child care licensing regulations related to nutrition, physical activity, and media use for preschool-aged children in the United States. *Preventing Chronic Disease, 6*(1), A11.

Kennedy, K. I., Fortney, J. A., Bonhomme, M. G., Potts, M., Lamptey, P., & Carswell, W. (1990). Do the benefits of breastfeeding outweigh the risk of postnatal transmission of HIV via breast milk? *Tropical Doctor, 20*, 25–29.

Klesges, R. C., Stein, R. J., Eck, L. H., Isbell, T. R., & Klesges, L. M. (1991). Parental influence on food selection in young children and its relationships to childhood obesity. *American Journal of Clinical Nutrition, 53*, 859–864.

Koplan, J. P., Liverman, C. T., & Kraak, V. I. (2005) *Preventing Childhood Obesity: Health in the Balance.* National Academies Press: Washington, DC.

Kotz, K., & Story, M. (1994). Food advertisements during children's Saturday morning television programming: Are they consistent with dietary recommendations? *Journal of the American Dietetic Association, 94*, 1296–1300.

Kurinij, N., Shiono, P. H., Ezrine, S. F., & Rhoads, G. G. (1989). Does maternal employment affect breast-feeding? *American Journal of Public Health, 79*(9), 1247–1250.

Landhuis, C., Poulton, R., Welch, D., & Hancox, R. (2008). Programming obesity and poor fitness: The long-term impact of childhood television. *Obesity, 16*(6), 1457–1459.

Laraia, B. A., Siega-Riz, A. M., & Evensen, K. R. (2004). Self-reported overweight and obesity are not associated with concern about food among adults in New York and Lousiana. *Preventive Medicine, 38*, 175–181.

Laraia, B. A., Siega-Riz, A. M., Kaufman, J. S., & Jones, A. (2004) Proximity of supermarkets is positively associated with diet quality index for pregnancy (DQI-P). *Preventive Medicine, 39*(5), 869–875.

Laraia, B. A., Siega-Riz, A. M., Gundersen, C., & Dole, N. (2006). Psychosocial factors and socioeconomic indicators are associated with household food insecurity among pregnant women. *Journal of Nutrition, 136*(1), 177–182.

Laraia, B. A., Siega-Riz, A. M., Dole, N., & London, E. (2008). Pregravid weight is associated with prior dietary restraint and psychosocial factors during pregnancy. *Obesity, 17*, 550–558.

Li, R., & Grummer-Strawn, L. (2002). Racial and ethnic disparities in breastfeeding among United States infants: Third National Health and Nutrition Examination Survey, 1988–1994. *Birth, 29*, 251–257.

Li, R., Zhao, Z., Mokdad, A., Barker, L., & Grummer-Strawn, L. (2003). Prevalence of breastfeeding in the United States: The 2001 National Immunization Survey. *Pediatrics, 111*(5, Pt. 2), 1198–1201.

Lyons, A. A., Park, J., & Nelson, C. H. (2008). Food insecurity and obesity: A comparison of self-reported and measured height and weight. *American Journal of Public Health, 98*(4), 751–757.

Martin, K., & Ferris, A. (2007). Food insecurity and gender are risk factors for obesity. *Journal of Nutrition Education and Behavior, 39*(1), 31–36.

Matheson, D., Varady, J., Varady, A., & Killen, J. (2002). Household food security and nutritional status of Hispanic children in the fifth grade. *American Journal of Clinical Nutrition, 76*(1), 210–217.

McCann, M. F., Baydar, N., & Williams, R. L. (2007). Breastfeeding attitudes and reported problems in a national sample of WIC participants. *Journal of Human Lactation, 23*(4), 314–324.

McGinnis, J. M., Gootman, J. A., Kraak, V. I., eds. *Food marketing to children and youth: threat or opportunity?* Washington, D.C.: National Academies Press, 2006.

Mokdad, A. H., Serdula, M. K., Dietz, W. H., Bowman, B. A., Marks, J. S., & Koplan, J. P. (1999). The spread of the obesity epidemic in the United States, 1991–1998. *Journal of the American Medical Association, 282*, 1519–1522.

Moore, L., & Diex Roux, A. (2006). Associations of neighborhood characteristics with the location and type of food stores. *Am J Public Health, 96*, 325–331.

Moore, L., Diez Roux, A., Nettleton, J., & Jacobs, D. (2008). Associations of the local food environment with diet quality–A comparison of assessments based on surveys and geographic information systems. *American Journal of Epidemiology, 167*(8), 917–924.

Monteiro, C. A., Moura, E. C., Conde, W. L., & Popkin, B. M. (2004). Socioeconomic status and obesity in adult populations of developing countries: A review. *Bulletin of the World Health Organization, 82*(12), 940–946.

Morland, K., Diez Roux, A.V., & Wing, S. (2006) Supermarkets, Other Food Stores, and Obesity. The Atherosclerosis Risk in Communities Study. *American Journal of Preventive Medicine, 30*(4), 333–339.

Morrison, J. A., Sprecher, D. L., Barton, B. A., Waclawiw, M. A., & Daniels, S. R. (1999). Overweight, fat patterning, and cardiovascular disease risk factors in black and white girls: The National Heart, Lung, and Blood Institute Growth and Health Study. *Journal of Pediatrics, 135*(4), 458–464.

Mykerezi, E., & Mills, B. (2010). The impact of Food Stamp Program participation on household food insecurity. *American Journal of Agricultural Economics, 92*(5), 1379–1391.

National School Lunch Program. (2011). *U.S. Department of Agriculture,* Retrieved March 30, 2011 from http://www.fns.usda.gov/cnd/lunch.

Nelson, K., Brown, M. E., & Lurie, N. (1998). Hunger in an adult patient population. *Journal of the American Medical Association, 279*, 1211–1214.

Nestle, M. (1993). Food lobbies, the food pyramid, and US nutrition policy. *International Journal of Health Services, 23*, 483–496.

Nestle, M. (2011, February 6). Dietary Guidelines try not to offend food industry. *Food Politics,* Retrieved March 20, 2011 from http://www.foodpolitics.com/2011/02/more-on-dietary-guidelines-san-francisco-chronicle.

Nestle, M., & Guttmacher, S. (1992). Hunger in the US: Rationale, methods, and policy implications of state hunger surveys. *Journal of Nutrition Education, 24*, 18S–22S.

Newman, J. (1990). Breastfeeding problems associated with the early introduction of bottles and pacifiers. *Journal of Human Lactation, 6*, 59–63.

Nord, M., Coleman-Jensen, A., Andrews, M., & Carlson, S. (2010). *Household food security in the United States, 2009* (No. EER-108). Washington, DC: U.S. Department of Agriculture.

Nord, M., & Golla, A. (2009). *Does SNAP decrease food insecurity? Untangling the self-selection effect* (No. EER-85). Washington, DC: U.S. Department of Agriculture.

Oberrieder, H., Walker, R., Monroe, D., & Adey-anju, M. (1995). Attitudes of dietetics students and registered dietitians toward obesity. *Journal of the American Dietetic Association, 95*(8), 9146.

Ogbuanu, C., Glover, S., Probst, J., Hussey, J., & Liu, J. (2011). Balancing work and family: Effect of employment characteristics on breastfeeding. *Journal of Human Lactation,* Epub ahead of print. DOI: 10.1177/0890334410394860.

Ogden, C. L., Carroll, M. D., Curtin, L. R., Lamb, M. M., & Flegal, K. M. (2010). Prevalence of high body mass index in US children and adolescents, 2007–2008. *Journal of the American Medical Association, 303*(3), 242–249.

Olson, C., & Strawderman, M. (2008). The relationship between food insecurity and obesity in rural childbearing women. *Journal of Rural Health, 24*(1), 60–66.

Olson, C. M. (1999). Nutrition and health outcomes associated with food insecurity and hunger. *Journal of Nutrition, 129,* 512S–524S.

Parsons, T. J., Manor, O., & Power, C. (2008). Television viewing and obesity: A prospective study in the 1958 British birth cohort. *European Journal of Clinical Nutrition, 62,* 1355–1363.

Pérez-Escamilla, R., Pollitt, D., Lonnerdal, B., & Dewey, K. G. (1994). Infant feeding policies in maternity wards and their effect on breast-feeding success: An analytical overview. *American Journal of Public Health, 84,* 89–97.

Pinhas-Hamiel, O., Dolan, L. M., Daniels, S. R., Standiford, D., Khoury, P. R., Zeitler, P., et al. (1996). Increased incidence of non-insulin-dependent diabetes mellitus among adolescents. *Journal of Pediatrics, 128*(5, Pt. 1), 608–615.

Poppendieck, J. E. (1992). Hunger and public policy: Lessons from the Great Depression. *Journal of Nutrition Education, 24,* 6S–11S.

Poti, J. & Popkin, B. (2011) Trends in energy intake among US children by eating location and food source, 1977–2006. *Journal of the American Dietetic Association. 211(8),* 1156–1164.

Powell, L. M., Chaloupka, F. J., & Bao, Y. The Availability of Fast-Food and Full-Service Restaurants in the United States: Associations with Neighborhood Characteristics *American Journal of Preventive Medicine, 33(4),* S240–S245.

Prentice, A. M. (2006). The emerging epidemic of obesity in developing countries. *International Journal of Epidemiology, 35,* 93–99.

Price, J. H., Desmond, S. M., Krol, R. A., Snyder, F. F., & O'Connell, J. K. (1987). Family practice physicians' beliefs, attitudes, and practices regarding obesity. *American Journal of Preventive Medicine, 3*(6), 339–345.

Puhl, R. M., & Latner, J. D. (2007). Stigma, obesity, and the health of the nation's children. *Psychological Bulletin, 133*(4), 557–580.

Puhl, R. M., Moss-Racusin, C. A., & Schwartz, M. B. (2007). Internalization of weight bias: Implications for binge eating and emotional well-being. *Obesity (Silver Spring), 15*(1), 19–23.

Radimer, K. L., Olson, C. M., Greene, J. C., Campbell, C. C., & Habicht, J. P. (1992). Understanding hunger and developing indicators to assess it in women and children. *Journal of Nutrition Education, 24,* 36S–44S.

Rassin, D. K., Markides, K. S., Banowski, T., Richardson, C. J., Mikrut, W. D., & Bee, D. E. (1993). Acculturation and breastfeeding on the United States-Mexico border. *American Journal of Medical Science, 306,* 28–34.

Rees, G. A., Richards, C. J., & Gregory, J. (2008). Food and nutrient intakes of primary school children: A comparison of school meals and packed lunches. *Journal of Human Nutrition and Dietetics, 21*(5), 420–427.

Rideout, V. J., & Hamel, E. (2006). *The media family: Electronic media in the lives of infants, toddlers, preschoolers and their parents* (No. 7500). Menlo Park, CA: Henry J. Kaiser Family Foundation.

Schwartz, M. & Brownell, K. (2007) Actions necessary to prevent childhood obesity: Creating the climate for change. *Journal of Law, Medicine & Ethics, 35*(1), 78–89.

Seligman, H., Bindman, A., Vittinghoff, E., Kanaya, A., & Kushel, M. (2007). Food insecurity is associated with diabetes mellitus: Results from the National Health and Nutrition Examination Survey (NHANES) 1999–2002. *Journal of General Internal Medicine, 22*(7), 1018–1023.

Seligman, H. K., Davis, T. C., Schillinger, D., & Wolf, M. S. (2010). Food insecurity is associated with hypoglycemia and poor diabetes self-management in a low-income sample with diabetes. *Journal of Health Care for the Poor and Underserved, 21*(4), 1227–1233.

Seligman, H. K., Laraia, B. A., & Kushel, M. B. (2010). Food insecurity is associated with chronic disease among low-income NHANES participants. *Journal of Nutrition, 140*(2), 304–310.

Singh, A. S., Mulder, C., Twisk, J. W. R., Van Mechelen, W., & Chinapaw, M. J. M. (2008). Tracking of childhood overweight into adulthood: A systematic review of the literature. *Obesity Review, 9,* 474–488.

Slopen, N., Fitzmaurice, G., Williams, D. R., & Gilman, S. E. (2010). Poverty, food insecurity, and the behavior of childhood internalizing and externalizing disorders. *Journal of the American Academy of Child and Adolescent Psychiatry, 49*(5), 444–452.

Stunkard, A., & Burt, V. (1967). Obesity and the body image: II: Age at onset of disturbances in the body image. *American Journal of Psychiatry, 123,* 1443–1447.

Swami, V., Chan, F., Wong, V., Furnham, A., & Tovee, M. (2008). Weight-based discrimination in occupational hiring and helping behavior. *Journal of Applied Social Psychology, 38*(4), 968–981.

The US Weight Loss and Diet Control Market (11th edition). Tampa, Fla: Marketdata Enterprises Inc; 2011.

Thulier, D. (2009). Breastfeeding in America: A history of influencing factors. *Journal of Human Lactation, 25,* 85.

Townsend, M. S., Peerson, J., Love, B., Achterberg, C., & Murphy, S. P. (2001). Food insecurity is positively related to overweight in women. *Journal of Nutrition, 131,* 1738–1745.

Troy, L., Miller, E., & Olson, S. (2011). *Hunger and obesity: Understanding a food insecurity paradigm: Workshop summary.* Washington, DC: National Academies Press, Prepublication Copy: Uncorrected Proofs.

U.S. Congress. (1945). House of Representatives 49th Congress 1st Session, Hearings Before the Committee on Agriculture on H.R. 2673, H.R. 3143 (H.R. 3370 Reported), Bills Relating to the School-Lunch Program, March 23-May 24, 1945, testimony of Major General Lewis B. Hershey.

U.S. Department of Agriculture. (2010, February 6). Nutrient availability. Retrieved March 29, 2011 from http://www.ers.usda.gov/data/foodconsumption/nutrientavailindex.htm.

U.S. Department of Agriculture. (2011a). ChooseMyPlate.gov. Retrieved June 23, 2011, from www.choosemyplate.gov.

U.S. Department of Agriculture. (2011b). MyPyramid.gov. Retrieved March 8, 2011, from www.mypyramid.gov.

U.S. Department of Agriculture. (2011c, March 2). SNAP Annual Summary. Washington, DC: USDA, Food and Nutrition Service. Retrieved March 30, 2011 from http://www.fns.usda.gov/pd/SNAPsummary.htm.

U.S. Department of Agriculture. (2011d, March 8). Supplemental Nutrition Assistance Program. (March 8, 2011). Washington, DC: USDA, Food and Nutrition Service. Retrieved March 10, 2011 from www.fns.usda.gov/snap.

U.S. Department of Agriculture & U.S. Department of Health and Human Services. (2010). Dietary guidelines for Americans, 2010 (7th Ed.), Washington, DC: U.S. Government Printing Office. Retrieved March 28, 2011 from http://www.cnpp.usda.gov/DGAs2010-PolicyDocument.htm.

U.S. Department of Health and Human Services. (1992). *FDA Consumer, 26*(6), July–August.

U.S. Department of Health and Human Services. (2010). *Healthy People 2020: Nutrition and weight status objectives.* Retrieved March 10, 2011 from www.healthypeople.gov/2020.

U.S. Senate Select Committee on Nutrition and Human Needs. (1977). *Dietary goals for the United States.* Washington, DC: U.S. Government Printing Office.

Vozoris, N. T., & Tarasuk, V. S. (2003). Household food insufficiency is associated with poorer health. *Journal of Nutrition, 133,* 120–126.

Wadden, T. A., & Stunkard, A. J. (1985). Social and psychological consequences of obesity. *Annals of Internal Medicine, 103,* 1062–1067.

Webb, A., Schiff, A., Currivan, D., & Villamar, E. (2008). Food stamp program participation but not food security is associated with higher adult BMI in Massachusetts residents living in low-income neighborhoods. *Public Health Nutrition, 11*(12), 1248–1255.

Wells, H., & Buzby, J. (2008). *Dietary assessment of major trends in U.S. food consumption, 1970–2005* (Economic Information Bulletin No. EIB-33. Washington, DC: U.S. Department of Agriculture, Economic Research Service.

Whitaker, R., & Orzol, S. (2006). Obesity among US urban preschool children: Relationships to race, ethnicity, and socioeconomic status. *Archives of Pediatrics & Adolescent Medicine, 160*(6), 578–584.

Wilde, P. E., & Peterman, J. N. (2006). Individual weight change is associated with household food security status. *Journal of Nutrition, 136*(5), 1395–1400.

Wilde, P. E., & Ranney, C. K. (2000). The monthly food stamp cycle: Shopping frequency and food intake decisions in an endogenous switching regression framework. *American Journal of Agricultural Economics, 82*, 200–213.

Winicki, J., & Jemison, K. (2003). Food insecurity and hunger in the Kindergarten classroom: It's effect on learning and growth. *Contemporary Economic Policy, 21*(2), 145–157.

World Health Organization and United Nations International Children's Emergency Fund. (1989). *Protecting, promoting and supporting breast-feeding: The special role of maternity services. A joint WHO/UNICEF statement.* Geneva: WHO Press.

World Health Organization. (2008). *HIV transmission through breastfeeding: A review of the evidence.* Geneva: WHO Press.

World Health Organization. (2010). *Guidelines on HIV and infant feeding 2010: Principles and recommendations for infant feeding in the context of HIV and a summary of the evidence.* Geneva: WHO Press.

Yutang, L. (1937). *The importance of living.* New York: William and Morrow Company.

Zagorsky, J., & Smith, P. (2009). Does the U.S. Food Stamp Program contribute to adult weight gain? *Economics and Human Biology, 7*(2), 246–258.

Zoumas-Morse, C., Rock, C. L., Sobo, E. J. & Neuhauser, M. L. (2001) Children's patterns of macronutrient intake and associations with restaurant and home eating. *Journal of the American Dietetic Association 101*(8), 923–925.

15

CHILDREN'S ORAL HEALTH

Jessica Y. Lee and William F. Vann, Jr.

INTRODUCTION

Oral health is a critical component of a child's overall health. C. Everett Koop (former Surgeon General) recognized the relationship between oral health and overall health and coined the often repeated quote "You're not healthy without good oral health." It has been reported that dental disease is the most prevalent unmet healthcare need of poor children of all ages (Newacheck, et al., 2000). Untreated caries is concentrated disproportionately in children of the lowest family income and declines as income increases (Vargas, Crall, & Schneider, 1998). Dental disease has far-reaching effects beyond the consequences of decayed teeth. Children with cavities are significantly more likely to weigh less than 80% of their ideal body weight and to suffer from failure to thrive (Acs, 1992). Not only does tooth decay affect a child's overall health; it also has social ramifications including children's hours lost from school and parents' hours lost from work. Gift and colleagues reported 117,000 hours of school were lost per 100,000 school-age children during 1 year because of dental issues. This translates to children losing more than 51 million school hours annually. The lost hours from school disproportionately affect lower income, minority, and noninsured children (Gift, Reisine, & Larach, 1992).

This chapter covers national trends in oral health, oral health issues, and prevention strategies, and it also discusses access to dental care in the context of the role of maternal and child health programs.

NATIONAL TRENDS IN THE ORAL HEALTH OF CHILDREN

Over the past 25 years the oral health of children in the United States has improved dramatically, with the prevalence of permanent tooth caries declining precipitously. However, during this same time frame the prevalence of dental caries in primary teeth has remained the same nationally and increased among the most vulnerable children. Dental caries is now considered the most prevalent chronic childhood disease. Today dental caries in preschool-aged children is a major U.S. public health problem. This issue has come under scrutiny recently by policymakers, physicians, and researchers (Vargas, et al., 1998).

The prevalence of early childhood caries and lack of access to dental care for young children was a major impetus for the Year 2000 Surgeon General's Conference, workshops, and report being dedicated to children's oral health issues (U.S. Department of Health and Human Services, 2000).

Current reports on the status of oral health for America's children include the following facts:

- Tooth decay is the most common disease of childhood in the United States. Data from the National Health and Nutrition Examination Survey (NHANES) (1999–2002) indicated that 41% of children aged 2 to 11 had dental caries in primary teeth and 42% of those aged 6 to 19 had caries in their permanent teeth (Beltran-Aguilar, et al., 2005).
- Early childhood caries (ECC) has a much higher prevalence among children from low-income families. For example, of Head Start children aged 3 to 5 years of age, the prevalence of ECC has been reported to be as high as 90% (Edelstein, 1995; O'Sullivan & Tinanoff, 1996).
- Up to 50% of tooth decay in children from low-income families remains untreated, often resulting in problems of chronic pain that affects a child's ability to chew food, thrive, and speak, and can lead to poor appearance, which may in turn reduce a child's ability to succeed (Centers for Disease Control, 2011; Jones, et al., 2000).
- Dental caries continues to decrease in the permanent dentition for youth, adolescents, and most adults. However, the prevalence of dental caries in the primary dentition for youth aged 2 to 5 years

increased between 1988 to 1994 and 1999 to 2004 (Dye, et al., 2007).

CHILDREN'S ORAL HEALTH ISSUES

An Overview of Developmental Stages of Children's Oral Health

The most authoritative framework (Pinkham, et al., 2005) for conceptualizing the pediatric oral health life cycle relies on four stages:

1. Conception to age 3
2. The primary dentition years—ages 3 to 6
3. The transitional dentition years—ages 6 to 12
4. Adolescence—ages 12–21

Stage One: Conception to Age 3

Although the concept of infant, baby, and toddler dental care has been firmly established in the pediatric dental community since the late 1980s (Goepferd, 1987), only in the last decade has this concept captured the interest of the wider dental community and the medical profession. The major rationale for the concept of infant dental care is based on the fact that many children get cavities before age 3, and to prevent all decay, prevention must be initiated before or commensurate with the eruption of the first primary teeth. Although there is considerable variability in their eruption times, typically children's primary (baby) teeth begin to erupt between 5 and 7 months. The first primary teeth to emerge usually are the front lower ones called the incisors. These are followed by the upper front primary incisors and successively by the remaining top and bottom teeth in the front and back.

Before and during tooth eruption children often experience a "teething process," wherein the gums may become redder and slightly swollen in response to the pressure of the newly emerging tooth. Sometimes this phenomenon leads to a localized area of inflammation or "sore spot," which can lead to a child's increased fussiness/irritability. In an effort to soothe the localized inflammation, some infants place their hands, fingers, or objects in their mouths. Increased saliva flow often results from this oral stimulation. Over-the-counter topical preparations should be avoided to prevent against over ingestion of anesthetics and other potential harmful medications for babies. Parents should be advised that commercially available one-piece teething toys are excellent for teething children, especially the toys that can be refrigerated, because cold teeth toys may help soothe the sore gums. Parents should be cautioned that teething does not cause an elevated temperature (Wake, et al., 2000) and such a finding should signal the need for a physician visit because the child could have an ear infection or other systemic condition that may be mistaken for teething symptoms.

The first visit to the dentist should occur during this stage. There is unanimity among professional organizations (e.g., American Academy of Pediatric Dentistry, 2010; American Academy of Pediatrics, 2008) catering to very young children that the first dental visit should occur near the time of the eruption of the first tooth and no later than age 1. This visit will include an oral examination and the structuring of an individualized plan of prevention and follow-up care that can help parents raise a cavity-free child. One hallmark of the follow-up plan is the reliance on oral health anticipatory guidance similar to the time-honored well-baby checks. Like their medical counterparts, dentists counsel parents to provide the best possible oral health using age-related developmental milestones that parents might anticipate before their next visit.

Stage Two: The Primary Dentition Years—Ages 3 to 6

Long ignored as "just baby teeth," the primary teeth are in fact the foundation for healthy permanent teeth in the future. They help facilitate eating and speaking during early childhood, and their early loss can set the stage for crooked and crowded permanent teeth. Cavities in primary teeth also lead to cavities in permanent teeth (Gray, Marchment, & Anderson, 1991). For all these reasons, this stage is critical. Most children ages 3 to 6 will need parental assistance to clean their teeth effectively.

Stage Three: The Transitional Years—Ages 6 to 12

Starting around age 6, the permanent teeth will begin to emerge, usually beginning with the lower and then the upper incisors, which will replace the primary incisors. Also at about age 6, children will get their upper and lower 6-year molar teeth. At the time of their emergence, the 6-year molars will be the most posterior teeth in the mouth. As this stage indicates, for the next 5 to 7 years the child will be in constant flux with the exfoliation of primary teeth and eruption of new permanent teeth. The fact that some key posterior primary molar teeth do not exfoliate until as late as age 12 underscores the importance of the primary teeth as natural space maintainers for the permanent teeth.

During this stage most children will assume the responsibility for their oral hygiene. This is also a stage when many children will be undergoing orthodontics, and most will take a keener interest in their overall aesthetics, particularly their smiles.

Stage Four: Adolescence

It has been said that adolescents are no longer children, yet they are not yet adults. During this stage children will establish a permanent tooth dentition of 14 upper and 14 lower permanent teeth or 28 permanent teeth in total. A few may experience the eruption of third molars or wisdom teeth during this stage. Some will have insufficient space for the four wisdom teeth.

This is a stage that has long been overlooked by the dental profession. Parents and dentists must be highly vigilant to reinforce good prevention as children progress through adolescence. Poor dietary habits, such as soda fetishes, are not uncommon during this stage, and such conditions can turn a cavity-free child into an adolescent with a mouthful of cavities.

Major Oral Health Problems of Childhood

There are three major oral health problems that affect children and adolescents: (1) dental caries (tooth decay, cavities), (2) periodontal disease (gum disease), and (3) malocclusions (crooked bite or defective bite).

Dental Caries

Dental caries (i.e., tooth decay) is an infectious, transmissible disease whereby bacteria in dental plaque metabolize sugars and other fermentable carbohydrates from the diet. The acid that is produced as a metabolic by-product dissolves the hard surfaces of the teeth. This disease may cause the loss of minerals from the teeth, known as demineralization. This occurs when exposure to the acid is prolonged and exceeds the natural ability of the teeth to remineralize or heal. The bacteria then can penetrate the surface of the teeth and attack the dentin and soft pulp tissue, leading to cavities (Centers for Disease Control, 2001).

Early childhood caries (ECC), also known as baby bottle tooth decay, refers to early and severe tooth decay in infants and pre-school-age children. A common cause of ECC is giving a child a bottle containing milk, formula, juice, soda, or any drink with sugar for extended periods of time to encourage sleep, comfort, and/or to calm the child. For example, children may be given a bottle when put to bed or be allowed to carry a bottle around with them during waking hours. The sugary drink pools in the child's mouth and becomes a breeding ground for bacteria that may result in cavities. If a child has ECC, his/her teeth may appear chalky white or brown or have yellow spots or cavities, and some

teeth may be partially broken. Estimates indicate that 24%–28% of all children experience ECC, and children in poverty are most affected (Dye, et al., 2007).

Periodontal Disease

Periodontal disease includes both gingivitis and periodontitis. Gingivitis is a disease of the gums that may occur among children. The first signs of gingivitis are red, swollen gums and bleeding while brushing. Often, however, there are no physical symptoms of gingivitis, and regular dental visits can be the only way to detect gingivitis in its early stages (American Dental Association, 2004). Periodontitis, the disease of the gums and supporting bone, is rare in healthy children. If a child has periodontitis, it may be an indication of an underlying condition, and the child should be referred to a physician for evaluation. Both gingivitis and periodontitis can be prevented and controlled by using plaque-removing techniques such as brushing and flossing (Casamassimo, 1996). However, flossing is generally not indicated until a child's teeth begin to touch one another (usually around age 3). Until that time, monitored and thorough brushing is sufficient.

Adolescence can be a critical period in the human being's periodontal status. Pubertal changes can affect the gum tissue of young adolescents, with an increase in inflammation, which in most cases can be managed through oral hygiene and regular dental care. Adolescents have a higher prevalence of gingivitis than adults or prepubertal children. The rise of sex hormones during adolescence is suspected to be the cause of the increased prevalence (Beck & Arbes, 2006).

Malocclusions

Malocclusion refers to the improper alignment of the jaws and teeth. Malocclusions can be either skeletal, when the upper and lower jaw do not align in relation to the skull, or dental, when the teeth in either jaw do not align properly. Many malocclusions are genetically determined. However, a common preventable form of malocclusion occurs as a result of nonnutritive sucking habits (e.g., sucking fingers, thumb, or pacifier). For this reason, sucking habits should be discouraged by age 2, or before permanent teeth erupt. Another common form of malocclusion occurs when a primary tooth is lost prematurely and a nearby permanent tooth shifts into the space, leaving inadequate room for the permanent replacement tooth. Many malocclusions are primarily aesthetic concerns, can interfere with oral functions, contribute to poor oral health and should be evaluated when appropriate.

KEY PREVENTION STRATEGIES

Prevention is the cornerstone for cost-effective dental care. Prevention for children of all ages is best delivered through a reliance on a dental home, a dentally healthy diet, the use of fluoridated water and other fluoride products, the use of dental sealants, and injury prevention.

The Dental Home

The dental home concept for children was first proposed some years ago by Nowak and Casamassimo (2002). Based on the medical home model, the dental home is an environment for focusing preventive, treatment, and referral services to optimize children's oral health. If the child's dental home can be established sufficiently early, it can provide an opportunity for non-threatening preventive services, such as the teaching of proper brushing techniques and application of topical fluorides, while examining for early signs of tooth decay. The dental home is also a perfect setting for parental counseling for a wide variety of dental matters, especially aimed at home care and diets that will assist in raising a cavity-free child.

In summary, the establishment of a dental home should provide children with accessible and compressive dental care. As mentioned previously, it is recommended that the dental home be established no later than 12 months of age.

A Dentally Healthy Diet (National Training Institute, 2010)

The best nutrition for children's oral health is the same as that for their general health: a healthy balanced diet consisting of a variety of foods. See http://www.mypyramid.gov for tips on a daily balanced diet for children.

The age range 0 to 3 years is a particularly vulnerable time. Parents need to pay close attention to dietary factors, because preventing early childhood caries is a dominant theme during this stage, and this challenge is totally under the control of the caregivers. This checklist (National Training Institute, 2010) will reduce ECC:

- Eliminate bottles at bedtime/naptime. If this is not practical, fill the bottle with water, and hold the child until he or she falls asleep.
- Explore alternative methods for calming a child and getting him/her to sleep, such as reading a book or listening to music.
- Clean the child's teeth and gums each day with a toothbrush that has a small head and soft bristles.
- Offer the child drinks with a cup as soon as he/she can sit up alone.
- Eliminate use of bottles after 1 year of age.
- Avoid unlimited or frequent access to milk or sugary drinks (from either a bottle or cup) throughout the day. After eruption of the first tooth, children should be given only fruit juice at mealtimes (no more than four to six ounces per day for 1 to 6 year olds).

For children in the stages older than age 3, the most harmful foods from the dental perspective include those that contain sugars as well as starches essential for a healthy diet. Accordingly, an effort must be made to limit sugar-laden foods, especially those that are sticky and tend to remain in contact with the teeth for long periods of time. Because sugars in foods are ubiquitous, it is acknowledged that they cannot be eliminated but rather selected and served wisely. Some specific suggestions include (National Training Institute, 2010):

- Avoid sweets, including sweetened soft drinks and other sugary liquids. When sweets are eaten it is preferable that they be included with a meal rather than eaten as a snack.
- At meals the combination of foods eaten helps to dilute the sugar concentration and wash the sugars away. Also, children are more likely to brush their teeth after a meal than after a snack.
- At snack time, limit sticky, starchy foods (raisins, crackers, bananas) that cling to the teeth for relatively long periods of time and are not easily washed away.
- After snacking, if brushing is not feasible, rinse the mouth with water.
- Avoid snacking before bedtime or naptime, since the potential for foods to adhere to the teeth surfaces for a longer period of time increases and salivary flow decreases.
- Limit the frequency of snacks. Although children need snacks, every time they eat they are exposing their teeth to potential decay. Providing larger snacks with less frequency will reduce the total number of exposures.

Tooth Brushing

Tooth decay (often referred to by the biological term *dental caries*) is a process that involves the demineralization or dissolution of tooth enamel. Demineralization is caused by bacterial plaque that accumulates naturally on the teeth. Beginning in infancy, almost all children are colonized with decay-causing bacteria, typically through transmission from their mother or primary caregiver (Caufield, 1997). Brushing serves to remove bacterial plaque, and without plaque there can be no demineralization and therefore no cavities. Simply stated, a clean tooth cannot get a cavity. Bacterial plaque on teeth can also lead to irritation of the gingival tissues (gums), leading to gingivitis.

Another major function of tooth brushing is the delivery of fluoride to the tooth surface. The fluoride in toothpaste helps facilitate remineralization or a reversal of the cavity-causing dissolution of the enamel. In short, the application of fluoride via toothpaste makes tooth enamel harder and less prone to acid dissolution leading to decay.

Tooth Brushing for Children Ages 0 to 3

Parents should be urged to begin cleaning the infants' gums regularly during the first months of life before the primary teeth begin to erupt. Using a damp washcloth or gauze, the gum pads should be gently rubbed and cleaned. Some parents like to combine this cleaning with bath times or after diaper changes to help establish a routine that the child will come to expect. In addition to cleaning bacteria and food debris from the mouth, this routine will ready the infant for tooth brushing when the primary teeth begin to emerge.

Upon the eruption of the first tooth, parents should begin brushing the infant's teeth using an infant-sized brush with small head and soft bristles. Brushing instructions are detailed in Table 15–1. Beginning with the eruption of the first tooth, parents should use a tiny "smear" of fluoridated toothpaste—smaller than a pea—a smear about the size as a grain of rice. This precaution is necessary because the infant will not be able to spit out excess toothpaste. The fluoride is highly desirable for the teeth but only a small amount is needed.

Parents should continue to take full control of tooth brushing during this stage. Brushing two times daily—morning and night—is recommended. The nighttime brushing should be

Table 15–1 Basic Brushing Techniques for Children[1]

- Use a soft, polished bristled, straight handle toothbrush.
- Squeeze a pea-size amount of fluoride toothpaste on the toothbrush.
- Place the head of the toothbrush at a 45-degree angle toward the gumline.
- Brush the front (cheek side) of each tooth, top and bottom, using gentle circular scrubbing motions.
- Brush the backs (tongue side) the same way, top and bottom.
- Then scrubbing back and forth gently brush the chewing surfaces of the teeth.
- Hold the toothbrush up and down to brush the insides of the teeth. Use the front tip of the brush and move it up and down.
- Finally, brush the tongue by rolling the toothbrush back to front, or by gently scrubbing back and forth. This may tickle the child at first, but with practice it will become easy.

[1]National Training Institute for Child Care Health Consultants. (2010). *Caring for children's oral health.* Training Module version 5. Chapel Hill (NC): University of North Carolina at Chapel Hill, National Training Institute for Child Care Health Consultants, Department of Maternal and Child Health.

just before bedtime, and after this brushing the child should have no food or liquids other than water. The nighttime before-bed brushing is critically important because it is highly desirable for the teeth to be plaque free during the sleeping hours, a time when salivary flow is diminished. Because saliva helps buffer the teeth against demineralization, it is important that they remain free of plaque during nighttime sleeping hours.

Parents should be aware that children in this stage will want to be independent and brush their own teeth, but children at this stage will not have the manual dexterity to brush effectively. If parents want to foster independence, they can allow the child to brush alone, checking behind them to make sure the teeth have been cleaned well. Another strategy to foster independence is to assign the morning brushing to the child with the nighttime before-bed brushing to the parent or caregiver.

The use of dental floss during this stage will not be needed for most children because the teeth are usually well spaced. However, the dentist will make the final recommendation on flossing during this stage, considering individual findings for the given child.

Tooth Brushing for Children Ages 3 to 6

Most children in this stage will continue to need close parental support with brushing. In general, children will not have the manual dexterity to brush effectively before they can tie their shoes, and this will vary by child. Although there may be some modifications by the dentist and her/his clinical team, the brushing techniques will remain the same as described in Table 15–1.

The use of fluoridated toothpaste remains important. Toward the end of this stage children may be able to spit effectively. If so, they can graduate from a smear-sized to a pea-sized amount of toothpaste. Recommendations for flossing at this stage will be made by the dentist, depending on the child's dental spacing and the child's risk for cavities. When flossing is recommended, the dental team will teach the parent how to floss the child's teeth because children in this stage will not have the manual dexterity to floss for themselves.

Tooth Brushing for Children Ages 6 to 12 and Adolescence

Beginning at age 6, most children will be able to brush their teeth unsupervised, but parents will need to make sure that a routine is established for brushing at least two times daily using fluoridated toothpaste. Although this concept will be emphasized by the dental team, parents will need to oversee the twice daily brushings to make sure children/adolescents are brushing for at least 2 minutes. It takes at least 2 minutes to clean all surfaces of the teeth effectively, and the twice daily 2-minute application of fluoride via toothpaste is also highly beneficial. Two-minute egg-timers are good to use as reminders, and older children might be asked to brush for the length of a song on their personal music players.

Although the dental team is likely to recommend modifications as children get older and more adept with manual dexterity, the basic brushing technique will remain the same as described in Table 15-1. During the 6 to 12 year age range and extending through adolescence, the dental team will begin to teach children how to floss, often using special floss-holding devices that will help complement manual dexterity. Children in these stages may be wearing dental appliances, and the dental staff will also work with children on an individual basis to help them master oral hygiene that can be compromised by dental appliances.

Depending on the individual child/adolescent and his or her proficiency with daily tooth brushing, cavity experience, the risk for new cavities, and the presence of dental appliances, the dentist will often recommend additional fluoride products such as daily fluoride mouth rinses. These are discussed more in the next section.

Fluoride Use (National Training Institute, 2010)

The widespread use of fluoride in the United States is the primary factor in preventing dental caries among both children and adults. As noted previously, fluoride works to prevent cavities in two ways: it increases the resistance of tooth enamel to demineralization and it enhances remineralization of early cavities.

Children may receive fluoride systemically and/or topically. Systemic fluoride is ingested into the metabolic system through fluoridated drinking water or through fluoride supplements (tablets or drops). Topical fluorides, which reach the teeth directly, include fluoridated water (washing over the tooth surface), fluoride toothpastes, fluoride mouth rinses, and fluoride treatments applied professionally. Current research indicates that the topical application of fluoride is the more important of the two methods in preventing decay.

The most common source of fluoride is water. Fluoride occurs naturally in some water, but in most major municipalities it is added to the water as a public health measure to help prevent tooth decay. In these communities, fluoride will be present in the drinking water and in all foods and liquid drinks produced with added water. When adequately fluoridated drinking water is **not** available, dental and medical professionals should prescribe fluoride supplements (fluoride vitamins, drops, tablets) for children and adolescents. In cases where it is not clear as to whether or not a water system is adequately fluoridated, the local and state health departments may be requested to test the water. Fluoride supplements should **not** be given if the primary water source is already adequately fluoridated. The dental team will help oversee these decisions based on the nuances of the family's water sources.

Home water filters have increased in popularity, and many families rely on bottled water for drinking because they believe it provides greater purity than tap water. However, some home filters may remove fluoride from water, and in general, tap water is more rigorously controlled and monitored than bottled water and thus more likely to be optimally fluoridated. Unless bottled water specifies the level of fluoride supplementation, consumers will not have access to this information. Bottled water specifically for young children, often referred to as "nursery water," contains the same dosage of fluoride supplementation as fluoridated tap water but is much more expensive. Children from families who rely on home filters and/or bottled water for drinking and cooking (i.e., as their primary water source) may not receive the appropriate amount of daily fluoride. The home water filter phenomenon, coupled with the recent craze for bottled water, has opened the door for a drastic reduction in access to fluoridated water for children, an outcome that has a potentially serious downside for children's oral health. This is also an area of great confusion for parents but one that is well understood by the dental team. Parents can look to them for advice and recommendations.

Fluoride supplements provided by health professionals are sold in many forms. For example, fluoride drops are available for young children 6 months of age and older; whereas older children and adolescents may be given chewable tablets with or without vitamins. There are limits in the amount of fluoride a child should be given. Too much fluoride during the period of active enamel calcification can cause enamel fluorosis (harmless discoloration or mottling) on unerupted permanent teeth. Most cases of enamel fluorosis result from children taking fluoride supplements when their drinking water is already optimally fluoridated. For example, a physician or dentist may prescribe fluoride supplements for a child who relies predominantly on well water, assuming the water is underfluoridated. However, some well water is naturally fluoridated. In general, testing of children's primary source of drinking water should occur prior to supplementation. Information about natural water fluoride levels can often be found at city or county health departments, but this is another confusing area for which the dental team will have good advice and recommendations.

Fluoride Varnish

Fluoride varnish is a topical fluoride preparation that deserves special mention because it is a relative newcomer as a preventive agent in the United States. Although used widely in Europe and Canada for over 30 years with an impressive record of effectiveness and safety, it did not become available in the United States until 1995 (Miller & Vann, 2008). Fluoride varnish is a very sticky, gelatinous product that is painted directly onto the teeth. It adheres to the outer surface of the enamel where it is slowly released and absorbed into the tooth enamel for approximately 24 hours. It can prevent decay on both the smooth surfaces and the biting (or grooved/fissured areas) of the teeth.

The most novel feature of fluoride varnish is that unlike other topical fluoride products that have been used for the past 30 years in the United States, varnish can be applied safely in children under age 4 (Miller & Vann, 2008). For this reason, in a short span of time fluoride varnish has because the standard of care for children 0 to 6 and is quickly becoming the topical fluoride of choice for children of all ages.

Because of its safety and the relatively quick and easy method of application, fluoride varnish is the first topical fluoride product to be used in the medical setting. The first widespread application of such use was in North Carolina's Into the Mouths of Babes Program (IMB), an oral health education, screening, and referral program that relies on fluoride varnish application in the medical office setting for children from low-income families covered by Medicaid (Rozier, et al., 2003). IMB began out as a pilot program in North Carolina in 2000 and soon went statewide. Now half the states have adopted similar programs aimed at improving the oral health of low-income children ages 0 to 36 months (Rozier, Stearns, Pahel, Quinonez, & Park, 2010).

Dental Sealants (National Training Institute, 2010)

Dental sealants are thin plastic coatings that can be applied to the deep grooves and fissures that often dominate the chewing surfaces of children's back teeth. Although sealants can be used for primary teeth under some circumstances, more often they are used for the four all-important 6-year molars and the four 12-year molars, so named because four molars erupt around age 6 and four more around age 12. These eight teeth are the important bookends in both the top and bottom jaws and often involve a tremendous amount of cost in remedial dental care over an individual's lifetime.

The application of dental sealants is faster, less costly, and less invasive than the placement of fillings, and sealant application will be one of the frontline preventive recommendations of the dental team. The grooves and fissures of teeth are the most vulnerable surfaces, contributing to about 90% of the cavities in a typical adolescent (National Center for Health Statistics, 2004). For this reason, the timeliness of sealant application is a very important consideration and another reason for children to be well situated in a dental home at an early age so sealants can be placed when needed and maintained on a regular basis when children are seen for routine examinations and other preventive needs. When placed properly and maintained regularly, sealants can last well into the young adulthood (Feigal, 1998).

Injury Prevention

Common oral injuries include crown fractures and tooth loss from sockets, as well as fractures of the jaw and alveolar process (the ridge-like border of the upper and lower jaws containing the sockets of the teeth). The types of injuries that commonly occur depend upon the developmental stage and age of the child. Very young children are most likely to suffer injury from falls, which often result in damage to the incisors or front teeth.

Injury Prevention in Children Ages 0 to 3 (National Training Institute, 2010)

- Remove low furniture with sharp edges (e.g., coffee tables) or install bumper guards around them.
- Cover doorstops with bumper guards or heavy foam rubber to prevent falls to toddlers while exploring behind doors.
- Place baby gates at both the top and the bottom of stairs.
- Put safety mechanisms on windows and cabinet doors.
- Use electrical socket covers.
- Place infants and toddlers in properly installed safety seats when in a motor vehicle.
- Ensure that children who are passengers on bikes or who ride bikes wear helmets and safety pads.
- Place a safety belt on children riding in shopping carts.

Injury Prevention in Children Ages 3 to 6

- Many of the previous recommendations will apply to children in this stage, especially those involving safety belt use.
- Although athletic mouth guards are used most often for children with permanent dentition, the dental team may have suggestions on this question for child athletes in this stage.

Injury Prevention for Children Ages 6 through Adolescence

- Children and adolescents should be encouraged to wear seat belts at all times.
- Children and adolescents should be encouraged to wear protective helmets for biking, skateboarding, and downhill skiing.
- Sports-related dental trauma can be a devastating phenomenon that sets the stage for a lifetime of expense and time commitment to manage the immediate injury and future needs. Parents should consult with the dentist for counseling about athletic mouth guards as an effective method of primary prevention for student athletes.

ACCESS TO DENTAL CARE FOR CHILDREN

Inadequate access to dental care is common among children of families living in poverty. This has been documented by numerous national and state reports including the U.S. General Accounting Office (2000) and the Surgeon General (U.S. Department of Health and Human Services, 2000). Since the early 1990s, low-income parents and racial and ethnic minorities have identified access to oral health services as their number one child health concern (Jones, et al., 2000). A national study found that 66% of children between the ages of 2 to 4 years had not had a dental visit during the preceding year (National Center for Education in Maternal and Child Health, 1998). Results from the 2003–2004 National Survey of Children's Health indicated that 13% of white children, 18% of Latino children, and 12% of African American children aged 0 to 17 did not have a dental visit in the previous year (Flores & Tomany-Korman, 2008).

The major barrier low-income parents face in obtaining needed oral treatment for their children is lack of financial resources (National Center for Education in Maternal and Child Health, 1998). Other reasons include low numbers of dentists accepting Medicaid patients, lack of experience among general dentists in treating children, lack of pediatric dentists, long waiting periods for appointments, extensive travel time to appointments in rural areas, and parents and families lack of awareness about dental care needs (Edelstein, 2000; Jones, et al., 2000). The Medicaid Early Periodic Screening, Diagnosis, and Treatment (EPSDT) program recommends a screening and referral for oral health care for all children by age 3. Regrettably, EPSDT has fallen short of this goal. Less than one-third of children under age 5, in many states such as Wisconsin, Pennsylvania, Wyoming, South Dakota, and Utah received dental services in FY 2007 (Centers for Medicare and Medicaid Services, 2009). Identifying low-income children and oral health problems

is important for both the overall health of the child and the cost associated with treating young children with severe decay.

The estimated annual dental bill in the United States to restore children's dental caries exceeds $2 billion, making it one of the most expensive if not the single most expensive uncontrolled disease of childhood (Kanellis, Damiano, & Momany, 2000). However, research documenting the total cost from this condition is limited. Cost estimates for individual children based on a review of dental records in an academic setting in 1992 ranged from $170 to $2,212 per child, and treatment costs increased greatly if care was provided in a hospital operating room under general anesthesia (Ramos-Gomez, Huang, Masouredis, & Braham, 1996). In another study hospitalizations increased the cost as much as $6,000 per patient (Weinstein, 1996). Griffin and colleagues (2000) found the cost of dental treatment for children who had received care in a hospital operating room setting was far greater than for those who had not. These children consumed a disproportionate share of Medicaid dental resources, with a reimbursement per hospitalized child that was 15 times greater than that of a nonhospitalized child ($1,508 vs. $104).

It has been documented that Medicaid alone is not enough to improve access to oral health care for young children, but that when Medicaid is partnered with another public health program, access to oral care can be greatly improved. These programs offer a variety of food, nutrition, and health education and referral services. Workers in the Special Supplemental Nutrition Program for Women, Infants, and Children (WIC) were surveyed about the benefits of WIC. An overwhelming majority listed referral for health care and social services among the top benefits. It is expected that WIC and Head Start (HS) screen children for oral health risk criteria and then refer them into the healthcare system for care. Creation of partnerships to help facilitate this access can ensure timely and appropriate treatment.

Understanding the role of maternal and child health programs and access to care should resonate with policy makers and providers. It is well documented that children on Medicaid have limited access to care and low utilization of dental services. There is evidence that Medicaid alone is insufficient to improve access and utilization of oral health care for high-risk preschool children. Community programs such as WIC and HS may be the first public programs to reach a population of high-risk low-income mothers and children under 5 years of age. Findings indicate that participation in community-based programs increases this low participation. An explanation for such an increase is that the enormity of the crisis, the collective and complementary talents of public health agencies, federal programs and social services organizations are vital in improving access to oral health care for young children (U.S. Department of Health and Human Services, 2000).

A study conducted by Schuster and colleagues (1998) examined the influence of care coordinators who visited families at home to assist with access to well-baby checks. They tracked utilization of well-baby visits as a measure of realized access. Using a randomized design they compared a sample of infants and children who received care coordination to those who did not. Their results indicated that care coordinators increased the number of well-baby visits by 21%. They also found that involvement in public programs (including WIC and Head Start) increased access to care. In many instances staff in community programs act as care coordinators. Identifying children from low-income families and those with oral health problems is important for both the overall health of the child and the cost associated with treating young children with severe dental caries. Community program staff are well positioned to identify children at high risk for dental caries and make appropriate referrals for early management.

Research indicates that children who participated in WIC, HS, and other community programs are more likely to have had a dental visit, thus increasing their access to oral health care. Because inadequate access to dental care is common among children of families living in poverty and because early childhood caries has become a childhood public health problem, community programs can serve as a vehicle to increase access to the oral healthcare system. Furthermore, children on Medicaid are a high-risk population who often need more frequent and extensive dental services than the general population. Evidence suggests that children participating in community-based programs may have a better connection to the health care system, and this may allow their care to be more planned and less urgent. This is consistent with the fact that an important goal of these programs is to make appropriate referrals to health and social services. Additionally, appropriate referrals may also lead to decreased costs of care. Because of its first and early contact, these programs can serve as a vehicle for oral health anticipatory guidance as well. For these reasons, the strategy for developing partnerships between WIC, HS/Early HS, and other community-based programs for the improvement of oral health is sound public health policy and has been shown to generate positive outcomes for preschool children enrolled in Medicaid. These partnerships should be expanded and strengthened in the future.

References

Acs, G. (1992). Effects of nursing caries on body weight in a pediatric population. *Pediatric Dentistry, 14,* 302–305.

American Academy of Pediatric Dentistry. (2010). Policy on the dental home. *Reference Manual, 33*(6), 24–25. Retrieved May 15, 2011 from http://www.aapd.org/media/Policies_Guidelines/P_DentalHome.pdf.

American Academy of Pediatrics, Section on Pediatric Dentistry and Oral Health. (2008). Preventive oral health intervention for pediatricians. *Pediatrics, 122*, 1387–1394.

American Dental Association. (n.d.). Oral health topics A–Z: Periodontal (gum) disease. Retrieved October 19, 2011 from http://www.ada.org/3063.aspx.

Beck, J. D., & Arbes, S. J., Jr. (2006). Epidemiology of gingival and periodontal disease. In: M. G. Newman, H. H. Taki, P. R. Klokkevold, & F. A. Carranza (Eds), Carranza's clinical periodontology (10th ed., pp. 117–119). St. Louis: Saunders Elsevier.

Beltrán-Aguilar, E. D., Barker, L. K., Canto, M. T., Dye, B. A., Gooch, B. F., Griffin, S. O., Hyman, J., Jaramillo, F., Kingman, A., Nowjack-Raymer, R., Selwitz, R. H., & Wu, T. (2005). Surveillance for dental caries, dental sealants, tooth retention, edentulism, and enamel fluorosis—United States, 1988–1994 and 1999–2002. *MMWR Surveillance Summaries, 54*(3), 1–44.

Casamassimo, P. (1996). *Bright futures in practice: Oral health.* Arlington, VA: National Center for Education and Child Health. Retrieved May 10, 2005 from http://www.brightfutures.org/oralhealth/about.html.

Caufield, P. W. (1997). Dental caries—a transmissible and infectious disease revisited: A position paper. *Pedriatric Dentistry, 19*, 491–498.

Centers for Disease Control and Prevention. (2001). Recommendations for using fluoride to prevent and control dental caries in the United States. *Morbidity and Mortality Weekly Report, 50*(RR14), 1–42. Retrieved May 15, 2011 from http://www.cdc.gov/mmwr/preview/mmwrhtml/rr5014a1.htm.

Centers for Disease Control and Prevention, National Center for Chronic Disease Prevention and Health Promotion, Division of Oral Health. (2011). Children's oral health. Retrieved May 15, 2011 from http://www.cdc.gov/oralhealth/topics/child.htm.

Centers for Medicare & Medicaid Services. (2009). *2008 national dental summary.* Washington, DC: U.S. Department of Health and Human Services. Retrieved May 15, 2011 from http://www.cms.gov/MedicaidDentalCoverage/Downloads/natdensum011209.pdf.

Dye, B. A., Tan, S., Smith, V., Lewis, B. G., Barker, L. K., Thornton-Evans, G., Eke, P. I., Beltran-Aguilar, E. D., Horowitz, A. M., & Li, C.-H. (2007). Trends in oral health status: United States, 1988–1994 and 1999–2004. National Center for Health Statistics. *Vital and Health Statistics, 11*(248).

Edelstein, B L. (1995). Dispelling the myth that 50% of U.S. schoolchildren have never had a cavity. *Public Health Reports, 110*, 522–530.

Feigal, R. (1998). Sealant and preventive restoration review: Review of effectiveness and clinical changes for improvement. *Pediatric Dentistry, 20*, 85–92.

Flores, G., & Tomany-Korman, S. C. (2008). Racial and ethnic disparities in medical and dental health, access to care, and use of services in U.S. children. *Pediatrics, 121*, e286–e298. DOI: 10.1542/peds.2007-1243.

Gift, H. C., Reisine, S. T., & Larach, D. C. (1992). The social impact of dental problems and visits. *American Journal of Public Health, 82*(12), 1663–1668.

Goepferd, S. J. (1987). An infant oral health program: The first 18 months. *Pediatric Dentistry, 9*, 8–12.

Gray, M. M., Marchment, M. D., & Anderson, R. J. (1991). The relationship between caries experience in the deciduous molars at 5 years and in first permanent molars of the same child at 7 years. *Community Dental Health, 8*, 3–7.

Griffin, S. O., Gooch, B. F., Beltrán, E., Sutherland, J. N., & Barsley, R. (2000). Dental services, costs, and factors associated with hospitalization for Medicaid-eligible children, Louisiana 1996–97. *Journal of Public Health Dentistry, 60*(1), 21–27.

Jones, C. M., Tinanoff, N., Edelstein, B. L., Schneider, D. A., DeBerry-Summer, B., Kanda, M. B., et al. (2000). Creating partnerships for improving oral health of low-income children. *Journal of Public Health Dentistry, 60*(3), 193–196.

Kanellis, M. J., Damiano, P. C., & Momany, E. T. (2000). Medicaid costs associated with the hospitalization of young children for restorative dental treatment under general anesthesia. *Journal of Public Health Dentistry, 60*, 28–32.

Miller, L. E. K., & Vann, W. F., Jr. (2008). The use of fluoride varnish in children: A critical review and treatment recommendations. *Clinical Pediatric Dentistry, 32*, 258–264.

National Center for Education in Maternal and Child Health. (1998). *Oral disease: A crisis among children in poverty.* Washington, DC: U.S. Department of Health and Human Services, Health Resources and Services Administration, Public Health Service, Maternal and Child Health Bureau.

National Center for Health Statistics, Centers for Disease Control and Prevention. National Health and Nutrition Examination Surveys 1999–2004. Retrieved May 15, 2011 from http://www.cdc.gov/nchs/nhanes.htm.

National Training Institute for Child Care Health Consultants. (2010). Caring for children's oral health. Training Module version 5. Chapel Hill, NC: University of North Carolina at Chapel Hill, National Training Institute for Child Care Health Consultants, Department of Maternal and Child Health.

Newacheck, P. W., Hughes, D. C., Yun-Yi Hung, Y.-Y., Wong, S., & Stoddard, J. J. (2000). The unmet health needs of America's children. *Pediatrics, 105*(4, Pt. 2), 989–997.

Nowak, A. J., & Casamassimo, P. S. (2002). The dental home: A primary care oral health concept. *Journal of the American Dental Association, 133*, 93–98.

O'Sullivan, D. M., & Tinanoff, N. (1996). The association of early dental caries patterns with caries incidence in preschool children. *Journal of Public Health Dentistry, 56*(2), 81–83.

Pinkham, J. R., Casamassimo, P. S., Fields, H. W., Jr., McTigue, D. J., & Nowak, A. (2005). *Pediatric dentistry: Infancy through adolescence* (4th ed.). St Louis, MO: Elsevier Saunders.

Ramos-Gomez, F. J., Huang, G. F., Masouredis, C. M., & Braham, R. L. (1996). Prevalence and treatment costs of infant caries in Northern California. *Journal of Dentistry for Children, 63*(2), 108–112.

Rozier, G. R., Sutton, B. K., Bawden, J. W., Haupt, K., Slade, G. D., & King, R. S. (2003). Prevention of early childhood caries in North Carolina medical practices: Implications for research and practice. *Journal of Dental Education, 67*, 876–885.

Rozier, R. G., Stearns, S. C., Pahel, B. T., Quinonez, R. B., & Park, J. (2010). How a North Carolina program boosted preventive oral health services for low-income children. *Health Affairs, 29*, 2278–2285.

Schuster, M. A., Wood, D. L., Duan, N., Mazel, R. M., Sherbourne, C. D., & Halfon, N. (1998). Utilization of well-child care services for African American infants in a low-income community: Results of a randomized, controlled case management/home visitation intervention. *Pediatrics, 101*, 999–1005.

U.S. Department of Health and Human Services. (2000). *Oral health of America: A report of the Surgeon General*. Rockville, MD: U.S. Department of Health and Human Services, National Institutes of Dental and Craniofacial Research, National Institutes of Health.

U.S. General Accounting Office. (1992). Early intervention: Federal investments like WIC can produce savings, Document HRD 92-18. Washington, DC: Author.

Vargas, C. N., Crall, J. J., & Schneider, D. A. (1998). Sociodemographic distribution of pediatric caries: NHANES III, 1988–1994. *Journal of the American Dental Association, 129*, 1229–1238.

Wake, M., Hesketh, K., & Lucas, J. (2000). Teething and tooth eruption in infants: A cohort study. *Pediatrics, 106*, 1374–1379.

Weinstein, P. (1996). Research recommendations: Pleas for enhanced research efforts to impact the epidemic of dental disease in infants. *Journal of Public Health Dentistry, 56*, 55–60.

16

GLOBAL MATERNAL AND CHILD HEALTH

Kavita Singh, Sian Curtis, and Shelah Bloom

(1) Everyone has the right to a standard of living adequate for the health and well-being of himself and of his family, including food, clothing, housing and medical care and necessary social services, and the right to security in the event of unemployment, sickness, disability, widowhood, old age or other lack of livelihood in circumstances beyond his control. (2) Motherhood and childhood are entitled to special care and assistance.

(United Nations General Assembly, 1948.
Article 25 of The UN Declaration of Human Rights)

INTRODUCTION

About 6.8 billion people now live on earth, the majority of whom live in less developed countries. In 2010, about 27% of the world's population were less than 15 years old, and approximately 26% were women of reproductive age (15 to 49 years old) (U.S. Census Bureau, 2010). Women and children are often the most vulnerable members of society, and the health of this population serves as a marker for wider development. Maternal and under-5 mortality are often viewed as indicators of both health and development. Under-5 and maternal mortality remain high in many parts of the world, fueled by poverty, political instability, environmental degradation, gender discrimination, economic crises, poor public infrastructure, inadequate health systems, and diseases such as HIV/AIDS. At the same time, considerable progress has been made in many countries in improving health conditions for mothers and children.

BACKGROUND, CONTEXT, AND INTERNATIONAL ORGANIZATIONS

The global nature of health thus has created a relatively new term, "global health," which is derived from the terms "public health" and "international health," which in turn came from the terms "tropical medicine" and "hygiene." During the colonial period there was a focus on understanding diseases that were new to Europeans and growth in world trade lead to concerns about sanitation, hygiene, and disease outbreaks. Several schools of tropical medicine were established in Europe and policies regarding sanitation at ports were implemented. Public health became a focus in the United States and Europe during the mid-19th century as part of social reform and as part of increasing knowledge concerning disease and disease transmission. "Public health is the science and art of protecting and improving the health of communities through education, promotion of healthy lifestyles, and research for disease and injury prevention" (Association of Schools of Public Health, n.d.). The term international health relates to practices, policies, and systems in countries other than one's own, and the term global health relates to achieving health equity among all people. Global health is focused on health issues and concerns that transcend national borders, class, race, and ethnicity and that require a collective action (Koplan, et al., 2009). Thus in a sense the term global health encompasses both the terms public health and international health but is unique in its focus on the communal aspect of health.

There are several international agencies that have taken the lead in providing programmatic and policy guidance in the area of global health. The United Nations was created in the aftermath of World War II as a vehicle for peace and conflict resolution among nations. The political institutions of the United Nations dealt with security, whereas the specialized agencies attached to it fostered cooperation necessary to address common problems in specialized areas. The World Health Organization (WHO) and the United Nations International Children's Emergency Fund (UNICEF) both were founded in 1948. UNICEF was created to assist the thousands of orphans and abandoned children resulting from the war in Europe. UNICEF now focuses on improving health and well-being for children all over the world. The WHO was established to promote and protect the health of all people. It is intended to function as an intergovernmental institution with the World Health Assembly as the supreme decision-making body. The Assembly generally meets each year in May in Geneva and is attended by delegations from all 192 member states. Its main function is to determine the policies of the organization. The Secretariat of the WHO has the responsibility to implement the resolutions and to deliver appropriate technical assistance to achieve common goals.

Many of the bilateral aid agencies were also established in the post-World War II era,

including the United States Agency for International Development (USAID), which was created by President John F. Kennedy under the Foreign Assistance Act in 1961. The history of USAID goes back to the Marshall Plan's reconstruction of Europe after World War II and the Truman Administration's Point Four Program. USAID is now one of the world's largest bilateral agencies focused on improving health and development around the world.

Recent developments such as increasing globalization have profound health implications that can be broadly summarized as increased mobility and health transfer risks between countries, increased exchanges of goods and information between countries in response to health problems, and changing roles of national governments and international organizations in the health sector. Recent illustrations of the truly global nature of health threats in today's world include the emergence and global spread of Severe Acute Respiratory Syndrome (SARS) in 2003, swine flu in 2009, the reemergence of tuberculosis (TB) as a growing public health threat in the industrialized world, the HIV/AIDS pandemic, and increasing levels of obesity in both developed and developing countries. In addition many new funding mechanisms are multilateral, such as the Global Fund to Fight AIDS, Tuberculosis, and Malaria and the Global Alliance for Vaccines and Immunization (GAVI). Many bilateral agencies are also using the global health terminology. In May 2009, President Obama announced the Global Health Initiative (GHI), which aims to improve health outcomes through the improvement in health systems with a focus on partnerships and in-country ownership in achieving goals.

THE MILLENNIUM DEVELOPMENT GOALS

The member nations of the United Nations unanimously adopted the Millennium Declaration at the conclusion of the Millennium Summit held in New York in September 2000. The Millennium Declaration contains

Table 16–1 Millennium Development Health Goals.

Goal 4: Reduce child mortality

Target for 2015:

Reduce by two-thirds the mortality rate among children.

Goal 5: Improve maternal health

Targets (5a) for 2015:

Reduce by three-quarters the ratio of women dying in childbirth.

Target (5b) for 2015:

Achieve universal access to reproductive health.

Goal 6: Combat HIV/AIDS, malaria and other diseases

Targets for 2015:

Halt and begin to reverse the spread of HIV/AIDS.

Achieve, by 2010, universal access to treatment for HIV/AIDS for all those who need it.

Halt and begin to reverse the incidence of malaria and other major diseases.

Source: United Nations Millennium Goals (2010). http://www.un.org/millenniumgoals/. Accessed September 26, 2011.

a statement of values, principles, and objectives for the international agenda for the 21st century and includes deadlines for collective action. Accompanying the Millennium Declaration is a set of clearly defined goals and associated targets to be achieved by 2015. The eight Millennium Development Goals (MDGs) cover a broad definition of development. Although all of the Millennium Development Goals are relevant to global MCH, three of the goals explicitly refer to health. These three goals and associated targets are listed in Table 16–1.

GLOBAL MCH PROGRAM STRATEGIES

Global MCH program strategies can be broadly split into two categories: disease-specific interventions or vertical programs and broad community-based strategies or horizontal programs typified by primary health care (PHC) initiatives (Claeson & Waldman, 2000). Vertical programs are highly focused and aim to have a dramatic impact on a single disease or group of diseases. Examples of disease specific programs include the Global Campaign to Eradicate Smallpox, the current Polio Eradication Campaign, and efforts to eradicate malaria from the 1950s–1970s. The campaign to eradicate smallpox resulted in what is often considered the greatest public health achievement to date—in 1979 the world was declared smallpox free. This devastating disease would no longer plague humankind. Global attempts to eradicate polio have achieved tremendous success though eradication is still elusive. In 1988, when the Global Campaign to Eradicate Polio was initiated, there were 125 endemic countries and 350,000 cases of polio. In 2008 there were only four endemic countries (Afghanistan, India, Nigeria, and Pakistan) and fewer than 2,000 cases. The campaign to end malaria began in 1955, but by 1978 only 37 of 143 countries were free of malaria. (Twenty-seven of the 37 countries were in Europe or North America.) The campaign was abandoned by the mid-1970s, because of the difficulty of eradicating malaria in the very countries most affected by the disease and a shift from eradication strategies to control strategies. Recently the President's Malaria Initiative (PMI) is beginning to broach a discussion of whether there should once again be plans to eliminate the disease in localized contexts.

Dissatisfaction with highly vertical disease-focused interventions fueled by the failure of the malaria eradication program led to a shift toward a broader, community-based primary health care (PHC) strategy in the late 1970s. The seminal concept of "health for all by the year 2000," achieved through PHC, was proclaimed at a conference convened by WHO and UNICEF in Alma Atta in 1978. PHC emphasizes the provision of universal MCH services, family planning, improved sanitation, and clean water supplies, achieved through equitable distribution of resources, community participation, emphasis on preventive rather than curative services, and a multisectoral approach.

Subsequent debates about the feasibility of achieving PHC objectives with limited resources led to the emergence of "selective primary health care" (SPHC) (Warren, 1988). SPHC aims to prioritize health problems that have a high impact in terms or mortality or morbidity and for which cost-effective interventions that can be applied in resource-poor environments are available. They were advocated as an interim strategy to improve the health of the largest number of people in the short to medium term. One of the early examples of a SPHC program was UNICEF's GOBI program (growth monitoring, oral rehydration, breastfeeding, and immunization). SPHC programs use available technology but also recognize that in order to be successful, such programs require functioning health structures at all levels and community acceptance and participation.

Other examples of broad-based programs include the Safe Motherhood Initiative (SMI) and the Integrated Management of Childhood Illness (IMCI) program—both of which are discussed later in this chapter. Both of these programs take a comprehensive approach to maternal health and under-5 health, respectively. Other programs, such as PMI, the Global Fund to Fight AIDS, TB, and Malaria and the President's Emergency Plan for AIDS Relief (PEPFAR), have been more vertical in nature. Clearly both vertical and horizontal programs have a place and are needed in global maternal and child health programs. The section on child survival compares a vertical program, the Expanded Program on Immunization (EPI), with the IMCI program. In addition to vertical and horizontal programs, the global health community is focused on overall health systems strengthening as needed to sustain improvements achieved by health programs.

THE STATE OF GLOBAL MCH

The availability of good-quality information on MCH globally is an ongoing challenge. Therefore, the quality of data is an important concern, especially when making comparisons between countries or over time within a country because variations in data collection procedures, definitions, and data quality can significantly distort conclusions. In developed countries, vital registration systems provide the data required to monitor mortality levels, causes of death, and fertility rates. Such systems are typically not completely functional in most developing countries. Coverage is very incomplete and tends to be biased toward the more affluent and educated segments of the population who also tend to experience better health outcomes. Even when data are available, they are often not reported in a timely manner and may be of poor quality. Sample vital registration systems provide improved data in some countries such as India and China, but such systems are not widely available. Therefore, population-based surveys such as the Demographic and Health Surveys (DHS) and UNICEF's Multiple Indicator Cluster Surveys (MICS) remain an important source of information on MCH globally. The widespread implementation of good-quality household surveys since the 1970s has allowed global trends in MCH outcomes and behaviors to be documented and greatly added to the global MCH knowledge base. Nevertheless, household surveys suffer from several limitations, and many significant knowledge gaps remain. Table 16–2 shows four key indicators of MCH for different regions of the world.

These regional estimates mask large variations among countries within regions but serve to illustrate the magnitude of global inequity in MCH. Maternal mortality ratio (MMR) estimates vary from 14 deaths per 100,000 live births in industrialized countries to 640 deaths per 100,000 live births in sub-Saharan Africa. Similarly, the under-5 mortality rates vary from 6 deaths per

Table 16–2 Selected Indicators of MCH by Region

Region	MMR	Under-5 Mortality Rate	Stunting Prevalence	Total Fertility Rate
Sub-Saharan Africa	640	129	42	5.3
Middle East and North Africa	170	41	32	3.1
South Asia	290	71	48	3.0
East Asia and Pacific	88	26	22	1.9
Latin America and Caribbean	85	23	14	2.4
CEE/CIS and Baltic States	34	21	NA	1.7
Industrialized countries	14	6	NA	1.7
Developing Countries	290	66	34	2.8
Least developed countries	590	NA	45	4.7
World	260	60	34	2.6

MMR: Number of maternal deaths per 100,000 live births. Figures are for 2008.
Under-5 Mortality Rate: Number of deaths of children under 5 years of age per 1,000 live births. Figures are for 2009.
Stunting Prevalence: Percentage of children under 5 years old whose height is below two standard deviations from the median height for age of the WHO recognized international reference population. Estimates are for 2003 to 2008.
Total Fertility Rate: Expected number of life-time births at current fertility rates. Estimates are for 2006. NA: not available.

Source: MMWR Data from: World Health Organization, 2010. Trends in Maternal Mortality 1990–2008. Geneva: WHO.
Under-five Mortality Data from: UNICEF, 2010. Levels and Trends in Child Mortality, Report 2010. New York. UNICEF.
Stunting Data from: UNICEF, 2009. State of the world's children. Geneva: UNICEF.
Total Fertility Rate data from: UNICEF, 2008. Progress for Children. A Report Card on Maternal Mortality. Number 7, September 2008. New York. UNICEF.

1,000 live births in industrialized countries to 129 deaths per 1,000 live births in sub-Saharan Africa. Sub-Saharan Africa typically has the poorest MCH outcomes, followed by South Asia, whereas industrialized nations have the best outcomes. MCH outcomes are highly correlated with economic development both between and within countries.

Maternal Health

Global maternal health has been evolving in earnest since the Safe Motherhood Conference in Nairobi in 1987 (Cohen, 1987). In 2000, it was estimated that 529,000 women died from maternal causes (AbouZahr & Wardlaw, 2000). The World Health Organization (WHO) estimated 358,000 maternal deaths in 2008, while the Institute of Health Metrics and Evaluation had a similar estimate at 342,900 (Hogan, et al., 2010; WHO, 2010). Though progress has been made, many developing countries are still not on target to reach a two-thirds reduction in maternal mortality (MDG5) by 2015. It is estimated that adequate maternal health care could prevent 90% to 95% of maternal deaths (Ransom & Yinger, 2002). For every woman who dies from a pregnancy-related cause, an estimated 20 women experience some kind of injury, infection, disease, or disability, resulting in an estimated 10 million women who suffer from maternal morbidity worldwide (Nanda, Swirlick, & Lule, 2005). Though many factors have an impact on maternal health, the provision of adequate health services is seen as the key to decreasing pregnancy-related morbidity and mortality (Campbell, et al., 2006; Koblinsky, 1995).

The International Classification of Diseases defines a maternal death as the death of a woman during pregnancy or within 42 days of its termination, regardless of the duration and site of the pregnancy, from any cause related to or aggravated by the pregnancy or its management, but not from accidental or incidental causes (WHO, 2007). Direct obstetric deaths, accounting for approximately 80% of maternal deaths, are those resulting from complications of pregnancy and birth. Indirect obstetric deaths are caused by an underlying illness or one that developed during pregnancy that was aggravated by the physiologic effects of pregnancy (WHO, 1993).

The most common measure of maternal death is the maternal mortality ratio, defined as the number of maternal deaths during a given time period per 100,000 live births during the same time period. The MMR indicates the risk of death to a woman once pregnant. Another key measure is the maternal mortality rate, which is the number of maternal deaths in a given time period per 100,000 women during the same time period. It reflects the frequency that women are exposed to the risk of death through fertility as well as the obstetric risk associated with each pregnancy. The lifetime risk of maternal death is based on the probability of becoming pregnant along with the probability of dying as a result of pregnancy across a woman's reproductive years. For example the lifetime risk of a maternal death is 1 in 31 for women in sub-Saharan Africa and 1 in 4,200 for women in Europe (WHO, 2010).

Monitoring maternal health status itself has been problematic because of the difficulty in measuring its key indicators. In developing countries many women give birth and are treated for complications outside of medical facilities and so many deaths and complications go unreported. In addition, because a maternal death is a relatively rare event, even in areas where the risk is high, obtaining a sound estimate requires a study population so large that it is often impractical. A number of field and statistical methods have been devised in recent years to improve the accuracy of measures of the risk and level of maternal death (Hill, AbouZahr, & Wardlaw, 2001; Hogan, et al., 2010; WHO, 2010). Generally, the MMR is not used to monitor and evaluate maternal health programs because of the potential difficulties in obtaining accurate estimates (Buekens, 2001).

Given the difficulties in measuring maternal mortality, process measures are often recommended to monitor progress of programs toward the goal of reducing maternal death and disability. Two measures have been proposed to act as a proxy for the level of maternal death and disability. These are the proportion of births attended by a skilled birth attendant (SBA), meaning a doctor, nurse, or midwife (not including traditional birth attendants—TBAs), and the proportion of births delivered by cesarean section. The proportion of women delivering with a skilled attendant has increased somewhat from 54% to 62% between 1995 and 2005. In South Asia and Sub-Saharan Africa, less than half of women deliver with a skilled attendant, whereas in East Asia 89% of women deliver with a skilled attendant (UNICEF, 2008). Although cesarean section can be a life-saving procedure when medically indicated, in cases in which it is not, the procedure unnecessarily increases the health risks for both the mother and baby, as well as the costs associated with childbirth. Cesarean section rates higher than 15% are generally thought to indicate that the procedure is being overused. Studies by the WHO found cesarean section rates to be 46% in China (Lumbiganon, et al., 2010) and a median of 33% in the eight Latin American countries studied (Villar, et al., 2006). On the other hand, cesarean section rates are below 5% in many sub-Saharan African countries

(Buekens, Curtis, & Alayon, 2003). This indicates the procedure may not be available to all women who need it. In resource-strained settings such as sub-Saharan Africa, increased access to cesarean section will improve maternal health outcomes, whereas in regions such as Latin America and in China, an overuse of cesarean section can drive up the rate of maternal morbidity.

Despite the problems with measurement, estimates of the magnitude of maternal mortality are still considered vital to the field of maternal health because they call attention to one of the largest ongoing health tragedies of the present era. The risk of maternal death represents the greatest health disparity between developed and less developed countries. For example, the MMR in several European countries is 5/100,000 or less whereas in Somalia the MMR is 1,200/100,000, and in Afghanistan the MMR is 1,400/100,000 (WHO, 2010). Within countries there also are often disparities in the MMR by urban/rural residence and socioeconomic status/wealth.

Variation exists by region and setting in the proportion of deaths due to each cause, but globally, direct obstetric deaths most commonly result from hemorrhage (25%), infections (15%), hypertensive disorders of pregnancy (16%), obstructed labor (8%), and unsafe abortions (18%). Most indirect maternal deaths result from aggravated conditions such as malaria, anemia, cardiovascular diseases, diabetes, and HIV/AIDS (WHO, 2005a). The majority of pregnancy complications arise during labor, delivery, or the immediate postpartum period. The majority of pregnancies progress normally, and assessing who is at risk for a complication is often not possible. Many complications cannot be predicted beforehand, and some such as postpartum hemorrhage can be fatal within hours if not treated. Thus, ensuring that all women have access to Emergency Obstetric Care (EmOC) is seen as crucial in reducing deaths from maternal causes. Facilities that provide basic EmOC have the ability to provide the (1) administration of antibiotics, oxytocin and anticonvulsants,

(2) manual removal of the placenta, (3) removal of retained products following miscarriage or abortion, and (4) assisted vaginal delivery with forceps or vacuum extractor. Comprehensive EmOC includes the four basic functions plus the ability to provide cesarean sections and safe blood transfusions. WHO recommends that for every 500,000 people there should be four facilities offering basic EmOC and one facility offering comprehensive EmOC. To manage obstetric complications a facility must have trained staff and a functional operating theater and must be able to administer blood transfusions and anesthesia.

Maternal morbidity conditions—illnesses or injury arising from pregnancy, birth, or its management—result from the same set of causes linked to mortality and can be acute or chronic in nature (Ashford, 2002). Measuring maternal morbidity is also very difficult, as many women do not enter the formal healthcare system. During the 1990s, many studies were undertaken to estimate the magnitude of maternal morbidity based on women's self-reports and to determine the validity and reliability of these estimates. Although some conditions such as eclampsia and severe bleeding could be reliably measured by asking a specific algorithm of questions on a survey, findings generally indicated that the sensitivity and specificity for the majority of morbidity conditions were low, making it inadvisable to use self-reports (Tsui, Wasserheit, & Haaga, 1997).

Accessing prompt and high-quality care is an obstacle for many women in developing countries. Thaddeus and Maine (1994) posited this in a conceptual model defining three phases of delay in obtaining appropriate maternal health care: the delay in the decision to seek care, the delay in getting to a facility, and the delay encountered once reaching the facility. Perceived quality of services and socioeconomic status are often barriers in the decision to seek care. Delays in getting to facilities are often due to difficulty in obtaining transportation and distance to the nearest equipped facility. Delays once at the facility include lack of supplies and trained staff. Because many women in rural areas do not live close to a facility providing emergency obstetric care, good referral and transport networks need to be in place to ensure access to care. Though research on the ability of TBAs to reduce maternal mortality has been mixed, it is important to integrate them into the referral and transport systems of the formal medical infrastructure. In addition to better referral and transport networks, more community-based approaches are needed to reduce maternal mortality. For example, research on community-based interventions using misoprostol has shown promising results regarding the reduction of maternal deaths from postpartum hemorrhage (Rajbhandari, et al., 2010; Walraven, et al., 2005).

In addition to the provision of EmOC, several other strategies are important in reducing maternal deaths and improving maternal health. Access to family planning services will reduce unintended pregnancies and lower women's lifetime risk for pregnancy-related death and disability by lowering fertility and reducing the need for abortion. Safe abortion services can be provided with relatively simple technology and will reduce complications of abortion. Postpartum and postabortion care (PAC) will ensure that the complications developed after birth and abortion—whether safe procedures are available or not—will be managed properly (Ashford, 2002). Finally, though many complications cannot be predicted during antenatal visits, such visits offer women many benefits. The provision of antenatal care allows an opportunity for the testing, treatment, and management of sexually transmitted infections (STIs) including HIV, malaria, hypertension, anemia, and other conditions that may arise, as well as for educating women about family planning, nutrition, and child care (WHO, 2004).

The Safe Motherhood Initiative (SMI) was launched at the 1987 Nairobi conference by a host of international organizations. The SMI mission was to draw attention to the magnitude of maternal mortality. Over the years, the SMI has become a global partnership of governmental and nongovernmental agencies, donors, and women's health advocates. Recommendations have been evidence based and now include the prevention and management of unwanted pregnancy and unsafe abortion, the need for every woman to have skilled care during pregnancy and childbirth, and the importance of access to referral care when complications arise. The Making Pregnancy Safer Initiative is a recent offshoot of the SMI, becoming an integral component of its missions and implementation. It aims to prevent maternal deaths that occur each year by reducing unwanted pregnancies and unsafe abortion, implementing best practices in the care of pregnant women, increasing the proportion of women assisted by a skilled birth attendant as part of an efficient referral system, reducing neonatal mortality and stillbirth rates, and establishing and providing access to facilities providing EmOC (WHO, 2004). The Lancet Maternal Survival Series steering group has also supported the importance of EmOC as part of intrapartum care that needs to be available to all women with a focus on the normality of the birth process and intervention only when necessary (Campbell, et al., 2006). In addition the steering group has also endorsed the importance of antenatal care, postpartum care, family planning, and safe abortion.

Child Health

Mortality is the definitive indicator of poor child health outcomes. Childhood mortality is commonly reported for different age ranges: early neonatal (0 to 6 days), neonatal (0 to 27 days), postneonatal (28 days to 11 months), infant (0 to 11 months), child (1 to 4 years), and under 5 years (0 to 4 years). The exact method used to calculate childhood mortality varies depending on the data sources available. For many developing countries the measures of mortality are calculated as the number of deaths occurring in the age interval in a given period divided by the number of children entering the age interval. For infant and under-5 mortality rates, this is the number of deaths under the age of 1 year or under the age of 5 years, respectively, divided by the number of live births. These two measures represent the probability that a newborn child dies before their first and fifth birthdays, respectively. As under-5 mortality declines, deaths at older ages (1 to 4 years) typically fall first. Therefore, in high mortality settings, there will tend to be a large difference between the infant and under-5 mortality, whereas in low mortality settings, the two measures will be quite similar because deaths among 1- to 4-year-olds are relatively few. Within infant mortality, many countries are struggling to reduce the number of deaths during the critical neonatal period.

Under-5 mortality is viewed as the key indicator for children's health and is considered not just an indicator of health but also an indicator of a country's development. UNICEF ranks countries by their estimated under-5 mortality in its annual State of the World's Children publications.

Considerable progress has been made in reducing under-5 mortality over the last several decades; however, the decline has not been as great as expected and has not been uniform across regions. The estimated global under-5 mortality rate has declined from almost 200 deaths per 1,000 live births in 1960 to 60 deaths per 1,000 live births in 2010 (Figure 16–1). However only four regions of the world—East Asia and the Pacific, Latin America and the Caribbean, CEE/CIS and Baltic States, and Industrialized Countries—are on track to meet MDG4. The two regions of the world where under-5 mortality is highest, Sub-Saharan Africa and South Asia, are unlikely to meet this goal. Fifty percent of under-5 deaths occur in Sub-Saharan Africa, and 33% occur in South Asia (UNICEF, 2010).

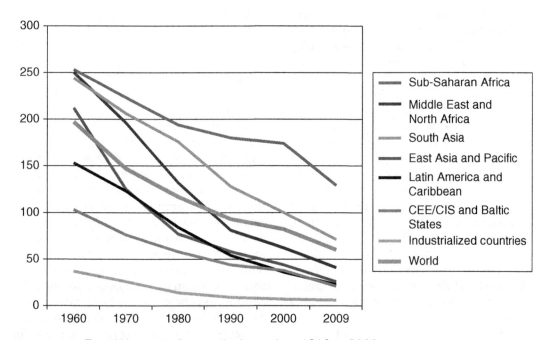

Figure 16–1 Trends in under-5 mortality by region, 1960 to 2009.

Source: UNICEF. (2010). Levels and trends in child mortality. Report 2010. New York: Author.

Between 1960 and 1990, under-5 mortality declined by 2.5% per year, whereas between 1990 and 2001 the rate of decline was only 1.1% per year (Black, Morris, & Bryce, 2003). Rates of decline have now increased to 2.1% in the 20-year period from 1990 to 2010, and if we focus on 2000 to 2009 the rate of decline has increased to 2.8% (UNICEF, 2010), but as mentioned earlier this will not be enough for all regions of the world to reach MDG4. The reasons for the prior deceleration varied across countries. In some areas (e.g., industrialized countries), mortality rates were very low, and thus, further reductions were difficult to achieve. Of concern were countries in which the pace of mortality decline was slowing at high levels of mortality, most notably in sub-Saharan Africa. Though under-5 mortality remains high in many parts of the world, the increase in the current rate of decline (likely due to a renewed commitment to child survival and expansion of programs and interventions) is promising.

According to UNICEF the global under-5 mortality rate of 60 deaths per 1,000 live births translates into approximately 8.1 million deaths of children under 5 years annually. The Institute of Health Metrics and Evaluation had a similar estimate of 7.7 million for 2010 (Rajaratnam, et al., 2010). These deaths are concentrated in developing countries, with approximately 98% occurring in developing countries and 70% of them occurring in 15 countries (UNICEF, 2010). The largest numbers of child deaths occur in India, Nigeria, the Democratic Republic of the Congo, Pakistan, Ethiopia, and China, and the highest under-5 mortality occurs in Chad (209/1000), Afghanistan (199/1000), the Democratic Republic of the Congo (199/1000), Guinea-Bissau (193/1000), Sierra Leone (192/1000), and Mali (191/1000). In contrast in Liechtenstein and San Marino, under-5 mortality is 2/1000.

What is most tragic about the 8.1 million under-5 deaths is that at least two-thirds could have been easily prevented. On a global level the major causes of death are neonatal causes (41%), pneumonia (14%), diarrhea (14%), malaria (8%), injuries (3%), HIV/AIDS (2%), and measles (1%). The main causes of neonatal deaths are preterm birth complications (12%), birth asphyxia (9%), sepsis (6%), and pneumonia (4%) (Black, et al., 2010). Under-nutrition is a contributing factor in an estimated one-half of under-5 deaths. Low birth weight is a contributing factor in 60–80% of neonatal deaths (Lawn, et al., 2005). Cause of death varies by region and by the level of mortality. Malaria is a significant cause of death in some countries, mostly in sub-Saharan Africa. AIDS deaths among children are concentrated in Eastern and Southern Africa. However, in countries with relatively high levels of under-5 mortality, diarrhea, pneumonia, and neonatal causes account for the majority of deaths. These have been the main causes of death in developing countries for decades. As mortality declines, deaths from infectious diseases such as diarrhea, pneumonia, and vaccine-preventable diseases such as measles tend to fall first. This pattern results in an increasing concentration of deaths in the neonatal period and a shift in the cause of death profile toward neonatal causes. In low child mortality settings, under-5 deaths are mostly due to neonatal conditions (e.g., congenital anomalies, conditions arising in the perinatal period) and injuries.

Preventive measures and treatments to address most of the main causes of under-5 mortality are known and relatively inexpensive. For example, pneumonia can be treated with antibiotics, diarrhea can be treated at home with ORS (unless the child is severely dehydrated in which case IV fluids would be needed), malaria can be treated with antimalarials (though resistance to some antimalarials is an issue), and measles can be prevented with immunization. HIV/AIDS is a relatively new challenge for many countries, and addressing neonatal causes of death is seen as crucial in furthering declines in under-5 mortality. Simple interventions to reduce neonatal mortality are being promoted such as kangaroo care (a method of holding a baby that involves skin-to-skin contact), postnatal checkups within the first days and week of life, and methods to resuscitate babies using a bag and mask.

Many proven prevention and treatment interventions to improve child survival can be implemented in resource-poor environments. These include exclusive breastfeeding; immunization; micronutrient supplementation (particularly vitamin A and zinc); complementary feeding; antibiotics for pneumonia, dysentery, and sepsis; oral rehydration therapy for diarrhea; antimalarial drugs and insecticide-treated bednets. Jones, Steketee, Black, Bhutta, and Morris (2003) estimated that achieving global coverage of existing interventions could prevent approximately 63% of the under-5 deaths that occur each year. Why, then, are children dying of preventable causes of death? A key issue is that interventions often do not reach the poorest individuals or individuals in rural and remote areas of developing countries. Later in this chapter the influence of poverty as a distal determinant is discussed. There is a clear need for better delivery strategies to get interventions to the people who most need them. The challenge is to achieve global coverage with these interventions in resource-poor environments with weak public health infrastructure. Coverage of key child survival interventions was only approximately 50% globally in 2003 (Jones, et al., 2003). The barriers to scaling up child survival interventions to achieve high coverage are the same as those for other health interventions in these settings: high staff turnover, poor management and supervision, weak and inadequate funding to name a few. Furthermore, in populations in which contact with health services is infrequent, delivery strategies that focus only on the delivery of services without addressing demand for services at the community level will be ineffective in achieving high coverage.

Many global initiatives have been aimed at reducing under-5 mortality and morbidity.

The WHO Expanded Programme on Immunization (EPI) is among those considered to have been effective in achieving high coverage and measurable impacts on mortality (Bryce, et al., 2003; Claeson, Gillespie, Mshinda, Troedsson, & Victora, 2003). EPI was launched in 1974, focused on immunizing children against six major infectious diseases (diphtheria, pertussis [whooping cough], tetanus, tuberculosis, polio, and measles) before their first birthday. Coverage of these vaccines was estimated to be less than 5% when the initiative was launched but had reached 82% for DTP3 (third dose of diphtheria-tetanus-pertussis) vaccine and 83% for measles by 2008 (WHO & UNICEF, 2009). Nevertheless, approximately 24 million infants did not receive DTP3 in 2008. Over 70% of these children lived in just 10 countries, indicating that in some countries EPI has the potential to save many more lives.

EPI is considered a vertical program, focused on specific diseases. Some programs are horizontal or focused on health issues in a broader sense—an example is the Integrated Management of Childhood Illness (IMCI) program. IMCI was launched by WHO and UNICEF in 1995 and as of 2003 was being implemented in more than 100 countries. The strategy is based on the fact that most sick children presenting at health facilities have signs and symptoms related to at least one of the major conditions that account for most of the under-5 deaths in a particular country. The IMCI strategy has three main components: (1) improvements in the case management skills of health staff through the provision of locally adapted guidelines and activities to promote their use, (2) improvements in the health system to support effective management of childhood illnesses, and (3) improvements in family and community practice. A multicountry evaluation of IMCI in five countries—Bangladesh, Brazil, Peru, Tanzania, and Uganda—has shown mixed results. For example, health workers trained in IMCI performed better on several measures than non-IMCI trained health workers

(Gouws, et al., 2004), but a study focused on Uganda found that although IMCI health workers provided better care, overall quality was still low (Pariyo, et al., 2005). A study in Tanzania found limited effect of IMCI on the impact indicators of nutritional status and anemia (Armstrong Schellenberg, et al., 2004). A challenge often lies in implementing all three components effectively and nationally within a country. Overall, it has been found that in order to implement IMCI effectively, a country needs a strong health system to begin with. Thus it is important to focus on both short-term and long-term solutions.

There has been a growing recognition that further large reductions in under-5 mortality will require large reductions in neonatal mortality. As noted previously, 41% of under-5 deaths (or 3.3 million deaths each year) globally are associated with neonatal causes, and deaths become increasingly concentrated in the neonatal period as under-5 mortality declines. The number of stillbirths is estimated to be similar to the number of neonatal deaths. In poor populations, many neonatal deaths are associated with poor maternal nutritional status and maternal infections during pregnancy (such as malaria and syphilis), which contribute to low birth weight and increased risk of preterm delivery. Unsafe delivery care and inappropriate care of the newborn after delivery also contribute significantly to preventable newborn deaths. About 70% of neonatal deaths occur because known and effective interventions are not reaching those who need them (Knippenburg, et al., 2005). Despite the impression that neonatal care involves high technology, many simple and low-cost interventions can be delivered in high mortality settings with weak health infrastructure using a combination of delivery strategies—outreach, family/community and facility-based care (Darmstadt, et al., 2005). These include antenatal care, birth preparedness, safe delivery care (including attendance by a SBA), postnatal care for the newborn, and kangaroo care. Postnatal care of the newborn should include prevention and management of hypothermia by drying and wrapping the entire baby right after delivery, encouraging immediate breastfeeding, clean cord care, and timely management and antibiotic treatment of infections. Kangaroo care is a simple intervention to keep babies warm, which is particularly important for low birth weight babies. Family planning is also an important newborn health intervention, as it increases the intervals between births and reduces births to very young and very old mothers whose newborns are at particular risk. Integrating essential newborn care into existing safe motherhood and child health initiatives is key to improving newborn health and survival and ultimately achieving sustained reductions in under-5 mortality.

Reproductive Health

The changing landscape of human reproduction in the latter half of the 20th century and at the turn of the millennium has been characterized as a global "reproductive revolution." This revolution has been marked by dramatic declines in fertility rates around the world and equally remarkable increases in the use of contraception. The world's total fertility rate (TFR) has declined from an estimated 4.95 from 1950 to 1955 to 2.52 from 2005 to 2010 (United Nations [UN] Department of Economic and Social Affairs, 2010). In 1960 just 9% of married women of reproductive age in developing countries were using a contraceptive method. According to the UN Department of Economic and Social Affairs (2010), global contraceptive use of any method was 73% and 56% for modern methods in 2009 (UN Department of Economic and Social Affairs, 2011).

There has been considerable variation between and within regions in fertility decline and the adoption of contraception. The TFR in sub-Saharan Africa was 6.7 children per woman between 1970 and 1975, 6.1 between 1990 and 1995 and 5.1 from 2005 to 2010. In contrast, the TFR in Latin

America and the Caribbean has declined from 5.0 children per woman between 1970 and 1975 to 3.0 between 1990 and 1995 to an estimated 2.3 children per woman between 2005 and 2010. Industrialized countries, countries with an already low TFR of 2.2 between 1970 and 1975, have also shown a decline in fertility with a TFR of only 1.7 children per woman between 2005 and 2010 (UN Department of Economic and Social Affairs, 2010). Replacement-level fertility is considered to be a TFR of 2.1 children per woman, a level of fertility below which no region fell before 1960. Today, East Asia and all regions in Europe are experiencing below replacement fertility.

Trends in contraceptive use show similar variation across world regions. In developing countries, contraceptive prevalence varies from a low of 21.8% in sub-Saharan Africa to a high of 72.9% in Latin America and the Caribbean, a rate comparable to the industrialized country average (UN Department of Economic and Social Affairs, 2011). The popularity of different contraceptive methods also varies across regions. The four most popular methods of contraception in developing countries are female sterilization (the most popular method in Asia and Latin America and the Caribbean), oral contraceptives, injectables (the most popular method in sub-Saharan Africa), and the intrauterine device (the predominant method in Western Asia/Middle East). Together, these four methods comprise 79% of all methods used in less developed regions (UN Department of Economic and Social Affairs, 2011). Female sterilization and to a lesser extent the intrauterine device, are especially good methods for limiting family size, whereas injectables or oral contraceptives can be used to limit or space births. Method selection is a function of regional variations in method availability, social norms, method costs, and awareness of different methods. Cultural and political contexts can also affect method use. Until relatively recently, many former Soviet countries relied predominantly on legal and

institutionalized abortion as a means of fertility regulation, at least partly as a result of a lack of widespread and efficient distribution of contraceptives under the Soviet regime.

International policy regarding fertility and contraceptive use has also changed over time, although it is difficult to be sure how much these policies incited change as opposed to merely reflecting trends that were already established.

In the late 1960s and 1970s, policy makers became concerned about the specter of global overpopulation. This period saw the establishment of the first national population policies designed to curtail population growth. The controversy in policy circles at the time was a question of whether there was a "population problem" and if so how best to bring about a decline in fertility (Sinding, 2000). One suggested method was a focus on economic growth and development that would lower fertility preferences and postpone marriage. A second strategy was the widespread introduction of contraception. Over time, as contraceptive use has skyrocketed and fertility plummeted, the focus has increasingly been on access to family planning on a voluntary basis, moving away from demographic targets, and offering family planning as part of a comprehensive reproductive health program. The focus on economic development and growth has shifted to an emphasis on gender equality and the empowerment of women and girls (McIntosh & Finkle, 1995).

This shift can be plainly seen in the changing policy language coming out of the United Nations' world population conferences. At the 1974 World Population Conference in Bucharest, developing countries joined with the Soviet bloc to protest the global demographic goals proposed by Western nations. At Bucharest also, arguments began about appropriate means for encouraging fertility decline, development or family planning. In 1984 in Mexico City, at the International Conference on Population, the debate became less polarized, with Western countries and the developing world agreeing, or at least being neutral, to the idea that rapid population growth could impede development and that family planning was an appropriate response to unwanted fertility. This watershed conference set the stage for what is often referred to as the Cairo "consensus," or the Program of Action, set forth in the 1994 International Conference on Population and Development (ICPD) in Cairo, Egypt. Cairo was a defining moment in international population policy. For the first time, development and population linkages were specifically addressed in the title of the conference. Furthermore, a heavy feminist involvement at Cairo shifted the focus from overall economic growth to gender inequalities (McIntosh & Finkle, 1995). Traditional development schemes, it was argued, ignore and can be harmful for women. Furthermore, there was concern that family planning programs in concert with demographic targets are unfair to women and that family planning should be offered on a voluntary basis together with comprehensive reproductive health services. Today the focus remains on providing services within a human rights framework and increasing access to contraceptives, safe abortion, and treatment for sexually transmitted infections (STIs).

Population and reproductive health remain politically controversial areas. Changes in the global political environment after the 1994 ICPD resulted in reproductive health being left out of the original Millennium Development Goals (Crossette, 2005). However, the MDGs were modified to include "achieve universal access to reproduce health" as a target under MDG5 in 2005 following recommendations in the UN Millennium Project Report (UN Development Programme, 2005), which made the case that population and reproductive health contribute in cross-cutting ways to the achievement of all of the MDGs. For example, the promotion of family planning in countries with high fertility rates has the potential to avert 32% of maternal deaths and 10% of childhood deaths (Cleland, Bernstein, Ezeh, Faundes, Glasier, & Innis, 2006). The inclusion of a reproductive health target in the MDGs has helped to refocus attention on the importance of reproductive health and family planning. This increased focus on reproductive health and family planning is needed. Although enormous progress has been made, it is estimated that every year 120 million couples have an unmet need for family planning resulting in 80 million unintended pregnancies including 45 million abortions (Glasier, Gulmezoglu, Schmid, Morena, & Van Look, 2006).

HIV/AIDS

The Joint United Nations Programme on HIV/AIDS (UNAIDS) estimates that worldwide, there were 33.4 million people living with HIV/AIDS, 2.7 million new infections, and 2 million AIDS deaths in 2008. Sub-Saharan Africa is by far the worst affected region of the world, with approximately 22.4 million people estimated to be living with HIV/AIDS and approximately 1.4 million AIDS deaths in 2008. HIV prevalence in sub-Saharan Africa was estimated to be approximately 5.2% in 2008 compared with approximately 0.8% globally. Within sub-Saharan Africa, adult HIV prevalence is estimated to range from less than 1% in Niger to almost 25% in Botswana (UNAIDS & WHO, 2009).

Considerable uncertainty surrounds estimates of HIV prevalence and AIDS mortality due to data issues in most countries. Estimates of HIV prevalence in populations with generalized epidemics are routinely obtained from antenatal surveillance systems, in which pregnant women in selected sites are anonymously tested for HIV. The quality and coverage of these systems vary across countries and over time within countries, complicating comparisons. However, even if there were no data quality issues in these systems, estimating the prevalence of HIV in the general adult population, which includes all men and women, not just women who happen to be pregnant, is problematic. Mathematical models have been developed to address this, but estimates have often been found to be very different from community or national prevalence studies. Increasingly, countries are including HIV testing in population-based surveys such as the DHS. These surveys have the advantage of wider representation of the population, including men, and typically better representation in rural areas than antenatal surveillance systems. However, they can be subject to high nonresponse rates for HIV testing, which has serious implications for the quality of the estimates obtained, especially if nonresponse is associated with HIV status. Estimates of HIV prevalence therefore should be interpreted cautiously, but they still provide an essential basis for tracking the epidemic and identifying general patterns and trends.

The HIV/AIDS epidemic has numerous implications for global MCH. First, HIV directly affects many of the populations of most interest in MCH: women of reproductive age, adolescents, and children. Approximately 16 million of the estimated 33.4 million people living with HIV/AIDS are women. In many parts of the world, the epidemic is becoming increasingly feminized, meaning that the ratio of new infections among women to men is increasing. New infections occur disproportionately among young adults aged 15 to 24 years, and in sub-Saharan Africa, new infections occur disproportionately among girls and young women (UNAIDS & WHO, 2009). In epidemics driven by heterosexual transmission, women are particularly vulnerable to HIV infection because of the underlying gender inequality in society. They are often infected by husbands or other stable partners in situations in which it is acceptable for men to have multiple partners. HIV infection is also strongly linked to experience of gender-based violence, with violence being a risk factor for infection, and infection itself being a risk factor for violence (Dunkle, et al., 2004; WHO, 2010). Women are also biologically more vulnerable to HIV infection; the rate of male-to-female transmission is estimated at approximately twice that of female-to-male transmission.

HIV is associated with an increased risk of child mortality and morbidity through both direct and indirect mechanisms. Mother-to-child transmission of HIV can occur during pregnancy, childbirth, or breastfeeding. Available evidence indicates that in the absence of antiretroviral therapy approximately 30% of children born to HIV-positive mothers will be infected and that 60% of infected children will die before their fifth birthday (Spira, et al., 1999). Indirect effects are many and varied, but most prominently involve illness and death of parents, which in turn are associated with reduced parental care and support, reduced food production at the household level, reduced access to health services for children, and dissolution of households when death occurs. In low-resource settings, already weak health services are further strained by the burden imposed to treat HIV-infected patients, reducing staff and financial resources for other services, including MCH services. At the same time, HIV/AIDS affects working-age adults, resulting in increased staff shortages in health facilities as qualified staff become sick and unable to perform their duties. A cross-national review of DHS and HIV prevalence data found that most countries in sub-Saharan Africa with high HIV prevalence (5% or more of adults seropositive) also experienced increased under-5 mortality rates (Adetunji, 2000).

The political and financial commitment to fighting HIV/AIDS has increased in the early part of the 21st century through initiatives such as the Global Fund to Fight AIDS, TB, and Malaria, the United Nations General Assembly Special Session on HIV/AIDS declaration, the U.S. government's PEPFAR program, and the WHO "3 by 5" Initiative. Several of these initiatives include an emphasis on providing antiretroviral (ARV) treatment, care, and support to individuals living with HIV/AIDS. For example, the WHO "3 by 5" Initiative aimed to put 3 million HIV-infected people on ARV therapy by 2005, whereas PEPFAR I aimed to provide treatment to 2 million HIV-infected people and to provide care to 10 million people infected by HIV/AIDS (including orphans and vulnerable children) by 2008. PEPFAR I provided ARV-treatment for 2.1 million men, women, and children (Office of the U.S. Global AIDS Coordinator, 2008). Targets for PEPFAR II are to provide treatment for 4 million people, prevent 12 million new infections, provide care to 12 million people living with or affected by HIV/AIDS (including 5 million orphans), provide at least 80% of the target population with prevention of maternal to child transmission (PMTCT) services, and ensure that children receive treatment relative to the proportion infected. Prevention efforts focus on the "ABC" messages (Abstinence, Be faithful, Correct and Consistent Condom use), along with voluntary counseling and testing (VCT) and PMTCT. The WHO PMTCT framework takes a holistic view of PMTCT and includes four main strategies: (1) primary prevention of HIV in young women; (2) avoidance of unintended pregnancies among HIV-infected women; (3) provision of ARVs targeted at preventing HIV transmission from HIV-infected women to their infants, safe delivery, counseling, and support for safer infant feeding practices; and (4) providing care and support for mothers and their families.

The increased emphasis on HIV/AIDS globally has both positive and negative implications for broader MCH programs. Certainly, the attention to HIV/AIDS is urgently needed given the very high levels of HIV infection throughout the world and the potential for emerging epidemics in areas such as the Caribbean, China, India, Central Asia, and Eastern Europe to explode. PMTCT programs are clearly linked to wider maternal and newborn health services such as antenatal care, safe delivery care, and family planning, with the potential to improve these services for all women, not just those infected with HIV. However, in severely resource-constrained settings, the heavy emphasis on a single disease could draw human and financial resources away from other health areas. For example, in 2003 and 2004, the U.S. government

reduced budgets for international MCH while increasing funds for AIDS, TB, and malaria. Although fighting HIV/AIDS is clearly a burning global health priority, meeting global targets in MCH will require more than fighting a single disease (Claeson, et al., 2003; Walker, Schwartlander, & Bryce, 2002). Recent efforts such as PEPFAR II and the Global Fund have broadened their HIV programs to cover other aspects of maternal and child health.

INEQUALITIES IN GLOBAL MCH

A recurrent theme throughout this chapter is the striking regional variation in global MCH outcomes. However, stark differentials in health outcomes exist between and within the countries in each of these regions. For example, Africa, which accounts for 14% of the world's population, accounts for 51% of under-5 deaths (UNICEF, 2010) and 58% of maternal deaths (WHO, 2010). Within Africa, under-5 mortality varies from 12/1000 in the Seychelles to 220/1000 in Angola (UNICEF, 2010). Similarly, maternal mortality varies from 36/100,000 in Mauritius to 1200/100,000 in both Chad and Somalia (WHO, 2010). India is an example of a country with large differentials in under-five mortality both regionally and by socioeconomic status. Under-5 mortality varies from 16.3/1,000 in Kerala State in the south to 96.4/1,000 in Uttar Pradesh in the north. Under-5 mortality also varies from 33.8/1,000 for children in the highest wealth quintile to 100.5/1000 for children in the lowest wealth quintile (International Institute for Population Sciences & Macro International, 2007). In this section, we briefly discuss some sources of inequality in health outcomes within and among countries worldwide, with a particular focus on three major factors: socioeconomic status, education, and gender.

Socioeconomic Status

In virtually every country in the world, the poor have a lower use of antenatal and delivery care, lower rates of contraceptive use, and higher fertility. Poor women are also more likely than wealthy women to have complications from an unsafe abortion. Poor women and children are at greater risk for disease as a result of poor sanitation, crowding, and undernutrition. Furthermore, poor women and children are less likely than their wealthy peers to receive either preventive health services or appropriate and timely treatment for illness and complications (Shiffman, 2000; Victora, et al., 2003). Socioeconomic differentials in MCH outcomes are not limited to the poorest, least industrialized countries and regions in the world. Data from 19 of the wealthiest countries in the world show that wage inequalities within a country are positively and significantly correlated with the infant mortality rate (Macinko, Shi, & Starfield, 2004).

Education

Education, particularly female education, is strongly and consistently associated with MCH outcomes. Educated women and their children are less likely to die than their less educated counterparts, with higher levels of education conferring additional advantage. The pathways by which female education influences MCH outcomes have not been conclusively identified, but several hypotheses are generally accepted. Education is thought to provide women with information and the ability to obtain and act on information on their and their children's health, resulting in improved domestic health care and hygiene and increased use of health services. It is also thought that education may enable women to communicate and negotiate more effectively with health providers. Education increases the status of the woman, strengthening her position within the household and her ability to obtain resources for herself and her children. It also increases the socioeconomic status of the woman both by allowing her to make a more favorable marriage and to work

in higher paid occupations (Cleland & van Ginneken, 1988). A recent study estimated that 51.2% of the reduction in under-5 deaths between 1970 and 2009 could be attributed to maternal education (Gakidou, Cowling, Lozano, & Murray, 2010).

Gender

There has been a recent call by policy makers on the global and national levels to address gender-related issues in health programs and policies. In most areas of the world women are at a disadvantage because of traditional gender norms. In regions such as Asia, cultural norms dictate both a low status for women and a strong preference for sons. This is translated in some areas into differences in survival between boy and girl children. The selection for boy children can take two major forms. The first is through sex-selective abortion made possible through ultrasound technologies. Abnormally high sex ratios at birth have been observed in Northern India, China, and parts of East Asia, indicating the use of sex-selective abortion in these populations. The second is through infanticide and neglect of female children, which leads to a higher mortality rate. Evidence for these practices has been found, for example, in India, where a girl is 40% more likely to die before her fifth birthday than a boy (Victora, et al., 2003). In the absence of strong gender preferences, girls are typically less likely than boys to die in childhood. Even within India there are important regional variations, with female child mortality being higher in North India, where women have lower status and a dowry tradition makes girl children more expensive.

Low status for women creates health risks for females throughout their lifetimes (Blanc, 2001; Shiffman, 2000). Women have typically less access to education and economic assets, less power of decision making and freedom of movement, all of which are associated with lower health outcomes (Bloom, Wypij, & Das Gupta, 2001). In a

WHO multicountry study of women's health and domestic violence, reporting of physical and sexual violence by ever-partnered women ranged from 15% to 71% across the 10 countries studied (WHO, 2005b). Low status also confers a greater risk for maternal mortality, in part due to a lower likelihood for receiving appropriate health care, lower contraceptive use, higher fertility, and an earlier age at marriage (Shiffman, 2000). Women who have less power in sexual relationships are less likely to have the power to negotiate safe sexual practices and are at greater risk for sexually transmitted infections such as HIV (Dunkle, et al., 2004).

Reducing Inequities

Obviously, socioeconomic standing, women's status, and female education are neither mutually exclusive nor exhaustive explanations for global disparities in MCH outcomes. Research about the role of these factors in health outcomes is complicated by the fact that socioeconomic status and gender roles are difficult constructs to measure and model, as they are often relative and culturally determined.

Other key factors are political commitment and conflict. Sri Lanka has much lower under-5 and maternal mortality than countries at the same per capita income, largely because of a social and political commitment to women and children. Many of the countries with the highest under-5 and maternal mortality such as Afghanistan, the Democratic Republic of the Congo and Sierra Leone are countries that have experienced significant civil conflict. Conflict leads to direct deaths from war itself and also indirect deaths due to undernutrition, lack of basic health services, and a breakdown of civil and social structures.

Institutional factors also play a role in reducing inequality in MCH outcomes. The majority of maternal and child deaths are preventable if women and children receive appropriate and timely healthcare interventions (Bryce, et al., 2003; Jones, et al., 2003;

Shiffman, 2000). How do poor countries, and for that matter rich countries, ensure that essential health care is available and used by all people—rich and poor, male and female, educated and uneducated? What is the best way to allocate scarce resources to maximize the efficiency of the existing healthcare infrastructure? How do we deliver the interventions to the people who are hardest to reach? Answers to these questions may sometimes vary by region, by country, or even by districts within countries. Though much remains unanswered the research literature is becoming richer with examples of programs and strategies that are working. Continued efforts to carefully address these questions are needed to see further improvements in maternal and child health and reproductive health.

CONCLUSION

This chapter provides a broad overview of global MCH. Considerable progress has been achieved in the latter part of the 20th century and early 21st century, but much remains to be done. At the current rate of progress, the millennium development goals listed in Table 16–1 will not be achieved by many countries, particularly those in sub-Saharan Africa. In addition, inequities in health outcomes exist not just between countries but also within countries. Addressing these challenges will not be easy. It will require leadership, sustained political will and financial commitment, and an emphasis on building strong health systems, as well as fighting specific diseases. The early part of the 21st century has seen large increases in international political commitment and resources for maternal and child health and reproductive health. Though much work remains to be done, these increased commitments have translated into improvements for mothers and children around the world. We expect to see these commitments continue to improve health outcomes for mothers and children around the world.

References

AbouZahr, C., & Wardlaw, T. (2000). *Maternal mortality in 2000: Estimates developed by WHO, UNICEF, and UNFPA*. Geneva: World Health Organization.

Adetunji, J. (2000). Trends in under-5 mortality rates and the HIV/AIDS epidemic. *Bulletin of the World Health Organization, 78*, 1200–1206.

Armstrong Schellenberg, J., Bryce, J., de Savigny, D., Lambrechts, T., Mbuya, C., Mgalula, L., & Wilczynska, K. (Tanzania IMCI Multi-Country Evaluation Health Facility Survey Study Group). (2004). The effect of integrated management of childhood illness on observed quality of care of under-fives in rural Tanzania. *Health Policy and Planning, 19*(1), 1–10.

Ashford, L. (2002). *Hidden suffering: Disabilities from pregnancy and childbirth in less developed countries*. Washington, DC: Population Reference Bureau.

Association of Schools of Public Health. (n.d.). What is public health? Retrieved May 20, 2011 from http://www.whatispublichealth.org/.

Black, R., Cousens, S., Johnson, H., Lawn, J., Rudan, I., Bassani, D., Campbell, H., Walker, C., Cibulskis, R., Eisele, T., Liu, L., & Mathews, C. for the Child Health Epidemiological Reference Group of WHO and UNICEF. (2010). Global, regional, and national causes of child mortality in 2008: A systematic analysis. *Lancet, 375*(9730), 1969–1982.

Black, R. E., Morris, S. S., & Bryce, J. (2003). Where and why are 10 million children dying every year? *Lancet, 361*, 2226–2234.

Blanc, A. K. (2001). The effect of power in sexual relationships on sexual and reproductive health: An examination of the evidence. *Studies in Family Planning, 32*, 189–213.

Bloom, S. S., Wypij, D., & Das Gupta, M. (2001). Dimensions of women's autonomy and the influence on maternal health care utilization in a North Indian city. *Demography, 38*, 67–78.

Bryce, J., el Arifeen, S., Pariyo, G., Lanata, C., Gwatkin, D., & Habicht, J. (2003). Reducing child mortality: Can public health deliver? *Lancet, 362*, 159–164.

Buekens, P. (2001). Is estimating maternal mortality useful? *Bulletin of the World Health Organization, 79*, 179.

Buekens, P., Curtis, S., & Alayon, S. (2003). Demographic and health surveys: Caesarean section rates in sub-Saharan Africa. *British Medical Journal, 326*, 136.

Campbell, O., & Graham, W., on behalf of The Lancet Maternal Survival Series steering group. (2006). Strategies for reducing maternal mortality: Getting on with what works. *Lancet, 368*, 1284–1299.

Claeson, M., & Waldman, R. J. (2000). The evolution of child health programmes in developing countries: From targeting diseases to targeting people. *Bulletin of the World Health Organization, 78*, 1234–1245.

Claeson, M., Gillespie, D., Mshinda, H., Troedsson, H., & Victora, C. (2003). Knowledge into action for child survival. *Lancet, 362*, 323–327.

Cleland, J., Bernstein, S., Ezeh, A., Faundes, A., Glasier, A., & Innis, J. (2006). Family planning: The unfinished agenda. *Lancet, 368*, 1810–1827.

Cleland, J. G., & van Ginneken, J. K. (1988). Maternal education and child survival in developing countries: The search for pathways of influence. *Social Science & Medicine, 27*, 1357–1368.

Cohen, S. (1987). The Safe Motherhood Conference. *International Family Planning Perspectives, 13*, 68–70.

Crossette, B. (2005). Reproductive health and the Millennium Development Goals: The missing link. *Studies in Family Planning, 36*(1), 71–79.

Darmstadt, G., Bhutta, Z., Cousens, S., Adam, T., Walker, N., & de Bemis, L., for the Lancet Neonatal Survival Steering Team. (2005). Evidence-based cost-effective interventions: how many newborn babies can we save? *Lancet, 365*, 977–988.

Dunkle, K. L., Jewkes, R. K., Brown, H. C., Gray, G. E., McIntyre, J. A., & Harlow, S. D. (2004). Gender-based violence, relationship power, and risk of HIV infection in women attending antenatal clinics in South Africa. *Lancet, 363*, 1415–1421.

Gakidou, E., Cowling, K., Lozano, R., & Murray, C. (2010). Increased educational attainment and its effect on child mortality in 175 countries between 1970 and 2009: A systematic analysis. *Lancet, 376*, 959–974.

Gillespie, D. G. (2004). Whatever happened to family planning and, for that matter, reproductive health? *International Family Planning Perspectives, 30*, 34–38.

Glasier, A., Gulmezoglu, A., Schmid, G., Morena, C., & Van Look, P. (2006). Sexual and reproductive health: A matter of life and death. *Lancet, 368*, 1595–1607.

Gouws, E., Bryce, J., Habicht, J. P., Amaral, J., Pariyo, G., Schellenberg, J. A., & Fontaine, O. (2004). Improving antimicrobial use among health workers in first-level facilities: Results from the Multi-Country Evaluation of the Integrated Management of Childhood Illness strategy. *Bulletin of the World Health Organization, 82*(7), 509–515.

Hill, K., AbouZahr, C., & Wardlaw, T. (2001). Estimates of maternal mortality for 1995. *Bulletin of the World Health Organization, 79*, 182–193.

Hogan, M., Foreman, K., Naghavi, M., Ahn, S., Wang, M., Makela, S., & Murray, C. (2010). Maternal mortality for 181 countries, 1990–2008: A systematic analysis of progress towards Millennium Development Goal 5. *Lancet, 375*(9726), 1609–1623.

International Institute for Population Sciences (IIPS) and Macro International. (2007). National Family Health Survey (NFHS-3), 2005–06: India: Vol. I. Mumbai: IIPS.

Jones, G., Steketee, R. W., Black, R. E., Bhutta, Z. A., & Morris, S. S. (2003). How many child deaths can we prevent this year? *Lancet, 362*, 65–71.

Knippenberg, R., Lawn, J., Darmstadt, G., Begkoyian, G., Fogstad, H., Walelign, N., & Paul, V. for the Lancet Neonatal Survival Steering Team. (2005). Systematic scaling up of neonatal care in countries. *Lancet, 365*, 1087–1098.

Koblinsky, M. A. (1995). Beyond maternal mortality: Magnitude, interrelationship, and consequences of women's health, pregnancy-related complications and nutritional-status on pregnancy outcomes. *International Journal of Gynecology & Obstetrics, 48*, S21–S32.

Koplan, J., Bond, C., Merson, M., Reddy, K., Rodriguez, M., Sewankambo, N., & Wasserheit, J. for the Consortium of Universities for Global Health Executive Board. (2009). Towards a common definition of global health. *Lancet, 373*, 1993–1995.

Lawn, J., Cousens, S., & Zupan, J. for the Lancet Neonatal Survival Steering Team. (2005). 4 million neonatal deaths: When? Where? Why? *Lancet, 365*, 891–900.

Lumbiganon, P., Laopaiboon, M., Gulmezoglu, A., et al. (2010). Method of delivery and pregnancy outcomes in Asia: The WHO global survey on maternal and perinatal health 2007–08. *Lancet, 375*, 490–499.

Macinko, J. A., Shi, L. Y., & Starfield, B. (2004). Wage inequality, the health system, and infant mortality in wealthy industrialized countries, 1970–1996. *Social Science & Medicine, 58*, 279–292.

McIntosh, C. A., & Finkle, J. L. (1995). The Cairo conference on population and development: A new paradigm. *Population and Development Review, 21*, 223–260.

Nanda, G., Switlick, K., & Lule, E. (2005). *Accelerating progress towards achieving the MDG to improve maternal health: A collection of promising approaches.* Washington, DC: World Bank.

Office of the U.S. Global AIDS Coordinator, U.S. Department of State. (2008, December 1). *Celebrate Life: Latest PEPFAR Results.* Retrieved May 21, 2011 from http://www.pepfar.gov/documents/organization/112594.pdf.

Pariyo, G. W., Gouws, E., Bryce, J., & Burnham, G. with Uganda IMCI Impact Study Team. (2005). Improving facility-based care for sick children in Uganda: Training is not enough. *Health Policy and Planning, 20*(Suppl. 1), i58–i68.

Rajaratnam, J. K., Marcus, J. R., Flaxman, A. D., Haidong, W., Levin-Rector, A., Dwyer, L., & Murray, C. J. (2010). Neonatal, postnatal, childhood, and under-5 mortality for 187 countries, 1970–2010: A systematic analysis of progress towards Millennium Development Goal 4. *Lancet, 375*(9730), 1988–2008.

Rajbhandari, S., Hodgis, S., Sanghvi, H., McPherson, R., Pradhan, Y., Baqui, A., & Misoprostol Study Group. (2010). Expanding uterotonic protection following childbirth through community-based distribution of misoprostol: Operations research study in Nepal. *International Journal of Gynecology and Obstetrics, 108*, 282–288.

Ransom, E., & Yinger, N. (2002). *Making motherhood safer: Overcoming obstacles on the pathway to care.* Washington, DC: Population Reference Bureau.

Shiffman, J. (2000). Can poor countries surmount high maternal mortality? *Studies in Family Planning, 31*, 274–289.

Sinding, S. W. (2000). The great population debates: How relevant are they for the 21st century? *American Journal of Public Health, 90*, 1841–1845.

Spira, R., Lepage, P., Msellati, P., Van De Perre, P., Leroy, V., Simonon, A., Karita, E., & Dabis, F. (1999). Natural history of human immunodeficiency virus type 1 infection in children: A five-year prospective study in Rwanda. *Pediatrics, 104*, e56.

Thaddeus, S., & Maine, D. (1994). Too far to walk: Maternal mortality in context. *Social Science & Medicine, 38*, 1091–1110.

Tsui, A. O., Wasserheit, J. N., & Haaga, J. G. (1997). *Reproductive health in developing countries: Expanding dimensions, building solutions.* Washington, DC: National Academy Press.

United Nations (UN). (2010). *The Millennium Development Goals.* Retrieved November 15, 2010 from http://www.un.org/millenniumgoals/.

United Nations Department of Economic and Social Affairs, Population Division. (2010). World population prospects: The 2010 revision: Volume I:

Comprehensive Tables. Retrieved May 21, 2011 from http://esa.un.org/unpd/wpp/Excel-Data/fertility .htm.

United Nations Department of Economic and Social Affairs, Population Division. (2011). World contraceptive use 2010. Retrieved May 21, 2011 from http://www.un.org/esa/population/publications/ wcu2010/Main.html.

United Nations Development Programme. (2005). The Millennium Development Goals. Messages from the UN Millennium Project Reports. Washington, DC: Author.

United Nations General Assembly. (1948). *Universal Declaration of Human Rights*, 10 December 1948, 217 A (III), Retrieved May 19, 2011 from http:// www.un.org/en/documents/udhr/.

UNAIDS and WHO. (2009). AIDS epidemic update, 2009. UNAID/09.36E. Geneva: UNAIDS.

UNICEF. (2008, September). *Progress for children. A report card on maternal mortality*. Number 7. New York. Geneva: UNICEF.

UNICEF. (2009). *State of the world's children*. Geneva: UNICEF.

UNICEF. (2010). *Levels and trends in child mortality*, Report 2010. New York: UNICEF.

U.S. Census Bureau. (2010). World population by age and sex. Retrieved DATE from http://sasweb.ssd .census.gov/idb/worldpopinfo.html.

Victora, C. G., Wagstaff, A., Schellenberg, J. A., Gwatkin, D., Claeson, M., & Habicht, J. P. (2003). Applying an equity lens to child health and mortality: More of the same is not enough. *Lancet, 362*, 233–241.

Villar, J., Valladares, E., Wojdyla, W., et al. (2006). Caesarean delivery rates and pregnancy outcomes: The 2005 WHO global survey on maternal and perinatal health in Latin America. *Lancet, 267*(9525), 1819–1829.

Walker, N., Schwartlander, B., & Bryce, J. (2002). Meeting international goals in child survival and HIV/AIDS. *Lancet, 360*, 284–289.

Walraven, G., Blum, J., Dampha, Y., Sowe, M., Morison, L., Winikoff, B., & Sloan, N. (2005). Misoprostol in the management of the third stage of labour in the home delivery setting in rural Gambia: A randomized controlled trial. *BJOG: An International Journal of Obstetrics and Gynaecology, 112*, 1277–1283.

Warren, K. S. (1988). The evolution of selective primary health-care. *Social Science & Medicine, 26*, 891–898.

World Health Organization (WHO). (1993). *International statistical classification of diseases and related health problems* (Vol. 2, 10th ed.). Geneva: Author.

World Health Organization (WHO). (2004). Safe motherhood and making pregnancy safer.

World Health Organization (WHO). (2005a). *Making every mother and child count*. Geneva: Author.

World Health Organization (WHO). (2005b). *Multi-country Study on Women's Health and Domestic Violence against Women*. Geneva: Author.

World Health Organization (WHO). (2007). *International Classification of Disease, 10th Revision. Clinical modification* (2nd ed.). Geneva: Author.

World Health Organization (WHO) & UNICEF. (2009). Global immunization data. Retrieved October 19, 2011 from http://www.who.int/immunization_ monitoring/Global_Immunization_Data.pdf.

World Health Organization (WHO). (2010). *Trends in maternal mortality 1990–2008*. Geneva: Author.

MATERNAL AND CHILD HEALTH SKILLS

17

RESEARCH ISSUES IN MATERNAL AND CHILD HEALTH

Martha S. Wingate, Karen Williams, Joseph Telfair, and Russell S. Kirby

THE NEED FOR RESEARCH IN MATERNAL AND CHILD HEALTH

Maternal and child health (MCH) is the field that focuses on the determinants, mechanisms, and systems that promote the health, safety, well-being, and appropriate development of children and their families (Alexander, 2003; Alexander, et al., 2002). Research is an essential cornerstone of the MCH field. MCH, a collaborative, multidisciplinary specialty area of public health, uses the research and practice tools of epidemiology, biostatistics, health behavior, environmental health, and health policy to focus on the health and well-being of children and families. This multidisciplinary field also draws from other social science and public administration disciplines (including health services research, medical sociology, geography, and demography) to (1) explore the etiology, determinants, and distribution of disease, injury, disability, and death; (2) assess needs, along with expanding crucial surveillance and data systems; (3) develop cost-effective prevention and intervention approaches; (4) plan for and monitor the implementation, administration, and functioning of systems of care; (5) evaluate the process and outcomes of programs and policies; and (6) guide effective, responsible advocacy and the dissemination of information and new knowledge.

Although public health and MCH research are traditionally valued for increasing our understanding of the determinants of the health status and healthcare utilization of the MCH population, this research further offers well-established methods to identify priorities among potential needs, to select an appropriate course of action among alternative interventions, and to assess the cost-effectiveness and impact, both intended and otherwise, of our chosen response. As rooted as the MCH field is in public health practice, MCH professionals must continually assess the evolving needs of the MCH population in light of ongoing developments in our healthcare and social service systems and the changing physical and social environments. In order to make needed policy and programmatic decisions regarding the allocation and targeting of limited resources, MCH professionals must become evidence-based practitioners, relying on scientifically rigorous and defensible data to guide their choices, thereby ensuring accountability and maintaining credibility. Research provides the means to distinguish effective, evidence-based practices from those with insufficient evidence to support their being touted as best practice. Indeed, the hallmark of responsible advocacy to inform the choices of the public and policy makers is its strict reliance on research-based evidence.

Pressing Research Needs

The MCH field faces numerous pressing research needs, some ongoing and others emerging. In recent times, MCH leaders have realized the need for an understanding of MCH population health that transcends single snapshots of time and narrow categories of causal criteria. Taking a broader, more longitudinal view of health for the MCH population requires further research into the factors affecting health throughout life, from the proximal to the macro level and from the local to the international level, and involves the application of new models, analytical strategies, and statistical techniques. Although any list of the most critical MCH research needs is open to debate and may quickly become outdated, our leading candidates on the list of pressing MCH research need areas follow.

Life Course Perspective

Simply stated, the life course perspective flows from the recognition that experiences very early in life, including the in utero experience and even experiences of prior generations, have a lasting influence on health outcomes. Rather than focusing on single periods of development, the life course perspective uncovers contributing factors in previous years, extending back into past generations; because maternal health heavily influences child health, the exposures and experiences of mothers are important to consider when studying child health (Braveman & Barclay, 2009; Lu & Halfon, 2003). MCH research within this framework considers health factors across time and generations. Empirical data and statistical frameworks to support this research are becoming more widely available, but more needs to be done to develop data collection methods and measures that can capture accurate information about previous experiences. The old adage "that which can't be measured can't be changed" underscores the importance to MCH of expanding the boundaries of our view and improving our research measurement capacity and thereby improving its ability to assess health status and healthcare use needs more completely.

Measuring Key MCH Concepts

MCH is rich in the use of highly abstract concepts to describe desired approaches to caring for the needs of children and families. Abstract terms frequently employed in MCH such as "systems," "cultural competency," "family centered," "community based," "medical home," "food insecurity," "gestational age," and "underinsurance" remain to be defined with the specificity required for research purposes. MCH researchers can assist practitioners and policymakers in the understanding and more scientific use of these concepts by conducting research examining their measurement, complexity, and nuances in both general application and specific contexts.

Research measurement approaches are invaluable to MCH in order for the field to document progress and assess the performance of its programs, policies, and practitioners. Our ability to advocate for and ensure coordinated, comprehensive, and continuous systems of care depends in part on our ability to measure current levels of health status and utilization and to track changes that we propose will result from specified policies and leadership efforts.

Assessing Needs, Evaluating Solutions, and Monitoring Performance

Within the statutory requirements of Title V of the Social Security Act, every state and territory must complete and report a 5-year needs assessment (PL 74-271, 1935; PL 101-239, 1989). Beyond the 5-year needs assessment, state MCH programs should engage in ongoing needs assessments as part of a rational planning cycle linked to policy development, program design, budgets, resource allocation, and evaluation (Maternal and Child Health Bureau, 2004). Despite the importance of needs assessment to MCH, the scientific knowledge base necessary to inform program leaders about the most rigorous, productive, and cost-effective approaches to address persistent need areas remains underdeveloped (Alexander & Petersen, 2004). There is a critical need to evaluate rigorously the current intervention and prevention programs and to expand the evaluation literature relevant to MCH in order to increase the effective use of available resources to affect health status and healthcare use most favorably. Similarly, in response to the Government Performance and Results Act of 1993 and various performance-based budgeting initiatives within states, state MCH programs must be prepared to articulate a set of performance measures that capture the depth and breadth of their efforts in ways that are reasonable and realistic but not potentially detrimental to the viability of the programs (PL 102-63, 1993). This becomes a delicate balancing act, fraught with challenges, including how to handle mandated programs, how to address politically sensitive activities, how to consider politically popular programs, and how to maintain focus on fundamentally important areas of MCH that are no longer in vogue. Although needs assessment methods continue to develop, the science of performance monitoring has also evolved. Nevertheless, performance measurement

and monitoring deserves increased attention from researchers interested in supporting the capacity of programs not only to survive but also to lead responsibly and effectively.

Assessing Child Health and Development at the Population Level

The vital records system in the United States provides an extraordinary resource for researchers interested in events surrounding perinatal health. However, for many years public health has not had a source for similar information extending through childhood and adolescence providing information beyond mortality and hospitalization-related illness or injury. However, the National Children's Study, authorized by the Children's Health Act of 2000 and funded by Congress, promises to provide a wealth of new information on health factors from prior to conception to the 21st birthday. The study's 105 planned data collection sites across the country will gather data on environmental and genetic factors and incidence of disease among a broad cohort of children (Kuehn, 2010). Although this provides an exciting opportunity for researchers to have data conducive to analysis from the life course perspective (Braveman & Barclay, 2009; Fine & Kotelchuck, 2010), it will be many years before the full potential of the National Children's Study can be realized. Capitalizing on full potential of this data will be important for MCH. In the meantime, the National Survey of Children's Health (NSCH) and the National Survey of Children with Special Health Care Needs (NSCSHCN) provide data for research on systems, programs, and children's health outcomes at the population level. Although these tools and the National Children's Study represent important strides towards population-wide surveys and research on children's health parameters, much more needs to be done to understand the lifestyle and physical factors that contribute to children's health outcomes, particularly the growing prevalence of obesity and chronic diseases. Detailed information about the design of both the NSCH and NS-CSHCN is available at www.nschdata.org.

Evaluating the Effects of Healthcare Reform

Recent progress on comprehensive healthcare reform at the federal level promises to have significant implications for the MCH population. As the details and the long-term effects of policy change, including the Patient Protection and Affordable Care Act of 2010, remain in debate, MCH researchers can play a unique role in determining how proposed agendas will influence MCH access to primary and obstetric and gynecologic care and which options will be most cost effective for families and communities. All actual and proposed changes demand vigorous scrutiny by MCH professionals and advocates and require a rich repository of research evidence for their scientific assessment.

Investigating Determinants of Health Disparities

Despite advances in health care in recent decades and improvements in health status for many, health disparities persist within the United States and across the globe. Within the United States, significant racial disparities continue for many perinatal outcomes. The infant mortality rate for black babies is well over twice as high as the rate for non-Hispanic whites, and the rate of preterm birth for blacks is also significantly higher than the rate for whites (Behrman & Butler, 2007). It is important to note that health disparities of current importance go beyond just racial and ethnic disparities. They also include nativity, socioeconomic status, and rural/urban differences, to name a few. Disparities span the perinatal period, childhood, and adulthood. There is a large body of literature that focuses on health disparities in outcomes and in healthcare services.

The United Nations' Millennium Development Goals (Bhutta, et al., 2010) have focused concerted international effort on reducing maternal mortality by three-fourths and child mortality by two-thirds by 2015. Monitoring these objectives has uncovered substantial differences in health status and improvement among regions of the world. Addressing these disparities requires understanding the many social determinants of MCH. Much research is necessary to determine the causes behind these disparities and the systemic and familial social determinants that most influence these and other MCH health outcomes.

International Issues

MCH researchers need to develop better ways to measure and report health outcomes in low-resource areas and to streamline definitions. Despite efforts, it is still very difficult to gather complete or representative data sets for countries without stable political and social systems. Additionally, saving and improving the lives of mothers and children requires developing cost-effective, feasible, evidence-based interventions for low-resource settings. MCH researchers should lead efforts to create and test policies and programs that will reduce or eliminate the social determinants that produce dangerous MCH outcomes. Working toward this goal requires international cooperation. Globalization has contributed to the growth of international cooperatives focusing on sharing health information and working together to combat disease. For example, the goal of the EURO-PERISTAT project is to develop valid and reliable indicators that can be used to monitor and evaluate perinatal health in the European Union (Zimbeck, Mohangoo, & Zeitlin, 2009). The European Surveillance of Congenital Anomalies (EUROCAT) is another example of a longstanding collaboration between European counties to conduct surveillance of congenital anomalies (Boyd, et al., 2011). MCH research needs to continue to explore opportunities for greater international collaboration on MCH issues, especially in light of the easy spread of epidemics across the globe and the increasing focus on the Millennium Development Goals.

FUNDAMENTAL CONCEPTS OF SCIENCE AND RESEARCH

Measurement, Order, and Classification

From a philosophical point of view, research and the scientific method are used to understand better the workings of the world around us (e.g., understanding the mechanisms underlying the distribution and spread of disease) and to better predict the probability of events to come. Testing and falsification are the hallmarks of this approach, Researchers propose research questions such that, through experimentation, they can find evidence, within the limitations of our study design and empirical data, that argues against (rejects) or does not refute (fails to reject) preconceived notions (hypotheses and theories) about reality. Fundamental to this research process is the classification or ordering of events and observations into identifiable categories of likes and dislikes (Bronowski, 1967). Practically speaking, research measurement entails our ability to identify cases from controls correctly, those with disease from those without, those who use healthcare services from those who do not, and those with specific risk characteristics from those who may be free of those attributes. The precise definition and measurement of ideas, concepts, or variables are critical steps in all scientific research. As such, the importance and value of studies that seek to develop new or refine existing measurement approaches should not be overlooked, particularly in a research field as relatively new as MCH. Furthermore, studies conducted on MCH-related topics require the same rigor and necessity of solid measurement as any other scholarly discipline.

Validity and Reliability of Measurement

To bring order to concepts about health problems, risk factors, and at-risk populations, observations are typically categorized using various measurement approaches. The basic ways of ordering include categorical and continuous measures. Categorical measures consist of dichotomous (two mutually exclusive categories), nominal (more than two mutually exclusive categories), ordinal (ordered qualitative categories), and interval (categories with a "natural," equal interval between values). Continuous variables are those with an interval scale with a true zero point so that ratios between values are meaningful (Isaac & Michael, 1995).

Errors in the classification of individuals or observations into one group or another are inherent to the process of grouping data and call into question the validity of the measurement approach employed. *Validity* of measurement asks this question, "Is this measuring what it claims?" In the strictest sense, to be valid, the measures should reflect true differences among groups on the characteristics or concepts that are measured and not be result of systematic or nonrandom errors in classifying. Validity of measurement is concerned with several types of validity, including criterion validity (also known as predictive validity), which asks whether the measure is a good predictor or "validator" of an outcome or criterion of interest; content validity, involving questions about breadth and adequate coverage of what it claims to measure; and construct validity, which asks whether the concept under measurement truly exists and whether the measure is really measuring it (Carmines & Zeller, 1979; Isaac & Michael, 1995; Nunnally, 1978).

The *reliability* of measurement is an equally important consideration in research and is directed at identifying measurement errors, mainly random or chance errors, related to the consistency and stability of scoring observations in a series of measurements. In other words, it entails assessing the accurate repeatability of a measurement approach or the agreement between multiple measurement approaches, that is, the yielding of the same results. Various methods are available for assessing the degree of reliability, all involving comparisons between multiple measures, for example, retest, alternate forms, and split-halves method (Carmines & Zeller, 1979; Isaac & Michael, 1995; Nunnally, 1978). In relationship to validity, a measure may be reliable but not valid, that is, an invalid result (one that does not appropriately measure the given concept, etc.) yet can be repeated (Isaac & Michael, 1995).

The assessment of measurement validity and reliability is a primary starting point for developing and assessing any research study. For example, studies about preterm birth should clearly describe the measurement of gestational age, including identification and addressing of out-of-range or implausible data, the treatment or imputation of missing data, and the combination of various approaches for measuring gestational age (e.g., last menstrual period, first trimester ultrasound, obstetric vs. pediatric methods). Appropriately, there is a considerable body of literature directed at reliability and validity of measurement, and the indicated references provide a starting point for further reading about these essential measurement issues (Carmines & Zeller, 1979; Isaac & Michael, 1995; Nunnally, 1978).

Causality, Association, and Chance

Beyond bringing order to observations, scientific research seeks to reveal the mechanisms that underlie the way the world works, for example, what causes asthma, low birth weight, or preterm delivery. By better understanding the relationships between occurrences and characteristics, researchers are better able to describe the flow of events that are around them and predict with greater accuracy the expected consequences of actions. Moreover, researchers are better able to develop effective interventions and understand how modifying the environment, behaviors, and conditions might change the course of future events and thereby improve

the future for children and their families. Nevertheless, the utility of science to reveal the causal nature of the surrounding environment and universe at large has been subject to ongoing debate.

Beyond the scope of this chapter, grounding in the philosophy of science is instructive to understand better the language of research and the distinct attention that is paid to the cautious use of the term "causality" (Bronowski, 1967; Popper, 1965; Rothman, Greenland, & Lash, 2008). Causality is generally used to indicate that a relationship exists between two concepts or events and that one is believed to determine the specific occurrence of the other. At issue with this notion is the recognition of chance and probability, the belief that, although future events may for the most part be predictable within an interval of confidence, there is always some uncertainty. In research, there is always some component of chance for which we use statistics to assess the probability of relationships and outcomes.

Recognizing the role of chance in science, researchers have taken a more circumscribed approach to the use of the term "causality" to describe research on hypothesized relationships. Various benchmarks have been advanced to differentiate whether an association should be considered causal versus noncausal, including (1) biological plausibility, (2) a time-sequenced relationship (the predictor always precedes the outcome), (3) the strength and type of the association (strong, dose-response), and (4) a necessary (nonsubstitutable), sufficient, and consistent relationship between predictor and outcome (Hill, 1965; Rothman, Greenland, & Lash, 2008). Although the development of absolute criteria for causality continues to be as elusive as the scientific search for "truth," these benchmarks do emphasize the need for prudence in the interpretation of research findings. It cannot be stressed enough that science does not prove what is and will always be true. It instead offers a pathway for lifelong learning, relearning, and intellectual adaptation in an uncertain and changing world.

In MCH, much of the research conducted is epidemiologic in nature and seeks to find potential risk factors and associations of particular characteristics with a given disease or outcome. Rarely is the intent of MCH research to reveal causal associations. For example, research on teen pregnancy typically reveals that infants born to mothers who are less than 18 years of age are at increased risk of being low birth weight. This association is well established, although it may not exist in every population and could possibly change in terms of the strength of the association. For very young teens, less than 15 years old, there may be biologically plausible reasons why young, still-developing mothers are more likely to have smaller babies. Nevertheless, it is important to note that a teen mother is not the cause of a low birth weight infant, and most infants born to teen mothers are not low birth weight.

BUILDING BLOCKS OF RESEARCH

Theories, Hypotheses, and Operational Definitions

Theories are used to drive the direction of research and scientific inquiry. Theories are sets of interrelated propositions that are collectively used to explain some aspect of reality. They may have stated boundaries, for example, populations and time frames that circumscribe the limits of the theory. They are neither true nor false and are useful only to the extent that they are accurately descriptive or predictive. Theoretical development typically begins with logical descriptions of phenomena and progresses to testable hypotheses, using empirical measures. Findings from these empirical studies can only support theories, not prove them.

Hypotheses and operational definitions are the empirical bases for examining theories and exploring whether there are relationships between two or more concepts. Hypotheses are used to test theories at the empirical level, and as they are used for testing, they

must provide propositional statements that are falsifiable. To be further useful, hypotheses should have available operations to measure variables and collect data in concrete situations (Miller & Salkind, 2002). Hypotheses are generally stated in the "null" form and suggest that there will be no difference or change in one concept variable, given a variation on another. Similar to theories, boundary statements may be used to define the populations, time period, or geographic area to which the hypothesis is limited.

Operational definitions are used to measure concepts found in hypotheses. In order to make sense of a concept, one must operationalize it so that it will be evident to others. For example, for a study on child abuse (a concept), a measurement tool must be developed to assess if it occurred and to which study participants. The measurement tool, possibly a survey, interview form, or case report, documents to other researchers the definition and procedures used to determine child abuse cases. Therefore, operational definitions employ empirical indicators, for example, questions, a scale, and test scores, to define and measure the existence and extent of observable events or characteristics that measure the concepts used in the hypothesis. Operational definitions require a level of abstraction that supports their use in different time and space settings while still providing a sufficient description of measurement procedures to be replicable and therefore to help standardize research. Within the MCH field, commonly used operational definitions employed for research include such concepts as use of prenatal care, premature birth, and unintended pregnancy. Conventions have been developed for measuring these concepts; for example, the Revised-Graduated Prenatal Care Utilization Index (R-GINDEX) has been employed to measure adequacy of prenatal care use (Alexander & Kotelchuck, 2001), and the use of these measurement conventions facilitates comparing research results and synthesizing of the current evidence on a particular topic.

Modeling Hypothesized Relationships

Modeling is a useful technique for organizing thoughts while developing research ideas and for visually describing the proposed relationships between concepts used in hypotheses. Modeling provides a visual depiction of the relationships of predictor variables to the outcome variables of interest. Variables are the primary components of hypotheses, and before constructing a theoretical model, the dependent and independent variables need to be identified. Dependent variables measure the outcome(s) of interest. Implicit in their label, change in the values of the dependent variable will depend on the values of the independent variables. Independent variables are the proposed predictors of the outcome, the variables that are potentially associated with changes in the dependent variable's values. For the purposes of modeling and developing stated hypotheses, two types of independent variables can be differentiated: the main independent variable(s), whose relationship with the dependent variables are of primary interest, and the other independent variables, which will be taken into account or controlled for in the analysis because of their perceived relationship with the main independent variables and the dependent variables. The example given in Figure 17–1 is simplified in order to present the basic components of theoretical models. However, there are a variety of references that provide further and more complete explanations of theoretical models (Rothman, Greenland, & Lash, 2008). This basic approach is elaborated in more complex research designs and analysis plans.

The following is a schematic example for a theoretical model (Figure 17–1).

The three types of variables are identified, and the directions of the relationships among the variables are specified by the directions of the arrows. Pluses or minuses could be noted by each arrow to signify a possible positive or negative association. The example model provides a boundary statement and indicates that there will be a relationship between the independent variable and the dependent variable after controlling for the potential confounders. Extraneous factors or variables that contribute to or influence the relationship between the independent and dependent variables are called confounders. Using the example in Figure 17–1, maternal smoking can influence birth weight (extraneous to prenatal care utilization) and would be considered a confounder.

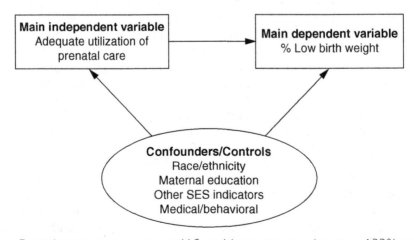

Figure 17–1 Boundary statement: among U.S. resident women who are < 133% poverty.

This model depicts the following formally stated null hypothesis. Among U.S. resident women at less than 133% of poverty (boundary statement): "There will be no change in the proportion of women delivering a preterm infant (dependent variable) by adequacy of prenatal care utilization (main independent variable), after taking into account maternal race/ethnicity, education, socio-economic status and medical and behavioral risk factors (control independent variables)." In order for this hypothesis to be tested, the variables listed in the model still require specific concrete operations definitions, for example, the percentage of low birth weight (less than 2,500 grams), adequate use of prenatal care (R-GINDEX), maternal education (less than 12 years, 12 years, or more than 12 years), etc. (Piper, Ray, & Griffin, 1990).

TYPES OF RESEARCH

Choosing an appropriate design for a research study is critical. This early decision can influence the overall conclusions that can be drawn from research findings. For much MCH research, study designs fall into three general categories: nonexperimental, experimental, and health services research. In addition, qualitative and mixed methods research will be discussed briefly. Each of these is described in greater detail later in this chapter. There are a number of texts that provide greater detail and depth to these types of research (Bowling, 2009; Campbell & Stanley, 1963, 1966; Creswell, 2008).

Nonexperimental Designs

Research that only observes and does not manipulate variables has a nonexperimental design (Bordens & Abbott, 2002). Epidemiologic studies, both descriptive and analytic, fall into this category of research designs. Descriptive studies are concerned with general distributions of disease and health status. Case studies are indepth studies of

single cases (Miller & Salkind, 2002), such as a summary of the influence of a parenting home intervention for teen mothers on a single mother/infant dyad (Stiles, 2010). Case series use a number (series) of cases in which the disease/outcome of interest is observed in order to evaluate whether any common features are shared. These observations, often obtained through questionnaires, data from records, etc., can be retrospective or prospective (Miller & Salkind, 2002). A study that follows nine infants after birth to document the developmental profiles that are markers for autism is an example of a case series (Bryson, et al., 2007). Both case studies and case series are useful to generate hypotheses and develop new measurement strategies, and are very common in the clinical research literature in obstetrics, perinatology, and pediatrics (Miller & Salkind, 2002).

Cross-sectional studies and screening surveys, both based on a representative sample questioned or evaluated at one point in time, are also descriptive studies. A cross-sectional study aims to assess the prevalence of a disease or condition and associated factors. Screening surveys are useful to potentially identify individuals or populations at high risk for some disease or condition so that some healthcare intervention or promotion can be implemented. Examples in public health of some interest to MCH include the Behavioral Risk Factor Surveillance System (BRFSS), the Youth Risk Behavior Survey (YRBS), the National Health Interview Survey (NHIS), and the National Health and Nutrition Examination Survey (NHANES).

Ecological studies aim to assess the relationship between an exposure and disease/mortality. The unit of study is a group of people (Bowling, 2009). Units of analysis may be administrative (five-digit ZIP Codes, census tracts or block groups, counties, states, nations), clinical settings (most commonly, hospitals), or educational (school districts). Research that considers whether government spending on health care and health policies that target the poor affect aggregate under-5 mortality and inequality in under-5 mortality within developing countries uses an ecological method (Kruk, Prescott, de Pinho, & Galea, 2011). With studies such as these, no inference can be made about individual behaviors and outcomes. In the aforementioned study, for example, the researchers do not know whether specific poor families that received more health care from the government experienced less under-5 mortality; they consider only whether mortality rates change in the entire population. Care must be taken in applying the results from ecological studies to the level of the individual (Robinson, 2009; Schwartz, 1994).

Analytic studies include case-control and cohort studies that, although nonexperimental, are concerned with the cause and prevention of disease. These types of studies typically compare population groups based on exposure to a given risk factor or disease/condition. They often use databases built from large surveys such as the Pregnancy Risk Assessment Monitoring System (PRAMS), the National Immunization Survey (NIS), and the National Survey of Children with Special Health Care Needs (NS-CSHCN). The case-control study starts by identifying a group with a condition/disease of interest and comparing it with a reference group (controls) to determine whether there is a difference in exposure to a hypothesized risk factor or factors. The aim of this type of study is to assess which factors occur more or less often among cases compared to controls in order to identify potential means of reducing risk factors for disease or increasing protective factors. This analysis allows for calculation of an odds ratio, an approximation of relative risk (in the case of a rare outcome), which can measure the association of a risk factor and a disease. The case-control study always has a retrospective approach, whether subjects are accrued prospectively or obtained from secondary sources, as the focus is on risk factors observed at a previous point in time among the cases and the selected controls

(Bowling, 2009; Hulley, Cummings, Browner, Grady, & Newman, 2006). Research in Nigeria that compared information on infants who had died (cases) and infants who remained alive (controls) after the neonatal period to determine whether delivery by a skilled birth attendant affected the risk of mortality is a case-control study (Lawoyin, Onadeko, & Asekun-Olarinmoye, 2010).

Cohort studies are longitudinal or "follow-up" studies of the occurrence of disease in a group of subjects exposed to a risk factor of interest compared to the occurrence of disease in a group of people not exposed to the risk factor. They are intended to assess the incidence of disease and the potential causative agents. The division into the "exposed" and "unexposed" groups often occurs naturally, with no manipulation (Bowling, 2009; Handler, Rosenberg, Kennelly, & Monahan, 1998; Miller & Salkind, 2002). Longitudinal cohort studies are prospective in nature, as the focus is on the occurrence of a disease or health state at some point after the initial time point under study. There are, however, retrospective cohort studies in which the exposure and subsequent development of disease have occurred in the past. The difference between prospective and retrospective cohort studies is the manner in which the study or project is conducted. Project Viva is an example of a prospective observational cohort study of pregnancy outcomes and health. This cohort has been used to examine a variety of questions, including whether maternal feeding restriction predicts childhood obesity (Rifas-Shiman, Rich-Edwards, Rifas-Shiman, Lieberman, Kleinman, & Lipshultz, 2011). These nonexperimental designs are frequently applied to descriptive or cross-sectional data sets. For example, a study of risk factors for placenta previa by race of mother using national public use birth certificate files is a case-control design of a cross-sectional study population.

Table 17–1 described designs for nonexperimental research.

Table 17–1 Research Designs: Nonexperimental; No manipulation of Variables; Observational Only.

Types of Research		Research Design	Description
Epidemiologic	Descriptive	Case study	Studies a single case in depth and is useful for generating hypotheses.
		Case series	Observes a series of cases with certain characteristics/conditions to determine any shared features; it is useful for generating hypotheses.
		Screening surveys and case finding	Detects individuals or populations at high risk for disease/condition through questionnaires and other screening tools.
		Cross-sectional survey	Considers a sample or subsample of a population and questions it at one point in time.
		Ecological	Assess exposure and disease/mortality using aggregate data from the population level (not from the individual level).
		Qualitative	Uses interviews, focus groups, and observations to explore issues and their perceived meanings and to develop hypotheses.
	Analytical	Case-Control	Involves comparing a group that has a condition/disease or has been exposed to a risk factor (cases) with a group that does not have the condition/disease or has not been exposed to the risk factor (controls). The aim is to identify things that occur more or less often in the cases than in the controls that could explain the difference in outcome between the two groups.
		Cohort	Divides a single group into "exposed" and "unexposed" groups naturally (without manipulation) and then determines which group develops the condition/disease and which group does not; intended to assess the incidence of disease and the potential causative agents of a disease.

Experimental Designs

Experimental designs manipulate the main independent variable and the control of other independent, confounding, or covariate variables. Table 17–2 describes the more common experimental research designs.

Randomized controlled trials are true experimental designs involving two or more randomly assigned groups. In the most basic form of randomized controlled trial, the experimental group receives the treatment, and the control group, although handled exactly like the experimental group in every other way, does not receive the treatment (Hulley, et al., 2006). Randomizing pregnant women into one group that is given micronutrient supplementation and another group that receives only iron-folic acid supplementation to determine which have better pregnancy outcomes is an example of an experimental study (Bhutta, et al., 2009). Quasi-experimental designs include natural, field, and community-intervention experiments. Natural experiments are those in which an independent variable is manipulated by natural or human-made occurrences not under the control of the investigator

Table 17–2 Research Designs: Experimental; Manipulation of Main Independent Variable and Control of Other Independent, Confounding, or Covariate Variables.

Type of Research	Research Design	Description
True experimental	Randomized controlled trial	Randomly assigns people to two groups and then treats each group differently; the investigator must have control over treatment and group assignment.
Quasi-experimental	Natural experiment	Assess a situation in which the investigator or natural causes manipulate the independent variable.
	Field experiment	Assess a situation in which the investigator or natural causes manipulate the independent variable.
	Community intervention experiment	Involves a community-wide intervention on a collective basis, rather than an individual basis.

(Isaac & Michaels, 1995). A classic public health example is the Dutch Famine Winter of 1944 to 1945 for studies of nutrition and pregnancy outcome (Painter, et al., 2008; Stein, Susser, Saenger, & Marolla, 1975). Field experiments, or clinical trials, are research studies occurring in a natural situation in which one or more variables are manipulated by the researcher(s). Studies using these designs typically examine individuals in relationship to some preventive health measure targeted at individual health behaviors (Friis & Sellers, 1999). This differs from community intervention experiments with a collective or community focus rather than an individual basis. The overall goal of the experiment or research is to assess the impact on the community as a whole. (See Table 17–2.)

HEALTH SERVICES RESEARCH AND EVALUATION

Table 17–3 describes some types of research applicable to MCH but outside of the epidemiologic or experimental realm.

These study types include those relevant to leadership, administration, and management. Needs assessment aims to gather information about the health of a population or community. It serves as the foundation for developing programmatic and policy directives and also helps allocate resources to achieve strategic objectives. This is the initial step in developing or establishing objectives for an organization or agency (Kettner, Moroney, & Martin, 1990; Petersen & Alexander, 2001). Systems evaluation documents the elements of systems that involve interrelated components working toward a common goal or outcome objective. This area of research continues to grow in both public health and MCH. An additional field that requires extensive use of systems evaluation is that of public health systems research (PHSR), defined as "a field of study that examines the organization, financing, and delivery of public health services within communities, and the impact of these services on public health" (Mays, Halverson, & Scutchfield, 2004 in Scutchfield, Marks, Perez, & Mays, 2007, p. 169). More MCH

Table 17-3 Research Designs: Health Services Research

Type of Research	Research Design	Description
Needs Assessment	Needs Assessment	Gathers information about the health of a population or community that will guide development of programs and policies; is the initial step in establishing objectives for a program or policy.
Evaluation	Process evaluation	Investigates to ensure the specific objectives of a program or intervention are met; considers both the nature and scope of activities conducted.
	Outcome evaluation	Investigates whether a program or intervention achieves the desired outcome or meets the overall goal of the program; assess results of program activities.
	Performance monitoring	Assesses progress/performance of programs or policies against stated objectives; performance measures are measurable outcomes sometimes linked to funding sources.
	Systems evaluation	Documents and assesses the elements of systems that work toward a common goal or outcome objective; is an emerging area in public health.
	Policy analysis	Assess the impact of policies on individuals and communities and works to make the public policy processes more effective.
Economic	Financial and service delivery use analysis	Includes a number of specific research study designs that focus on use and service delivery (resource allocation; cost-forecasting, and cost reduction impact assessment; cost-effectiveness and benefit assessment; quality assurance; risk adjustment; patient flow and satisfaction).
Action	Community-based participatory	Responds to community demand and addresses locally identified needs; communities are active participants in the research process.

focus is needed in this field. Additionally policy analysis, which can greatly enhance the policy process, aims to assess the impact of policy development. Financial and service delivery use analysis focuses on resource allocation (also linked to needs assessment), cost forecasting and cost-reduction impact assessment, cost-effectiveness and benefit assessment, quality assurance, risk adjustment, and patient flow/satisfaction.

Another research type described in Table 17-3 is action research, specifically, community-based participatory research, "a collaborative process of research involving researchers and community representatives; it engages community members, employs local knowledge in the understanding of health problems and the design of interventions, and invests community members in the processes and products of research. In addition, community members are invested in the dissemination and use of research findings and ultimately in the reduction of health disparities" (Agency for Healthcare Research and Quality, 2001). This partnership approach to research equally involves community members, organizational members, and researchers in all aspects of the research process. Partners guide the process with their expertise and share responsibility in order to improve the health of the community (Cargo & Mercer, 2008; Eisinger & Senturia, 2001; Felix-Aaron & Stryer, 2003; Freudenberg, 2001; O'Toole, Feliz-Aaron, Chin, Horowitz, & Tyson, 2003). A study of children's playground violence that actively involved and included the perspectives of parents and an elementary school principal in addition to researcher observation demonstrates use of a community-based, participatory research model (Drabick & Baugh, 2010).

Multi-level Models

Although many studies in MCH continue to be conducted across individuals (mothers, infants) or across ecological units (hospitals, counties, census tracts), statistical methods that account for variation in dependent variables across levels have become increasingly available. These models enable the researcher to model hypothetical relationships between variables measured across individuals, families, neighborhoods or communities, or states in analyses that more closely reflect theoretical frameworks such as Bronfenbrenner's (1979) socioecological model. Multi-level methods can be applied to most epidemiologic study designs in MCH, including cross-sectional, case-control, and cohort designs.

For example, in analyzing factors associated with nonmedically indicated induction of labor among pregnant women in a state, a researcher might design a multi-level analysis that accounts for individual variables

(demographics, reproductive history, events associated with the current pregnancy), physician or attendant at delivery variables, hospital-level variables, and state policy variables. This analysis would demonstrate whether the higher-level variables influence the associations found at the individual level, or whether factors measured across physicians, hospitals, or states contribute statistically to our understanding of what variables increase or reduce a woman's likelihood of nonmedically indicated labor induction.

MCH professionals interested in utilizing multi-level methods will find numerous texts (e.g., Gelman & Hill, 2006; Luke, 2004; Raudenbush & Byrk, 2002) and methods review articles (e.g., Bingenheimer & Raudenbush, 2004; Culhane & Elo, 2005; Diez Roux, 2000) in the literature. Statistical programs for multi-level modeling are also increasingly available. These models can be analyzed in SAS, SPSS, and Stata, as well as with more specialized software including HLM, MLwiN, and routines in WinBUGS, and R, and MPlus.

Geographical Information Systems and MCH Research

Geographic Information Systems (GIS) have come into increasing use in the field of MCH. GIS software combines automated software capabilities with relational database functionality in an environment that also provides an increasing array of spatial analytical features. The application of GIS to public health is described in a recent textbook (Cromley and McLafferty, 2011). Most data in public health databases supports geocoding to latitude-longitude coordinates or to spatial administrative units (census blocks, census tracts, ZIP codes or ZIP Code Tabulation Areas [ZCTAs], municipalities, counties, states) that can be mapped. Although GIS analyses in MCH are most likely to involve cross-sectional or ecological study designs, GIS is also used to support multi-level analyses through the classification of individual observations to larger spatial units.

The Practice of Evaluation

Evaluation is equally critical to the success of any public health or MCH program. Evaluation is studying a program to decide whether it achieved measurable, clearly stated goals and objectives and whether it completed its activities. Process evaluation investigates whether the specific program achieves its objectives. It studies both the scope and nature of the activities conducted. Outcome evaluation considers whether the program or intervention achieves the decided outcomes or meets the overall goal of the program (Rossi & Freeman, 1993; Shadish, Cook, & Leviton, 1991; Weiss, 1972). Performance monitoring is rooted in the basic concept of evaluation, because it aims to assess progress and/or performance against stated objectives. Many MCH programs, particularly Title V, use performance measures, which are measurable outcomes linked to funding sources (Petersen & Alexander, 2001).

MCH program evaluation has a twofold definition: (1) the application of evaluation approaches, techniques, and knowledge to systematically assess and improve the planning, implementation and effectiveness of programs (Chen, 2005; McDavid & Hawthorn, 2006) and (2) the systematic application of this evidence to inform the decision-making process of the development, implementation, or continuation of a program or service activity (Fitzpatrick, Sanders & Worthen, 2004; Patton, 2008; Rossi, Lipsey, & Freeman, 2004a, 2004b; Wholey, Hatry, & Newcomer, 1994). This definition implies that MCH program evaluation is primarily concerned with two substantive activities: (1) the assessment of the effectiveness of MCH program interventions and (2) the outcome data from these assessments and the use of these data to influence program and policy development and change. Program evaluation in MCH is the systematic and scientific approach to: (1) plan and document program inputs; (2) plan and assess program activities; (3) identify gaps and

challenges; (4) troubleshoot resolutions on an ongoing basis; (5) collect program data; and (6) report program outputs (Chen, 2005; McDavid & Hawthorn, 2006; Patton, 2008).

In MCH practice, evaluative emphasis is on activities and approaches that will provide information needed to make judgments about a program. These determinations are made with consideration of the social, political, and cultural contexts in which programs are developed and implemented, as well the nature and scope of collaborations with other agencies and programs and the level of participation of stakeholders (Parker, Eng, Schulz, & Israel, 1999; Peoples-Sheps & Telfair, 2005; Springett & Wallerstein, 2008; Telfair, 2005; Telfair & Mulvihill, 2000). As such, the practice of program evaluation in MCH is a product that is partly social, partly political, and only partly technical (Chelimsky, 1997; Herman, Morris, & Fitz-Gibbon, 1987).

MCH program evaluation is by definition a longitudinal process involving assessment of service or intervention efforts—be they policy-based or practice-based—at the local, state, national, or global levels (Chelimsky, 1997; Fitzpatrick, Sanders & Worthen, 2004). As such there is a focus on process and short/intermittent/long-term outcome indicators and measures (Schalock, 2001b; Steckler & Linnan, 2002) and those elements that influence development, utilization, and implementation (Bartholomew, Parcel, Kok, & Gottlieb, 2001; Wholey, Hatry, & Newcomer, 1994). These elements are well covered in other parts of this chapter. MCH practitioners must make program evaluation a key component of activities in order to address anticipated and existing challenges. As a critical activity practitioners need to view evaluation as a part of the service delivery/intervention process by maintaining on staff a person or persons with at least elementary evaluation skills, focusing on the use of evaluation results to inform program decision making, and viewing evaluators as collaborators (Telfair, 2005). Policy efforts, both development and utilization, must be rigorously evaluated in both the short and long term, particularly because outcomes of these policies can and do influence their broader application and program decisions that affect specific or targeted populations (Bartholomew, et al., 2001). Unfortunately many times such rigor is not part of the policy review process. Thus, for those engaged in setting policies and planning programs to be implemented at the local community and even state levels and for program administrators being faced with new demands for more rigorous accountability (e.g., Centers for Medicare and Medicaid Services), this reality is very frustrating.

What is needed is to challenge the existing reality by engaging in evaluation at the program level that allows for the needs of all involved (clients, staff members, administrators, planners, and policy makers) to be met without feeling they are at risk of giving something up (e.g., staff members taking time away for providing services) or of losing something (e.g., planners not having the opportunity to get information that would help in long-term decision making).

Evaluation research addresses the social and political accountability issues inherent in applied work. Many programs are instituted with the hope that they will effectively ameliorate a specific problem (e.g., teenage pregnancy) or address a long-standing issue. Nonetheless, the basis for assessing the short- and long-term outcomes of these programs is not always clearly defined or agreed on by those involved, the stakeholders. This dilemma requires that the evaluation endeavor be comprehensive and flexible enough to anticipate and address a number of key accountability issues that define MCH programs (Telfair & Mulvihill, 2000; Springett & Wallerstein, 2008). These would include the following:

1. To ensure that the policy-based or service-based intervention is adequate for addressing the problem that it was designed to target
2. To ensure that the target program, with its cluster of services, is achieving maximum effectiveness

3. To ensure that the program's or agency's mechanism for accountability is functioning as it should (such as meeting the requirements of its funders)
4. To influence policy and other decision makers
5. To ensure that policies are understood by those they are intended
6. To enhance the standing of the target agency/program
7. To provide evidence that allows for staff and stakeholders to understand and appreciate the extent and effectiveness of the services provided to clients

Both process and outcome evaluation can be used to address these challenges. Process evaluation (McDavid & Hawthorn, 2006; Steckler & Linnan, 2002) focuses on documentation of proposed activities, targeted outcomes, and its linkages to corresponding goals and objectives of the program in a systematic manner. Process evaluation provides opportunities to identify issues related to the planned activities, troubleshoot, and revise and/or modify programmatic efforts to best fit the linked goals and objectives, assessment of short-term and intermittent outcomes (summative evaluation), as well as measurement of gaps between actual and expected levels of achievement (Steckler & Linnan, 2002; McDavid & Hawthorn, 2006). Process evaluation allows for continuous tracking of progress towards achievement of goals and objectives and assessment of qualitative and quantitative indicators of program achievement and verification of what program aspects were delivered and to whom and if they were delivered at the intended level (Steckler & Linnan, 2002; McDavid & Hawthorn, 2006). Process evaluation also allows for an assessment of the variations in program delivery and provides information on which components contribute to the short-term, intermediate, and long-term outcomes of recipients compared to nonrecipients (Chen, 2005).

Outcome evaluation involves assessment of all outcome-related program components

(Schalock, 2001a, 2001b). Outcome evaluation focuses on the assessment of short-term and intermediate program outputs and requires a comparative measurement and analysis of program achievements of its goals and objectives. Comparison can be temporal (pre, post, and follow-up), behavioral (skills), cognitive/intellectual (knowledge), or perceptual (qualitative) changes (Mertens, 2005; Rossi, Lipsey, & Freeman, 2004a, 2004b). Outcome evaluation has a macroscopic focus on a programmatic effects and impacts and is not ongoing as it is conducted annually, or at the end of a designated program period. Rigorous outcome evaluation is conducted for the purposes of assessing or proving (providing evidence for) programmatic sustainability and justification for its support. Outcome evaluation does include assessment and evaluation of qualitative and quantitative statistical indicators associated with individual and comparative service or policy assessments (Rossi, Lipsey, & Freeman, 2004b). The concurrent triangulation (mixed methods) approach inherent in outcome evaluation is used to confirm, cross-validate, and corroborate findings from the assessments (Brunner & Guzman, 1989; Springett & Wallerstein, 2008; Schalock, 2001a).

The advantage of the integrated use of both process evaluation and outcome evaluation in MCH program evaluation is the use of separate methods serves as a means to offset the weakness inherent within one method with the strengths of the other. This becomes important when examining core MCH issues such as family-centered care; health disparities; delivery of culturally competent services; community-based collaboration and services delivery; assessment of access, utilization, and quality of services and programs; and so forth.

Methodologically, this integrative approach requires that the quantitative and qualitative data collection is concurrent, implemented simultaneously during the evaluation. The results of the two methods are especially useful in policy assessment because it assures a more informative and participatory effort during the analysis, interpretation and reporting of results (Mertens, 2005; Rossi, Lipsey, & Freeman, 2004a; Schalock, 2001b).

QUALITATIVE AND MIXED METHODS RESEARCH

Qualitative Studies

Qualitative research focuses on understanding the meanings behind phenomena. Although quantitative research begins with a hypothesis that is then measured and analyzed with statistical methods, qualitative research starts with the goal of deeply exploring an issue and gathers information to construct a hypothesis (Greenhalgh & Taylor, 1997). Many research questions focus on phenomena that are not amenable to scientific study using quantitative approaches. In the field of MCH, some examples include resilience, racism, and satisfaction with group model prenatal care. Qualitative research is particularly useful in gaining understanding about new topics when there is not already enough existing knowledge to formulate a hypothesis for quantitative analysis (Patton, 2002). The three most common qualitative methods are participant observations, in-depth interviews, and focus groups. (See Table 17–4).

Samples for qualitative research are often selected purposefully, rather than randomly. Information about an issue is then gleaned through focus groups, semi-structured interviews, study of narrative documents, and observation. Observation can be either passive, in which the researcher watches a situation, or participatory, in which the researcher becomes part of the environment under study and observes from the inside (Miller & Salkind, 2002; Patton, 2002). These tools can be altered and mixed throughout the information-gathering process (Greenhalgh & Taylor, 1997). Researchers often continue to pursue data until saturation is achieved, which is the point when further interviews, discussions, or observations fail to produce new information (Miller & Salkind, 2002; Patton, 2002).

Analyzing qualitative data involves coding and organization into major and minor themes

Table 17–4 Research Designs: Qualitative and Mixed Methods

Type of Research	Research Design	Description
Qualitative	Participant observation	Appropriate for gathering data in natural settings on subjects in their usual context
	Structured/in-depth interview	Optimal for collecting information on individual experiences, perspectives, personal histories
	Focus groups	Effective in obtaining the data on cultural norms and expectations in the community

that then become the basis for theories and typically requires the use of specialized software for qualitative data analysis. Researchers use several processes called "triangulation" to help ensure their findings are as close as possible to the truth. Data triangulation involves comparing data from a variety of sources to corroborate the stories heard. In methods triangulation, researchers compare information gathered through a variety of techniques to see if the messages remain consistent. Researcher triangulation involves multiple researchers coding and interpreting the data to see if they draw similar conclusions (Patton, 2002).

As an example of qualitative research, consider a study in which adolescent women participate in interviews to understand their decisions to begin and continue sexual activity. Researchers selected 10 late-adolescent women and recorded 45–60 minute interviews with each of them. Participants were allowed to review the interview to verify accuracy. Researchers then arranged the data into narratives with beginning, middle, and end; content analysis was used to identify and code themes that emerged in the narratives. For these women, curiosity, a college culture that encouraged sex, and feeling pressure from older, "experienced" male partners contributed to their sexual debut and continued sexual activity (Fantasia, 2011).

Mixed Methods Studies

Sometimes a research question is best answered with a mix of quantitative and qualitative techniques. Researchers may decide to use both methods in order to bolster the evidence for their conclusions, clarify their findings, and discover new information that can reframe their original research question. The overarching goal of mixed methods research is to draw on the strengths and minimize the weaknesses of qualitative and quantitative designs (Miller & Salkind, 2002). Several of the ways researchers combine qualitative and quantitative methods are gathering and analyzing qualitative data and then using it to develop a tool to collect quantitative data; gathering both qualitative and quantitative data simultaneously and combining results, and gathering qualitative data, studying it to determine themes, and then numerically counting these themes (Creswell, Fetters, & Ivankova, 2004).

For example, mixed methods were employed in one study to examine (qualitatively and quantitatively) differences between public and private insurance coverage types. In-depth interviews were conducted with a small cohort of the overall study population. The findings from these interviews were used to guide the quantitative analysis of existing data (DeVoe, Wallace, Selph, Westfall, & Crocker, 2010).

INTERNAL AND EXTERNAL VALIDITY

MCH researchers less frequently employ experimental research designs than nonexperimental, quasi-experimental, and qualitative or mixed methods designs. Nevertheless, experimental designs sit at the top of the hierarchy of research supporting evidence-based practice. Demand is growing for public health practitioners to improve the field's ability to make decisions by applying more rigorous analytical research methods and study designs (Brownson, Baker, Leet, Gillespie, & True, 2011). Meta-analyses and comprehensive, systematic reviews of experimental research designs provide the highest level of quantitative evidence, followed by experimental, well-controlled research studies (Campbell & Stanley, 1966; Petitti, 2000). Cohort studies and carefully conducted case-control studies sit lower in the hierarchy, with descriptive studies (case series, cross-sectional and ecological analyses, case-control study designs applied to administrative or single center databases) still lower in the hierarchy of evidence.

Regardless of the design of a study, researchers must take pains to ensure study validity, both internal validity (scientific integrity of research protocol implementation) and external validity, or validity of inference (relevance of study conclusions to other populations and settings).

In quantitative research, internal validity depends on the statistical methods used to analyze the data and the accuracy of the interpretation of statistical results. Internal validity in qualitative research depends on use of triangulation to make sure that researchers are interpreting data consistently and with minimal influence of bias. External validity of quantitative research largely rests on how representative the study sample is of the entire target population. It also depends on the research method chosen. Generally, research designs at higher levels of evidence tend to provide more valid results. Typically, experimental research designs make some sacrifice of external validity in the zeal to make the strongest possible case for the internal validity of their findings. Cross-sectional study designs often provide limited internal validity, but their results, within the

context of the study questions posed, can be generalized more broadly. External validity for qualitative research is more of a challenge because the sample chosen is usually not randomized and is often much smaller than the sample size for qualitative research. However, qualitative research's ability to explore questions about meaning and underlying cause make it an essential research tool.

At state and local public health levels, MCH practitioners, in order to address myriad emerging need priorities, are routinely faced with selecting an intervention strategy from a host of highly touted "best practices" and must rely on the professional literature to provide a rational basis for their decision making. Assessing each report's study design for potential threats to validity of inference is an accepted approach (Cooper, 1989). Applying experimental research designs to MCH studies and completing well-structured meta-analyses and systematic reviews to address pressing issues of health policy and risk factor epidemiology will ensure that public health actions are based on scientific evidence and thereby increase accountability.

DATA: TYPES AND SOURCES

A crucial step in the development of a research or evaluation design is the selection of the data source(s). Researchers must decide whether to collect their own data or to use an existing database. Good quality secondary databases, covering in detail a wide array of MCH populations and topics, are increasingly available to researchers at a time when research funding for primary data collection is constrained (Boslaugh, 2007). Not only must researchers choose between using primary and secondary data, they must also justify their choice in terms of data acquisition costs, study duration costs, the quality, completeness and availability of needed data elements, and the potential validity and broad generalizability of results.

Secondary data for research is attractive for several reasons. It saves time that would be required for collecting primary data, and it lowers the cost that would be associated with this process (Stewart, 1984). To the extent that a secondary database can answer the same research question more quickly and at lower cost, the funder of the research receives better value for the research investment. Moreover, secondary databases can often provide extensive information on a large number of cases. Population-based secondary data, such as vital records, provide multiyear data on entire populations. The National Longitudinal Study of Adolescent Health (AddHealth) (http://www.cpc.unc.edu/projects/addhealth) and the Early Childhood Longitudinal Study-Birth Cohort (ECLS-B) (http://nces.ed.gov/ecls/birth.asp) are examples of representative surveys or studies that offer extensive collections of variables. The results of studies using these databases have broad generalizability compared with the more limited representativeness of studies using primary data collected from a single, local population. A list of secondary databases and potential sources of secondary data is provided in Table 17–5.

Notwithstanding these attributes, several problems are associated with the use of secondary data. Being restricted to the variables contained on the data set is a basic limitation of secondary data. The primary collection of data affords researchers the opportunity to select their own variables of interest and to decide how these variables will be measured, collected, and coded. This allows researchers to proceed from a theoretical or conceptual model to the determination of the operational definitions that will be employed to collect specific data elements or values from each individual case. In contrast, researchers using a secondary database must work with the data elements that are available. This presents a scientific and creative challenge.

At the international level, procuring secondary data useful for comparison and analysis is challenging because of incomplete surveillance in low-resource and conflict settings and because of differences in definitions and measurement tools. For example, the World Health Organization publishes data on neonatal mortality rates across the globe. However, many of these numbers are generated by mathematical model predictions rather than actual counts. (World Health Organization, 2010). In addition, the Demographic and Health Surveys (DHS) are nationally representative household surveys that provide data for various population, health, and nutrition indicators in developing nations.

Researchers using secondary data must start from a theoretical base with specific research hypotheses in mind. Being unable to specify the operational definitions of their research constructs, they must move backward from the available data elements to determine whether the existing variables can be used, manipulated, or combined in such a manner as to provide conceptually valid indicators that will be useful for their own research purposes. This task involves both science and ingenuity. For example, the reported biological age initially collected on a database can be reformulated in a secondary analysis as a measure of legal status or age of majority. Income and occupation variables can be combined into a measure of status inconsistency. The art of secondary data analysis entails the creative reconceptualization and manipulation of existing variables into cogent new measures. When elegantly done, it would almost appear that the original data elements were collected for the specific purpose of the secondary analysis.

Bias and Threats to Valid Interpretation of Data and Results

Secondary databases can be very important for research, planning, evaluation, and needs assessment in MCH. These databases can provide powerful evidence for new policy initiatives or justification for ongoing program activities. However, the use of these databases entails complex measurement issues.

Table 17–5 MCH-Related Secondary Data Sources*

A. National Vital Records (National Center for Health Statistics [NCHS])
   1. Live Births
   2. Fetal Deaths
   3. Induced Abortions
   4. Infant Deaths
   5. Marriages
   6. Divorces
   7. Linked Live Birth-Infant Death Files
   8. Matched Linked Multiple Pregnancy Files
   9. Maternally linked/transgenerational birth outcomes files

B. National Health and Medical Records Surveys (NCHS)
   1. National Hospital Discharge Survey
   2. Family Planning Reporting Survey

C. National Population-Based Surveys (NCHS)
   1. National Health Interview Survey
   2. National Health and Nutrition Examination Survey
   3. Hispanic Health and Nutrition Examination Survey
   4. National Survey of Family Growth
   5. Ambulatory Medical Care Survey
   6. Nursing Home Survey
   7. Medical Care Utilization and Expenditure Survey
   8. National Survey of Children's Health
   9. National Survey of Children with Special Health Care Needs
   10. National Immunization Survey

D. Other Sources of National Data
   1. Census Bureau
   2. Centers for Disease Control and Prevention
      a. Pregnancy Risk Assessment and Monitoring System
      b. Developmental Disability Surveillance
      c. Teenage Pregnancy Surveillance
      d. Birth Defects Surveillance
      e. Assisted Reproductive Technology
      f. State and Local Area Integrated Telephone Survey
      g. Youth Risk Behavior Surveillance System
   3. Consumer Product Safety Commission
   4. FBI: Uniform Crime Reports
   5. National Institute for Occupational Health and Safety
      a. Traumatic Occupational Fatality
      b. Fatal Accident Circumstances
   6. United States Department of Agriculture
      a. Special Supplemental Food Program for Women, Infants, and Children
      b. Pregnancy Nutrition Surveillance System
      c. Pediatric Nutrition Surveillance System
   7. Indian Health Service

E. State and Local Data Sources
   1. State Vital Records
      a. Live Births
      b. Fetal Deaths

(Continued)

Table 17–5 (Continued)*

---

    c. Induced Abortions
    d. Spontaneous Losses
    e. Infant Deaths
    f. Marriages
    g. Divorces
  2. State and local health and social service programs
    a. Prenatal Care Programs
    b. Special Supplemental Food Program for Women, Infants, and Children
    c. Immunization
    d. Child Abuse Reporting
    e. Foster Care
    f. Juvenile Corrections
    g. Social Services
    h. Adoptions
    i. Child Health
    j. Newborn Screening and Hearing Screening
    k. Children with Special Health Care Needs
    l. Child Lead Exposure
  3. State Medical Societies
  4. State Hospital Associations
  5. School Systems
  6. Community Health Centers
  7. Poison Control Centers
  8. State Registries: Tumor, cancer, birth defects, head trauma, spinal cord injury, pregnancy-associated mortality
  9. State Medicaid
  10. State Vital Records
  11. Medical Registry Boards
  12. Police and Fire departments
  13. Wildlife, Hunting, and Boating departments

F. Other Data Sources
  1. Insurance Companies
  2. Private medical records
  3. Hospital and Health Maintenance Organization medical records

G. Sources for International Data
  1. World Health Organization Global Health Observatory
  2. World Bank World Development Indicators
  3. United Nations Children's Fund (UNICEF)
  4. Demographic and Health Surveys
  5. National Ministries of Health or Health Departments in foreign countries

---

*Some of these datasets are limited to only selected states or countries

---

Knowledge of the database and the coding of the variables they contain are essential to prevent simplistic and erroneous interpretations of the data. Discussing inherent problems in secondary databases like vital records should not dampen enthusiasm for their use. These data are extremely useful. In particular, vital record data sets may offer benefits not available in hospital or medical record databases because of their coverage of entire populations over time and the increasing application of error checking programs by states.

Using and interpreting data elements that have been collected, coded, and recoded by others is one of the major difficulties in using secondary data. To analyze secondary data appropriately or to interpret the results of such analyses, a good working knowledge of the database is essential. This includes understanding variable definitions, reporting completeness and accuracy, and variable recoding strategies. As decisions about data measurement may produce unexpected biases, the credible use of secondary data for research and policy requires an indepth assessment of the data, a careful and detailed documentation of the data coding procedures, and a cautious interpretation of the results (Ananth, 2005; Kirby, 2001).

Several challenges threaten accurate interpretation of secondary data. Although also complicating the processing and analysis of primary data, the "finished" appearance of a secondary database or analysis might make them less apparent. The remainder of this section is devoted to a discussion of the fundamental threats to the accurate interpretation of these data. These include:

- Missing data
- Out-of-range data
- Bivariate inconsistency
- Interpreting small and large numbers
- Concept validity
- Equating risk or association with cause

Several state vital record databases will illustrate examples of these threats. State vital record data, specifically, Certificates of Live Birth and Infant Death, are commonly used data for MCH research, evaluation, and needs assessment efforts. Although many questions have been raised regarding their accuracy, these vital record data continue to be widely used for MCH program planning and evaluation.

Missing Data

The first threat to accurate data interpretation involves the completeness of data reporting and the treatment of missing data. Missing or incomplete data can create major interpretation problems because it is uncertain whether cases with missing data are similar to or markedly different from those with completely recorded information. Researchers must consider whether calculating rates and percentages only from existing data is appropriate. There are good reasons to assume that cases with missing data are different from those with complete data. For example, several studies have noted that women whose birth certificates are missing gestational age data are more likely to have lower educational attainment and other indicators of lower socioeconomic status (Buekens, Delvoye, Wollast, & Robyn, 1984; David, 1980; Taffel, Johnson, & Heuser, 1982; Wenner & Young, 1974). As these women may have a higher risk of preterm delivery, we may suspect that cases with missing gestational age information may actually have a different gestational age distribution than those with reported gestational age information.

Sometimes the ways in which data are combined or presented obscure the issue of missing data. A notable example is the Institute of Medicine's "Index of Adequacy of Prenatal Care" (Kessner, Singer, Kalk, & Schlesinger, 1973). In this index, cases with missing prenatal care data were traditionally classified as receiving inadequate prenatal care, whereas cases with missing gestational age data were excluded from the index. Using Minnesota data from 1990 to 1991 (Table 17–6), we observed that, depending on the treatment of missing cases, the proportion of infants with mothers adequately using prenatal care is either 62.9% or 74.5%.

If the 15.7% with missing data have the same pattern of prenatal care use as those with completed data, then the 74.5% figure may be a good estimate of adequate

Table 17-6 Adequacy of Prenatal Care, 1990–1991 Minnesota Live Births

All Cases	Only Complete Cases
62.9% Adequate	74.5% Adequate
21.4% Less than adequate	25.5% Less than Adequate
15.7% Missing	

prenatal care use. However, if cases with missing data are less likely to adequately use prenatal care, then the 75% would be an overestimate.

Having missing data on the date of last normal menses (DLNM), a key variable needed to calculate the gestational age interval, which in turn is used to compute adequacy of prenatal care indices, is a well-recognized problem. Nationwide, an appreciable percentage of birth certificates have missing or incomplete DLNM data. A state-level report indicated variations in missing DLNM data ranging from approximately 5% to 30% (Alexander, Petersen, Tompkins, Zinzeleta, & Jones, 1990). Reporting varied by year. In South Carolina, the percentage of missing DLNM data was 31% in 1974 but less than 3% by 1990 (Alexander, Tompkins, & Cornely, 1990). Because the percentage of missing adequacy of prenatal care data will exceed the percentage of missing gestational age data, an abrupt change in the proportion missing DLNM data, or major differences in the percentage missing between population groups can lead to the misinterpretation of prenatal care statistics (Alexander, Tompkins, Petersen, & Weiss, 1991). In secondary analyses, researchers must give careful attention to the proportion of cases with missing values and the treatment of these cases when computing new variables and the effect of missing data on the resulting indices should be clearly reported.

Out-of-Range Data

Out-of-range data present another fundamental problem for secondary data analysis. The proportion of out-of-range data is often not reported because conventions for defining such data may not exist or are variable specific. Out-of-range data are those considered biologically implausible or those outside the normally expected range. This problem primarily concerns continuous variables. The problem with defining out-of-range data is determining the specific values that define the limits of the valid range. For example, although 10 to 50 years may seem like a reasonable range to use to define valid ages of mother, recent reports of live births to an 8-year-old and to women in their 50s or older have increased the difficulty in selecting these cutoff points. Because some health status measures are typically described in terms like "less than 2500 grams" for low birth weight or "less than 37 weeks" for preterm delivery," improbable and clearly erroneous values may be inadvertently included in the calculation of percentages of low birth weight and preterm delivery. If cases with out-of-range values are included in the calculation of percentages and rates, for example, preterm and very low birth weight, the resulting rates may be inflated. Setting precise limits that define the data values considered plausible can prevent this error.

Out-of-range data are a particular concern for investigations of cases at the extreme tails of distributions, for example, very low birth weight, macrosomia, very preterm and postterm delivery, preteen pregnancy, and intrauterine growth restriction. When secondary data are used for investigations of these topics, decisions made regarding the treatment of out-of-range data should be well documented.

Bivariate Inconsistency

A data value may appear accurate until compared with another; then it may become apparent that one is incorrect. This threat to accurate data interpretation is known as bivariate inconsistency. A fairly typical example of this is a case with a birth weight of 3,700 grams and a gestational age of 22 weeks. Such combinations are virtually impossible. Tables have been developed to identify cases with implausible or inconsistent birth weight and gestational age values (e.g., Alexander, Himes, Kaufman, Mor, & Kogan, 1996). Other combinations of variables that can be checked for inconsistency include maternal age and parity or age and education. Checking for bivariate inconsistency is a good strategy when employing a secondary database and can reveal important information about the potential accuracy of the data that would not be evident from merely assessing the proportion of data that is missing or out of range.

Interpreting Small and Large Numbers

The next threat to accurate data interpretation involves large and small numbers. Vital record databases are attractive because they represent entire populations and, as such, contain a large number of cases from which to draw inferences. Nevertheless, despite large sample sizes, many of the health status indicators monitored are relatively rare events. For example, infant death rates, either based on a small number of births or a small number of deaths, are subject to considerable fluctuation. Highs and lows may not reflect prevailing trends.

Large numbers are also a problem. Reliance on statistical tests can interfere with the appropriate interpretation of the data. Statistical testing is most useful for samples. For large populations such as national U.S. birth certificate files, the majority of statistical comparisons will be significant based on large numbers alone; although "significant," they may not signify a meaningful public health or clinical concern. For example,

Table 17–7 Infant Mortality Rates by Military Status and Ethnicity, 1979–1989, Single Live Births to Adult, Married Hawaii Resident Women

	White	Black
Military	6.8	9.7
Nonmilitary	5.1	16.8
Significance	p < 0.01	NS
N	52,720	5,333

using data from Hawaii (Table 17–7), we note that the infant mortality rates vary significantly by military status among whites, although the actual difference is relatively moderate.

Among African Americans, the difference in infant mortality rates by military status is quite marked but is not significant. The differences in the number of live births among military status and ethnic groups underlie the results of the significance tests.

Construct Validity

The selection of a health status indicator for research, evaluation, or needs assessment involves a good conceptualization about what the indicator measures. At issue here is construct validity, a fundamental predicament in interpreting data. For example, gestational age refers to a unit of time between conception and birth, but this term is commonly used to refer to a host of other measures of fetal and newborn physical and neurologic maturity that are highly correlated with, but conceptually distinct from, gestational age (Alexander, Tompkins, Hulsey, Petersen, & Mor, 1995; Wilcox, 2010). Furthermore, using neonatal and postneonatal time periods to differentiate endogenous–exogenous causes of death has been a hallmark in perinatal research but has been soundly criticized as no longer conceptually valid (Kirby, 1993).

Sometimes the stated title of the indicator may seem out of line with the strategy employed to measure it. The term teen pregnancy is a good example of a health status indicator without a well-established measurement convention. Thirteen to 19 years of age are technically the teenage years, but younger than 18, the age of majority, is often used in research. As seen in the U.S. national data presented in Table 17–8, the risk of low birth weight to the infant of a 19-year-old mother is quite distinct from that of a 13 year old.

The inclusion of 18- and 19-year-old mothers in the teenage group greatly inflates the numbers and percentages of teenage mothers while reducing the level of the associated risks observed to the group.

Investigating the impact of prenatal care often involves discussing the conceptual premise for the indices used to describe prenatal care (Alexander & Kotelchuck, 1996, 2001). In Table 17–9, low and very low birth weight percentages are displayed by two different indices: (1) a modification of the original Institute of Medicine (IOM) index developed in the 1960s and (2) an updated version of this index using the latest standards for prenatal care visits recommended by the American College of Obstetrics and Gynecology.

The strength of the relationship between adequacy of prenatal care and birth weight is

dependent on the index used. The American College of Obstetricians and Gynecologists (ACOG) index results in a lower proportion of cases in the adequate category, and the adequate category no longer has the lowest percentage of moderately low birth weight infants. Neither index shows a strong relationship to very low birth weight.

Table 17–8 Low Birth Weight by Age of Mother, 2000–2002, Single Live Births to U.S. Residents.

Age of Mother	Number	Percentage of Low Birth Weight
11	17	28.8
12	104	17.0
13	586	15.1
14	2,428	12.0
15	6,724	11.2
16	14,301	10.6
17	23,409	9.8
18	35,133	9.5
19	44,810	8.7
< 18	47,569	10.4
< 20	127,512	9.5

Table 17–9 Very Low (VLBW) and Moderately Low Birth Weight (MLBW) Percentages by Two Measures of Adequacy of Prenatal Care U.S., 2001–2002, Single Live Births to U.S. Residents.

	MODIFIED IOM*			ACOG†		
	Percent	%VLBW	%MLBW	Percent	%VLBW	%MLBW
Adequate	71.88	0.93	4.36	46.64	1.42	5.81
Intermediate	17.61	1.16	6.12	38.95	0.53	3.53
Inadequate	4.08	0.87	7.30	7.98	0.50	5.31
No care	1.00	6.26	13.31	1.00	6.26	13.31
Missing	5.43	2.43	6.24	5.43	2.43	6.24
	100.00			100.00		

*IOM (Institute of Medicine)
†ACOG (American College of Obstetricians and Gynecologists

Construct validity should not be confused with content validity. Some indices or measures do not provide full coverage of the concept they measure. For example, prenatal care use indices address only the quantity of visits and do not consider the quality or content of care received. These indices may also exclude other forms of prenatal care.

Equating Risk or Association with Cause

Another threat to data interpretation is improperly distinguishing causal factors from risk factors. Rarely are causal relationships being investigated, for example, a relationship where a variable is a direct biological precursor. Most investigations focus on risk factors, for example, factors that are associated with an increased chance of a poor outcome. Although a characteristic may be a risk factor, not all individuals with that factor will experience negative outcomes.

These national data (Table 17–10) examine low birth weight percentages by age of mother and prenatal care use.

Teen mothers (less than 18 years of age) have a higher percentage of low birth weight (9.56%) than adult mothers (5.95%). Nevertheless, nearly 95% of total low birth weight births occur to adult mothers. Eliminating all teen pregnancies would reduce the number of total low birth weight infants by only 6%.

Similarly, note the higher low birth weight percentages to mothers with no or inadequate prenatal care. Over 80% of the low birth weight infants are to mothers with adequate or intermediate use of prenatal care. Certainly, the young age of mother and no prenatal care use, as measured here, are associated with a low birth weight. Still, it cannot be concluded that even eliminating both of these risk factors will reduce as much as 10% of the low birth weight problem.

ETHICS

Although research should follow the highest ethical standards, public health research in the United States has not historically met that goal. Research, concerned as it is with the pursuit of knowledge and truth, must be equally concerned with the integrity and purity of the research process. Ethical considerations must be paramount in all phases of the research process from conceptualization through study design, data gathering,

Table 17–10 Low Birth Weight (LBW) by Age of Mother and Prenatal Care, 2001–2002, Single Live Births to U.S. Residents.

Age of Mother	% Distribution	% LBW*	% LBW Distribution
< 18	3.79	9.56	5.96
18+	96.21	5.98	94.04
Prenatal Care			
Adequate	71.88	5.29	62.49
Intermediate	17.61	7.28	21.07
Inadequate	4.08	8.18	5.48
No care	1.00	19.57	3.22
Missing	5.43	8.67	7.74

*LBW (low birth weight: < 2500 grams)

analysis, and reporting of results. Although all researchers should maintain vigilance in ensuring the highest ethical quality of their own work to retain credibility in individual studies, for the sake of the entire field of science research should be conducted in the most scrupulous manner in order to contribute accurate information to the larger knowledge base in a way that it will be believed and ultimately used in the promotion of health and quality of life.

Because of the importance of research in MCH, research must be undertaken within accepted standards of ethical conduct. Unethical conduct in research includes falsifying data, deliberately misclassifying study subjects and controls, deliberately mishandling data, and failing to disclose fully how data were manipulated (e.g., how missing or outlier variables were handled). Mistakes can happen in research, and even these can call into question the credibility of the result. Deliberate misconduct such as withholding treatment or failing to disclose any increased risks due to participation in the research can cast doubt on the entire scientific enterprise and result in public reluctance to engage in future research or to accept research findings.

Several ethical concerns are specific to the field of MCH. Research involving children and pregnant women requires a higher degree of scrutiny because of the vulnerability of the population under study. Researchers must be very careful when considering how to assure informed consent with these populations, how to treat subjects justly, how to maintain the confidentiality of the data collected, and how to minimize harm to the research subjects. Institutional review boards pay particular attention to these issues when the research subjects include children or pregnant women because of the potential for harm from the research study itself, harm from the intentional or inadvertent disclosure of information, or harm from insufficient attempts to fully explain the nature of the study when seeking consent to participate. The fact that infants and children cannot consent for themselves makes them uniquely vulnerable to ethical lapses.

The issues surrounding research with human subjects are so important to the integrity of the research process that the National Institutes of Health (NIH), the largest government research entity in the country, has a website devoted to resources on bioethics in research and on the use of human subjects (bioethics.od.nih.gov/). Every federally funded research institution in the United States requires this education, and every institution maintains an active institutional review board designed to review thoroughly every research proposal generated within the institution for its adherence to research ethics and standards relating to human subjects in research.

REVIEWING THE LITERATURE

MCH practitioners, as well as students and faculty, often must make decisions based not on their own knowledge or research but solely on information available in the professional literature. Their ability to review and synthesize the literature is therefore a critical part of their decision-making process. Equally important is the quality of the literature itself. Here again, the MCH professional plays an invaluable role by serving as a reviewer for peer-reviewed, professional journals and by contributing manuscripts describing scientifically rigorous research.

A fundamental part of gaining research experience is reviewing the research of others. There are two main methods for conducting synthesis of existing research. One is a systematic review. Systematic reviews retrieve all of the literature on a specified topic and organize the results to determine the strength of evidence for or against a particular intervention or hypothesis. Systematic reviews may consider both qualitative and quantitative data (Riegelman, 2005).

Another kind of synthesis is a meta-analysis. Meta-analyses pool the sample populations from multiple studies by independent researchers on a specified topic and use statistical tests to draw conclusions about a hypothesis. Unlike systematic reviews, which offer qualitative comments on a body of literature, meta-analyses are mathematical syntheses (Miller & Salkind, 2002).

Research syntheses are beneficial because they provide a more conclusive picture of the truth about a particular issue by drawing from the results of multiple studies. They have several potential weaknesses, though. Publication bias distorts literature review results; it occurs when research that fails to find significant results is not published and thus is inaccessible to reviewers. A unique challenge for meta-analysis is diversity of sample populations. Combining sample groups for mathematical calculation can yield inaccurate or simply unhelpful results if the groups are not comparable. Researchers must take care to select studies based on defined criteria to overcome this obstacle.

The use of an organized approach to reviewing a scientific research article allows the reviewer to critically assess variable measurement issues, study design, statistical analysis, and ethics. It also provides a structure for the development of manuscripts that report research. There are a number of references that outline a structure for reviewing articles and organizing materials into a manuscript for submission for publication (Alexander, 2005; Vintzileos & Ananth, 2010).

CONCLUSION

Although MCH's traditional orientation to public health practice, policy, and advocacy lends an applied focus to MCH research, it is supported and given credibility by an underpinning of scientific evidence. In a culture that demands evidence-based accountability, the MCH practitioner and MCH researcher are interdependent and need a basic background in each other's domains in order for our research to be relevant and our practice to be cost effective. The importance of communication between MCH researchers and practitioners for the dissemination and application of scientific information is highlighted by the popular slogan "from data to action." This phrase describes part of a needed cycle of collaboration that can be drawn full circle for the benefit of the MCH population by adding "from action to research" to our vision to ensure that we evaluate what we do and continually refine and, as needed, retarget our practice and policy endeavors.

The fundamental elements of science and research (i.e., hypothesis testing, empirical data measurement, study design, statistical analysis) are the same for MCH as for any other field within public health. Advanced graduate-level training in the principles and tools of research is often initially compartmentalized by discipline with study design falling within epidemiology courses, statistical analysis techniques coming from biostatistics, and measurement theory sometimes being taught by health behavioral sciences. Nevertheless, these different elements of research are interconnected in the actual practice of research. Like legs of a tripod, a failure in one may seriously compromise the ultimate utility of a study. Strength in one area, for example, an experimental study designed to limit possible threats to validity of inference, cannot fully compensate for clear weakness in another area, such as poor reliability and validity of measurement of the key variables. Inevitably, no research study is without flaw. Thus, the strength of our scientific method comes from its emphasis on persistent testing and retesting. Occasionally, one study makes a breakthrough, but overall, lasting advances are based on the contributions of many researchers whose work at exploring, replicating, and refining new approaches may stretch across several careers from mentor to students to the next generation, all pursuing a similar research agenda.

The health status and healthcare use concerns facing MCH are so complex that it is unlikely these seemingly intractable problems will be resolved in one generation of research. For example, the topic of racial disparities in perinatal health is hardly new and has attracted research attention for more than a half-century. Such intractable problems highlight the need for the MCH field to maintain a strong emphasis on research and research training to ensure that there will be an ongoing cadre of investigators committed to the important research issues and health problems of the MCH population.

References

Agency for Healthcare Research and Quality. (2001). Background. In *Community-based participatory research: Conference summary*. Retrieved May 15, 2011 from http://www.ahrq.gov/research/cbpr/cbpr1.htm#backround.

Alexander, G. R. (2003). Maternal and child health. In, M. J. Stahl, (Ed.). *Encyclopedia of health care management*. Knoxville, TN: Sage Publications.

Alexander, G. R. (2005). A guide to reviewing manuscripts. *Maternal and Child Health Journal*, 9(1), 113–117.

Alexander, G. R., & Kotelchuck, M. (1996). A comparison of prenatal care indices: Classification of adequacy of prenatal care use. *Public Health Reports*, 111, 408–418.

Alexander, G. R., & Kotelchuck, M. (2001). Assessing the role and effectiveness of prenatal care: History, challenges, and directions for future research. *Public Health Reports*, 116, 306–316.

Alexander, G. R., & Petersen, D. J. (2004). MCH needs assessment capacity shows improvement; but, meager MCH evaluation capacity may impede performance (editorial). *Maternal and Child Health Journal*, 8, 103–105.

Alexander, G. R., Himes, J. H., Kaufman, R., Mor, J., & Kogan, M. (1996). A US national reference for fetal growth. *Obstetrics & Gynecology*, 87, 163–168.

Alexander, G. R., Petersen, D. J., Pass, M. A., Slay, M., Chadwick, C., & Shumpert. (2002). Maternal and child health/public health milestones, history and philosophy (Vol. I–XII). Birmingham, AL: University of Alabama at Birmingham Department of Maternal and Child Health, MCH Leadership Skills Training Institute. Retrieved May 19, 2011 from http://images.main.uab.edu/isoph/MCH/Tech_Reports/MCH_History/.

Alexander, G. R., Petersen, D. J., Tompkins, M. E., Zinzeleta, E., & Jones, M. D. (1990). *The DHHS Region III perinatal data and chart book*. Baltimore, MD: School of Hygiene and Public Health, Johns Hopkins University and Region III Perinatal Information Consortium, Bureau of Maternal and Child Health, U.S. Department of Health and Human Services.

Alexander, G. R., Tompkins, M. E., & Cornely, D. A. (1990). Gestational age reporting and preterm delivery. *Public Health Reports*, 105, 267–275.

Alexander, G. R., Tompkins, M. E., Hulsey, T. C., Petersen, D. J., & Mor, J. M. (1995). Discordance between LMP-based and clinically estimated gestational age: Implications for research, programs and policy. *Public Health Reports*, 110, 395–402.

Alexander, G. R., Tompkins, M. E., Petersen, D. J., & Weiss, J. (1991). Sources of bias in prenatal care utilization indices: Implications for evaluating the Medicaid expansion. *American Journal of Public Health*, 81, 1013–1016.

Ananth, C. V. (2005). Perinatal epidemiologic research with vital statistics data: validity is the essential quality. *American Journal of Obstetrics and Gynecology*, 193(1), 5–6.

Bartholomew, L. K., Parcel, G. S., Kok, G., & Gottlieb, N. H. (2001). Intervention mapping step 5: Planning for evaluation. In L. K. Bartholomew, G. S. Parcel, G. Kok, & N. H. Gottlieb. *Intervention mapping* (pp. 320–352). Mountain View: Mayfield Publishing Company.

Behrman, R. E., & Butler A. S. (Eds.). (2007). *Preterm birth: Causes, consequences, and prevention*. Institute of Medicine Committee on Understanding Premature Birth and Assuring Healthy Outcomes. Washington, DC: National Academies Press.

Bhutta, Z. A., Chopra, M., Axelson, H., Berman, P., Boerma, T., Bryce, J., & Wardlaw, T. (2010). Countdown to 2015 decade report (2000-10): Taking stock of maternal, newborn, and child survival. *Lancet*, 376(9743), 2032–2044.

Bhutta, Z. A., Rizvi, A., Raza, F., Hotwani, S., Zaidi, S., Hossain, M., & Bhutta, S. (2009). A comparative evaluation of multiple micro-nutrient and iron-folic acid supplementation during Pregnancy in Pakistan: Impact on pregnancy outcomes. *Food and Nutrition Bulletin, 30*(4, Supp.), S496–S505.

Bingenheimer, J. B., & Raudenbush, S. W. (2004). Statistical and substantive inferences in public health: Issues in the application of multilevel models. *Annual Review of Public Health, 25,* 53–77.

Bordens, K. S., & Abbott, B. B. (2002). *Research design and methods: A process approach* (5th ed.). Boston: McGraw-Hill.

Boslaugh, S. (2007). *Secondary data sources for public health: A practical guide.* Practical guides to biostatistics and epidemiology. New York: Cambridge University Press.

Bowling, A. (2009). *Research methods in health: Investigating health and health services* (3rd ed.). Berkshire, UK: Open University Press

Boyd, P. A., Haeusler, M., Barisic, I., Loane, M., Garne, E., & Dolk, H. (2011). Paper 1: The EUROCAT network—organization and processes. *Birth defects research. Part A, Clinical and molecular teratology, 91*(Suppl. 1), S2–S15.

Braveman, P., & Barclay, C. (2009). Health disparities beginning in childhood: A life course perspective. *Pediatrics, 124*(Suppl. 3), S163–S175.

Bronfenbrenner, U. (1979). *The ecology of human development.* Cambridge, MA: Harvard University Press.

Bronowski, J. (1967). *The common sense of science.* Cambridge: Harvard University Press.

Brownson, R. C., Baker, E. A., Leet, T. L., Gillespie, K. N., & True, W. R. (2011). *Evidence-based public health.* Oxford, UK: Oxford University Press.

Brunner, I., & Guzman, A. (1989). Participatory evaluation: A tool to assess and empower people. In R. F. Connor & M. H. Hendricks (Eds.). *New directions for program evaluation: International innovations in evaluation methodology* (no. 42, pp. 9–17). San Francisco: Jossey-Bass Publishers.

Bryson, S. E., Zwaigenbaum, L., Brian, J., Roberts, W., Szatmari, P., Rombough, V., & McDermott, C. (2007). A prospective case series of high risk infants who developed autism. *Journal of Autism and Developmental Disorders, 37,* 12–24.

Buekens, P., Delvoye, P., Wollast, E., & Robyn, C. (1984). Epidemiology of pregnancies with unknown last menstrual period. *Journal of Epidemiology and Community Health, 38,* 79–80.

Campbell, D. T., & Stanley, J. C. (1963, 1966). *Experimental and quasi-experimental designs for research.* Chicago, IL: Rand McNally.

Cargo, M., & Mercer, S. L. (2008). The values and challenges of participatory research: Strengthening its practice. *Annual Review of Public Health, 29,* 325–350.

Carmines, E. G., & Zeller, R. A. (1979). *Reliability and validity assessment: Quantitative applications in the social sciences series,* Number 07-017. Beverly Hills, CA: Sage Publications.

Chelimsky, E. (1997). The political environment of evaluation and what it means for the development of the field. In E. Chelimsky & W. R. Shadish (Eds.), *Evaluation for the 21st century* (pp. 53–68). Thousand Oaks, CA: Sage Publications.

Chen, H. (2005). *Practical program evaluation: Assessing and improving implementation and effectiveness.* Thousand Oaks, CA: Sage Publications.

Cooper, H. M. (1989). *Integrating research: A guide for literature reviews* (2nd ed.). Applied social research methods series (Vol. 2). Newbury Park, CA: Sage Publications.

Creswell, J. W. (2008). *Research design: Qualitative, quantitative, and mixed methods approaches.* Thousand Oaks, CA: Sage Publications.

Creswell, J. W., Fetters, M. D., & Ivankova, N. V. (2004). Designing a mixed methods study in primary care. *Annals of Family Medicine, 2,* 7–12.

Cromley, E. K. & McLafferty, S. L. (2011). *GIS and public health* (2nd ed.). New York: Guilford Press.

Culhane, J. F., & Elo, I. T. (2005). Neighborhood context and reproductive health. *American Journal of Obstetrics and Gynecology, 192,* 522–529.

David, R. J. (1980). The quality and completeness of birth weight and gestational age data in computerized birth files. *American Journal of Public Health, 79,* 964–973.

DeVoe, J. E., Wallace, L., Selph, S., Westfall, N., & Crocker, S. (2010). Comparing type of health insurance among low-income children: A mixed-methods study from Oregon. *Maternal and Child Health Journal, 15*(8), 1238–1248, Epub. DOI: 10.1007/s10995-010-0706-4.

Diez Roux, A. V. (2000). Multilevel analysis in public health research. *Annual Review of Public Health, 21,* 171–192.

Drabick, D. A. G., & Baugh, D. (2010). A community-based approach to preventing youth violence: What can we learn from the playground? *Progress in Community Health Partnerships, 4*(3), 189–196.

Eisinger, A., & Senturia, K. (2001). Doing community-driven research: A description of Seattle partners for healthy communities. *Journal of Urban Health, 78,* 519–534.

Fantasia, H. C. (2011). Influences of social norms and context on sexual decision making among adolescent women. *Journal of Midwifery and Women's Health, 56*(1), 48–53.

Felix-Aaron, K., & Stryer, D. (2003). Moving from rhetoric to evidence-based action in health care. *Journal of General Internal Medicine, 7,* 589–591.

Fine, A. & Kotelchuck, M. (2010). *Rethinking MCH: The life course model as an organizing framework concept paper.* Version 1.1. Washington, DC: U.S. Department of Health and Human Services, Health Resources and Services Administration, Maternal and Child Health Bureau. Retrieved May 18, 2011 from http://www.hrsa.gov/ourstories/mchb75th/images/rethinkingmch.pdf.

Fitzpatrick, J. L., Sanders, J. R., & Worthen, B. R. (2004). *Program evaluation: Alternative approaches and practical guidelines.* Boston, MA: Pearson Education, Inc.

Freudenberg, N. (2001). Case history of the center for urban epidemiologic studies in New York City. *Journal of Urban Health, 78,* 508–518.

Friis, R. H., & Sellers, T. A. (1999). *Epidemiology for public health practice* (2nd ed.). Gaithersburg, MD: Aspen Publications.

Gelman, A., & Hill, J. (2006). *Data analysis using regression and multilevel/hierarchical models.* Cambridge, New York: Cambridge University Press.

Gillman, M. W., Rich-Edwards, J. W., Rifas-Shiman, S. L., Lieberman, E. S., Kleinman, K. P., & Lipshultz, S. E. (2004). Maternal age and other predictors of newborn blood pressure. *Journal of Pediatrics, 144,* 240–245.

Government Performance and Results Act of 1993. PL 102-63. (1993). Retrieved May 18, 2011 from http://www.whitehouse.gov/omb/mgmt-gpra/gplaw2m.

Greenhalgh, T., & Taylor, R. (1997). Papers that go beyond numbers (qualitative research). *British Medical Journal, 315,* 740–743.

Handler, A., Rosenberg, D., & Monahan, C. (1998). *Analytic methods in maternal and child health.* Washington, DC: Health Resources and Services Administration, Maternal and Child Health Bureau. Retrieved May 18, 2011 from http://ask.hrsa.gov/detail_materials.cfm?ProdID-1566.

Herman, J. L., Morris, L. L., & Fitz-Gibbon, C. T. (1987). *Evaluator's handbook.* Newbury Park, CA: Sage Publications.

Hill, A. B. (1965). The environment and disease: Association or causation? *Proceedings of the Royal Society of Medicine, 58,* 295–300.

Hulley, S. B., Cummings, S. R., Browner, W. S., Grady, D., & Newman, T. B. (2006). *Designing clinical research* (3rd ed.). Philadelphia: Lippincott.

Isaac, S., & Michael, B. W. (1995). *Handbook in research and evaluation for education and the behavioral sciences* (3rd ed.). San Diego: EdITS.

Kessner, D. M., Singer, J., Kalk, C. W., & Schlesinger, E. R. (1973). Infant death: An analysis by maternal risk and health care. In *Contrasts in health status* (Vol. I). Washington, DC: Institute of Medicine, National Academy of Sciences.

Kettner, P. M., Moroney, R. M., & Martin, L. L. (1990). *Designing and managing programs: An effectiveness-based approach.* Newbury Park, CA: Sage.

Kirby, R. S. (1993). Neonatal and postneonatal mortality: Useful constructs or outdated concepts? *Journal of Perinatology, 13,* 433–441.

Kirby, R. S. (2001). Invited commentary: Using vital statistics databases for perinatal epidemiology: Does the quality go in before the name goes on? *American Journal of Epidemiology, 154,* 889–890.

Kruk, M. E., Prescott, M. R., de Pinho, H., & Galea, S. (2011). Equity and the child health Millennium Development Goal: The role of pro-poor health policies. *Journal of Epidemiology and Community Health, 65*(4), 327–333.

Kuehn, B. M. (2010). National Children's Study expands. *Journal of the American Medical Association, 304*(16), 1776.

Lawoyin, T. O., Onadeko, M. O., & Asekun-Olarinmoye, E. O. (2010). Neonatal mortality and perinatal risk factors in rural Southwestern Nigeria: a community-based prospective study. *West African Journal of Medicine, 29*(1), 19–23.

Lu, M., & Halfon, N. (2003). Racial and ethnic disparities in birth outcomes: a life course perspective. *Maternal and Child Health Journal, 7*(1), 13–30.

Luke, D. A. (2004). *Multilevel modeling.* Thousand Oaks, CA: Sage Publications.

McDavid, J. C., & Hawthorn, L. R. L. (2006). *Program evaluation & performance measurement: An introduction to practice.* Thousand Oaks, CA: Sage Publications.

Maternal and Child Health Bureau, Health Resources and Services Administration. (2004). Maternal and

Child Health Needs Assessment and State Performance Measures. DHSC Technical Assistance Workshop. Retrieved October 19, 2011 from http://128.248.232.90/archives/mchb/needs2004/index.htm and http://128.248.232.90/archives/mchb/needs2004/workshop.htm.

Mays, G. P., Halverson, P. K., & Scutchfield, F. D. (2004). Making public health improvement real: the vital role of systems research. *Journal of Public Health Management and Practice, 10*, 183–185.

Mertens, D. M. (2005). *Research and evaluation in education and psychology: Integrating diversity with quantitative, qualitative, and mixed methods* (2nd ed.). Thousand Oaks, CA: Sage Publications.

Miller, D. C., & Salkind, N. J. (2002). *Handbook of research design and social measurement* (6th ed.). Newbury Park, CA: Sage.

Nunnally, J. C. (1978). *Psychometric theory* (2nd ed.). New York: McGraw-Hill.

O'Toole, T., Felix-Aaron, K., Chin, M. H., Horowitz, C., & Tyson, F. (2003). Community-based participatory research: Opportunities, challenges and the need for a common language. *Journal of General Internal Medicine, 8*, 592–594.

Omnibus Reconciliation Act of 1989 PL 101-239. (1989). Title V, Subtitle C, MCH Block Grant Program. Retrieved May 19, 2011 from http://images.main.uab.edu/isoph/MCH/Tech_Reports/MCHLegislation.pdf.

Painter, R. C., Osmond, C., Gluckman, P., Hanson, M., Phillips, D. I. W., & Roseboom, T. J. (2008). Transgenerational effects of prenatal exposure to the Dutch famine on neonatal adiposity and health in later life. *British Journal of Obstetrics and Gynaecology, 115*, 1243–1249.

Parker, E. A., Eng, E., Schulz, A. J., & Israel, B. A. (1999). Evaluating community-based health programs that seek to increase community capacity. In J. Telfair, L. C. Leviton, & J. S. Merchant (Eds.), *Evaluating health and human service programs in community settings* (Vol. 83, pp. 37–53). San Francisco: Jossey-Bass Publishers.

Patton, M. Q. (2002). *Qualitative research and evaluation methods* (3rd ed.). Thousand Oaks, CA: Sage Publications.

Patton, M. Q. (2008). *Utilization-focused evaluation* (4th ed.). Los Angeles, CA: Sage Publications.

Peoples-Sheps, M. D. & Telfair, J. (2005). Maternal and child health program monitoring and performance appraisal. In J. B. Kotch (Ed.), *Maternal and child health: Programs, problems and policy in public health* (2nd ed., pp. 583–623). Sudbury, MA: Jones and Bartlett Publishers.

Petersen, D. J., & Alexander, G. R. (2001). *Needs assessment in public health: A practical guide for students and professionals*. New York: Kluwer Academic/Plenum Publishers.

Petitti, D. B. (2000). *Meta-analysis, decision analysis, and cost-effectiveness analysis: Methods for quantitative synthesis in medicine* (2nd ed.). Oxford: Oxford University Press.

Piper, J. M., Ray, W. A., & Griffin, M. R. (1990). Effects of Medicaid expansion on prenatal care and pregnancy outcome in Tennessee. *Journal of the American Medical Association, 264*, 2219–2223.

Platt, L. J., & Hill, I. (1995, June). *Measuring systems development in Wyoming: Instruments to assess communities' progress*. Washington, DC: Health Systems Research.

Popper, K. R. (1965). *The logic of scientific discovery*. New York: Harper & Row.

Raudenbush, S. W., & Byrk, A.S. (2002). *Hierarchical linear models: Applications and data analysis methods* (2nd ed.). Thousand Oaks, CA: Sage.

Riegelman, R. K. (2005). *Studying a study and testing a test: How to read the medical evidence* (5th ed.). Philadelphia, PA: Lippincott Williams & Wilkins.

Rifas-Shiman, S. L., Sherry, B., Scanlon, K., Birch, L. L., Gillman, M. W., & Taveras, E. M.. (2011). Does maternal feeding restriction lead to childhood obesity in a prospective cohort study? *Archives of Diseases in Childhood, 96*, 265–269.

Robinson, W. S. (2009). Ecological correlations and the behaviour of individuals. *International Journal of Epidemiology, 38*, 337–341.

Rossi, P. H., & Freeman, H. E. (1993). *Evaluation: A systematic approach*. Newbury Park, CA: Sage.

Rossi, P. H., Lipsey, M. W., & Freeman, H. E. (2004a). Assessing program impact. In *Evaluation: A systematic approach* (7th ed., pp. 265–300). Thousand Oaks, CA: Sage Publications, Inc.

Rossi, P. H., Lipsey, M. W., & Freeman, H. E. (2004b). Detecting, interpreting, and analyzing program effects. In *Evaluation: A systematic approach* (7th ed., pp. 301–330. Thousand Oaks: Sage Publications, Inc.

Rothman, K. J., Greenland, S., & Lash, T. L. (2008). *Modern epidemiology* (3rd ed.). Philadelphia: Wolters Kluwer.

Schalock, R. L. (2001a). Analyzing and interpreting outcomes. In *Outcome-based evaluation* (2nd ed., pp. 195–232). New York: Kluwer Academic/ Plenum Publishers.

Schalock, R. L. (2001b). Measuring outcomes. In *Outcome-based evaluation* (2nd ed., pp. 159–194. New York: Kluwer Academic/Plenum Publishers.

Schwartz, S. (1994). The fallacy of the ecological fallacy: The potential misuse of a concept and the consequences. *American Journal of Public Health, 84*(5), 819–824.

Scutchfield, F. D., Marks, J. S., Perez, D. J., & Mays, G. P. (2007). Public health services and systems research. *American Journal of Preventive Medicine, 33*(2), 170–171.

Shadish, W. R., Cook, T. D., & Leviton, L. C. (1991). *Foundations of program evaluation.* Newbury Park, CA: Sage Publications.

Social Security Act of 1935, PL 74-271. (1935). Title V: Grants to States for Maternal and Child Welfare. Retrieved May 19, 2011 from http://images.main .uab.edu/isoph/MCH/Tech_Reports/MCHLegisla- tion.pdf.

Springett, J., & Wallerstein, N. (2008). Issues in participatory evaluation. In M. Minkler & N. Wallerstein, (Eds.). *Community-based participatory research for health: From process to outcomes* (pp. 199–220). San Francisco: Jossey-Bass Publishers.

Steckler, A., & Linnan, L. (Eds.). (2002). *Process evaluation for public health intervention and research.* San Francisco, CA: Jossey-Bass Publishers.

Stein, Z., Susser, M., Saenger, G., & Marolla, F. (1975). *Famine and human development: The Dutch Hunger Winter of 1944–1945.* Oxford University Press, New York.

Stewart, D. W. (1984). *Secondary research: Information sources and methods.* Applied social research methods series (Vol. 4). Beverly Hills, CA: Sage Publications.

Stiles, A. (2010). Case study of an intervention to enhance maternal sensitivity in adolescent mothers. *Journal of Obstetric, Gynecologic, and Neonatal Nursing, 29*, 723–733.

Taffel, S., Johnson, D., & Heuser, R. (1982). A method of imputing length of gestation on birth certificates. U.S. Department of Health and Human Services. *Vital & Health Statistics.* Data Evaluation and Methods Research Series 2, No. 93.

Telfair, J. (2005). The practice of evaluation research. In J. Kotch (Ed.), *Maternal and child health: Programs, problems and policies in public health* (2nd ed., pp. 625–649). Sudbury, MA: Jones and Bartlett Publishers.

Telfair, J., & Mulvihill, B. A. (2000). Bridging science and practice: The integrated model of community-based evaluation. *Journal of Community Practice, 7,* 37–65.

Vintzileos, A. M., & Ananth, C. V. (2010). How to write and publish an original research article. *American Journal of Obstetrics and Gynecology, 202*(4), 344. e1-6.

Weiss, C. H. (1972). *Evaluation research.* Englewood Cliffs, NJ: Prentice Hall.

Wenner, W. H., & Young, E. B. (1974). Nonspecific date of last menstrual period: An indication of poor reproductive outcome. *American Journal of Obstetrics and Gynecology, 120,* 1071–1079.

Wholey, J. S., Hatry, H. P., & Newcomer, K. E. (Eds.). (1994). *Handbook of practical program evaluation.* San Francisco, CA: Jossey-Bass Publishers.

Wilcox, A. J. (2010). *Fertility and pregnancy: An epidemiologic perspective.* Oxford University Press: New York.

World Health Organization. (2010). *Part II: Global health indicators.* Geneva, Switzerland: World Health Organization.

Zimbeck, M., Mohangoo, A., & Zeitlin, J; EURO-PERISTAT Report Writing Committee. (2009). The European perinatal health report: delivering comparable data for examining differences in maternal and infant health. *European Journal of Obstetrics, Gynecology, and Reproductive Biology, 146*(2), 149–151.

18

Assessment and Program Planning in Maternal and Child Health

Mary D. Peoples-Sheps, Pam Dickens, Diane M. Calleson, and David Janicke

Planning remains at the nexus of health care policy and regulatory choices as we enter a new century. At its core, health planning promotes the active participation of stakeholders and the public in efforts to improve the system. Planning is not antithetical to the operation of competitive markets, for all successful markets rely upon some degree of public oversight. Rather . . . planners promote accountability and help to make visible community needs that might otherwise be obscured by market forces. Ultimately planning promotes efficiency, equity, and security by providing a voice for the uninsured and the underserved in our communities. The enduring challenge of making the health care system more accountable to ordinary citizens remains.

(American Health Planning Association, 2008)

INTRODUCTION

Assessment and program planning are MCH skills that draw upon a deep knowledge of the health problems of mothers and children and apply that knowledge to produce positive changes in health status. Regardless of political climate, economic context, organizational priorities, or cultural milieu, MCH professionals are called upon repeatedly to assess, plan, and implement interventions. Program assessment and planning are essential public health services (IOM, 2002; Turnock, 2009). Virtually all MCH professionals engage in assessment and planning processes at one time or another, some specializing in assessment or program planning, whereas others incorporate these tasks into their roles as health administrators, health-care providers, and epidemiologists.

In this chapter, the steps of the assessment and planning process are described and the connection of each step to evaluation is highlighted. Linking planning with evaluation early in the process and frequently as the plan unfolds provides opportunities for a significant focus on program improvement and monitoring of the program's short- and long-term outcomes.

OVERVIEW OF THE PROCESS

Assessment and planning are carried out through a series of integrated steps shown in Figure 18–1. The steps are presented in a circular format to demonstrate that the process—problem assessment, health services needs assessment, selection of interventions, development of a logic model and setting objectives, program implementation and evaluation—is sequential and continuous. These steps are also iterative; that is, there is movement back and forth among them as new information provides opportunity for revision and refinement of earlier steps. Iteration ensures that each step uniquely influences, and is influenced by, the steps that both precede and follow it.

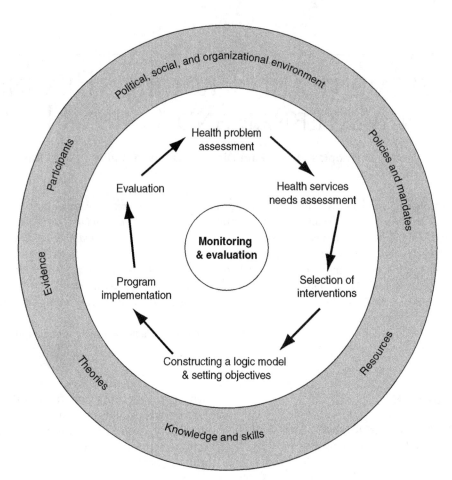

Figure 18-1 *MCH assessment and program planning.*

Evaluation is recognized at two points in the diagram. It is the final step in the overall planning process, through which information about the effectiveness of the program is generated and then used to inform the next round of assessment. Evaluation is also used throughout the planning process to monitor progress on development and implementation of the intervention and assist planners in making changes as needed.

THE CONTEXT

Figure 18-1 also identifies a number of factors that interact with the program planning process. The political, social, and organizational

environments in which planning is conducted influence whether and how a problem is perceived, the types of interventions that are acceptable, and the community assets available to synergize the entire planning endeavor (Issel, 2009; McKnight, 2000). It is critical to ensure that the program plan is congruent with the community's interests and priorities. Policies and mandates of the organizations involved in the process set parameters on acceptable planning activities and decisions. Financial resources are essential to support the planning process, including implementation of the selected interventions. Securing financial resources frequently involves applications for external support from funding agencies;

as a result, the standards and criteria of those agencies become extremely important to the planning process.

KNOWLEDGE AND SKILLS

Assessment and planning depend upon the application of a specialized set of knowledge and skills, including the public health measurement sciences, decision-making strategies, and state-of-the-art knowledge about health conditions. To understand health problems and design effective interventions, a strong working knowledge of theories of human and organizational behavior is required (Glanz, Rimer, & Viswanath, 2008). This knowledge is complemented by (1) an understanding of the evidence that links a health problem to potential interventions and (2) evidence of effectiveness generated by interventions designed to address similar health problems or the same problems in other environments (Brownson, Baker, Leet, & Gillespie, 2011). Planning also requires specialized interactive skills in group process, community development, and leadership, essential tools for working with communities, forging partnerships, and maintaining critical relationships.

PARTICIPANTS

The knowledge and skills required to address a specific health problem are obtained by assembling teams of carefully selected participants very early in the process. As needs for new information and points of view evolve, new members should be added to ensure the best possible program for the problem at hand. Participants in the planning process may include qualified representatives of public health organizations at the federal, state, and local levels, communities, academia, media, employers, and business (Issel, 2009; Petersen & Alexander, 2001; Turnock, 2009). All of these organizations and groups are stakeholders in the health of their populations.

ASSESSMENT OF HEALTH PROBLEMS

A health problem is identified when the level of a health condition in a population of mothers or children differs adversely from an expected level. A thorough assessment of the problem, including a systematic verification of incidence and prevalence and analysis of precursors and consequences, provides an essential foundation for the entire planning process.

Verification

Perception that a health condition may have reached a level of concern occurs in one or more ways:

- Routine surveillance of specific health indicators, often carried out to monitor progress on national or state-level health objectives, indicates an adverse trend. An excellent example of this process is the tracking of childhood overweight rates, which led to recognition that they were increasing rapidly.
- A statewide or community assessment reveals a problem. Health departments, community agencies, and advocacy groups carry out these assessments frequently. State-level MCH programs conduct needs assessments at least every 5 years to comply with MCH Block Grant application requirements (USDHHS, 2011a).
- An individual, community, or health service suspects an increase in an adverse health condition (e.g., several cases of an unusual birth defect in a neighborhood surrounding a site where potential carcinogens have been discarded). The actual level of the condition is compared with rates in the general population, and an unacceptable gap is identified.

Before taking action on a perceived problem, it is important to verify that the original perception is correct. Four characteristics of the perceived health problem are examined to determine whether observed levels really constitute a departure from expected levels:

- Incidence or prevalence of the health condition
- Variation across population groups and geographic areas
- Duration of the observed level of the problem and how it has changed over time
- Expected future course of the problem if no intervention takes place

The existence of a health problem is supported if the incidence or prevalence of the condition is worse in the population of concern than it is in the general population or in another group serving as a standard for comparison (e.g., a subpopulation or a neighboring population group). Additional evidence of a problem is found if the condition has worsened or has been at the same unacceptable level for some time and/or if it is likely to worsen in the future. For example, the National Health and Nutrition Examination Survey (NHANES) 2007–2008 estimated that 16.9% of children and adolescents were obese. When one considers that the rate had been at this level for a relatively short duration because it has been increasing steadily since the early 1970s, the expected future course of the problem assumes even greater concern. Between 1976 to 1980 and 2007 to 2008, the prevalence of obesity among children aged 6 to 11 years increased from 6.5% to 19.6% and for adolescents aged 12 to 19 years, the increase was 5.0% to 18.1%. Finally, increasing rates over the past 4 decades have been observed for all race/gender combinations, but non-Hispanic black and Mexican American children showed troubling variations from the total population, with rates ranging from 10.7% to 29.2% (Ogden & Carroll, 2010). Thus, a review of duration, expected course, and variations in prevalence of obesity in children and adolescents suggests that the problem is real and that it harbors a distressing future if the trend is not reversed.

Problem Analysis

Once the existence of a health problem is verified, a thorough understanding of the problem's determinants and consequences, as well as the direction and strength of the relationships among them, is needed. This analysis of the problem is essential to creating and implementing effective interventions.

There are many ways to analyze public health problems, but they all share a special concern for the interconnections among innate, behavioral, social, and broader environmental domains. Figure 18–2 is a diagram of the social-ecological model (Dahlgren & Whitehead, 1991), a visual presentation of these domains as they affect health. This model offers a broad framework that encourages a comprehensive problem analysis by guiding planners to domains where determinants for specific problems may be found. For many public health problems, the search identifies scientifically tested causal relationships among the determinants, and between determinants and the problem, and suggests where well-respected theories of behavior might provide further illumination.

Figure 18–3 is an example of how the social-ecological levels can guide analysis of a specific MCH problem, in this case, childhood overweight and obesity. Some of the precursors are directly related to the biological processes that lead to the problem. Others are not as directly linked; instead, they influence the precursors that have a more direct effect. Still others are associated with the problem statistically, but they are considered markers for other unknown or unmeasured phenomena.

Starting at the top of Figure 18–3, socioeconomic, cultural, and environmental factors that are associated with overweight among children include low income, unsafe neighborhoods, neighborhoods not conducive to walking or other exercise, marketing practices and school policies. These factors, in turn, influence living and working conditions, like both parents employed and

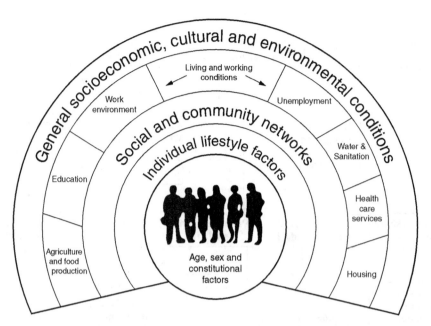

Figure 18–2 *A guide to thinking about the determinants of population health.*
Source: Dahlgren G, Whitehead M. 1991. Policies and Strategies to Promote Social Equity in Health. Stockholm, Sweden: Institute for Futures Studies.

working long hours, limited access to play-grounds, limited physical education classes, and inappropriate meal options in schools.

Family, social, and community factors include the stresses related to living and working conditions, children being at home and unsupervised after school, and parents having inadequate time to prepare meals at home. Individual lifestyle factors contribute to behaviors that have become prevalent among children in the past 2 decades: low levels of physical activity and unhealthy eating practices. The innate factors represent biological characteristics that may predispose to overweight and demographic groups in which the problem is most significant.

Identifying the linkages among precursors and between the precursors and the problem requires familiarity with the analytic epidemiology literature (Brownson, et al., 2011) and an understanding of the concept of relative risk.[1] Measures of relative risk can help in determining the potential impact of intervening with a specific precursor. For example, if overuse of video games and other sedentary recreation has a higher relative risk for overweight than eating meals outside of the home, an intervention intended to shift attention from video games to outside play would potentially have more of an impact on the problem than an intervention focused on eating at home.

The diagram shown in Figure 18–3 may be derived from published literature. It is a solid beginning but not a finished product. A complete problem analysis is refined by discussions with people involved with the problem and by examination of the incidence/prevalence, duration, and likely future course of the precursors in the population affected by the health problem. This process allows

[1]Relative risk, which is measured by an odds ratio, is an indicator of the strength of association between a risk factor and a health problem. It is the ratio of the incidence of the problem in the population of people with the risk factor to the incidence in the population without the risk factor (Gordis, 2009).

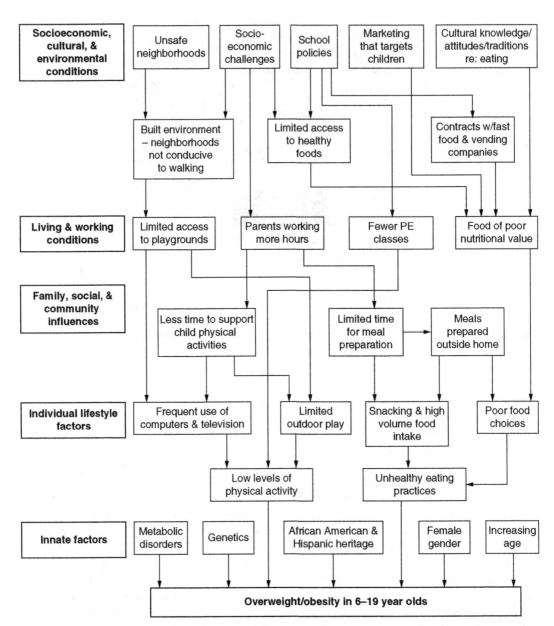

Figure 18–3 Diagram of selected precursors of overweight and obesity in children 6 to 19 years of age.

Sources: Data from Brownell and Horgan (2004). Brownell (2004). Fields & Higgins (2008). Goodman (2008). Gorin & Crane (2008). Mali, Schulze, & Huk (2006). Sallis & Glanz (2006). Vartanian, Schwartz, & Brownell (2007).

identification of precursors that are especially prevalent in the population of concern as well as those that do not apply.

In summary, a thorough analysis of the problem

- constitutes a framework for identifying alternative interventions to modify the risk factors or compensate for those that cannot be modified,
- identifies the relationships from which a logic model is developed,
- links the assessment phases of planning to program design and implementation, and
- provides part of the evidence base for the remaining steps of the program planning process.

Moreover, by analyzing a broad range of precursors from different domains, programs with multiple interventions can be devised to address precursors in different social-ecological domains simultaneously. These multilevel approaches often harbor greater probabilities of success than single component interventions. They can assume even greater precision when directed toward target populations defined by innate precursors, such as age, race/ethnicity, and gender.

Consequences

Analysis of the problem provides the base from which program planning unfolds. Identifying and quantifying the consequences of the problem, such as effects on individuals, families, and society, serve a different but equally important function. A full description of the consequences encourages recognition of the importance of the health problem and forms a rationale that may help convince policy makers and funding agencies that the problem must be addressed. In the situation described in Figure 18-3, children who are overweight or obese are at risk for self-image problems, social discrimination, serious medical problems and continuing weight gain into adulthood. These effects, in turn, limit quality of life and contribute to chronic diseases and disabilities, both of which influence rates of premature deaths (Koplan, Liverman, & Kraak, 2005). Demonstrating these effects through incidence and prevalence rates is an important component of establishing the relative priority of the problem for subsequent action.

SOURCES OF DATA FOR ASSESSING HEALTH PROBLEMS

Often the data required for assessment of health status problems are available from federal sources, such as the Centers for Disease Control and Prevention (CDC) *Data and Statistics* (CDC, 2011a) online data sources and the U.S. Department of Health and Human Services *Gateway to Data and Statistics* (USDHHS, 2011b). Data sources that are specific to states and local areas may be identified by state centers for health statistics. If data of acceptable quality are not available, collection of primary data should be considered. This is a decision that should be made carefully and in consultation with experts in qualitative and quantitative data collection, because collecting data is expensive and producing data of high quality depends on well-conceived and carefully executed methods.

HEALTH SERVICES NEEDS ASSESSMENT

The second major step in the program planning process is identification and analysis of needs for services that address specific precursors of the health problem. This assessment examines the adequacy of existing services to prevent the problem by ameliorating its precursors directly or compensating for their effects. Unfortunately, no single measure captures unmet need. Instead, needs are usually assessed from two or more of the following five perspectives (Bradshaw, 1972; Peoples-Sheps, 2001a):

1. Availability of recommended services
2. Relative availability of services
3. Demand for services

4. Use of services by populations at risk

5. Perceptions of service needs

Availability of Recommended Services

The starting point for considering health service needs is an assessment of the extent to which appropriate services are available to prevent or ameliorate modifiable precursors of the health problem. Needs are met when recommended services are available and the needs are unmet when they are not. This assessment has three steps: (1) identifying effective interventions that could or should be available, (2) identifying interventions that are available, and (3) comparing the two lists to identify services that are not available. The last set represents unmet needs for services.

Because prevention must be directed toward the modifiable precursors of a problem, it is important to examine the problem diagram closely before attempting to locate appropriate interventions. For many MCH problems, recommendations for effective interventions have been developed. Public health and other professional organizations that focus on maternal and child health, such as the American College of Obstetricians and Gynecologists and the American Academy of Pediatrics, often promulgate these recommendations to foster adequacy and quality of care. For broader programmatic interventions, the CDC and the Health Resources and Services Administration (HRSA) in the U.S. Department of Health and Human Services are excellent resources. These agencies develop interventions for emerging problems and sometimes offer funding to communities to implement them. Other recommendations are available from *The Guide to Community Preventive Services*, an Internet-based document developed by the independent Task Force on Community Preventive Services (2011). It summarizes current information about effectiveness and costs of a variety of population-based interventions. The goal of this process is to identify interventions that have strong evidence bases.

Recommendations by professional organizations may be supplemented by recommendations developed by the local health planning group, which should have a good sense of the community's culture and assets. By considering each precursor in light of local assets and issues, this group may identify viable interventions that would not be appropriate in other areas and important variations on the recommendations of professional groups. For example, one recommended approach to combating childhood overweight is for children to walk or bike to school (CDC, 2011b). However, in a community where there are no crosswalks spanning major roads, walking or biking to school, even with adults, may not be safe. In this case, the local planners may suggest building crosswalks or overpasses as a way of addressing this impediment in their community.

With a set of recommendations for interventions compiled, the next challenge is to inventory resources that are actually available. Most communities have published inventories of community services. These guides are often general, however, and may not provide information of sufficient detail about interventions for specific health problems. As a result, some supplemental information may need to be collected through interviews with key informants, such as directors of relevant community agencies.

The final step in assessing availability of services involves comparing recommended with available interventions. The interventions that are recommended but not available to the population at risk, or are available only in part, represent unmet needs.

Relative Availability of Services

Sometimes it is informative to assess service needs of the population of concern by comparing what is available to that group with the situation of another comparable population, such as those with a similar risk profile in another area. With a focus on equity, unmet needs are defined as services available to the comparison population and not available to the population of concern.

Demand for Services

The first two ways of assessing needs focus on availability of services. Whether available services are used is another question, addressed in part by an assessment of demand for services. With this measure, needs are reflected by the number of people who seek the recommended and available services. Those who receive the service are counted in utilization rates. The assumption underlying this perspective is that receipt of services signifies that needs are met. Those who do not receive the service presumably continue to have unmet needs. This approach has the appeal of producing an easy-to-understand proportion:

$$\frac{\text{Number of individuals not served}}{\begin{array}{c}\text{Number of individuals who requested}\\\text{the service}\end{array}}$$

Although the simplicity of measuring demand is attractive, it harbors some important limitations. First, those who do not seek services are omitted from this estimate. This group may not even know that appropriate interventions exist. In the case of overweight children, for example, parents may not seek help because they assume that being overweight is part of a stage their child is going through rather than a condition that puts him or her at risk for many subsequent health and social problems. Second, it is often difficult to access data on individuals not served because this type of "waiting list" information is not consistently retained by healthcare organizations.

Because of the second limitation, an alternative estimate of demand is in use. This involves comparing actual use of services to the maximum capacity of a service. If the service is consistently booked to capacity, it may be assumed that additional services would be used, if they were available. However, this conclusion should be tempered by recognition of the tendency of service use to expand to meet the level of available services.

Use of Services by Populations at Risk

The fourth approach to measuring need is a variation on the demand measure. In this case, needs are considered met for the population at risk who receive a given intervention and they are unmet for those who do not. The population at risk is characterized by precursors in the problem diagram. Then the number of this group using (or not using) the service can be calculated as a proportion of the total number with a given risk factor. For example, if a school has developed a segment of the health curriculum that encourages children to be more active in their daily routines, the following proportion could measure the extent to which needs of the population at risk (e.g., those involved in sedentary activities) remain unmet:

$$\frac{\begin{array}{c}\text{Number of children who spend}\\> 3 \text{ hours/day in sedentary activities but}\\\text{do not receive the curriculum}\end{array}}{\begin{array}{c}\text{Number of children who spend}\\> 3 \text{ hours/day in sedentary activities}\end{array}}$$

Perceptions of Service Needs

Perceived needs are the services people say they need to prevent a health problem. Needs are unmet if the people are not receiving those services. Information about perceived need can be gathered through surveys, interviews, and focus groups (Issel, 2009; Witkin & Altshuld, 1995), which can be designed to tap several important dimensions. People at risk, people with the health condition, service providers, and community leaders may identify needed services that do not emerge through other means of assessing needs. They may also provide insight regarding the importance of some unmet needs in comparison to others and in identification of barriers to use of services. Barriers may be related to how the services are delivered or to cultural beliefs or expectations that inhibit use of services by the populations at risk.

Information derived from perceptions of relevant informants personalizes health service assessments and makes the resulting information specific to the population and its community. Like the other perspectives of need, however, perceptions may harbor some limitations. The expectations of the individuals from whom perceptions are solicited can affect their responses. Needs may be underestimated if individuals are not aware of options that could be available to address the problem. They may be overestimated if the perceptions are based on unreasonable expectations.

Assessment of Community Assets

Equally important and often invaluable to understanding health-related needs are informants' insights about community assets (e.g., infrastructure, organizations, associations, and individual talents) that can help to modify the deficits documented in needs assessments and serve as bases for launching interventions or as catalysts to make them successful (Issel, 2009). Assessments of the strengths of a community or population usually involve collection of primary data. Appropriate questions can be included in the protocols for assessing perceived needs.

Assessing Other Characteristics of Services

Availability and use of services are the basic characteristics to examine in a needs assessment. Information about other qualities of services, however, can provide much deeper insight into service needs (Keppel & Freedman,

1995; Petersen & Alexander, 2001). Characteristics such as accessibility, acceptability, appropriateness, coordination, effectiveness, cost, and insurance coverage can be explored for further illumination of why certain deficiencies in availability and use exist.

Summary of Unmet Needs

In the absence of a single measure of service need, planners must consider which of the alternative approaches to estimating need will generate the most useful information for their situations, with the fewest limitations. In general, it is rarely feasible to examine needs from all perspectives and rarely adequate to use only one. The wise approach is to use at least two perspectives, chosen carefully to generate the most useful information about the problem at hand.

Because the resulting set of unmet needs is generated from different perspectives/ measures, some contradictory findings usually emerge. An assessment of recommended services, for example, may document numerous after-school programs offering outdoor activities in the community, but the perceived needs assessment may indicate that most parents think there is an unmet need for such programs. Contradictions such as this provide an opportunity to explore the needs for service in greater depth. In this case, the true shortcomings may be in terms of knowledge about available programs, referrals to them, and/or financial coverage of those services.

Setting Priorities among Unmet Needs

If the list of unmet needs is long, it can be rendered more helpful to the planning process by prioritizing the options. This process involves considering the relative priority of each unmet need (or intervention) on the list, with highest priority given to interventions with:

- High prevalence of the precursor to which the service is addressed

- Strong relationships between the precursor and the problem
- Relatively large extent of unmet need for the service

This prioritized list completes the health services needs assessment and serves as the starting point for the next step in the planning process.

DEVELOPMENT AND SELECTION OF INTERVENTIONS

The third step in the planning process is development and selection of interventions. By this stage, the planning team has a good understanding of unmet needs for services to address the health problem. Services that are recommended but not available at all have been identified, as well as others that are in the community but not functioning well, or functioning well but covering only a portion of the people in need.

For many MCH problems, the set of unmet needs generated by a detailed needs assessment is a strong and adequate base from which to develop intervention options, since the set was derived from a spectrum of evidence-based recommendations and the opinions of invested parties. However, a needs assessment does not always generate a complete list of alternative interventions. In some situations, interventions for key precursors may not be developed to the point of inclusion in professional recommendations or in the perceptions of involved individuals.

Development of Interventions

Development of interventions begins with a systematic review of modifiable precursors, followed by a review of the literature for specific interventions designed to address them and for which clear evidence of effectiveness has been generated. Table 18–1 shows how precursors and evidence-based interventions can be linked and categorized by social-ecological model levels.

Program theories also guide the search for potentially effective interventions. The Stages of Change, Health Belief Model, Social Cognitive, and Community Organization theories are a few of the most frequently used (Glanz, et al., 2008). Different theories will have a better fit for each program plan based on the intended level of change.

The childhood overweight/obesity problem offers an example of how a theory could be applied to design an intervention intended to promote healthy behavior. To develop the

Table 18–1 Modifiable Precursors of Childhood Overweight/Obesity and Evidence-Based Interventions

Social-Ecological Model Level	Modifiable Precursors	Evidence-Based Interventions
Socioeconomic, cultural, and environmental conditions	Unsafe neighborhoods, not conducive to outside physical activities	After-school dance classes targeted to high-risk girls (GEMS)[1]
Living and working conditions	Fewer PE classes; food of poor nutritional value	Enhanced physical education and health education in school[2]
Family and lifestyle factors	Sedentary activities (computers and TV), poor food choices, inadequate meal preparation	Group meetings of parents and children focused on knowledge and behavior change[3]

[1]Robinson, et al., 2003.
[2]Gortmaker, et al., 1999.
[3]Janicke, et al., 2008.

content of an educational message the planners want to deliver to parents about physical exercise, they could use the Health Belief Model (Glanz, Rimer, & Viswanath, 2008; Rosenstock, 1974), which involves addressing each of six factors that influence a person's decision to take a preventive action:

1. Perceived susceptibility: Belief by the parents or caregivers that their children are susceptible to getting a health problem (like overweight/obesity).

2. Perceived severity: Belief that the health condition and its sequelae are serious.

3. Perceived benefits: Belief that a proposed preventive action will reduce the risk and seriousness of the health problem.

4. Perceived barriers: Perception of few tangible and psychological costs to taking the preventive action.

5. Cues to action: Reminders, thank-you notes, rewards, and recognitions that may be needed to prompt the activity.

6. Self-efficacy: Confidence in ability to take action.

According to the Health Belief Model, the program's interventions would address each of these factors in order to motivate parents to allow and encourage their children to increase their physical activity. Some factors would be addressed through educational materials in various media and others through personal contacts.

Interventions derived from theory offer great opportunity for improving health problems. However, if they have also been evaluated for effectiveness in reducing the problem at hand, they hold even greater value when compared with other options (Brownson, et al., 2011).

Once a solid list of interventions that have been empirically tested and/or theoretically derived is compiled, further development of each option can begin. If the list is fairly long, perhaps more than five or six options, it is helpful to reduce the size of the pool.

The basic idea here is to retain options that are most likely to be selected for implementation. Planners may consider retaining interventions that are:

- Linked to precursors that are strongly associated with the problem,
- Capable of serving the population most at risk,
- Built on community strengths, interests, and priorities,
- Considered essential in professional recommendations,
- Consistent with mandates of agencies, organizations, and associations represented on the planning team,
- Capable of showing effects sooner rather than later, and
- Likely to correspond with funding priorities.

Although reducing the list of options is the goal, it is nevertheless wise to retain one or more interventions that address each level of the precursors in the problem diagram, Figure 18–3. This permits a range of final options, as well as opportunity to combine options for multifaceted programs.

For the options retained, key characteristics must be identified. This description is a tool that informs the next several planning tasks. It should include major characteristics of the program (e.g., what the program will do, where activities will occur, who will be served), evidence of effectiveness in improving the health problem and in affecting other relevant outcomes, cost, administrative requirements, technical requirements, and any political controversies that may be anticipated. Descriptions of interventions that have been tested in other settings can usually be obtained from their developers.

Criteria for Selection of an Intervention

The success of a public health program, of course, depends on its ability to ameliorate the health problem in the population or community in which it exists. The efficacy of the intervention is crucial. In addition to efficacy, this criterion should account for expected penetration of the target population, the time that might elapse before any effects are seen, and side effects. Ideally, effectiveness is estimated from evaluation studies of the effectiveness of this or a similar program on a similar population. If interventions were derived from professional recommendations, evidence of effectiveness should be available from the same source. However, if the health problem is emerging and the intervention is a new recommendation or one developed by the planning group alone, evidence of effectiveness will not be available. In this case, estimates should be made, based upon the known strength of the relationship between the targeted precursor and the health problem, and of the estimated influence of the program on the precursor. If an intervention is based on one or more behavioral theories, research from applications to similar health problems may also inform estimates of effectiveness.

It is important to avoid overestimating effectiveness. New programs should be developed with sound theoretical underpinnings, implemented as small-scale demonstration projects, and then evaluated with rigorous research methods before they are applied to large population groups. As a result, new programs serving small populations may not be able to produce competitive estimates of population effectiveness when compared with programs that can be dispersed to larger groups. As a rule, limiting intervention options to those with clear evidence of effectiveness is preferred.

Effectiveness is a necessary criterion for selecting an intervention, but not a sufficient one. Even the most efficacious intervention cannot achieve its goals if staffing is inadequate, the clients and staff speak different languages, costs of services are beyond the means of intended recipients, or access is impeded by protesters around the building in which the services are offered. All of these issues and many more must be considered, including another option that might be equally successful at a lower cost.

The five criteria shown in Table 18-2 are basic to most decisions. Another criterion of growing importance when addressing complex problems is the extent to which a program fosters organizational collaboration or partnerships among public agencies or between public and private organizations. MCH agencies and programs also place emphasis on the ability of the intervention to encourage development of systems of care, especially for children with special healthcare needs. If financial support from a third party is desirable, it is imperative to incorporate the funding agency's priorities into the criteria for selecting an intervention.

Assessment of Program Alternatives According to the Criteria

Applying the criteria to program alternatives in order to select one for implementation is the third activity in this step of the planning process. There are many ways to do this, ranging from highly interactive discussions through highly quantitative analytic procedures. The most important ingredients for a sound decision are a systematic process and participation from relevant stakeholders. The criteria-weighting method (Peoples-Sheps, 2001b; Spiegel & Hyman, 1991) promotes systematic consideration of each criterion, weighted according to its relative importance. And the process can be structured so that it encourages participation but allows verbal dominance to be controlled.

Table 18-2 is an example of criteria weighting. The criteria identified previously are listed in the left column of the matrix. Each criterion has been assigned a set of scores ranging from 1 (least consistent with the criterion) to 4 (most consistent). The next column indicates the weight assigned to each criterion. Weights are used when one or more criteria are considered more important than the others. In this case, the weights

Table 18–2 Criteria Weighting Method for Selecting a Program to Prevent Overweight and Obesity in Children

| | | Programs | | | | | |
| | | After-school dance classes | | Enhanced physical education and health education in school | | Family-based weight control | |
Criteria[1]	Weight[2]	Raw Score	Wtd. Score	Raw Score	Wtd. Score	Raw Score	Wtd. Score
Effectiveness	3	2	6	2	6	3	9
Cost	3	4	12	3	9	3	9
Administrative feasibility	2	3	6	2	4	4	8
Political feasibility	2	4	8	2	4	4	8
Technical feasibility	1	4	4	3	3	4	4
Total		17	36	12	26	18	38

[1]**Criteria:**

Effectiveness:

4 = Highly effective, long-lasting
3 = Effective, duration of effects uncertain
2 = Good chance of improving the problem
1 = 50% chance of improving the problem

Cost:

4 = Very inexpensive
3 = Affordable
2 = Expensive
1 = Very expensive

Administrative feasibility:

4 = Fits easily in existing administrative unit
3 = Minor modifications in administrative unit required
2 = Difficult to administer
1 = Impossible to administer

Political feasibility:

4 = Acceptable to all constituents
3 = Acceptable to most constituents; little active opposition
2 = Acceptable to some constituents; little active opposition
1 = Unacceptable to most constituents

Technical feasibility:

4 = Technology and human resources readily available
3 = Technology available; human resources not available
2 = Technology not available; human resources available
1 = Technology and human resources not available

[2]**Weights:**

3 = Most important
2 = Very important
1 = Important

range from 1 (important) to 3 (most important). In this example, technical feasibility is weighted 1 whereas both effectiveness and cost have been assigned higher weights of 3.

The next section of the matrix identifies programs under consideration. Each program has two columns. The first includes a raw score on each criterion. A definition for each score, which can be modified according to the data available on each option, is given at the bottom of the table. The second column under each program consists of weighted scores; that is, the product of the weight of each criterion and the corresponding raw score.

The scores in Table 18–2 suggest that a family-based weight control program would be the best choice. To increase the probability of success in improving a health problem, however, one might decide to combine interventions to address two or more precursors in a multifaceted program. This approach is consistent with the social-ecological model (Figure 18–2) and the corresponding problem diagram (Figure 18–3). It presents opportunities to affect several levels of precursors through a coordinated intervention strategy. With regard to childhood overweight/obesity, the planning team could decide to address the problem on two or even three fronts by combining the interventions in Table 18–2 into one coordinated program (Janicke, et al., 2008).

Making a decision about which program to implement is one of the most important aspects of the planning process, on a par with defining the problem correctly in the first place. Regardless of whether a single intervention is selected or a few alternatives are ultimately combined into a broader spectrum initiative, the criteria-weighting method provides a useful framework for organizing the discussions that are essential to the ultimate decision.

LOGIC MODEL AND OBJECTIVES

Constructing a logic model and setting objectives for the program are conducted concurrently and result in a solid framework, or blueprint, for the program. A logic model describes the conceptual framework, and objectives specify activities and indicators that permit measurement and monitoring.

Logic Model

A logic model is a visual representation of how the program plan will work to bring about the desired change in health status. It is a useful tool for systematic thinking about the plan, then planning, describing, and evaluating the program (W.K. Kellogg Foundation, 2004). A logic model promotes many key elements of the planning process, including:

- Specification of program activities, outputs, and outcomes

- Identification of factors that may affect the success of the program
- Anticipation of data and resources that will be needed to implement and evaluate the program
- Providing a roadmap for all program stakeholders
- Ensuring that the intervention reaches its intended outcomes and impact over time

At least three major types of logic models have proven to be particularly helpful to planners and program managers. A logic model may be derived from the theory of change that has influenced the design of the program. It provides a rationale for the program and illustrates how and why planners think the program will work. This model is built upon the types of theories described in the previous section. An outcome-based logic model focuses on the early aspects of program planning and serves to connect the resources and activities with the desired results of the program. These models often include short- and long-term outcomes and anticipated impacts as a result of program activities, thus offering a framework for evaluation at each level. An activities-based logic model provides the details required to implement the program. It is a very useful tool for program monitoring and management.

Often, a single type of model does not align with a project's requirements, so planners must decide what they want to achieve with the logic model and then build it to meet their needs, usually combining parts of each of the main types described above. As the program plan grows and develops, so does its logic model. A program logic model is a snapshot of a program at a point in time rather than the program's actual flow of events. It is a work in progress and can be refined as the program plan develops.

Table 18–3 is a logic model for a family-based weight control intervention, using the "outcomes approach" described previously. The left-hand column identifies the resources or inputs that will potentially enable or limit

Table 18–3 Logic Model for a Family-Based Weight Control Intervention

	Outputs		Outcomes		
Inputs	**Activities**	**Participants**	**Short Term**	**Medium Term**	**Long Term**
Trained interventionists	Conduct weekly group sessions for parents and children on diet and exercise, setting goals, self-monitoring of food intake, and pedometer monitoring of physical exercise	Parents of students enrolled in the school	Reduce intake of foods with high calories, fat, sugar, and salt	Increase time spent in physical activity each week	Reduce rates of overweight and obesity in children in the school
Recruiters					
Financial resources					
Pedometers		Students at risk for overweight/obesity	Increase intake of vegetables and fruits	Improve balance of daily intake of healthy vs. unhealthy foods	
Diaries for self-monitoring					
Educational materials					
Facilities for meetings		Students who are overweight or obese	Increase physical exercise	Reduce BMI levels of parent and child participants	

Source: Centers for Disease Control and Prevention (2012). DASH Funded Partner Site, Program Management, 801 Tools and Resources: Logic Model Template. http://www.cdc.gov/DASH/program_mgt/docs_pdfs/Logic_Model_template.pdf. Page last modified February 22, 2012. Accessed April 5, 2012.

the program's effectiveness. Next the program activities—the tasks the program will complete in order to produce its outcomes—are listed. Activities may include processes, techniques, tools, events and actions of the plan, such as educational curricula, series of training sessions, and development of infrastructures. In this example, the activities are weekly group sessions for parents and children, daily self-monitoring of food intake, and daily pedometer-monitoring of physical activity. The participants' column specifies who will be reached by the program. In Table 18–3, this applies to parents and two groups of children.

Next, the logic model includes three levels of outcomes: short, medium, and long term. Short-term outcomes are specific changes in attitudes, skills, behaviors, knowledge, or level of functioning expected to result from the program activities. Medium-term outcomes include decisions, policies, social action, and other expected results of accomplishment of the short-term outcomes. Finally, the logic model includes long-term outcomes, impacts, or organizational, community, or system-level changes expected to result from program activities, such as improved health conditions at a larger population level, increased capacity, or changes in policy.

Setting Objectives

A carefully developed logic model guides development of a program's objectives. Each of the items listed under outputs and outcomes in the logic model can be restated in the form of one or more objectives. Objectives should be SMART: Specific, Measurable, Attainable, Realistic, and Time-Sensitive (Issel, 2009). Table 18–4 shows examples of the components of several objectives that could be developed from the logic model in Table 18–3. The table shows specific and

Table 18–4 Selected Objectives of a Family-Based Weight Control Intervention Program

Specific and Measurable Indicator	Population	Target	Time Frame
% with gender and age-specific BMI (body mass index)[1] within normal range	Children in the school	85%	1 year
Mean % of recommended daily servings of fruits and vegetables	Parents and children receiving the intervention	70%	6 months
Mean # minutes engaged in physical activity/week	Parents and children receiving the intervention	90 minutes	3 months, 6 months
Mean # steps/day	Parents and children receiving the intervention	Men 7,000 Women 5,000 Children 3,500	3 months, 6 months
Mean # servings of potato chips and other salty high-calorie foods/week	Parents and children receiving the intervention	2/week	3 months, 6 months
Mean # servings of vegetables and fruits/day	Parents and children receiving the intervention	9 servings	3 months, 6 months
% enrolled in the program	Eligible children Parents of eligible children	55%	4 weeks, 16 weeks
One hour group sessions		Weekly	16 weeks

[1]Body Mass Index: Body weight in kilograms divided by height in meters squared (kg/m^2).

measurable indicators with one or more targets and time frames for each objective.

Creating meaningful objectives involves choosing a numeric value as the target of the objective. Target values should not be selected at random. They can be derived from published results of studies of similar interventions, data sets from organizational or marketing assessments, community assessments, professional standards, national goals such as *Healthy People 2020* (USDHHS, 2011c), state goals, or surveillance data.

Availability of baseline data is another important factor to consider when setting targets. Setting an absolute target, such as 85% for the measure "% children with gender and age-specific body mass indices (BMI) within normal range" does not indicate a starting point. The task is much larger if the current percentage is 40% than if it is 80%. A more informative approach may be setting the target as an amount of change from the baseline. Data for baseline comparisons should be available from the problem and needs assessments. If they are not available, baseline data can be collected before the program starts or early in its operational phase.

Other factors to consider in setting targets include the speed with which the program will become fully operational, whether some negative effects are expected before seeing positive ones (e.g., often programs that rely on reporting of cases see an increase in cases reported because the intervention is available before they see a decrease due to the intervention itself), and if there is a reason to set targets particularly high or low. In the end, the levels selected for targets are usually derived from a synthesis of the data and information available at the time.

The time frame that accompanies each measure and target must also be carefully considered. Medium and long-term outcome objectives are often written for the life of the program; whereas output and short-term outcome objectives may have shorter time frames. This is because program activities may change from year to year by design or because of developments encountered as the program is implemented. For example, a program may be designed so that recruitment of clients is a major activity in year 1, replaced in year 2 with service delivery activities. Alternatively, it may be found that by the end of year 1, recruitment has not been as productive as expected, so different recruitment activities are added in year 2. In both cases, the output objectives would change from year 1 to year 2.

Program objectives provide a blueprint for a program plan. They are also used as standards for comparison when assessing the program's progress. The resulting information can guide management decisions about program activities and resource allocation. If progress on one objective is poor, but other targets are met, resources may be diverted to improve performance on the lagging objective. If poor performance persists, either the activities or the targets may need to be modified. Thus, objectives are a framework around which the program is constructed and amended.

An evaluator can play a central role in working with a program planner to create measurable objectives. Although a trained program planner will have a strong skill set in creating SMART objectives, a good evaluator can work with the planner to determine whether the objectives can be measured with well-designed evaluation methods.

Logic models and SMART objectives are excellent tools for program planners and evaluators to facilitate discussions about the program. Conversations about how the program's objectives and activities are linked with the defined outputs and outcomes in the logic model strengthen the entire process and encourage development of effective programs. By working together as a team early in the process, obvious gaps can be addressed and changed to fit the ideal goals of the program and can strengthen the design and methods of the evaluation process. Flexibility is essential, though, and the logic model and the objectives are simply tools that may need to be revisited as changes are needed in development and implementation of the program.

PROGRAM IMPLEMENTATION

After the program's objectives are developed, the next step is to design the program in detail and develop the implementation plan. Through the processes of selecting interventions, constructing a logic model, and setting objectives, a blueprint for the program takes shape. Now, the challenge is to harness those ideas into an operational program that will encourage achievement of each program objective, by describing exactly how the program will function over time. Program operations and implementation must be detailed in a way that the funders and/or grant reviewers can understand exactly what the program entails.

Program Design

Describing an operating program parallels the logic model and involves careful attention to four major design elements:

- Program activities
- Client characteristics
- Organizational infrastructure
- Human resources

The program should be developed by individuals with the knowledge and skills to incorporate relevant theories and practice standards appropriately. Often these individuals are members of the professions that will deliver the intervention. Hence, health educators may be best qualified to design behavior modification interventions because they are trained in this area; public health nurses are in a similar position with regard to infant healthcare interventions; and health administrators are likely to have greater expertise in efforts to modify organizational behavior. To change federal or state policies, laws, or regulations, experts in the specific change processes required should play major roles (Issel, 2009; Petersen & Alexander, 2001).

Program Activities

Every detail of the program's operations should be considered at this point. If the intervention is to be offered in an agency setting, this would include space and scheduling issues. Interventions that are regulatory in nature, such as efforts to change laws or modify federal regulations would involve collaborating with key change agents, proposing the exact wording of the new regulation or law, and shepherding the proposal through appropriate channels. For the family-based weight control program depicted in the logic model, Table 18–3, identification and recruitment of eligible families, timing and location of weekly sessions, and design of the content curriculum for each session would be among the topics for discussion and decision.

Although each of these points may seem like common sense, the planners of this program may not have considered them specifically without consideration of the theories underlying each of the program activities and evidence from similar interventions implemented with other population groups. If the chosen intervention is one that has been developed and recommended by a public health source, like CDC or HRSA, its theoretical foundation should already be developed. The planner's role in this case may be limited to choosing activities that fit best with the population's circumstances.

To specify details of program activities, it is helpful to consider when each activity will occur and where and how it will be done. Two tools that are helpful at this stage are written procedures and flowcharts.

- Written procedures are clear and concise statements about activities to be done, including exactly what tasks are involved, the sequence they should follow, and who is responsible for them.
- Flowcharts offer another way of accomplishing the same result. These charts show the sequence of activities in diagrammatic form. They are especially

useful when depicting several parallel sets of activities.

For a program to function smoothly components must work together; thus, coordination of the program's activities is as important to this description as detailing them. For example, the personnel department and service delivery units, each providing a different type of service, must have specific mechanisms for ensuring unimpeded interactions. These mechanisms should be detailed as procedures for routine coordination, like referral procedures from one set of providers to another. In addition, there should be a procedure for handling the atypical problems that will arise.

Client Characteristics

The program must fit with the characteristics of the clients in order for it to function well. If the first language of the target group is not English, then bilingual providers or interpreters should be hired. If the intervention is targeted to mothers of young children, provisions for child care should be taken into account. If the target group is school-age children, marketing materials should be designed to correspond with the interests and reading levels of that age group in its geocultural setting. Many of these characteristics were identified when the health problem was analyzed, but a more detailed understanding may require interviews or focus group discussions with members of the target population as the full program is designed. The goal is for the activities to match the target audience.

Organizational Infrastructure

When selecting an intervention, consideration was given to feasibility, both administrative and technical. The issue at that stage was whether or not the administrative structure and technical capability to carry out the program existed or could be developed. Now, these capabilities must be operationalized so that appropriate administrative

support and control is available to ensure that program objectives can be met. An organizational chart is the universal tool for depicting the structure of an organization and subunits within it (Breckon, 1997). Most MCH programs are set up within existing agencies, where the location of a new program can facilitate or impede day-to-day operations. One possible location is within an existing organizational unit. There is often some economic advantage to this approach, and it is a useful method for promoting sustainability of a program over time, but there is also a risk that the program will become indistinguishable from the other programs in the unit.

An alternative is to structure the program as a demonstration project by setting it up as an organizationally distinct, short-term initiative. One reason to take a demonstration project approach is to retain the totality of the intervention so that it can be rigorously evaluated. From an administrative perspective, demonstration projects often have high visibility, are not tied to the peculiarities of an ongoing bureaucracy, and are allowed considerable organizational autonomy. All of these characteristics tend to encourage creativity within the project. On the other hand, there are disadvantages of demonstration projects. Since they may require the same types of staff as ongoing units, functions may be duplicated and, thus, become wasteful and inefficient. Demonstration projects sometimes become elitist and entrenched in their own institutional culture, thereby losing the creativity and flexibility for which they are best known.

Traditionally, MCH programs have been offered in either the public or the private sector. As new types of healthcare organizations dominate the field and as public-private partnerships are encouraged from many sides, new challenges for organizational structure have emerged. In situations where staff members are shared by partnering organizations, chains of authority and responsibility present emerging challenges.

Human Resources

With the program's activities and organizational structure specified, the types and numbers of personnel needed to implement the intervention—the activities, monitoring, and leadership—can be determined. The planning team should discuss alternative types of providers so that the final selection represents the best fit of provider training and experience with the job to be done (Charns & Lockhart, 1997). Supervisory responsibilities and time commitments are taken into account when estimating expected productivity of staff members. These estimates should be calculated as carefully as possible since underestimates could cause serious delays in delivery of program activities. These delays, in turn, will have adverse effects on outcome objectives.

The universal tool for linking staff members to program activities and to organizational structure is the position description (Breckon, 1997). Most organizations and agencies have standard formats for position descriptions, which include job title, minimum and desired qualifications, chain of command, and job functions and responsibilities. Because position descriptions reflect many decisions made in the process of program design, they are critical links in the planning process. They can also serve an important role for the individuals who fill the positions in that they link those individuals to the program's specific objectives.

Implementation Planning

Implementation refers to a set of activities conducted in the time period between formal approval of the program and the program's actual start date. Implementation planning is the process of (1) identifying what needs to be done during that period of time and (2) scheduling those activities so that the program can be launched smoothly to reach the objectives. The resources and activities required to implement a program are different from the design elements of an operating program (i.e., program activities, client characteristics, organizational infrastructure, and human resources). The resources required for implementation include personnel, equipment, supplies, organizational permissions, and other items included in the "inputs" column of the logic model. Implementation activities are the tasks that must be done in order to have the resources available to start the program (Spiegel & Hyman, 1991).

As shown in Table 18–4 for a family-based weight-control program, ongoing program activities include holding weekly sessions with families and teaching them how to self-monitor food intake and to monitor exercise with a pedometer. Resources needed to carry out these ongoing activities include facilities, diaries, and pedometers. Implementation activities are the tasks required to have these resources when and where they are needed. Parents must be contacted and recruited. The facility must be scheduled and supplies ordered and received.

Scheduling implementation activities to meet program start dates can be challenging. For each activity, the length of time required for completion and its sequence relative to the other activities must be determined. In addition, responsibilities for each activity should be assigned. If many people are working on implementation, several chains of activities can be carried out concurrently. If the number of implementation activities is relatively small (about –20-40), they can be easily organized in a timeline, a visual strategy that shows at a glance when each should start and be completed. Separate chains of activities can be shown, even those that are concurrent. More complex implementation plans require readily available project management software.

Unanticipated events between a program's approval date and actual start date can produce delays and additional implementation activities. As a result, it is wise to allow for extra time during the implementation period.

BUDGETING

The budget is one of the most essential components of the planning process. If the budget is omitted or poorly executed, all of the preceding work amounts to no more than wishful thinking. Like the logic model and program objectives, the budget provides a blueprint of the plan. A budget includes costs of the program's planned activities and all the details that support these activities. It can help to clarify responsibilities and to contribute to cost awareness among the participants in the process. Working through budget details may produce fresh ideas or new perspectives on other parts of the plan, thus providing another opportunity for iteration.

Most organizations and funding sources have required formats for budgets. In general, the budget has two parts: personnel and nonpersonnel. The personnel section includes entries for each position, percentage of time devoted by each one to the program, annual salary, and benefits. Nonpersonnel items include detailed information about costs for equipment, supplies, travel, communication, contracts, and other items specific to the program.

Both personnel and nonpersonnel costs are considered direct costs. That is, they include items that can be identified specifically with the program and will be expended to carry out the program's activities.

Estimating the cost of each item is fairly straightforward. The key is to obtain costs from the correct source; for example, the personnel department of the organization is usually the best source for salaries and benefits, whereas distributors are more reliable sources for nonpersonnel items. Cost estimates should be detailed for each item and then multiplied by the quantity required of that item. For multiyear budgets, changes in costs over the budget period, such as salary raises and airfare increases, must be built into the estimates. Some costs that may not be immediately obvious are: (1) items that

will be needed later in the budget period for phased-in services, (2) costs of evaluation, and (3) implementation expenses. All of these should be included in the budget. Table 18–5 is a sample budget for a family weight-control program, showing the categories mentioned previously.

Programs also incur indirect costs, funds required to support sponsored activities but cannot be directly identified with a specific program. The costs result from shared services such as libraries, physical plant operation and maintenance, utilities, administrative expenses, and depreciation for buildings and equipment. The indirect cost dollars received are not extra dollars for direct expenses, but are part of the budget and are fully used to make the system work. Without them, research laboratories and service delivery facilities cannot be built and maintained. Each organization has specific amounts required for indirect costs, which may vary across funders.

It is sometimes necessary to distinguish between requested funds and donated funds. This distinction is used when a proposal for the program is being submitted to an outside funding source for consideration. Funding sources are often interested in the extent to which the applicant organization will support the program. The term "donated" refers to the applicant's contributions. "Requested" funds are those the applicant is requesting from an outside source.

The budget itself, like the one shown in Table 18–5, is supplemented and explained by a budget justification in narrative form. This is a matter of briefly justifying each expense and must be consistent with the program description and the implementation plan. For example, if three interventionists are required to deliver the program, the justification includes information about why three individuals are needed and what their credentials are. This information should conform exactly to the "human resources" component of the program description.

Table 18–5 Sample Budget for a Family-Based Weight-Control Intervention

Personnel	Title	Quantity	% Effort	Base Salary	Salary	Fringe Benefits	Total
TBA	Program director	1	30%	52,000	15,600	4,680	20,280
TBA	Interventionist	3	10%	85,000	25,500	7,650	33,150
Consultant	Curriculum designer	1	10%	65,000	6,500	NA	6,500
Nonpersonnel							
Equipment							
	Laptop computer	3 @ $800					2,400
Supplies							
	Pedometers	100 @ $10					1,000
	Diaries	100 @ $5					500
	Educational materials	50 sets @ 12					600
Travel	Map miles	1,000 @ 0.35					350
Communications	Telephone	10% agency bill					600
Printing							
Total Direct							**$65,380**
Indirect @ 10%							**$6,538**
TOTAL							**$71,918**

EVALUATION PLANNING

Evaluators work with planners during the development of the program to create an evaluation plan. The evaluation plan builds from the objectives and logic model, and focuses on measuring the program's outputs, short-, medium-, and long-term outcomes. In the early stages of a program, the evaluation focuses on whether program activities are operating as planned and how they can be improved. As the program moves forward evaluators work with programmers to assess short-term outcomes. Ideally, the evaluation is also funded in order to determine if the long-term health outcomes are attained. Evaluation results inform the next round of planning, identify if adjustments should be made to the program, and produce information useful for decision-making by managers, policy makers, funding agencies, and the public.

CONCLUSION

For MCH professionals, the systematic steps of the assessment and program planning process sometimes seem to get lost amid continually changing resources, legislative mandates, and administrative red tape. In the face of these realities of everyday life in busy agencies, however, mothers and children are encountering complex and multifaceted health problems. The challenge to MCH professionals is to develop and implement strategic, well-thought-out programs to prevent those problems. MCH assessment and program planning methods provide a socioecological perspective and a problem-solving analytic framework for meeting this challenge. They promote deliberate decision making and development of creative and responsive programs using well-tested theories and evidence from other interventions, while operating comfortably in a social and political context. In addition, they use many of the analytic, interactive and managerial techniques available to the field of public health, thus serving as a bridge between research and practice. MCH assessment and health program planning are strengthened with a rigorous evaluation and monitoring focus.

The process and methods discussed in this chapter can be used at any jurisdictional level (e.g., local, state, federal) and for any system of care (e.g., public health systems,

managed care organizations, regional planning agencies). The process is dynamic, involving continuity and iteration, as well as the development of program plans that are intended to be changed. Over many years, MCH professionals have found that assessment and program planning skills are indispensable tools in their efforts to improve the health of mothers and children.

ACKNOWLEDGMENTS

Parts of this chapter are examined in more detail in a series of self-instructional manuals available for review or download at www.shepscenter.unc.edu/trainingMaterials.html. We are grateful to the co-authors of the manuals whose unique skills and perspectives have enriched our understanding of program planning in countless ways. We would also like to extend special appreciation to the Public Health Leadership Program at UNC Gillings School of Global Public Health and to the College of Public Health and Health Professions at the University of Florida.

References

American Health Planning Association. (2008). Mission statement. Washington, DC: Author. Retrieved May 8, 2011 from http://www.ahpanet.org/Mission.html.

Bradshaw, J. (1972). The concept of social need. *New Society, 30*, 640–643.

Breckon, D. J. (1997). *Managing health promotion programs: Leadership skills for the 21st century.* Gaithersburg, MD: Aspen Publishers, Inc.

Brownell, K. D. (2004). Fast food and obesity in children. *Pediatrics, 113*, 132.

Brownell, K. D., & Horgen, K. B. (2004). *Food fight: The inside story of the food industry, America's obesity crisis, and what we can do about it.* New York: McGraw-Hill.

Brownson, R. C., Baker, E. A., Leet, T. L., & Gillespie, K. N. (2011). *Evidence-based public health.* New York: Oxford University Press.

Centers for Disease Control and Prevention. (2011a). *Data and statistics.* Retrieved February 14, 2011 from http://www.cdc.gov/datastatistics/.

Centers for Disease Control and Prevention. (2011b). *Kidswalk-to-school.* Retrieved February 14, 2011 from http://www.cdc.gov/nccdphp/dnpa/kidswalk/.

Charns, M. P., & Lockhart, C. A. (1997). Work design. In S. M. Shortell & A. D. Kaluzny (Eds.), *Essentials of health care management.* New York, NY: Delmar Publishers.

Dahlgren, G., & Whitehead, M. (1991). *Policies and strategies to promote social equity in health.* Stockholm: Institute for the Futures Studies.

Fields, D., & Higgins, P. (2008). Physiological mechanisms impacting weight regulations. In E. Jelalian & R. G. Steele (Eds.), *Handbook of childhood and adolescent obesity* (pp. 109–126). New York: Springer Publishing Company.

Glanz, K., Rimer, B. & Viswanath, K. (2008). *Health behavior and health education: Theory, research and practice* (4th ed.). San Francisco: Jossey-Bass Publishers.

Goodman, E. (2008). Socioeconomic factors related to obesity in children and adolescents. In E. Jelalian

& R. G. Steele (Eds), *Handbook of childhood and adolescent obesity* (pp. 127–144). New York: Springer Publishing Company.

Gordis, L. (2009). *Epidemiology* (4th ed.). Philadelphia: Saunders Elsevier.

Gorin, A. A., & Crane, M. M. (2008). The obesogenic environment. In *Handbook of childhood and adolescent obesity* (pp. 145–162). New York: Springer Publishing Company.

Gortmaker, S. L., Peterson, K., Wiecha, J., Sobol, A. M., Dixit, S., Fox, M. K., & Laird, N. (1999). Reducing obesity via a school-based interdisciplinary intervention among youth. *Archives of Pediatrics and Adolescent Medicine, 153,* 409–418.

Institute of Medicine (IOM). (2002). *The future of the public's health in the 21st century.* Washington, DC: National Academies Press.

Issel, L. M. (2009). *Health program planning and evaluation: A practical, systematic approach for community health.* Sudbury, MA: Jones and Bartlett Publishers.

Janicke, D. M., Sallinen, B. J., Perri, M. G., Lutes, L. D., Huerta, M., Silverstein J. H., & Brumback, B. (2008). Comparison of parent-only vs. family-based interventions for overweight children in underserved rural areas: Outcomes from project STORY. *Archives of Pediatrics and Adolescent Medicine, 162,* 1119–1125.

Keppel, K. G., & Freedman, M. A. (1995). What is assessment? *Journal of Public Health Management and Practice, 1,* 1–7.

Koplan, J. P., Liverman, C. T., & Kraak, V. I. (Eds.). (2005). *Preventing childhood obesity: Health in the balance.* Institute of Medicine. Washington, DC: National Academies Press.

Malik, V. S., Schulze, M. B., & Hu, F. B. (2006). Intake of sugar-sweetened beverages and weight gain: a systematic review. *American Journal of Clinical Nutrition, 84,* 274–288.

McKnight, J. L. (2000). Rationale for a community approach to health improvement. In T. A. Bruce & S. U. McKane (Eds.), *Community-based public health: A partnership model.* Washington, DC: American Public Health Association.

Ogden, C., & Carroll, M. (2010). Prevalence of obesity among children and adolescents: United States, Trends 1963-1965 through 2007-2008. *CDC Health E-Stats.* Retrieved May 23, 2011 from http://www.cdc.gov/nchs/data/hestat/obesity_child_07_08/obesity_child_07_08.htm.

Peoples-Sheps, M. D. (2001a). *Health services needs assessment.* Washington, DC: U.S. Department of Health and Human Services, Health Resources and Services Administration, Maternal and Child Health Bureau. Retrieved October 18, 2011 from http://www.shepscenter.unc.edu/data/peoples/healthservices.pdf.

Peoples-Sheps, M. D. (2001b). *Development and selection of interventions.* Chapel Hill: University of North Carolina at Chapel Hill, School of Public Health. Retrieved October 19, 2011 from http://www.shepscenter.unc.edu/data/peoples/development.pdf.

Petersen, D. J., & Alexander, G. R. (2001). *Needs assessment in public health: A practical guide for students and professionals.* New York: Kluwer Academic/Plenum Publishers.

Robinson, T. N., Killen, J. D., Kraemer, H. C., Wilson, D. M., Matheson, D. M., Haskell, W. L., Pruitt, L. A., Powell, T. M., Owens, A. S., Thompson, N. S., Flint-Moore, N. M., Davis, G. J., Emig, K. A., Brown, R. T., Rochon, J., Green, S., & Varady, A. (2003). Dance and reducing television viewing to prevent weight gain in African-American girls: the Stanford GEMS pilot study. *Ethnicity & Disease, 13,* S65–S77.

Rosenstock, I. M. (1974). The health belief model and preventive health behavior. *Health Education Monographs, 2,* 54–386.

Sallis, J. F., & Glanz, K. (2006). The role of built environments in physical activity, eating, and obesity in childhood. *Future Child, 16,* 89–108.

Spiegel, A. D. & Hyman, H. H. (1991). *Strategic Health Planning: Methods and Techniques Applied to Marketing and Management.* Norwood, NJ: Ablex Publishing Corporation.

Task Force on Community Preventive Services. (2011). *The guide to community preventive services.* Retrieved May 23, 2011 from http://www.thecommunityguide.org/index.html.

Turnock, B. (2009). *Public health: What it is and how it works.* Sudbury, MA: Jones and Bartlett Publishers.

U.S. Department of Health and Human Services, Health Resources and Services Administration, Maternal and Child Health Bureau (USDHHS). (2011a). *Maternal and Child Health Services Title V Block Grant Program: Guidance and forms for the Title V Application/Annual Report.* Retrieved May 23, 2011 from ftp://ftp.hrsa.gov/mchb/blockgrant/bgguideforms.pdf.

U.S. Department of Health and Human Services. (2011b). *Gateway to Data and Statistics.* Retrieved May 23, 2011 from http://www.hhs-stat.net/.

U.S. Department of Health and Human Services. (2011c). Healthy People 2020 Improving the

Health of Americans. Retrieved May 23, 2011 from http://healthypeople.gov/2020/topicsobjectives2020/default.aspx.

Vartanian, L. R., Schwartz, M. B., & Brownell, K. D. (2007). Effects of soft drink consumption on nutrition and health: a systematic review and meta-analysis. *American Journal of Public Health, 97,* 667–675.

W. K. Kellogg Foundation. (2004). *Logic model development guide.* Retrieved May 23, 2011 from http://www.wkkf.org/knowledge-center/resources/2006/02/WK-Kellogg-Foundation-Logic-Model-Development-Guide.aspx.

Witkin, B. R., & Altschuld, J. W. (1995). *Planning and conducting needs assessments.* Thousand Oaks, CA: Sage Publications.

19

Monitoring and Evaluation for Global Maternal and Child Health Programs

Ilene S. Speizer, Laili Irani, Joseph Telfair, and Ghazaleh Samandari

Not everything that can be counted counts, and not everything that counts can be counted.

(William Bruce Cameron, 1963)

INTRODUCTION

The field of maternal and child health (MCH) is driven by concerns about the effective delivery of services and the assessment of programs for women, infants, children, adolescents, and families. Such programs are designed and implemented at the village, community, or clinic levels; some are also implemented at the district, province, national, or international levels. Since MCH is primarily a service-based field, understanding the process, utility, and implications of program implementation are important to ensure that scarce resources are being used to meet vital MCH needs. The monitoring and evaluation (M&E) of MCH programs is important for marshaling and presenting objective evidence of the worth of a particular program or activity (Baker & Northman, 1981) and engaging key stakeholders in the decision-making process to support midcourse corrections and/or continuation of successful programs (Carter, 1994; Patton, 1997; Rossi,

Lipsey, & Freeman, 2004; Wholey, 1994). Program planning involves engaging numerous stakeholders; examining the social, political, cultural, and health system contexts within which programs will be implemented; and undertaking, when possible, evidence-based interventions for improving the health and well-being of mothers, infants, and children. Particularly for global health programs, data obtained from M&E efforts can provide evidence of program progress and outcomes in contexts where the available evidence is scarce or inadequate.

This chapter will provide a framework for the use of M&E data to inform program design and improvement and to measure program impact. Key themes covered in this chapter include: (1) the types of questions answered by monitoring and evaluation methods; (2) indicators for program monitoring and evaluation; (3) data sources to monitor and evaluate programs; (4) strength and utility of various evaluation designs; (5) selection of the evaluation design; (6) the importance of engaging stakeholders in all stages of M&E; and (7) M&E guidelines. We examine these themes through a small number of global MCH examples; however, all approaches presented are applicable to local, regional, national, and international MCH programs. Special attention is paid to an applied as opposed to a theoretical or a "how-to" approach to evaluation. A theoretical perspective of evaluation can be found in an excellent text by Shadish, Cook, and Leviton (1991). General texts on the "how-to" of evaluation are provided by Fitz-Gibbon and Morris (1987) and Isaac and Michael (1997). More specific global M&E guides include those on adolescent reproductive health programs by Adamchak, et al., (2000), HIV/AIDS by Rehle, Saidel, Mills, and Magnani (2006), and child health programs by Gage, Ali, and Suzuki (2005).

CONTEXT FOR THE PRACTICE OF MCH MONITORING AND EVALUATION

As previously mentioned, the practice of monitoring program activities and evaluating the effect of programs on health behaviors and health outcomes is important to ensure that scarce resources are being used appropriately. To implement program M&E activities, program managers need to engage an evaluator who is either part of the team (an internal evaluator) or external to the implementing organization (an external evaluator). In both cases, the evaluator must work with program implementers to ensure that the M&E findings are programmatically applicable and, ultimately, utilized. Where appropriate, other key stakeholders, such as funders, policy makers, and frontline workers (e.g., doctors, nurses, health educators, etc.) should be included in the M&E development and dissemination process; this will ensure that findings are used for program modifications and to support future program design efforts.

In many cases, program M&E is an afterthought, requested by a donor, policy maker, or project director after the program is already underway. Although post-hoc evaluations are possible, evaluations work best when their design is part of the program planning process. At the program design stage, the program objectives and logic model can be used to identify a program monitoring plan that can be implemented during project initiation. In addition, if baseline data are needed as part of the evaluation design, plans for collecting baseline data can be developed as part of the planning process.

Recently, the global health community has begun to recognize the importance of undertaking evaluations of pilot and larger-scale MCH programs. For example, at the United States Agency for International Development (USAID), there is an increased effort and emphasis to systematically document the achievements and shortcomings of all their field projects and to share this information with the key stakeholders (USAID, 2011). As the global MCH field competes for limited resources, being able to demonstrate the effectiveness of a particular strategy in a particular setting can temper reservations of international donors and local governments that may be cautious about testing new approaches. For example, as new contraceptive methods, such as emergency contraception, are introduced into countries, funding organizations need monitoring information that demonstrates that women will (1) hear about emergency contraception and know where they can get it, (2) have positive attitudes toward emergency contraception, and (3) use the method. Evaluation findings will be important to show that not only is the method being purchased but that its use is leading to a reduction in unintended pregnancies in the target populations. This type of M&E information on emergency contraception can be used by the pharmaceutical industry, local nongovernmental organizations (NGOs), international donors, and government policy makers to confirm their support and encourage adoption of emergency contraception into the standards of practice.

QUESTIONS THAT CAN BE ANSWERED BY M&E

From the outset, it is important to understand the fundamental difference between monitoring and evaluation. In particular, *monitoring is an approach to tracking changes in program performance over time.* For example, a program to promote the use of insecticide-treated bed nets for pregnant women and children in the Democratic Republic of Congo (DRC) may want to document how many outreach workers (or nurses or doctors) were trained in the use and retreatment of bed nets, how many bed nets were distributed, and how many bed nets were retreated (in the last month or some other period). In addition, *monitoring data can be used to track trends in key outcomes over time* such as the number of cases of malaria in children under one year of age that were reported to a health facility in the last 3 months.

Evaluation is a systematic approach to attribute changes in specific outcomes to program activities. Moreover, evaluation, as a form of applied research, is concerned with providing information that can be applied to social problems being addressed by MCH organizations and programs. As such, the focus of evaluation is the systematic use of social research methods and program outcomes "to judge and to improve the planning, monitoring, effectiveness and efficacy of health, education, welfare and other human service programs" (Rossi, et al., 2004, p. 21). For example, although monitoring data may show that the number of cases of malaria in infants in the DRC has declined over time, without a specific evaluation design, it is not possible to conclude that these declines in malaria cases are a result of direct program inputs for the use of treated bed nets. This is because the declines in malaria cases could have occurred because of other reasons, such as a local drought that resulted in the drying up of water sources or to another program that promoted the covering or removal of standing water. A rigorous evaluation design would make it possible to determine if the specific bed net intervention program *caused* the observed declines in malaria cases among infants under age 1.

Figure 19–1 provides a useful perspective on the types of questions that can be answered with M&E information as well as information from other types of assessments. This figure was specifically designed with human immunodeficiency virus (HIV) and acquired immune deficiency syndrome (AIDS) programs in mind; however, it is useful for considering how questions are framed at various levels in MCH and public health.

This figure is read from the lowest step upwards. The first four steps of this figure are related to the planning process. In particular, there are numerous data sources and approaches that can be used to determine:

- What is the maternal or child health problem;
- What are the contributing factors that lead to this problem;
- What interventions can work (or have worked previously); and
- What resources are needed for specific interventions?

All of these program planning steps are crucial to ensuring that program implementers are applying the appropriate intervention elements for the target audience. Notably, each question in this stepwise process also uses varying data sources and tools. For problem identification, it is important to understand the nature, magnitude, and extent of the problem using a variety of sources such as surveillance data or a situation analysis, perhaps gathered through key informant interviews or field observations. For example, if there are numerous new cases of cholera among children in Dhaka, Bangladesh, as observed from an increase in cases reported at a health facility (through routine health information systems), it may be necessary to conduct community informant interviews or field observations to better understand the water quality issues that

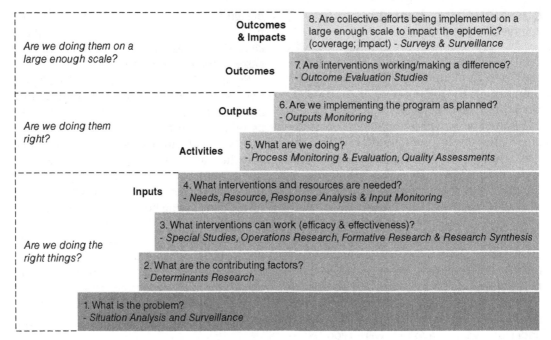

Figure 19–1 A public health questions approach to unifying HIV/AIDS monitoring and evaluation. *Source:* Adapted from Rugg, Peersman, & Carael, 2004.

may be affecting the risks of cholera among children. Following the identification of the problem, program planners, with assistance from their M&E experts, need to conduct a systematic review of factors that are directly related to the outcome (e.g., modifiers or proximate determinants) as well as an assessment of community assets. These formative activities will help the program managers or stakeholders to better understand why problems exist and provide community-level insights to inform program design.

Furthermore, in the planning process, program teams should review existing literature on effective program responses and may need to undertake special studies, operations research, and formative/qualitative studies to identify what the best response will be for each problem identified. Finally, the program planner will need to identify the inputs (e.g., financial, infrastructure, and personnel) needed to implement the target program. Based on the findings from these

first four steps in the process, the planner will develop program goals and objectives, as well as a logic model that describes the planned intervention approach. The logic model will clearly lay out the activities, outputs, outcomes, and impacts that the program intends to change over the life of the intervention; these activities, outputs, outcomes, and impacts are what the M&E team will examine to ensure that the program is undertaking activities as planned and if these activities are leading to the intended population-level outcomes and impacts.

Of note in the third step of the figure is the use of operations research (OR) to determine the efficacy of intervention models. OR is a process used to identify approaches to solve day-to-day challenges encountered by programs, using a controlled environment to test the efficacy of various options. For example, if the number of clients of antenatal services is low and there appear to be access barriers to the use of antenatal services, a small-scale

OR study might be used to test if changing clinic hours or training outreach workers to refer pregnant women to the clinic increases clinic use. OR is a continuous process with five key steps:

1. Identifying the problem
2. Selecting the intervention strategy
3. Testing and evaluating the strategy using a rigorous study design
4. Disseminating the findings
5. Using the lessons learned to improve the services

The types of study designs used for OR are similar to those that are discussed in the section on evaluation. The notable difference between OR and program evaluation is that generally, operations research is testing and validating whether an approach *can* work under controlled circumstances (efficacy) whereas program evaluation examines the effect of the approach under less controlled, or more "real-world" circumstances (effectiveness).

Steps five to seven in Figure 19–1 determine what the program is doing and whether the intervention is being implemented as planned. These are important monitoring steps in the process as the focus is on program activities (outputs) rather than on changes in behaviors (outcomes and impacts). An advantage of monitoring is that it allows for the understanding of the gap between actual and expected levels of achievement and when corrective action (such as the need to pay per diem to doctors and nurses to attend a training; otherwise, attendance will be lower than expected) may be warranted (Peoples-Sheps, 1997; Wholey & Hatry, 1992; Wholey & Newcomer, 1997). Monitoring includes activities such as process monitoring as well as quality assessments and output monitoring. Process monitoring tracks the implementation of program activities (e.g., when and where training sessions are happening and whether they are happening according to plan). Quality assessments examine the content and approach used in the implemented activities (e.g., is

the training curriculum being followed). Output monitoring keeps track of the number of activities implemented over the course of the program and whether they are happening in the quantity to cover the target population as intended. Through these monitoring approaches, program managers will be able to determine which activities are being implemented and which activities are not being implemented (e.g., instructors omitting lessons/activities they are uncomfortable administering). Moreover, the quality assessments will determine if the program is being implemented in a high-quality manner and if implementation is the same across sites and, if not, some of the key factors that are different across sites. Process monitoring and quality assessments provide information on what is actually happening. This information is useful when linked with an outcome evaluation to help explain unexpected findings. For example, differences by site (e.g., community, school, or health facility) might be attributed to the approach that was undertaken in the different settings for program implementation. Furthermore, using information from output monitoring such as the number of providers trained will permit programs to understand the level of coverage within a target area. For example, if only 5% of providers are trained in a community, the effect of the program is expected to be small as compared to another area where the percentage of providers trained is closer to 80–90%.

Process evaluations (included in step five in Figure 19–1) focus on changes in program-specific behaviors that are a direct result of program activities; they assess the variations in program delivery and provide information on what components contribute to the achieved short- and long-term outcome differences between recipients and nonrecipients. It is the latter focus on clearly identified short- and long-term outcomes based on key, targeted questions about recipients and nonrecipients that distinguish process evaluation from process or output monitoring (Scheirer, 1994). Process evaluations answer questions such as:

- What services are actually being delivered and to whom?
- Is there a discernible change in the persons trained by the program?
- Is this change as planned?

For example, as part of a process evaluation, the evaluator would want to know whether community workers who were trained to counsel pregnant women on the advantages of having a skilled birth attendant at delivery are indeed giving this information to pregnant women during each encounter. If these types of program-related changes are not occurring, there is no reason to expect that the program will have its intended impacts on maternal and infant health outcomes. It is part of step seven, outcome evaluation, where the evaluator will determine whether the activities of the community workers lead to population-level improvements in maternal and infant outcomes.

Step seven, the outcome evaluation (see Figure 19–1), answers the very basic, but often difficult, question of whether interventions are causing a change in the behaviors and health of the target population. That is, an outcome evaluation examines the result, effect, or impact (expected or unexpected, intended or unintended) that can be reasonably attributed to the activities or actions of a program. This includes an intermittent (short-term or ongoing) or an ultimate (long-term or end-of-program) outcome. To assess whether the intervention led to changes in behaviors requires an indepth understanding of the program design (often illustrated through the logic model). The logic model will help the evaluator (1) understand the kind of change desired and the means by which the change is to be brought about, (2) operationalize the definition of the desired change, (3) identify indicators appropriate for the identification and measurement of the change, and (4) determine the feasibility of the intervention

to produce the desired change (Fitz-Gibbon & Morris, 1987; Isaac & Michael, 1997; Telfair, 1999).

After evaluation research has demonstrated that a program is or is not causing changes in behaviors and health outcomes among the target population, the eighth and final step as shown in Figure 19–1 is to determine whether a program is having a population-level impact. Through large-scale surveillance and surveys, state- or country-wide programs can be examined to see if they are leading to the intended long-term changes (e.g., impacts) on population-level health and well-being, which is often measured in terms of morbidity, mortality, and improved quality of life. Questions about the cost effectiveness of programs are asked at this step and varying intervention options can be compared to determine which will be the most cost effective to be implemented at a larger scale. Cost-effectiveness analysis (CEA) provides an assessment of the monetary cost per unit of effectiveness (e.g., death or illness averted, or disability adjusted life year increased) (Jamison, et al., 2006; Philips, 2009). CEA is particularly useful for determining priorities in resource allocation across multiple interventions.

INDICATORS AND THEIR USE IN M&E

An indicator is a variable that measures one aspect of a program or project. In M&E, indicators are used to show that program activities are carried out as planned (monitoring) or that a program activity has caused a change or difference in a behavior or outcome (evaluation). Indicators that are useful to evaluators are those that are expected to vary over the course of the program and provide information on current conditions of program implementation (monitoring) and on behavior changes (evaluation). Useful indicators are measured in meaningful units for program management, such that they are appropriate for the program element being measured and can be compared to past and future values. Indicators must focus on a single aspect of a program or project such as an input, output, or overarching objective of the project and the related metric should be defined in a way that captures that programmatic aspect as precisely as possible. A complete and appropriate set of indicators for a given program should include at least one indicator for each significant aspect of program activities as laid out in a logic model.

Indicators need to be as relevant as possible to the program and context and should be useful to inform constructive change. Good indicators provide information useful for program decision making; are consistent with international standards and other reporting requirements; are defined in clear and unambiguous terms; are nondirectional (i.e., neither positive nor negative); have values that are easy to interpret and explain; and have values that are precise (i.e., accurately measures items), valid (i.e., corresponds to what is being measured), and reliable (i.e., gives the same results each time measured). Finally, good indicators are comparable across population groups, geography, and other program factors, as needed. Although it is tempting as a project evaluator to use indicators that state the expected direction of change (e.g., increased contraceptive prevalence rate), as mentioned in the list presented earlier, having indicators that are nondirectional (e.g., contraceptive prevalence rate) is more appropriate as this permits the evaluator to examine both expected and unexpected changes in the indicators. When a program manager is interested in a specific increase in an indicator (e.g., a 5% increase in the contraceptive prevalence rate), this is considered to be a target or objective, rather than a general indicator. A program's targets (and objectives) are important for evaluation purposes; however, for the evaluator, it is better to use a clear, nondirectional indicator for measurement purposes.

Process and output indicators are important for assessing whether the program is being implemented as planned. These indicators are often reported in the form of a number (e.g., the number of nurses trained to counsel on breastfeeding practices, the number of bed nets distributed, or the number of radio spots on condom use for HIV prevention aired). These indicators can be compared to targets to see if the trend is changing as expected (e.g., either rising or remaining constant). In some cases, to assess program implementation and program potential, evaluators will select coverage indicators that relate program performance to the target group for program implementation. For example, if the necessary data are available, a program manager could report the number of providers trained (from program records), the percentage of providers trained (assuming that a list of all providers in the target area is available), or the percentage of facilities with at least one trained provider (assuming that a list of facilities and the providers that work in the facilities is available). These coverage indicators provide more appropriate data for determining whether the program is being implemented at a large enough scale to potentially have a population-level impact. As discussed previously, a program that covers only 5% of providers versus a program that covers 85% of providers will have different population-level effects. Obtaining information on the relevant denominators to permit using coverage indictors is not always possible, but when these types of denominators are available, coverage indicators should be considered as part of process and output monitoring.

Outcome and impact indicators are generally reported at the population level and thus are reported as a percentage. Some common examples of outcome indicators in MCH programs include short-term outcomes such as the percentage of the population with knowledge of HIV/AIDS and the proportion of households storing drinking water safely, intermediate outcomes such as rates of intimate partner violence and percentage of women using modern contraception, and impact or long-term outcomes such as rates of unwanted or unintended pregnancies and the infant mortality rate. Often, information for outcome indicators comes from censuses, surveys, or surveillance systems where the data source provides both the numerators and the denominators. Useful resource documents for informing indicator selection are listed in Appendix 19–A.

DATA SOURCES FOR MONITORING AND EVALUATION

Data for monitoring and evaluation of MCH programs can come from numerous sources. Although many of the indicators used for program M&E come from quantitative data sources, qualitative data sources are also useful.

Quantitative Data

Quantitative data are based on information that is measured and expressed with numbers or percentages, as ranges or averages, and in tables and graphs. They tend to come from questions that are objective and closed ended such as, "Did you ever breastfeed [your last child]?" or questions that have specific response options to choose from such as, "Where did you give birth to [your last child]?", with a list of locations to choose from. The advantage of quantitative data is that they can be used to compare different groups or participants—girls and boys, clients from different socioeconomic or ethnic backgrounds, or clients in a program as compared to nonparticipants (as counts, values, percentages, rates) according to such indicators as health status, health-related knowledge, skills, behavior, and satisfaction with care. For quantitative long-term monitoring or process evaluations, one might assess the number of people who participate and how their composition (age, race, or economic class) compares with the composition of a particular community. The disadvantage of quantitative data is that when there

are unexpected findings (e.g., an effect that is counter to what was expected), it is difficult to explain why (or how) these patterns emerged.

Qualitative Data

Qualitative data are usually collected by document review, direct observation, and individual or group interviews. Qualitative data are useful to obtain greater depth on an individual or community's attitudes, norms, and behaviors. The information tends to be richer because individuals can expand on their thinking on a specific topic as compared to quantitative data that are more descriptive and presented through straightforward answers and numbers. Qualitative data are particularly useful as part of the formative program planning phase because they can help identify areas for expansion and focus by a specific program. They are also useful to help explain unexpected M&E findings. For example, if monitoring data show that, following the initiation of youth-friendly services that included training providers to counsel and treat youth clients for sexual and reproductive health needs, there is no increase in youth clients, it may be necessary to undertake focus group discussions in the community to better understand the community perceptions of the new program approach and whether the community approves of youth visiting these sites.

Notably, qualitative data can also be expressed in numbers. For example, interview responses can be tallied to report the number of participants who respond in a particular way (i.e., consensus statements, observations). Likewise, if indepth interviews are conducted to determine the ways women react to the threat of intimate partner violence at home, the responses can be quantified to determine what percentage of interviewees report one or another response, such as the percentage of respondents who did nothing, the percentage who reported to family members or the police, and the percentage who sought medical care.

Specific Data Sources

Often, monitoring data will come from program records such as training logs, distribution reports, and other programmatic sources that keep track of program implementation activities. At times, specific program monitoring tools will need to be developed to ensure that the program obtains a greater level of detail (e.g., a training log that includes the details on participants such as the clinic or school where they are based). The focus of the remainder of this section on data sources will be on indicators where the data source is not program records.

Data sources for M&E purposes come from both health-systems-level data as well as from population- or community-level data. Health-system-level data sources, their advantages and disadvantages, and the types of indicators that can be used for M&E of MCH programs with health-system-level-data are discussed first.

Health-System Data

Routine health information system (RHIS) or health management information system (HMIS) data are collected on a regular basis by facility staff as part of their routine activities; these data are compiled and sent on to higher administrative levels. The information available in RHIS and HMIS include service statistics such as the number of cases of specific diseases, number of births, number of vaccinations, number of antenatal visits, or number of postpartum visits. RHIS and HMIS data do not include details on the characteristics of the clients, with the exception of reporting of age and gender, specifically for the child visits. At times, RHIS and HMIS data are linked with population-level data to estimate the coverage of services (e.g., the percentage of the child population immunized), but these coverage indicators are often limited by outdated census data used in the denominators. The main advantage of RHIS data as part of an M&E plan is that the data are routinely collected so additional resources are not required to obtain and use these data. The disadvantage, as mentioned previously, is that the data often do not include important details such as the characteristics of clients, information on nonusers of the services, health worker performance, and quality of care (Gage, et al., 2005).

The second type of health system data come from health facility surveys; these surveys are often undertaken at the national level, funded by the World Health Organization/ United Nations or the USAID, and conducted every 5 or 10 years. These facility assessments tend to collect detailed information on the types of services offered, referral options, types of medicines available, and other factors related to quality of care and performance at public and private health facilities. Depending on the timing of the program evaluation and hence the availability of recent facility-level survey data, it may be possible to use a recent health facility assessment to inform program planning or for midcourse corrections. It is often difficult to design an evaluation around these types of data sources as they tend to be collected infrequently. In some cases, undertaking a facility-level survey as part of the M&E plan may be the most efficient approach; however, this would be smaller and more targeted than the larger national-level facility surveys. Facility surveys often include facility audits, provider surveys, exit interviews, and in some cases client-provider observations and/or mystery clients (i.e., sending a person to pose as a client to observe the quality of services provided). The selected indicators, as well as availability of resources for primary data collection, will determine whether undertaking facility surveys should be part of the M&E approach. In some cases, including a checklist of activities undertaken by providers (e.g., to monitor implementation of a new technique) is a rapid assessment tool for program monitoring and process evaluations. Alternatively, undertaking a full-scale facility-level survey to determine whether there are changes in quality of services over time becomes a larger endeavor contributing to the evaluation of an intervention.

Population-Based Surveys

There are a number of population-based surveys from developing and developed countries that can be used as part of program planning and outcome monitoring. Notably, for many MCH programs that take place at a community or district level, the data from large, population-based surveys are often not available at the level of the intervention (e.g., community, village, or district), limiting the utility for program evaluation. Moreover, since the data are usually available at multi-year intervals, it is difficult to time an evaluation so that the data will be available when needed. That said, using large survey tools to help design smaller scale community or district-level surveys will ensure that the measures and indicators used have already been validated in the country or region of interest.

The most frequent population-based surveys from developing countries are the USAID-funded Demographic and Health Surveys (http://www.measuredhs.com/). These are large, nationally representative surveys on MCH, reproductive health, HIV, morbidity, and mortality. In all countries, women of reproductive age are included and, in many countries, men are also surveyed. Another nationally representative survey from many developing countries is the UNICEF-Multiple Indicator Survey (MICS) (http://www.unicef .org/statistics/index_24302.html). These surveys provide information on MCH, reproductive health, and mortality. To learn about additional population-based survey methods, see Gage, et al., 2005.

In the United States, there are also similar, large-scale surveys that can be used for MCH program planning and outcome monitoring. These include the Pregnancy Risk Assessment Monitoring System (PRAMS; http://www.cdc.gov/PRAMS/), the National Survey of Family Growth (NSFG; http:// www.cdc.gov/nchs/nsfg.htm), the Youth Risk Behavior Surveillance System (YRBSS;

http://apps.nccd.cdc.gov/YouthOnline/App/ Default.aspx), and the Behavioral Risk Factor Surveillance System (BRFSS; http:// www.cdc.gov/brfss/) among others. Again, these data sources are useful for monitoring trends in key outcomes such as state-level teen pregnancy rates; however, they are generally less useful for evaluating the impact of smaller programs implemented at state or county levels.

Conducting population-based surveys focused specifically on the target population of an intervention is often the best approach to ensuring that the relevant data are available for program evaluation. As is discussed in the next section, in the ideal scenario, data are also collected in a site where the intervention is not being undertaken to provide a relevant counterfactual or comparison, that is, what would have happened in the absence of the program. For many evaluations of MCH programs, if the intervention is at the facility, school, or community level, then data collection is conducted at the same level. An important consideration for ensuring the rigor of the evaluation design is that the data collected are representative of the level that is being studied. For example, if a program is seeking to improve the quality of care of antenatal services in a district, then data should be collected either from all facilities or a representative sample of all facilities. Likewise, if information from clients is collected, the evaluator should seek to select a random sample of clients from each participating facility. Similarly, for an evaluation of a program at the school or community level, the objective of the evaluation should be to have a representation of the schools (or communities) included rather than to include only one school (or community) in the evaluation because it was "willing to participate." An indepth discussion of sampling and the effect of selection bias is beyond the scope of this chapter; however, it is important to keep these considerations in mind at the time of designing an evaluation and determining which data sources to use. A useful resource is an HIV/AIDS handbook by Rehle and colleagues (2006), in which the authors describe sampling strategies for monitoring HIV risk behaviors. It is advisable to engage a sampling expert as part of an evaluation team if the intention is to include a representative sample at the population or site level.

STUDY DESIGNS FOR EVALUATING MCH PROGRAM SUCCESS

Weiss (1991) stated, "Evaluations are used in many ways; one must do different things to facilitate different uses" (p. 179). To accommodate these "different uses," evaluation designs often use a broad range of methods and procedures (the evaluator's "toolbox") as discussed by Miller (1991), Morse (1991), Patton (1990), and Datta (1997). Determining an evaluation approach for MCH interventions must be based on a joint review and understanding of the goals and objectives of the program as well as the objectives of the evaluation—to inform midcourse corrections, to inform future funding, to inform program success/effectiveness, and/or to determine whether to scale up a program. This joint review should include various key stakeholders such as participants, program/agency staff, administrators, community leaders, funders, and the evaluator(s).

Evaluators are often asked to conduct summative evaluations that provide information to allow program/intervention planners, implementers, policy makers, and funders to assess the overall quality and impact of a program for the purposes of accountability and policy formulation. Summative evaluation requires examining whether an intervention led to changes in behaviors and health outcomes at the population level, rather than merely among a smaller group of program participants. This question involves the important concept of causality: whether one event (or an intervention in this case) produces another event (the outcome). Causality can help MCH program managers and funders be assured that

their scarce resources are producing the intended benefits. Thus, if a new intervention is developed, it is important to undertake a pilot test to demonstrate whether (or not) it is effective (i.e., leads to the intended outcomes). Efficacy studies require a study design that produces valid inferences about cause and effect. For example, if a pilot test with a rigorous study design demonstrates the intended effect, the findings can be used to request funding and programmatic support to expand the intervention or discontinue the intervention if it produces unintended or no effects.

As mentioned previously, the role of the evaluator is to demonstrate causality. Three requirements make it possible to demonstrate that an intervention caused the outcomes or impacts of interest:

1. The intervention began before the changes in the outcomes;
2. The outcome does not change in the absence of the intervention; and
3. The evaluator can rule out all other possible causes for the changes in the outcomes.

Outcome and impact evaluation designs differ in how they attempt to meet these three requirements. The second and third requirements are what pose the main evaluation challenge of demonstrating what would have happened in the absence of the program; this is called the counterfactual since it is the case that is not, in fact, observed. Different evaluation designs vary in how they address the counterfactual.

Randomized Experiments

The most rigorous evaluation design, a randomized experiment (also called experimental design), has the highest degree of validity to demonstrate causality between the intervention and the outcomes of interest. A randomized experiment requires that subjects, groups, or areas of study are randomly assigned to be in the intervention (or treatment) group or the control (nontreatment) group (Rossi & Freeman, 1993). For example, if an evaluator wants to test whether an intervention to counsel on prevention of mother to child transmission (PMTCT) of HIV leads to improved HIV-related birth outcomes, the program may offer counseling to a random sample of pregnant women in one clinic (or in multiple clinics). Those women who received the counseling would be in the intervention group and those women who did not receive the counseling would be in the control group. In this case, the randomization is at the individual level. An alternate strategy for the same intervention might be that in a district where there are 20 health facilities, half of the health facilities are randomly assigned to participate in the intervention (and all providers are trained on PMTCT counseling) and the other half of facilities are randomly assigned to serve as the control group. In this case, randomization is at the facility level. An additional component of randomized experiments is that it is also possible to test multiple interventions where three or more groups are randomly assigned (keeping one of the groups as the control group). For example, an evaluation in Western Kenya tested a multisectoral approach to educate adolescents and their parents on sexual and reproductive health (Askew, Chege, Njue, & Radeny, 2004). The program included a community-based component that involved engaging local civic and religious leaders as well as reaching out to inschool youth with peer educators; a facility-based component that involved training staff as well as creating adolescent-friendly spaces; and a school-based component that included holding meetings for the students, training teachers, and establishing extracurricular classes. The study was a randomized experiment and randomly selected test sites to receive the community- and facility-based intervention while additional randomly selected sites received all three components (the community, facility, and school-based interventions). In the randomly assigned control sites, none of the intervention components were administered.

The study involved a comparison of the three sites to see if one intervention led to fewer adolescent pregnancies over the follow-up period (Askew, et al., 2004).

The key feature of a randomized experiment is that the individuals or groups are randomly assigned. The objective of random assignment is that, with a sufficiently large sample, randomization will ensure that the intervention and the control groups are equivalent with respect to all factors other than exposure to the program that is being evaluated. In particular, the control group serves as the counterfactual of what would have happened in the absence of the program (Padian, et al., 2011). In the ideal scenario for a randomized experiment, baseline data on key indicators are collected prior to the intervention in both the intervention and the control groups. Then, an intervention is implemented with the intervention group only and following the intervention, another assessment of the key indicators is taken from both the intervention and control groups. Figure 19–2 demonstrates this classical randomized experimental design.

In this case, the program impact is the difference between the change in the intervention group between the second and first observations and the change in the control group between the two observations ([O2 – O1] – [O4 – O3] +/– error). Notably, while the randomization process is meant to assure that the intervention and control groups are equivalent, with baseline data it is possible to actually compare the groups prior

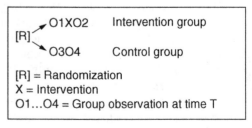

Figure 19–2 Classical randomized experimental design.

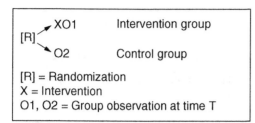

Figure 19-3 *Posttest only randomized experimental design.*

to program implementation. If significant differences are observed (e.g., one group is older or more educated), these differences can be controlled as part of the analysis. In this case, it is useful to have a statistician on the evaluation team to perform multivariate analyses as needed.

Sometimes a randomized experiment involves only post-test observations of the two groups. In this case, the groups are randomly assigned, but baseline data are not collected (possibly for reasons of costs or timing of program implementation). Figure 19-3 demonstrates this posttest only randomized experimental design. For a posttest only design, the observations between the intervention and comparison group are compared after the intervention and differences between the groups are assumed to be indicative of program effects. In this case, the program impact is again the difference between the intervention and control group after program implementation ([O1 − O2] +/− error). This is not the ideal scenario; without the baseline data it is not possible to confirm that randomization led to equivalence in the groups (i.e., the groups being the same). However, observed differences between the groups at posttest, such as demographic differences rather than program-related differences, can be controlled at the time of analysis.

Although the randomized experiment is considered the "gold standard" of impact evaluation designs, in many real-world scenarios,

randomization is not feasible. Reasons for this include the possibility that it is unethical to offer services to one group but not another and the potential difficulty of identifying enough facilities or locations that are similar and can be randomized into intervention and comparison sites. In addition, some interventions are intentionally placed in sites of either greater need or greater political will and thus there are not appropriate comparison sites with similar need or political will (Victora, Black, Boerma, & Bryce, 2011). Other constraints that make randomized experiments difficult include (1) the fact that randomized experiments require a high degree of control over where the program will be implemented and the types of activities that will be undertaken and this is not often appealing to decision makers; (2) the evaluator is brought in after the program is already underway, making randomization impossible; (3) the possibility for spillover or contamination whereby people in the comparison sites are exposed to the program as well; and (4) the risk of dropouts in the intervention or control areas that would bias the results. Under these constraints, the alternative design is a quasi-experimental design.

Quasi-Experimental Designs

Where randomization of individuals or groups is not feasible, the next best option for demonstrating the impact of an intervention on the outcomes of interest is to use a quasi-experimental design (Shadish, et al., 1991). The quasi-experimental design provides an approximation to a randomized experiment. This is a versatile method that can be used to measure results at the program and population levels. In addition, this method can provide evidence of an impact that is nearly as strong as a randomized experiment when it is properly designed, controlled, and analyzed.

The classical quasi-experimental design (Figure 19-4) is similar to the classical randomized experiment shown in Figure 19-2;

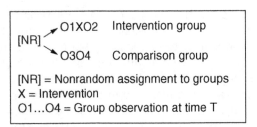

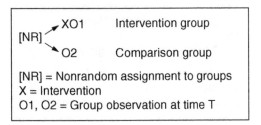

Figure 19–4 *Classical quasi-experimental design.*

Figure 19–5 *Posttest only quasi-experimental design.*

data are collected prior to the intervention and postintervention. The main difference is that the group (the intervention and comparison group[1]) assignment is non-random. Because of nonrandom assignment, it is not possible to assume equivalence between the groups; the evaluator must assess the differences between the groups at baseline. Any observed demographic or behavioral differences between the groups related to exposure to the intervention will need to be controlled for in the analysis. As part of a quasi-experimental design, the comparison group can be identified through matching, which is a process of identifying individuals or groups that are similar to the intervention participants or groups on all relevant characteristics. For example, if an intervention intends to improve the nutritional status of children in religious schools in Nigeria, an appropriate comparison group would be schools of the same religious denomination that are not receiving the program. Ideally, comparison schools would also be in the same district or region of the country to avoid other ethnic or cultural differences between the groups. The solution when matching is not possible is to propose and negotiate alternative strategies that allow for comparison group selection. One example of such a strategy is the delayed crossover design which requires that participants be assigned to either a group that initially receives the

intervention or the group that will "cross over" and receive the intervention after at least two periods of data collection (pre- and postintervention) have passed. In this case, the early group will be followed to determine the long-term effect of the intervention, and after at least two data collection periods, the latter group will also receive the intervention and be followed. It is critical that the evaluator, in partnership with the program staff, develop creative and scientifically sound strategies that allow for the attribution of program or service effectiveness. In addition, time and resources need to be planned at the time of program/evaluation design to ensure that the comparison group will receive the intervention as planned, assuming that the intervention had the intended impact.

An alternative to the pretest and posttest quasi-experimental design is the posttest only quasi-experimental design (Figure 19–5). In this case, data are collected only at the end of the program among participants (or groups) who received the program and among the comparison group. This is a weaker design and makes the use of matching approaches even more important; controlling for demographic and other differences observed at the time of posttest data collection will be important to help isolate the intervention effects.

A third alternative is to use a generic control group. In this design, data from the general population, such as from one of the large

---

[1]For the quasi-experimental design, the group without the intervention is called a comparison group (instead of a control group) to indicate that there was nonrandom assignment to the groups.

population-based surveys mentioned earlier, provide the basis to compare trends in the country (or district or community) against data in the intervention group over the life of the project. For this approach to succeed, it is important to have data from the generic control group from approximately the same time period(s) and with the same measurement methods as the intervention group. These requirements are a key limitation to using this approach for evaluating programs in developing countries.

Nonexperimental Designs

Evaluators may conduct a nonexperimental evaluation because of resource constraints, the inability to identify an appropriate comparison group, or if a program has full coverage and exposes the entire population to a program component, such as mass media. The nonexperimental design does not include a control or comparison group and is the weakest study design because it is difficult to determine what would have happened in the absence of the intervention. A key requirement for a nonexperimental evaluation design is a clear conceptual understanding of how the intervention is meant to influence the outcomes of interest. This means that the conceptual frameworks and logic models need to be well developed for use by evaluators at the program planning phase. Many evaluations are non-experimental, and there is a renewed emphasis on undertaking stronger evaluations in the MCH field (Center for Global Development, 2006; USAID, 2011).

There are two main types of nonexperimental study designs. The first is a time-series design that uses preintervention trends as a comparison to what happens following the introduction of the intervention in the population served by the intervention. In the ideal case, multiple observations are taken of the intervention group pre- and postintervention. Figure 19–6 demonstrates this ideal case.

The trends are analyzed to determine if the program led to changes in the direction

O1 O2 O3 X O4 O5 O6   Intervention group

X = Intervention
O1–O6 = Group observations at time T

Figure 19-6 Nonexperimental time series design.

or pattern of the trend. The next approach is to simply use pretest and posttest data with the intervention group and examine if there are changes between the beginning and the end. This design allows the documentation of changes in outcome indicators; however, it is not possible to attribute all of these changes to the intervention alone. Figure 19–7 demonstrates this simple nonexperimental design approach.

One way to strengthen this design is to measure the participants' level of exposure to the program, if feasible. The argument that the program led to changes will be strengthened if the analysis can show that those persons who had greater exposure to the program had greater change in the outcomes. However, an important limitation of the nonexperimental approach is selection bias. In this case, it is still possible that selection bias led to observed differences and could be a reflection of those persons who were exposed to the program being different in some systematic way from those who were not exposed to the program.

Another way to strengthen a nonexperimental evaluation design is to collect data from the same participants over time using a panel or longitudinal design. By following

O1 X O2   Intervention group

X = Intervention
O1, O2 = Group observations at time T

Figure 19-7 Nonexperimental pre- and posttest design.

the same individuals over time, they serve as their own controls; characteristics of an individual observed earlier can be controlled for in the analysis of changes in the outcomes of interest. For example, a study to examine contraceptive adoption following mass media programs that promote family planning and smaller family sizes could use longitudinal data for the evaluation. In this case, it would be useful to collect data prior to the mass media screening. For the evaluation, the goal would be to interview the same sample (and link the observations) that was interviewed previously. In this case, if some women were more motivated to use family planning, the analysis can control for this motivation prior to the program and examine the impact of the program controlling for motivational differences in the sample. Without the earlier longitudinal data, the program might demonstrate an impact but the observed impact may not be a true impact because those women who were more motivated to use family planning may have adopted it even in the absence of the new program. Longitudinal designs that follow the same individuals over time can be used as well with randomized experiments and for quasi-experimental designs; however, this adds cost and logistical issues to these already stronger designs.

CHOOSING AND IMPLEMENTING AN EVALUATION DESIGN

As mentioned earlier, the selection of an evaluation design will be based on project goals and objectives and clearly provided expectations from the project staff, administrators, funders, and policy makers (the key stakeholders). In addition, the scale of the project and the amount of resources available will also affect decisions on evaluation designs; a pretest and posttest nonexperimental design may be sufficient for small-scale pilot projects, but a larger scale program that is intended to be rolled out at the district or higher level may need a quasi-experimental design to demonstrate that resources are

being used appropriately. There are additional contextual factors that influence the selection of the evaluation design. First, the evaluation design should be reflective of a process that takes into account both the need for enough rigor to demonstrate the effectiveness of the program and the unique requirements of the sociocultural context in which the intervention is to be implemented. Second, the evaluation should be designed to measure the varying short- and long-term outcomes of interest to the key stakeholders as well as to the evaluation team. Third, the outcome evaluation should be closely tied to the monitoring and process evaluations to permit clear assessments of what worked, where, and why. Finally, at all stages of the evaluation process, the evaluation data should be used to inform program improvements, which requires close collaboration between the evaluators and the program implementers (Patton, 2011). Moreover, other key stakeholders should be engaged throughout the process so that they will be more likely to use the data to inform future programming. This can happen through various means (in person, print, and electronic) that provide information in a manner that is simple and straightforward, such as charts, graphs, storyboards, or simple tables.

Droitcour (1997), Cook (1991), Marcantonio and Cook (1994), and Rossi, et al. (2004) advise that independent of the research design chosen by the evaluator (e.g., randomized experiment or quasi-experimental), the validity and reliability of the design must be of primary concern. Concerns with ensuring validity must address two questions: (1) to what extent are the program or intervention effects due to the program or intervention rather than competing explanations (the key concern of causality)? and (2) to what extent can results be generalized to other situations? Considering these issues at the design phase will increase the likelihood that evaluation results will be used by the managers of the program being evaluated and by others seeking guidance on future MCH program design. In addition, threats to the internal and external validity, that is, problems with the design that make the study not meaningful for the target population or whether the study can be generalized beyond the study population must be addressed, particularly if a quasi-experimental design is chosen (Barnard, 2000; Miller, 1991). This is a reason to use, whenever possible, validated survey research tools and to select study populations that are representative of the target population.

THE IMPORTANCE OF ENGAGING STAKEHOLDERS

As discussed earlier, evaluation studies have a range of primary stakeholders that are invested in the products of its endeavors and are integral to the successful use of these products (Patton, 1997). Primary stakeholders should be kept informed and involved during the evaluation process and be made aware of the outcome of the evaluation (Brunner & Guzman, 1989; Rossi, et al., 2004). Examples of common stakeholders include policy makers and decision makers at the government and local levels whose approval can influence the support for a program to be instituted, continued, or expanded. Another important stakeholder is the target population comprised of persons, households, or other units who participate in the program and receive the intervention services under evaluation. Program staff that oversee and manage the implementation of the field programs should also be involved in all phases of the evaluation. Other public, private, and nongovernmental organizations serving the same target population should also be kept apprised of the study results so that they will use evaluation data to inform their activities. Lastly, it is beneficial to share results with the evaluation and research community at large, through peer-reviewed publications or external reports, because this will assist in dissemination of findings and improvement of programs in other areas.

Because of the emphasis on social and political accountability that surrounds the information produced by an evaluation, a number of logistical and reporting problems and issues arise. Evaluators usually find themselves confronted with individuals, groups, and/or agencies that have competing views on the use and appropriateness of the evaluation process and its results (Bicknell & Telfair, 1999; Patton, 1997; Rossi & Freeman, 1993; Schalock, 2001). In order to conduct their work with a reasonable degree of rigor and effectiveness, evaluators must understand their relationship with stakeholders and programs, as well as stakeholders' and program relationships with one another (Rossi & Freeman, 1993). Hence, it is imperative that the primary stakeholders agree to a fixed set of indicators and main program outcomes of interest before the evaluation begins. This can happen using the intervention logic model as a basis for discussion. Technical rigor remains a crucial part of the work of evaluators, particularly in determining and implementing the type of evaluation approach most suitable for addressing key program problems and issues.

To support the work of evaluators and program planners to engage stakeholders and to support evidence-based decision making, the MEASURE Evaluation project has designed a set of tools that can be used at varying phases of the process. (See http://www.cpc.unc.edu/measure/tools/monitoring-evaluation-systems/ddiu-tools/ddiu-strategies-and-tools.) These resources include a stakeholder assessment to identify key stakeholders, an instrument to analyze decision entry points, a stakeholder engagement tool to identify appropriate ways and times to engage specific stakeholders, a resource to identify constraints to data use, a decision calendar on when and how to use data to inform decisions, and approaches to targeted data use workshops. Details on these tools and their use can be found in a recent document by the MEASURE Evaluation project called *Data Demand and Information Use in the Health*

Sector: Strategies and Tools (Foreit, Moreland, & LaFond, 2006) (http://www.cpc.unc.edu/measure/publications/pdf/ms-06-16b.pdf).

MONITORING AND EVALUATION GUIDELINES

As previously discussed, obtaining information to inform programmatic decision making throughout program implementation (monitoring) and for future program planning (evaluation) is important for MCH programs that have finite resources and want to ensure that the resources are being used effectively. Given the applied nature of MCH M&E activities and the emphasis on identifying and obtaining data that are useful and relevant to key stakeholders connected to the program, it is important to delineate M&E guidelines (Patton, 1997). These guidelines follow from the discussions of key questions, indicators, data sources, and evaluation designs and are particularly important to keep in mind for work in developing country settings where collecting data can be difficult given financial, human resource, and other logistical constraints.

1. The data collected should serve the practical information needs of the intended users. In particular, the evaluator should focus data collection efforts on indicators that are most directly related to the program effects and are the most likely to show changes.
2. The evaluation should be designed in a realistic, prudent, diplomatic, and frugal manner. Notably, the gold standard evaluation approach (randomized experiment) is not appropriate for all evaluations. Thus, by understanding the key stakeholders' motivations for the evaluation, the evaluator will be better able to select the appropriate evaluation design to meet those needs.
3. M&E activities should be conducted legally, ethically, and with regard to those involved in and affected by the evaluation. Any evaluation that collects data from human subjects should be reviewed by an ethics review board to determine if the procedures being used are appropriate for the specific context; this includes in-country ethics review boards for those evaluations that take place in international settings.
4. M&E information should be accurate and reveal and convey technically accurate information. This means avoiding measures that are susceptible to cultural differences, historical events, or other factors that would prevent accurate calculation of indicators of interest to the program.
5. Evaluators should collect information to show that the program at least has done no harm to the target population. In some cases, there will be resistance to new program models (e.g., sexuality education in the schools) because of concerns that the program will lead to the behavior that it is meant to prevent (e.g., increased sexual activity among in-school youth). By collecting information on intended and unintended program impacts, ideally using a control or comparison group, the evaluator will be able to show the positive and negative impacts of the program.
6. The evaluator, especially one working in developing country settings, should be flexible in balancing the need for consistent measurement over time with a program manager's desire to make adjustments with the natural changes in the program setting. Developmental evaluation is a new form of evaluation that permits continued adjustments to program design throughout the process (Patton, 2011); in this case the evaluator is part of the program design team. Although not all evaluations in the global MCH context will be developmental evaluations, there is always a need for flexibility as changes are likely to take place, whether the evaluator likes it or not.

7. The evaluator should ensure that M&E findings are shared in a timely fashion with key stakeholders. It will often be necessary to present program findings in a less technical format for the non-evaluation community that will be the most likely to use the results for program and policy decision making.

CONCLUSION

The use of M&E information is dependent on the social, cultural, and political contexts in which the endeavor takes place. As with all forms of applied research, evaluators must be vigilant in appraising the environment of those involved with the work (stakeholders). Participation in the evaluation process by those being evaluated is a key tenet of global MCH practice. Furthermore, the use of M&E findings for decision making and program development must be of primary concern if changes in these programs are to reflect the needs of its participants (e.g., women, children, youth, and families) and if the changes are to have the desired effect.

References

Adamchak, S., Bond, K., MacLaren, L., Magnani, R., Nelson, K. & Seltzer, J. (2000). *A guide to monitoring and evaluating adolescent reproductive health programs. FOCUS on Young Adults.* Tool Series 5. Retrieved October 19, 2011 from http://www.pathfind.org/pf/pubs/focus/guidesandtools/PDF/Part%20I.pdf and http://www.pathfind.org/pf/pubs/focus/guidesandtools/PDF/Part%20II.pdf.

Askew, I., Chege, J., Njue, C., & Radeny, S. (2004). *A multi-sectoral approach to providing reproductive health information and services to young people in Western Kenya.* Kenya Adolescent Reproductive Health Project. Washington, DC: FRONTIER, Population Council.

Baker, F., & Northman, J. E. (Eds.). (1981). Helping: Human services for the '80s. St. Louis: C.V. Mosby Company.

Barnard, H. R. (2000). *Social research methods: Qualitative and quantitative approaches.* Thousand Oaks, CA: Sage Publications.

Bertrand, J. T., & Escudero, G. (2002). *Compendium of indicators for evaluating reproductive health programs* (Vol. 1–2). MEASURE Evaluation Project. Retrieved October 19, 2011 from http://www.cpc.unc.edu/measure/publications/pdf/ms-02-06-vol_1_title_page.pdf.

Bicknell, R. C., & Telfair, J. (1999). The process of selling a community evaluation to a community: The Cumberland County experience. *New Directions in Evaluation, 83,* 87–94.

Brunner, I., & Guzman, A. (1989). Participatory evaluation: A tool to assess and empower people. In R. F. Connor & M. H. Hendricks (Eds.), *New directions for program evaluation: International innovations in evaluation methodology* (no. 42, pp. 9–17). San Francisco: Jossey-Bass Publishers.

Carter, R. (1994). Maximizing the use of evaluation results. In J. S. Wholey, H. P. Hatry, & K. E. Newcomer (Eds.), *Handbook of practical program evaluation* (pp. 576–589). San Francisco: Jossey-Bass Publishers.

Center for Global Development. (2006). *When will we ever learn? Improving lives through impact evaluation.* Report of the Evaluation Gap Working Group. Washington, DC: Center for Global Development.

Cook, T. D. (1991). Clarifying the warrant for generalized causal inferences in quasi-experimentation. In, M. W. McLaughlin & D. Phillips (Eds.), *Evaluation and education: At quarter century,* 1991 Yearbook, National Society for the Study of Education. Chicago, IL: National Society for the Study of Education.

Datta, L. (1997). Multimethod evaluations: Using case studies together with other methods. In, E. Chelimsky & W. R. Shadish (Eds.), *Evaluation for the 21st century* (pp. 344–359). Thousand Oaks, CA: Sage Publications.

Droitcour, J. A. (1997). Cross-design synthesis: Concept and application. In E. Chelimsky & W. R. Shadish (Eds.), *Evaluation for the 21st century* (pp. 360–372). Thousand Oaks, CA: Sage Publications.

Fitz-Gibbon, C. T., & Morris, L. L. (1987). *How to design a program evaluation.* Newbury Park, CA: Sage Publications.

Foreit, K., Moreland, S., & LaFond, A. (2006), *Data demand and information use in the health sector: Strategies and tools.* MEASURE Evaluation. Retrieved May 15, 2011 from http://www.cpc.unc.edu/measure/publications/ms-06-16b.

Gage, A. J., Ali, D., & Suzuki, C. (2005). *A guide for monitoring and evaluating child health programs.* MEASURE Evaluation. Chapel Hill: University of North Carolina at Chapel Hill, Carolina Population Center. Retrieved May 15, 2011 from http://www.cpc.unc.edu/measure/publications/pdf/ms-05-15.pdf [cited] May 15, 2011.

Isaac, S., & Michael, W. B. (1997). *Handbook in research and evaluation* (3rd ed.). San Diego: EdITS.

Jamison, D. T., Breman, J. G., Measham, A. R., Alleyne, G., Claeson, M., Evans, D. B., Jha, P., & Musgrove, P. (Eds.). (2006). Cost–effectiveness analysis. In *Priorities in health* (pp. 39–58). New York: Oxford University Press. DOI: 10.1596/978-0-8213-6260-0/Chpt-3.

Marcantonio, R. J., & Cook, T. D. (1994). Convincing quasi-experiments: The interrupted time series and regression-continuity designs. In J. Wholey, H. Hatry, & K. Newcomer (Eds.), *Handbook of practical program evaluation* (pp. 133–154). San Francisco, CA: Jossey-Bass Publishers.

Miller, D. C. (1991). *Handbook of research design and social measurement* (5th ed.). Newbury Park, CA: Sage Publications.

Morse, J. M. (1991). Approaches to qualitative-quantitative methodological triangulation. *Nursing Research, 40,* 120–122.

Padian, N. S., Holmes, C. B., McCoy, S. I., Lyerla, R., Bouey, P. D., & Goosby, E. P. (2011, March). Implementation science for the U.S. president's emergency plan for AIDS relief (PEPFAR). *Journal of Acquired Immune Deficiency Syndrome, 56*(3), 199–203.

Patton, M. Q. (1990). *Qualitative evaluation and research methods* (2nd ed.). Newbury Park, CA: Sage Publications.

Patton, M. Q. (1997). *Utilization-focused evaluation* (3rd ed.). Thousand Oaks, CA: Sage Publications.

Patton, M. Q. (2011). Developmental evaluation defined and positioned. In M. Q. Patton, *Developmental evaluation: Applying complexity concepts to enhance innovation and use.* New York, NY: Guilford Publications.

Peoples-Sheps, M. D. (1997). Planning and monitoring maternal and child health programs. In J. B. Kotch (Ed.), *Maternal and child health: Programs, problems and policy in public health* (pp. 423–460), Gaithersburg, MD: Aspen Publishers.

Phillips, C. (2009). *What is cost-effectiveness?* (2nd ed.). London: Hayward Medical Communications. Retrieved May 15, 2011 from http://www.medicine.ox.ac.uk/bandolier/painres/download/whatis/Cost-effect.pdf.

Rehle, T., Saidel, T., Mills, S., & Magnani, R. (Eds.). (2006). *Evaluating programs for HIV/AIDS prevention and care in developing countries: A handbook for program managers and decision makers.* Durham, NC: Family Health International. Retrieved May 15, 2011 from http://www.fhi.org/en/hivaids/pub/archive/evalchap/index.htm.

Rossi, P. H., & Freeman, H. E. (1993). *Evaluation: A systematic approach* (5th ed.). Newbury Park, CA: Sage Publications.

Rossi, P. H., Lipsey, M. W., & Freeman, H. E. (2004). *Evaluation: A systematic approach* (7th ed.). Thousand Oaks, CA: Sage Publications.

Rugg, D., Peersman, G., & Carael, M. (2004, November). *Global advances in monitoring and evaluation of HIV/AIDS: From AIDS case reporting to program improvement.* In D. Rugg, G. Peersman, & M. Carael, *Global advances in HIV/AIDS monitoring and evaluation: New directions for evaluation,* No. 103. San Francisco: Jossey-Bass Publishers.

Schalock, R. L. (2001). *Outcome-based evaluation* (2nd ed.). New York: Kluwer Academic/Plenum Publishers.

Scheirer, M. (1994). Designing and using process evaluation. In J. Wholey, H. Hatry, & K. Newcomer (Eds.), *Handbook of practical program evaluation* (pp. 40–68). San Francisco, CA: Jossey-Bass Publishers.

Shadish, W. R., Cook, T. D., & Leviton, L. C. (1991). *Foundations of program evaluation: Theories of practice.* Newbury Park, CA: Sage Publications.

Telfair, J. (1999). Improving the prospects for a successful relationship between community and evaluator. *New Directions for Evaluation,* No. 83, 55–66.

United States Agency for International Development (USAID). (2011). Evaluation policy. Washington, DC: USAID. Retrieved October 20, 2011 from http://www.usaid.gov/evaluation/.

Victora, C. G., Black, R. E., Boerma, J. T., & Bryce, J. (2011). Measuring impact in the Millennium Development Goal era and beyond: A new approach to large-scale effectiveness evaluations. *Lancet. 377*(9759), 85–95.

Weiss, C. H. (1991). Linking evaluation to policy research. In W. R. Shadish, T. D. Cook, & L. Leviton (Eds.), *Foundations of program evaluation: Theories of practice* (pp. 179–224). Thousand Oaks, CA: Sage Publications.

Wholey, J. S. (1994). Assessing the feasibility and likely usefulness of evaluation. In J. S. Wholey, H. P. Hatry, & K. E. Newcomer (Eds.), *Handbook of practical program evaluation* (pp. 15–39). San Francisco, CA: Jossey-Bass Publishers.

Wholey, J. S., & Hatry, H. P. (1992). The case for performance monitoring. *Public Administration Review, 5,* 604–610.

Wholey, J. S., & Newcomer, K. E. (1997). Clarifying goals and reporting results. *New Directions for Evaluation,* No. 75, 91–98

Appendix 19-A
Useful Resources for Selecting Indicators

The validity and reliability of indicators is partly a function of the available data sources but also relate to their selection and definition. As described earlier, indicators need to be consistent with international standards, reported in clear and unambiguous terms, be nondirectional, and have values that are easy to interpret. A good starting point for selecting indicators is to use those that have been used previously for similar M&E activities.

In the global health field, there are numerous guides that include lists of validated indicators that can serve as reference documents for identifying MCH indicators. These include:

- A Guide for Monitoring and Evaluating Child Health Programs (http://www.cpc.unc.edu/measure/publications/pdf/ms-05-15.pdf)

- Compendium of Indicators for Evaluating Reproductive Health Programs (vol. 1 & 2) (http://www.cpc.unc.edu/measure/publications/html/ms-02-06.html)
- National AIDS Programmes: A Guide to Monitoring and Evaluation (http://data.unaids.org/Publications/IRC-pub05/jc427-mon_ev-full_en.pdf)
- A Guide to Monitoring and Evaluating Adolescent Reproductive Health Programs
- Part 1: (http://www.pathfind.org/pf/pubs/focus/guidesandtools/PDF/Part%20I.pdf)
- Part 2: (http://www.pathfind.org/pf/pubs/focus/guidesandtools/PDF/Part%20II.pdf)
- Violence Against Women and Girls: A Compendium of Monitoring and Evaluation Indicators (http://www.cpc.unc.edu/measure/publications/ms-08-30)

20

Advocacy and Policy Development in Maternal and Child Health

Donna J. Petersen, Catherine A. Hess, and Lewis Margolis

Never doubt that a small group of thoughtful, committed citizens can change the world. Indeed it is the only thing that ever has.

(Margaret Mead, 1901–1978)

INTRODUCTION

In this chapter we address an important skill area for maternal and child health (MCH) professionals, the skills of advocacy. Because children have special developmental and physical needs (that to a greater or lesser degree have been translated into positive rights by different communities and cultures), the fundamental value for child advocates would seem to be that goods and services ought to be distributed on the basis of need (Margolis & Salkind, 1996). We expand upon this discussion by focusing on actions that can be taken as part of the policy development process for the purposes of promoting and protecting the health and well-being of children and families. The mission of Title V of the Social Security Act (U.S. Congress, 1935), the legislative basis for MCH programs in the United States, to assure the health of all mothers and children, cannot be accomplished without maternal and child health professionals and constituents engaging in advocacy, although

that advocacy will take different forms consistent with the varying roles of professionals and constituents. As a public health program, MCH embraces the core functions of public health—assessment, policy development, and assurance (Institute of Medicine, 1988). Advocacy draws on the scientific knowledge base generated through assessment activities to inform, promote, and influence policy development. Advocacy can also be a tool for ensuring that policies are implemented effectively to achieve desired results. Advocacy is a fundamental element of nearly every essential public health service including mobilizing partnerships to identify and solve maternal and child health problems and providing leadership for priority setting, planning, and policy development (Grason, 1999).

Although assessment and assurance functions are explicitly included within the statutory responsibility of Title V MCH programs (HRSA, 2000), this legislation is less direct in speaking to the policy development role. The legislation's emphases on assessing need for and ensuring access to care support contemporary priorities of key stakeholders, the federal and state legislators interested in accountability and constituents interested in social justice in the form of equal access to resources and services to protect and promote health and prevent disease. Still, the history of MCH in this country has its roots in active advocacy for program and policy development aimed at improving child health and welfare more broadly (Alexander, et al., 2002; Hutchins, n.d.; Rosenbaum, 1983). Attention to advocacy and policy development remains important in current and future efforts to achieve maternal and child health's goals for the health and well-being of women, children, and families. In this chapter we define and discuss the nature of advocacy and policy development and why advocacy is an important MCH activity. We describe the nature of advocates and the various types of people and organizations that engage in advocacy. We then discuss the targets of advocacy efforts and how advocacy can be more successful while sharing some advocacy examples. We conclude with a brief overview of the policy development process and an encouraging word for those who might be willing to join with others in advocating for optimal maternal and child health.

WHAT IS ADVOCACY?

Definitions of child advocacy characterize the contemporary child advocate as operating at three levels:

1. On the individual or case level, an advocate is a person acting on behalf of a child . . . a defender, protector, mediator, supporter, investigator, negotiator, monitor, promoter, enabler, and/or counselor (Fernandez, 1980). Individual or case advocacy is the process of challenging an organization on behalf of an individual, a process in which an individual or group attempts to obtain more

responsive, adequate, and effective services for a child or a family.

2. On the organizational level, an advocate is a person or group attempting to alter and monitor legislative, budgetary, and administrative processes and, at times, monitor professionals and professionalism (Kahn & McGowan, 1972).

3. Systems or class advocacy is the process of reforming an organization or a system to benefit a group of people, cases, or users of the organization or system. Class advocacy may begin with action on behalf of one individual and then move its focus to all members of a class of cases. Often, individuals with similar motivations for case advocacy organize in order to take advantage of the power of numbers and combined resources. Advocacy on behalf of a class is often precipitated by an event with broad public exposure and emotional impact. For example, a fundamental change in Medicaid policy occurred in the early 1980s when the mother of Katie Beckett was able to impress on President Reagan the outrageous expenses resulting from the regulation that children with special health care needs be hospitalized for certain services when those same services could be provided less expensively and often more humanely at home (Roberts & Considine, 1997).

Advocacy in MCH is typically conducted in a policy development context and seeks to secure the authority, the resources and the direction to support efforts on behalf of the health of the population of interest to MCH, namely, women, children and youth (including those with special health care needs), and families. We advocate for the creation of new programs or policies that are needed for the benefit of the MCH population; we advocate for the elimination of policies and programs that are no longer needed or are potentially harmful; and we advocate for the amendment of existing policies and programs toward improving their reach, quality, or outcomes. Assuming the necessary legislative, or policy, basis exists for our desired programs, we can advocate for effective implementation, for necessary resources, or for appropriate interpretation and enforcement. We can advocate for changes in program direction, for improved collaboration and cooperation, or to inform relevant audiences about important MCH issues and MCH work. Common synonyms for the verb "to advocate" include to recommend, support, urge, lecture, or preach. For the noun "advocate" we find such synonyms as counselor, proponent, or counselor-at-law. These words help us understand the nature of advocacy and the role of advocates seeking change.

WHY IS ADVOCACY IMPORTANT IN MATERNAL AND CHILD HEALTH?

The mere assertion of rights is not sufficient to ensure that children's rights are satisfied. Inequities in the distribution of decision-making authority, economic resources, and information among different segments of a population behoove individuals and organizations to act as advocates for children in order to articulate their needs and interests, especially in the presence of opposition. As argued by Preston (1984), the older population, in contrast to children, has three willing cohorts of advocates for their interests—older persons themselves, the adult children of the older population who want assistance in the care of their parents, and nonelderly adults who see themselves as eventually becoming old and needing assistance.

The history of MCH is a chronicle of successful advocacy efforts on behalf of the nation's mothers and children. From the establishment of the early legislative basis for MCH (U.S. Congress, 1912, 1921, and 1935) to modern efforts to craft universal health insurance for children, MCH leaders have embraced advocacy as a fundamental responsibility and have viewed it as necessary to achieve MCH goals. Grace Abbott, Director of the Children's Bureau from 1921–1934, summed it up beautifully in this quote, now familiar to most in the MCH professions:

Sometimes when I get home at night in Washington, I feel as though I had been in a great traffic jam; the jam is moving toward the Hill where Congress sits in judgment on all the administrative agencies of the government. In that traffic jam there are all kinds of vehicles moving up toward the Capitol . . . there are all the conveyances that the Army can put in the street . . . there are the hayricks and the binders and the ploughs and all the other things the Department of Agriculture manages to put into the streets . . . I stand on the sidewalk watching it become more and more congested and more difficult, and then, because the responsibility is mine and I must, I take a very firm hold on the handles of the baby carriage and I wheel it into the traffic. Grace Abbott (Alexander, et al., 2002, p. 1)

Because the MCH population is typically composed of those who cannot speak for themselves, a voice is required, an advocate, someone speaking on behalf of children and their families to express their needs. Further justifications for advocacy in MCH include the vulnerability of the population, particularly during critical periods of growth and development; the dependence of children on families and institutions to ensure their well-being; the disproportionate representation of the underserved including minorities and the poor within the population of the nation's mothers and children; their persistent lack of representation in political arenas; and the known efficacy of preventive interventions directed at children in promoting healthy adulthood (Saunders, 1999). In spite of these truths, or perhaps because of them, we now have in the United States myriad programs designed to address various aspects of child growth and development, pregnancy and childbearing, family stability, and community empowerment. The advocacy efforts that led to the establishment of a national public school system and what we know today as the MCH Services Block Grant, or the development of such programs as Aid to Families with Dependent Children (now Temporary Assistance for Needy Families), Head Start, Medicaid, and child protection programs all had their roots in society's desire to give every child and family an opportunity to achieve their greatest potential.

These are successes primarily of *legislative advocacy*, working through the legislative process to create the foundation, the authorization, and the appropriation of funds for specific programs. Unfortunately, the resulting confusion over program eligibility, covered services, jurisdictional province, and fiscal responsibility has led to the development of a new kind of advocacy, *interagency* or *systems-level advocacy*. In this type of advocacy, MCH leaders work to forge partnerships across programs in order to lessen the administrative barriers so that resources and opportunities can be optimized. As an example of the distinction between the two, in the early 1990s in Minnesota, advocates were successful in securing legislative approval for the creation of a program within the state human services agency to provide mental health services to children. As the program was implemented, it quickly became apparent to advocates that unless the state departments of health and education contributed to the program by helping identify, screen, and refer children, the program would never achieve its stated goal of improving child mental health status in the state. Having the program created in statute and funded with state appropriations is an example of legislative advocacy. Encouraging other state agencies to collaborate with the new program in order to promote its success is an example of systems-level or interagency advocacy. A more recent example is the enactment, as part of the 2010 Affordable Care Act, of the new Section 511 of Title V authorizing and funding a Maternal, Infant, and Early Childhood Home Visiting program. At the federal level, the funds are administered jointly by the Administration for Children and Families and the Maternal and Child Health Bureau. States determine lead agencies to administer the program. The enactment of this provision in the national health care reform legislation was the result of legislative advocacy. Its successful implementation will hinge on the ability of different programs and agencies with different approaches to home visiting to collaborate on implementation that will improve the health and well-being of women and children.

The third type of advocacy in MCH is *judicial advocacy*. Judicial advocacy is invoked when legislative and systems-level advocacy efforts are exhausted, and the only remaining route of redress is through the courts. Judicial advocacy typically seeks to clarify the interpretation of a statute or a regulation, to force the implementation of a law, or to promote personal or group constitutional rights. For example, lawsuits have been filed in more than half of states to address a range of implementation issues with the Medicaid-based Early Periodic Screening Diagnosis and Treatment (EPSDT) program, from addressing provision of specific services such as screening for lead poisoning and community-based mental health services to more far-reaching issues with multiple aspects of the program (Peters, 2006). Another good example from the area of children with special health care needs is the case of the Pennsylvania suit by parents, which resulted in a ruling guaranteeing free public education for all handicapped children (*Pennsylvania Association for Retarded Children v. Pennsylvania*, 1971). It was only after this landmark ruling that Congress passed the Education for All Handicapped Children Act.

We need also mention here that although we typically think of MCH advocacy as being directed *at* government policy makers and program directors, advocates for MCH can operate *from within* government MCH programs as well. As advocacy and policy development are part of the leadership functions of MCH professionals, it is not uncommon for government agency staff to advocate for MCH issues within their own agencies as well as with other public agencies whose work affects the health of MCH populations. Ideally, advocates outside public institutions work in concert with advocates inside these public agencies toward a collective agenda. However, advocacy from within governmental agencies is controversial. The Centers for Disease Control and Prevention, for example, has supported advocacy institutes to teach individuals to influence policies regarding the use of tobacco by youth. These same institutes are roundly criticized by other government officials whose constituencies depend on the production and sale of tobacco products. Nevertheless, the 1970 White House Conference on Children called for a formal system of child advocacy (White House Conference, 1971). Quoting from the final report, "This Forum believes independent representation for children, a system of child advocacy, is urgently needed and should be immediately created" (White House Conference, 1971, p. 390). Citing such basic child needs as parental care, a secure home, moral guidance, proper nutrition, health, discipline, and education, the forum observed that "government should be responsive to these needs" (White House Conference, 1971, p. 389). Among its recommendations were a cabinet-level Department of Children and Youth, a National Advisory Council on Child Advocacy, an Office of Child Advocacy (specifically recommended for immediate establishment) within the new department, federally funded state advisory councils on child advocacy, and local advocacy boards, funded by the state councils, which would hire full-time, salaried child advocates to be responsible for children in a specific geographic region. Although these recommendations were never implemented, states and communities around the country have set up child advocacy agencies at the state and local levels.

Advocacy is important in MCH because the policy development process is so complex, and policy makers must respond to competing and often conflicting demands. As stated in a public hearing on April 9, 2004, by Lee Hamilton, former Congressman from Indiana and Vice-Chair of the 9/11 Commission, "policy makers face terrible dilemmas; information is incomplete, the in-box is huge, resources are limited, there are only so many hours in the day. The choices are tough, and none is tougher than deciding what is a priority and what is not." Advocates help ensure that the needs and desires of women, children, and families remain priority issues for policy makers.

WHO ARE ADVOCATES? WHO CAN BE AN ADVOCATE?

Anyone can be an advocate, and everyone in the field of MCH should be an advocate. It is difficult, if not impossible, to achieve improvements in health without urging change in factors that affect health. Although the Children's Bureau's charge at the time of its establishment in 1912 was "to investigate and report on all matters pertaining to child life and welfare among all classes of people" (U.S. Congress, 1912), it was the bureau's activist interpretation of that charge that led to success in areas such as national birth registration, the national school lunch program, and child labor laws (Hutchins, n.d.; Rosenbaum, 1983). That interpretation, using data or evidence to stimulate action, has been a continuous thread woven through maternal and child health success stories at local, state, and national levels over the past century.

Advocates come in all types, and organizations that engage in advocacy can take many forms. From the individual parent advocating in response to a personal tragedy (e.g., Megan's Law) and grassroots coalitions assembled to address the needs of specific classes of individuals (e.g., children with special health care needs) to large, well-established national organizations with broad and varying agendas such as the Children's Defense Fund, advocates share a desire to effect change. For some advocates, the role is a temporary one that can be abandoned once the pertinent situation is resolved. For others, like the parent advocates who organize locally to maintain a focus on children with special health care needs and who collectively comprise the national organization Family Voices, the nature of the advocacy work usually results in a lifetime commitment. These types of advocates have a personal stake, a clear self-interest, in the results of their advocacy work, though clearly their successes result in benefits to large numbers of people.

Further along the advocacy continuum are the organizations that identify advocacy as an essential component of their mission. It is useful to consider the various types of organizations that typically advocate for MCH and to assess their relative strengths and weaknesses as advocates (Johnson, 1999). One type of organization that engages in advocacy is the trade association. These are membership organizations of individuals or agencies that are involved in the same line of work. Examples relevant to MCH are state and national associations of clinicians such as the American Academy of Pediatrics (AAP), the American College of Obstetricians and Gynecologists, the American Academy of Family Practitioners, or the American College of Nurse Midwives and associations of provider organizations such as the National Association of Children's Hospitals (NACH) or state Primary Care Associations (PCAs). Other key associations focus on public health broadly including the American Public Health Association (APHA) and related state associations; the Association of State and Territorial Health Officials (ASTHO), the National Association of County and City Health Officials (NACCHO), and the National Association of Local Boards of Health (NALBOH). Still others focus on MCH specifically, including CityMatCH, the Association of Teachers

of Maternal and Child Health (ATMCH), and the Association of Maternal and Child Health Programs (AMCHP).

MCH professionals are eligible to join many of these trade associations and do so for purposes of professional development and affiliation or to benefit from opportunities to work with and learn from peers. Each of these associations also plays a key role in advocating for maternal and child health directly and providing an important vehicle and support for individual advocacy. Most of these organizations provide fact sheets, policy news briefs and updates, and legislative contact information. They offer training and other tools for advocacy and organize opportunities for advocates to join others in collaborative efforts to influence state legislatures or Congress. (See the References section at the end of this chapter for a list of relevant websites.)

These associations and others like them have played key and successful roles in advocacy at local, state, and national levels. Each brings with it the credibility of the expertise of its membership. These groups often serve as resources for policy makers seeking information and guidance on specific issues. On the other hand, these groups may be perceived as motivated by self-interest and therefore biased in the information they provide. We discuss ways to overcome these weaknesses in later sections of this chapter.

Another kind of organization that plays a key role in MCH advocacy is the voluntary organization. These organizations include groups like The Arc and the March of Dimes. Strengths of these organizations are the extensive volunteer base they enjoy and the passion they bring to the issues that affect them directly. On the other hand, their focus within MCH tends to be narrowed to very specific issues. The National March of Dimes in 2010 is focused on improving the health of infants and children by preventing birth defects, premature birth and infant mortality, and, in particular, the reduction or elimination of racial and ethnic disparities in these outcomes (www.marchofdimes.com), and the Arc strives for equity and equality for people with disabilities through public policy (http://thearc.org).

There are also organizations that are not membership/volunteer based but that are established for the sole purpose of representing or speaking on behalf of certain groups or causes. The Children's Defense Fund at the national level is an example, and most states have child advocacy organizations represented nationally by Voices for America's Children. The strengths of these organizations include the depth of their knowledge about the subject matter of interest to them, their knowledge about the policymaking process, and their highly professional approach to their work. Like trade associations though, these groups are believed to have strong political biases that may mute their overall effectiveness in the political arena.

Last but not least are public agencies. Although bound by official policies and procedures that often dictate who can advocate about what issues in public arenas, public agencies, their leaders, and staff carry an official mantle that carries its own weight in advocacy. For MCH professionals within public agencies, advocacy usually starts within with assembling the data, information, and arguments for the agency advancing certain policies and programs. When successful, such internal advocacy can result directly in new policies or programs, from those at the level of an administrative division to gubernatorial or legislative initiatives. When agency resources or political constraints impede action to advance specific policies and programs, the information and arguments may be picked up by external partners who often have had a role in shaping them. For public agencies, having strong family and consumer involvement is essential not only for effective internal policy and program development but also for creating a knowledgeable constituency that will advocate for key programs and policy positions when needed.

The strategic question may not be who can be an advocate, because anyone at any point in time can be an advocate whether operating alone, as part of a grassroots coalition, or as a member of a large organization. Rather, the more important question might be which type of advocate is more likely to be effective on a given issue with a particular target audience, or what combination of advocates as private individuals, as official agency representatives, as members of associations, or as volunteers at local, state, and national levels is required to achieve advocacy success.

WHERE ARE ADVOCACY EFFORTS DIRECTED?

As discussed earlier, MCH advocacy is aimed at achieving change to improve the health of women, children, and families. Where it is directed or targeted depends on who has the power to make the change, or who can influence those with that power. Advocates for the prevention and reduction of tobacco use have succeeded in securing national legislation prohibiting tobacco advertising in broadcast media, restricting the sale of tobacco products to underage youth, and requiring warning statements on tobacco packaging and on print advertisements. Advocates were also extremely important in the negotiations that led to the Master Settlement Agreement of 1998. Still these advocates know that it is unlikely that a national prohibition on the sale or use of tobacco products will ever be enacted by the U.S. Congress, and as such they have turned their attention to the state level where they have been effective in the establishment of Clean Indoor Air Laws in most states, in the banning of vending machines in many, and in the establishment of ever-increasing tobacco taxes. Another triumph at the state level is the case of preventing tap water burns. Dr. Murray Katcher, former Director of Maternal and Child Health for Wisconsin, and his colleagues (1989) successfully advocated for regulating the maximum setting of water heaters at 120°F in

Wisconsin. After a few other states joined ranks with Wisconsin, water heater manufacturers voluntarily agreed to a national standard that set the maximum temperature of new water heaters at the factory. Manufacturers realized that it would be in their best interest to have a single standard rather than 50 different standards, and advocates achieved a success without resorting to federal regulation.

In states where such efforts have been less successful, advocates have turned their focus to the community level, recognizing the truth in the old adage, "all politics is local" (attributed to Thomas P. "Tip" O'Neill, Jr., former speaker of the U.S. House of Representatives, 1977–1987[1]). In Prattville, Alabama, the city council was persuaded to enact a local smoking ordinance based on the work of a local youth group that conducted extensive public polling and interviews with restaurant and bar owners in order to demonstrate strong public sentiment for restrictions on smoking in public places. Spending the time clarifying objectives, assessing the likelihood of success, and securing the right blend of allies will determine the most appropriate target for advocacy work.

As another example, we can examine the goal of having all children insured. Some uninsured children are eligible for Medicaid or the State Children's Health Insurance Program (SCHIP) but are not enrolled, and some still do not qualify for any federal or state programs. This latter group includes certain immigrant children. If our advocacy goal is to increase the number of children with insurance, should we advocate at the local level, the state level, or the federal level? Should we target our efforts at legislators, the courts, or the agencies that operate at the systems level? Further analysis of the problem and potential solutions should help guide us, for in this instance and many others, action may

be appropriate and necessary at all levels in each of these arenas. If our concern is primarily focused on immigrant children, our efforts are probably best directed at the federal level where the prohibitions on their coverage originate. Although federal legislation sets the parameters for these programs and provides the first dollars, states must commit matching dollars in order to draw down federal funds and make many of the decisions on eligibility, coverage, and enrollment systems. Advocating with state legislatures may be needed to ensure that the state allocates the necessary resources and adopts state-level legislation authorizing federal requirements or selected options. If children in our community or state are eligible for SCHIP or Medicaid but are not enrolled, our efforts may best be directed at the level at which enrollment and outreach for enrollment occur. Because states vary on their approach to matters such as these, determining what is needed and how to ask for it is part of the assessment and strategy development process critical to successful advocacy.

Success in the legislative arena does not guarantee the changes necessary for children to realize the benefits. Advocacy involves continuing involvement during the rulemaking process. Advocates must now turn their attention to the administrative department charged with the responsibility of implementing the law. In order to influence and monitor the implementation of regulations that put the legislation into effect, meetings with administrative staff may be necessary. Proposed regulations must be publicized with an adequate period for public comment. Advocates need to keep the sponsoring legislator(s) informed of the implementation process, especially if it is not going well. In contrast, active advocacy through the Consumer Product Safety Commission has resulted in numerous regulatory bans of

---

[1]WGBH. (n.d.) Biography: Thomas P."Tip" O'Neill, in Jimmy Carter. The American Experience. Retrieved March 20, 2011 from http://www.pbs.org/wgbh/americanexperience/features/biography/carter-oneill/.

dangerous products such as unsafe toys, infant cribs with entrapment and strangulation hazards, and three-wheel all-terrain vehicles. In contrast to the popular impression of regulations as illegitimate violations of personal liberties, much public health regulation has enjoyed widespread public support. The most conspicuous examples come from auto safety regulation, but even in an era of suspicion of government, clean air and water regulations and even regulation of handguns and of access to tobacco products by minors can be successful, if opposition by well-funded special interests can be matched by the organized activities of child and public health advocates.

Regulatory authority for public health, as is the case for many other governmental functions in the United States, is divided among the three levels: federal, state, and local. Although most public health regulation resides at the state level, each level of government has a role to play. Advocates, therefore, need to be active at each level. Although the federal government is legitimately involved in actions and services that are in the public interest of the entire nation, especially in the case of conditions that do not respect state boundaries, it is at the state level that responsibility for assessment, assurance, and policy development is vested unless specifically assumed by the federal government. Child advocates with a national agenda may find the strategy of working up from the state level desirable. There are many examples of advocacy at the local level that not only succeeded in improving the health of children but also became precedents for action at the state level.

It is important to note that, regardless of the target of advocacy efforts, the involvement of professionals and constituents from the local level is critical to success at every level, be it local, state, or national. "Grassroots support" may be an overused term, but the underlying meaning suggests strength in numbers and true constituent/public support for the advocacy agenda. Professional advocacy

organizations and trade organizations have learned that the best way to get around the perceived bias they bring to their advocacy is to involve a broad-based coalition specific to the issue being addressed. The power of the scientific and content expertise of the professionals within the organization, coupled with the power of local constituent support, is a potent force for change in advocacy efforts. Child safety experts in the state of Maryland were not successful in securing passage of a child safety seat law until they engaged the help and support of the obvious constituency group, parents of young children. Policy makers find it hard to ignore the demands of large blocks of voters who are passionate about an issue. Of course this can work in the opposite direction as well. Despite the mounting scientific evidence in support of motorcycle helmet laws, several states have never enacted such laws or have repealed laws they had enacted, persuaded more by the hundreds of motorcycle enthusiasts who circle state capitol buildings and fill the hearing rooms than the testimony of the experts.

HOW IS ADVOCACY CONDUCTED? HOW CAN ADVOCACY BE MORE SUCCESSFUL?

Optimally, advocacy is an artful blend of education and action. Few problems in maternal and child health have only one best solution. Information and education lay important groundwork for identifying policy options and advocacy strategies. There are often various ways to approach a particular problem, and given that public health interventions may involve infringements on certain liberties (e.g., seat belt laws, compulsory vaccinations, etc.) or challenge prevailing wisdom or tradition (e.g., dietary recommendations, methods of child discipline, etc.), information and education can be critical in garnering support for policies that will be effective. Yet, as history and experience demonstrate, linking education with policy change at the legislative or regulatory levels can be more effective than public information campaigns alone. For example, seat belts and child auto safety restraints had been technologically feasible for decades before states began requiring their use. Before legislation, the percentage of child passengers using child auto safety restraints was in the teens. Today, in states such as North Carolina with vigorous enforcement of legislative mandates and loaner programs for poor families coupled with media campaigns, child auto safety restraint use may be as high as 80%.

The odds of success of advocacy efforts can be enhanced by discussion with a broad constituency about the problem and about which approach is likely to work and be acceptable to the public and elected or appointed officials. As such, the best advocacy is based on knowledge about a situation grounded in rigorous scientific data that leads to a shared understanding of the problem and an honest dialogue about the best approach for a particular community.

Common elements of successful advocacy include:

1. Sound assessment of the problem and possible solutions, sufficient to identify and justify the best clear alternative program or policy options that have strong odds of success in addressing the problem and improving outcomes
2. The clear articulation of both the problem *and* the suggested program and policy strategies for resolving or addressing the problem
3. The identification of key decision makers, those who can influence decision makers, other stakeholders, and constituents who have or should have interest in the problem, including both those who may agree and those who may disagree with the advocacy position
4. The development of a strategy for achieving the goals of the advocacy efforts that may include:
   i. Identifying an existing coalition or forming a new coalition to support the effort.
   ii. Developing and executing a communication strategy to reach and educate key players in the desired action and to anticipate and address issues that may be raised in opposition. Communication targets potentially include the decision makers, those who can influence them, other stakeholders, the media, and the general public.
   iii. Follow-up, follow-up, and more follow-up including reminders, thank-you notes and communication about the results/successes of the advocacy effort.

The intensity of any of these elements or whether they are included in an overall advocacy effort will depend upon the nature of the advocacy (legislative, systems, or judicial), the level at which it is being undertaken (federal, state, or local), and the scope of those involved in the advocacy (one individual, a few individuals, a small coalition, a large coalition). The extent to which each of these elements is used is also dependent on a realistic appraisal of the time frame and the political environment for action.

We mention the term "coalition" several times in this chapter. It is true that no matter what your advocacy objective, your chances of success will be enhanced if you partner with others. Forming coalitions, from informal alliances to formally organized groups, increases the odds for success in a number of ways. On a basic level, numbers matter. The more individuals and organizations that are working together to advocate, the more the effort may receive attention from certain target audiences, especially executive and legislative policy makers or the media that influence them. Partnering with others also increases the depth and breadth of expertise that is brought to bear on advocacy efforts. Further, the inclusion of specific individuals or organizations can enhance the credibility of the effort. It can also have the opposite effect, depending on the issue and the target audience you are trying to reach. In one state, having the Catholic Archdiocese join in advocacy efforts to increase family planning funding paid big dividends. On the other hand, when the Ku Klux Klan offered its support for the males-only membership policy of the Augusta National Golf Club, the club's response was less than enthusiastic. The larger and more diverse the coalition, the greater the effort necessary to organize the work, but the greater the ultimate success. Whether to form a coalition, whom to ask to join, and how it should operate are questions that should be considered in the context of the goal of the advocacy effort and a strategic analysis of the strengths, weaknesses, opportunities, and threats associated with this goal.

It may take decades to achieve some major policy changes, as it did with tobacco control efforts. Coalitions are important in sustaining energy and momentum in these instances. On the other hand, some policy actions can happen quickly, "in the dead of night" and with little public debate. The fact that policy change can happen quickly and without open discussion with stakeholders argues for the importance of ongoing information sharing and education of key decision makers, stakeholders, and constituents, that they may be armed with solid information before action is required. Standing coalitions and organizations with advocacy missions also need to be prepared to act quickly, proactively seizing opportunities and reactively addressing unanticipated counterproposals and actions.

In 1996, toward the end of the U.S. Senate's consideration of legislation to overhaul the welfare system, some new language was added to the massive bill by one senator. This provision, to authorize a new program within Title V of the Social Security Act of abstinence-only education, was added without public hearing or debate. Although some advocates for more comprehensive approaches to sex education did discover that the provision had been added to the legislation, there was no time or opportunity to promote a full consideration of the merits of this relatively small

provision within this major piece of legislation. Advocates succeeded only in changing the language to require new funding, rather than drawing funding away from core MCH programs, as was originally proposed.

An example of a successful, longer term effort at the national level was the advocacy that resulted in the 1997 enactment and the 2009 reauthorization of the State Children's Health Insurance Program (SCHIP). The foundation for the success of that advocacy can be traced back to the Maternal and Child Health Coalition formed in the 1980s to advocate for key programs providing health coverage and access to care, such as Title V, Medicaid, and Community Health Centers. Active leaders in this large coalition included the Children's Defense Fund, the March of Dimes, the Association of Maternal and Child Health Programs, the American Academy of Pediatrics, the National Association of Children's Hospitals, and the National Association of Community Health Centers. This coalition achieved advocacy successes in federal appropriations and in major legislative changes in Title V and Medicaid in the late 1980s.

When there seemed to be a real possibility of national health care reform in the early 1990s, the MCH Coalition and its members advocated for attention to the specific needs of children. Although the effort at national reform at that time ultimately failed, these organizations and their state and local counterparts had done much of the work necessary to advocate for improved health care coverage for children and learned some valuable lessons for future advocacy on behalf of SCHIP.

After mourning the loss of the national health reform opportunity and licking their individual and collective wounds, these groups formed a new coalition in the mid-1990s to advocate specifically and more narrowly for federal legislation to expand health coverage for children. From the previous advocacy efforts, the information on the problems of uninsured children was available, clear, and compelling. The new Child

Health Group also was clear about its objective: to secure federal legislation to increase the number of children with health care coverage. Although many of the organizations individually had well-developed positions about such important issues as the vehicle for coverage (Medicaid or not), the benefits package, the providers, and other policy options, the coalition was united in agreeing that there were multiple ways to achieve improved coverage. The coalition made it clear that it would work with and support the efforts of those in Congress who shared the overall goal. The coalition developed materials, held briefings, and invited congressional staffers from both houses and both parties to its meetings to inform and educate them about the problem of uninsured children and about important issues to consider in designing solutions.

Although the 1997 SCHIP law reflected the multiple compromises made to accommodate the various interests and political philosophies of those involved in its passage, today there is broad, bipartisan agreement that SCHIP has been a success. That consensus and the revitalized activities of the Children's Health Group helped in the ultimately successful effort to reauthorize the program, even after two vetoes by President George W. Bush in 2008, and some divisions between advocates for comprehensive health care reform and advocates for children in 2009. Many children's advocates at both state and national levels now are focused on ensuring that child and family needs continue to be attended to in implementing national health care reform that was enacted in 2010. All of the components of advocacy outlined previously came into play in this example, with coalition building, education, information sharing, and development and adjusting of strategy occurring over the course of nearly 2 decades.

Lessons learned from this example are that successful advocacy often takes time and that what may appear to be an advocacy failure may in the long run be viewed as an important contributing step toward later

success. Many major policy and systems changes have similar histories. At the very least, advocacy efforts communicate interest in an issue on the part of a group of concerned constituents, raise awareness of the level of interest in or concern for that issue, and encourage others to become involved. At their very best, such advocacy efforts enable policy and program creation or improvement toward the larger goals of promoting the health of women, children, and youth, those with special health care needs, and their families. Advocacy is an essential element in successful policy development, implementation, and evaluation. As such, it must be understood by all MCH professionals.

HOW DOES ADVOCACY RELATE TO THE POLICY DEVELOPMENT PROCESS?

Someone once said that laws were like sausages—no one should have to see how they are actually made. The truth is that the public policy process is indeed a messy one, but one in which we must be willing to engage if we are to succeed in effecting change for women, children, and families. There are many good websites available (www.house.gov) that describe the process of lawmaking at the national and state levels, and it is important that one become familiar with how this process works at the level that advocacy efforts will be targeted in order that opportunities to influence the process not be missed. How bills are created and introduced, the various committees that hear certain types of bills, how floor votes are handled, how conference committees are formed, the role of the political parties in the process, and the role of the executive branch and the governor are all things one must understand. Beyond the mechanics of these processes, though, lie the nuances of the traditions and the culture within which they are executed. It is equally important that one understand these subtleties of the policymaking process in a given state to avoid undermining advocacy efforts inadvertently. Which hearings are open to public testimony? How can one sign up to testify? How long should someone be prepared to speak? What are the "rules" for addressing the members of the committee and for responding to questions? Should advocates testify alone or should whole groups attend hearings? Should handouts be distributed? Can written testimony be provided in addition to or in lieu of oral testimony? Do the committees have staff assigned? Do the individual members have staff assigned? Is it better to meet with the legislator or his or her staff member? Where do people park? All of these are important to successful advocacy efforts.

It is always a good idea to visit the state capitol and determine the lay of the land and how to get around before venturing there in a mad rush during the legislative session. It is essential that advocates learn the structure of the legislature; identify the committees that are likely going to be key to their efforts (usually a health or health and human services committee, the finance and appropriations committees, possibly the education committee, or maybe a special or select committee dedicated to issues relating to children and families); and learn the names, backgrounds, and political affiliations of key members of each chamber (the senate and the house), each committee of interest to the advocacy agenda, and any special legislative commission. It is important to determine the level of staff infrastructure that exists within the state and whether those staff are assigned to political parties, chambers, committees, committee chairs, or individual members. Some states have very well-developed staff structures in place whereas in others the legislators operate with little to no staff support. It is also important to learn the location of the local offices of key legislators outside of the capitol. It is often easier to reach them there and to have more extensive conversations with them when the legislature is not in session.

It is also important to know the calendar for budget preparation and the process by which agencies develop their legislative agendas. Some states have biennial budgets whereas others do budgets annually. Most legislatures meet in the winter and spring. Agencies work on budgets and legislative agendas in the summer and fall. Clearly, advocacy is important year-round.

CONCLUSION

Although anyone and everyone can and should be an advocate, how one advocates and the strengths and weaknesses of one's advocacy vary by one's position, the type of advocacy, and its context. One can and should advocate as a private individual, separate from and regardless of any advocacy efforts that may be conducted in the context of one's work position. Advocating as an individual can be a way to build on or compensate for limitations on advocacy at work. Advocacy as an individual also can provide a vehicle for having an effect at a level different from that at which one generally works. For those MCH professionals working at the federal or national level, getting involved in advocacy at the local or state level can be a stimulating and rewarding effort, both for the individual and the issues on which he or she works. Similarly, for those working at a local or state level, national-level advocacy can be an invigorating and enlightening experience.

In any event, as an MCH professional engaging in advocacy, you should be prepared to follow a few simple rules to improve your chances of success while maintaining the integrity expected of your position.

1. Be prepared. Do your homework! It is your responsibility to bring the science base to advocacy efforts. Others will contribute plenty of politics, but as a professional, you must keep the advocacy responsible.
2. Never raise a problem without offering a solution, preferably a solution you believe will be effective, cost efficient, and acceptable to the public.

3. Be inclusive. Numbers matter, and various points of view strengthen your position. It is better to identify your opposition early and invite them to discuss issues with you directly rather than learn about them during a confrontation in front of the members of the legislature.

4. Be prepared for the long haul. Even at the state level it can take years to effect policy change. Be willing to engage in critical self-assessment in order to determine possible areas of weakness and modify your strategy accordingly.

5. Be consistent. If you have your facts lined up, your strategy prepared and your coalition assembled, it should be easy to stay on message and avoid confusion and contradiction. When you can, keep the message simple and direct.

6. Be respectful. Take the high road on the issues. Thank everyone who participates and contributes to your efforts. Respond to every enquiry. Follow up with everyone who helps you, who requests information or who may need a reminder.

Our legacy is one of strong leadership, advocating for the structures, systems, and services that women, children, and their families need to achieve their optimal potential. The 75-year history of Title V and the related programs it has helped foster over time are testimony to the endurance and many achievements of maternal and child health advocacy. Our future will be shaped by the advocacy efforts we undertake today to continue to support an agenda that values women, children, and families and that promotes maternal and child health. We are all advocates!

References

Alexander, G. R., Chadwick, C., Petersen, D. J., Pass, M. A., Slay, M., & Shumpert, N. (2002). *Maternal and child health/public health milestones*. Birmingham, AL: University of Alabama at Birmingham, Department of Maternal and Child Health, MCH Leadership Skills Training Institute.

Association of Maternal and Child Health Programs. (2010). *Celebrating the legacy, shaping the future: 75 years of state and federal partnership to improve maternal and child health*. Washington, DC: Author.

Fernandez, H. C. (1980). *The child advocacy handbook*. New York: The Pilgrim Press.

Grason, H., & Guyer, B. (1995). *Public MCH program functions framework: Essential public health services to promote maternal and child health in America*. Baltimore, MD: Johns Hopkins University, Child and Adolescent Health Policy.

Health Resources and Services Administration (HRSA). (2000) *Understanding Title V of the Social Security Act*. Rockville, MD: U.S. Public Health Service.

Hutchins, V. L. (n.d.). *Maternal and child health at the millennium*. Rockville, MD: Health Resources and Services Administration, Maternal and Child Health Bureau.

Institute of Medicine. (1988). *The future of public health*. Washington, DC: National Academy Press.

Johnson, K. (1999). Harnessing our energy: A counterpoint to "Breaking Away." *Maternal and Child Health Journal, 3*(1), 57–60.

Kahn, A., & McGowan, S. (1972). *Child advocacy: Report of a national baseline study*. HEW Publication #OCD 7318. Washington, DC: Columbia University School of Social Work and U.S. Department of Health, Education and Welfare, Office of Child Development, Children's Bureau.

Katcher, M. L., Landry, G. L., & Shapiro, M. M. (1989). Liquid crystal thermometer use in pediatric office counseling about tap water burn prevention. *Pediatrics, 83*, 766–771.

Margolis, L. H., & Salkind, N. J. (1996). Parents as advocates. *Journal for a Just and Caring Education, 2*, 103–120.

Pennsylvania Association for Retarded Children v. Pennsylvania, 334 F. Supp. 1257 E. D. Pa (1971).

Peters, C. P. (2006). *EPSDT: Medicaid's critical but controversial benefits program for children*. Issue Brief

No. 819. Washington, DC: George Washington University, National Health Policy Forum.

Preston, S. H. (1984). Children and the elderly: Divergent paths for America's dependents. *Demography, 21,* 435–457.

Roberts, B. S., & Considine, B. G. (1997). Public policy advocacy. In H. M. Wallace, J. C. MacQueen, R. F. Biehl, & J. A. Blackman (Eds.), *Mosby's resource guide to children with disabilities and chronic illness* (pp. 162–171). St. Louis, MO: Mosby.

Rosenbaum, S. (1983). The Maternal and Child Health Block Grant of 1981: Teaching an old program new tricks. *Clearinghouse Review,* National Clearinghouse for Legal Services, Inc., *17*(5), 400–414.

Saunders, S. E., Hess, C. A., Nelson, R., & Petersen, D. J. (1999). Health care reform and the MCH population. *Journal of Public Health Management and Practice_1*(1), 78–85.

U.S. Congress. (1912). *An act to establish in the Department of Commerce and Labor a bureau to be known as the Children's Bureau.* 37 US Statutes 79.

U.S. Congress 1921: An act for the promotion of the welfare and hygiene of maternity and infancy. US Statutes 42.

U.S. Congress. (1935). Grants to states for maternal and child welfare. *Social Security Act.* 49 US Statutes 633, Title V.

White House Conference on Children. (1971). Report to the President. Washington, DC: U.S. Government Printing Office, 1971.

Websites for Further Information

American Academy of Pediatrics: www.aap.org

American College of Nurse Midwives: www.midwife.org

American College of Obstetricians and Gynecologists: www.acog.org

American Public Health Association: www.apha.org

Association of Maternal and Child Health Programs: www.amchp.org

Association of Teachers of Maternal and Child Health: www.atmch.org

Association of State and Territorial Health Officials: www.astho.org

Children's Defense Fund: www.childrensdefense.org

Children's Defense Fund Action Council: www.cdfactioncouncil.org

CityMatCH: www.citymatch.org

Families USA: www.familiesusa.org

Family Voices: www.familyvoices.org

Maternal and Child Health Bureau, Health Resources and Services Administration, U.S. Department of Health and Human Services: www.mchb.hrsa.gov

National Association of Children's Hospitals: www.childrenshospitals.net

National Association of City and County Health Officials: www.naccho.org

National Association of Community Health Centers: www.nachc.com

National Association of Local Boards of Health: www.nalboh.org

National March of Dimes: www.marchofdimes.com

The Arc: thearc.org

Voices for America's Children: www.childadvocacy.org

INDEX

Numbers

1 to 4 year-olds. *see* preschool children
"3 by 5" Initiative, 385
3 to 6 year olds. *see* preschool children
5 to 9 year olds. *see* school-age children
5-year needs assessments, 397
6 to 12 year olds. *see* school-age children
13 to 20 year olds. *see* adolescent health
18-item food security scale, 334–335

A

AAP (American Academy of Pediatrics).
   see American Academy of Pediatrics (AAP)
Abbott, Grace, 479
"ABC" messages (Abstinence, Be faithful,
   Condom use), 386
Aber, L., 30
abortion
   adolescents and, 198–199
   family planning and, 90–97
   globally, 378
   right to, 260
   teen pregnancy rates and, 207
abstinence-only programs
   family planning and, 94

in MCH Services Block Grant, 487
   teen pregnancy and, 214, 220
abuse of children. *see also* neglect
   early medical findings on, 19
   gender differences in, 268
   history of protections against, 13
   mortality rates from, 149
   preschoolers, 149–150, 158–159
   school-age, 182–184
Academic Pediatric Association, 295
access to care
   adolescent health and, 211–212
   disparities in MCH and, 245–247
   for oral health, 367–368
   by preschool children, 150–151
   by school-age children, 176–178
ACE (Adverse Childhood Experiences) Study,
   74–75
ACOG (American College of Obstetricians and
   Gynecologists). *see* American College of
   Obstetricians and Gynecologists (ACOG)
acquired immunodeficiency syndrome (AIDS).
   see HIV/AIDS
ACS (American Community Survey), 42
action research, 407
activism. *see* advocacy

493